SECOND EDITION

# PUBLIC HEALTH LEADERSHIP

PUTTING
PRINCIPLES
INTO PRACTICE

## LOUIS ROWITZ

JONES AND BARTLETT PUBLISHERS

*Sudbury, Massachusetts*

BOSTON    TORONTO    LONDON    SINGAPORE

*World Headquarters*

Jones and Bartlett Publishers
40 Tall Pine Drive
Sudbury, MA 01776
978-443-5000
info@jbpub.com
www.jbpub.com

Jones and Bartlett Publishers
Canada
6339 Ormindale Way
Mississauga, Ontario L5V 1J2
Canada

Jones and Bartlett Publishers
International
Barb House, Barb Mews
London W6 7PA
United Kingdom

Jones and Bartlett's books and products are available through most bookstores and online book-sellers. To contact Jones and Bartlett Publishers directly, call 800-832-0034, fax 978-443-8000, or visit our website www.jbpub.com.

This publication is designed to provide accurate and authoritative information in regard to the Subject Matter covered. It is sold with the understanding that the publisher is not engaged in rendering legal, accounting, or other professional service. If legal advice or other expert assistance is required, the service of a competent professional person should be sought.

**Production Credits**
Publisher: Michael Brown
Production Director: Amy Rose
Associate Editor: Katey Birtcher
Editorial Assistant: Catie Heverling
Production Editor: Tracey Chapman
Marketing Manager: Sophie Fleck
Manufacturing and Inventory Control Supervisor: Amy Bacus
Composition: Auburn Associates, Inc.
Illustrator: Accurate Artists, Inc.
Cover Design: Kristin E. Ohlin
Cover Images: © Christine Kuehnel/ShutterStock, Inc.; © Christophe Rolland/ShutterStock, Inc.
Printing and Binding: Malloy, Inc.
Cover Printing: Malloy, Inc.

Library of Congress Cataloging-in-Publication Data
Rowitz, Louis.
  Public health leadership : putting principles into practice / Louis Rowitz. – 2nd ed.
     p. ; cm.
  Includes bibliographical references and index.
  ISBN-13: 978-0-7637-5050-3 (pbk.)
  ISBN-10: 0-7637-5050-6 (pbk.)
  1. Public health administration. 2. Leadership. I. Title.
  [DNLM: 1. Public Health Administration. 2. Leadership. WA 525 R882p 2009]
  RA427.R69 2009
  362.1′068–dc22

                                                              2008018042
6048
Printed in the United States of America
12 11 10 09 08   10 9 8 7 6 5 4 3 2 1

*To my wife, Toni, who inspires me and makes me laugh*

# CONTENTS

# PREFACE

## An Author's Reflections on Writing a Second Edition

When I finished the first edition of this book in 2000 and sent it to the publisher, I felt like I was sending my baby away from home for the first time. As a parent, I had done what I could do and now my baby had a life of its own. In the intervening years, I have talked to several hundred public health professionals from around the country who were trying to understand what leadership is and to become more effective as they took on higher levels of administrative responsibilities. I also talked to the parents—other directors and administrators—of public health leadership programs. We all were discovering that it takes a lifelong commitment to learning to master the tools of leadership. I have tried in this second edition to share the new ideas about leadership and the new areas of learning that my peers and I have discovered. This edition reflects this in revisions of all the original chapters and the addition of four new chapters. Many new exercises and case studies included as well.

I was asked a few years ago to reflect on the lessons I had learned from training public health leaders over the last 15 years. Here is my list:

- A critical task for public health leaders is to make their bosses, whoever they are, look good.
- No leadership position is forever, but a leadership mind-set is forever.
- The call to be a leader is often unexpected and affected by circumstances and context.
- You can lose your job even when you have done a good job—that's politics.
- Leadership is about passion, lifelong learning, ethics, enthusiasm, and optimism, but don't punish yourself if you occasionally get depressed. We are human after all.
- Do not sacrifice your home and family for any job. Family sustains us.
- In educating the public health workforce, watch for the "ah-ha" moments and write them down.
- Fight for your beliefs and use your leadership skills to put your beliefs into action.
- People would rather complain about problems than fix them.
- People who self-define themselves as leaders make leadership a self-fulfilling prophecy.

- Experience often brings an understanding and a maturity toolbox that can guide the future and grow the next generation of leaders.
- Leadership is about bringing order out of chaos.

Remember the important comment of Heraclitus in 500 BC:
"The only constant is change."

*Louis Rowitz*
Chicago, Illinois

## An Author's Vision—2001

During my career as a governmental mental health agency professional, as a researcher in a state-based research institute oriented to improving the quality of life of people with disabilities, as an associate dean in a school of public health, as a professor of public health, and as the director of the Mid-America Regional Public Health Leadership Institute for eight years, I have found that each set of experiences has added to my knowledge of leadership in public health. Two important facts have come to the forefront of my professional beliefs. First, public health affects us all. It is not a field that can go away in the future. There will always be a need for professionals to monitor the health of the public and create programs to enhance our health. Second, public health leaders are needed to make the whole public health process work.

It is possible to train the public health leaders who will strengthen the infrastructure of public health in our society. Leadership knowledge and tools can be taught. However, public health professionals need to put the knowledge and tools into action. It is through action that skills become developed. In addition, leadership needs to occur within the context of public health and the paradigms that guide the public health field. Public health leaders need to synthesize the comprehensive approaches to leadership by the business community with the special needs of the public health field. The outcome will be training and educational approaches unique to public health. Leaders exist at all levels of the public health system. Leadership is more than a place on the top of the organization chart. It is a strong belief that public health leaders will influence the public health landscape. Public health leaders gain tools and skills from strong public health mentoring. Our experienced colleagues offer much knowledge and many practice experiences. Mentoring puts leadership development into the real world and allows for the continuity of leadership over time.

Public health leaders not only function within the traditional public health organization; they also function across organizations. Transorganizational skills are critical. In addition, public health leaders practice their leadership within community settings. It is often through public health leaders that the validation of our community values and our beliefs in social justice occur. Leadership development is also a way to link academic public health with the practice of public health because information integrates research knowledge with the realities of public health practice.

During the 1990s, there was increasing evidence that leadership needed to come to public health. Through the support of the Public Health Practice

Program Office at the Centers for Disease Control and Prevention, a national public health leadership institute and a number of state-based or regional leadership institutes were developed. Public health professionals in 40 states now have access to a state or regional leadership institute. Almost 4,000 public health professionals have participated in a leadership development program.

Public health professionals at the top of their organization are eligible for training in the national institute. Public health leaders have taught us about practice and about the multilayered realities of leadership. Public health leadership programs need to be available to professionals in all of the nation's states and territories. The first decade of the 21st century will require the increasing need for leadership to guide the public health agenda in an ever-changing healthcare system.

My vision is to orient public health leaders to a better understanding of who they are, and how to use their public health leadership tools and skills. Leaders are committed to lifelong learning. If public health leaders take the leadership risk, they will greatly strengthen the public health system. Common paradigms of action will be blended with a flexibility required when change is a constant factor. Not only must the leader know what leadership is all about, but the leader must learn techniques that can be transferred into reality. It is important to look to the future and always be responsive to the world around us.

This book was written because I believe in the public health profession and I also believe in our ability to lead. Public health has always been oriented to solving the health problems of the present with a view to potential problems of the future.

In Part I, information is related to the knowledge associated with the theories and principles of leadership, leadership styles and practices, the public health system, and the five levels of public health leadership. The core functions model is presented and applied to public health leadership in Part II. Part III explores the leadership tools needed for the 21st century leader. Public health leaders continually develop their skills and put their skills to work on improving the health of the public. Part IV presents information on the personal evaluation of leadership and the evaluation of leadership programs. Part V looks to the future and presents some emerging public health trends.

Throughout the book, case studies written by public health leaders are presented. Public health leadership exercises can be found throughout the book. There are also discussion questions in each of the chapters of the book.

This is your chance to have a key role in defining the future of public health. Carpe diem! Seize the day!

# ACKNOWLEDGMENTS

I would first like to thank the 800 Fellows who have graduated from the Mid-America Regional Public Health Leadership Institute. Each one of these leaders has taught me much about the challenges facing public health. I have also learned much from my colleagues who over the years have struggled with the complex issues involved in leadership development. I especially want to thank Ann Anderson, Beth Quill, Mike Reid, Barney Turnock, Carol Woltring, and Kate Wright for our many discussions about leadership. I also wish to thank all the case study writers for their willingness to write the cases that help strengthen the public health leadership model presented in this book.

My colleagues and friends at the CDC or retired from the CDC who believed in public health leadership development over the years must be thanked: Ed Baker, Tom Balderson, Donna Carmichael, Steve Frederick, Joe Henderson, Stephanie Bailey, Dennis Lenaway, and Bud Nicola have battled to maintain a national focus on public health leadership development. During my study of public health leaders in 1996, the CDC supported my sabbatical.

I want to personally thank Gary Robinson and Gina Swehla of the Illinois Department of Public Health for supporting leadership development. Judith Monroe, Kathy Weaver, Jerry King, and Sue Hancock in Indiana; Margaret Schmelzer, Larry Gilbertson, and Terry Brandenberg in Wisconsin; and Dina Kurz in Michigan helped me move a leadership program in Illinois to a partnership with several other states.

I also need to thank my colleagues and friends at the University of Illinois School of Public Health: Barney Turnock, Patrick Lenihan, Ramon Bonzon, Geoff Downie, Sophie Naji, Rani Mishra, and Diane Knizner. My friend and former colleague Judy Munson and I still try to push the envelope to see where public health leadership development needs to go.

# PART I

# Leadership
# Theories and Principles

# CHAPTER 1

# THE BASICS OF LEADERSHIP

> In a society capable of renewal, [leaders] not only welcome
> the future and the changes it brings but believe they can have a
> hand in shaping that future.
>
> J. W. Gardner, *Self-Renewal*

The 21st century has not unsurprisingly increased the amount of attention paid to the concept of change. Yet change has always been and always will be a fact of life. For instance, the lack of substantive federal health care reform during the 1990s is no indication that the health care system remained static during the past decade and a half, nor that change will be unnecessary in the future. To cite two examples where change is demanded, large segments of the U.S. population remain under- or uninsured, and certain culturally diverse racial and ethnic groups have less access to health care than the populace as a whole.

Public health agencies and professionals are experiencing an identity crisis because of the recent reconfiguring of their roles and responsibilities since the terrorist events of September 11, 2001. Adding to the crisis is the public's lack of awareness of the nature of public health and the accomplishments of the public health system. Parents and friends still ask public health professionals what they do for a living. Of course, confusion about professional identity exists elsewhere in health care. Physicians who work for managed care organizations resist the restrictions placed on their ability to provide the tests and services they feel their patients require, not to mention the limitations on their salaries. The traditional caregiving roles of nurses are also changing as hospital bed utilization declines and many hospitals close their doors.

In order to manage the changes that are occurring, health care and public health professionals need to become involved in advocacy at the political and policy development level. They need to create their own vision of what personal health care and population-based health should be and to act in concert to realize that vision; and for these tasks to be accomplished, some of these professionals must acquire the full range of leadership skills and translate these skills into action. In 1988, *The Future of Public Health* made the argument that the creation of effective leaders must not be left to chance.[1] In line with this view, the report also stated a concern that schools of public health were not teaching the necessary leadership courses. This was reinforced in the 2003 report on *The Future of the Public's Health* where a recommendation was made that leadership training needs to be a requirement for public health professionals working in the governmental public health sector.[2] In 2007, the Institute of Medicine listed leadership development as one of the 16 critical public health content areas in the training of physicians for careers in public health.[3]

The training of future leaders is critical. Public health leaders will need training not only in the specialties of public health but also in the latest management techniques and tools. To support public health activities at the local, state, and federal level, they will require good communication, problem-solving, decision-making, and policy development skills, among others. Leaders must learn how their organizations function; how to work across organizations, which has been called meta-leadership; and how to integrate their organizations' activities into the communities they serve. In addition, the changing demographics of the U.S. population will lead to the need for ethnically diverse public health professionals to accept leadership positions in the governmental sector.

There is a major difference between managing change and leading change.[4] To lead change, leaders must be visionary and must be able to develop a vision to partially define the future. They must then get others to share their vision and help realize it. Of course, managing change is also important, for it keeps the system running smoothly.

Selling a vision to others can be especially difficult for people from ethnically diverse groups, people with disabilities, and women, for the vision they are trying to sell might well involve cultural, ethnic, community, and gender issues, and they will probably have to disseminate it to people who have a different background than they do.[5] Developing a vision that can be shared is critical in a society where diversity is the rule rather than the exception. Any vision will remain just a vision if it falls outside the belief system of the managers and the leaders.

In 1996, the Institute of Medicine released a report on the first year of its committee on public health. The report, entitled *Healthy Communities: New Partnerships for the Future of Public Health*,[6] reviewed the 1988 *Future of Public Health* report and concluded that progress had occurred in leadership development in the 1990s. Among other signs of progress was the creation of a national public health leadership program and a number of state and regional leadership development programs. The training of public health leaders needs to continue. Stress must be placed on the multidimensional aspects of leadership as well as the multidisciplinary approaches of the public health field as a whole. Building and strengthening the infrastructure of public health requires strong and effective leaders.

Note, however, that until now leadership development has been based on an industrial or agency paradigm of leadership.[7] Leaders of the 21st century must possess different skills with a systems thinking and complexity focus. They will also need to recognize that leading is a process in which they must pursue their vision through influencing others and the places they work. Leaders will find that advancing the skills of their workforce will increase the chance that their vision will become a reality. In addition, they will have to break down the barriers between organization and community to create an environment in which a shared value system and a shared vision for the future can come into being.

The remainder of the chapter comprises a short section containing a definition of leadership and a long section that discusses 16 important principles of public health leadership. As part of their effort to understand the nature of leadership, students should do Exercise 1-1, which provides an opportunity for students to express what they believe about leadership in general and public health leadership in particular. This exercise also presents the option of developing a journal to record ideas, leadership notes on papers or books read, and personal reflections on leadership experiences.

## Definition of Leadership

Leadership is creativity in action. It is the ability to see the present in terms of the future while maintaining respect for the past. Leadership is based on respect for history and the knowledge that true growth builds on existing strengths. Leading is in part a visionary endeavor, but it requires the fortitude and flexibility necessary to put vision into action and the ability to work with others and to follow when someone else is the better leader.

Public health leadership includes a commitment to the community and the values for which it stands. A community perspective requires a systems thinking orientation. Community refers not only to the local community in which a person works but also to the larger global community that can impact the health of the public over time. It also includes a commitment to social justice, but public health leaders must not let this commitment undermine their ability to pursue a well-designed public health agenda. In addition, public health leaders need to act within the governing paradigms of public health, but this does not mean that they cannot alter the paradigms. Leaders propose new paradigms when old ones lose their effectiveness. The major governing paradigm today relates to the core functions and essential services of public health. This paradigm is introduced in Chapter 7 and discussed in more detail in Chapters 8–10.

## Public Health Leadership Principles

One way of filling out the definition of public health leadership in particular is to consider some of the principles that public health leaders should use to guide their actions. Following is a list of 16 such principles. In the discussion of these principles (and elsewhere in this book), mention is made of a study of 130 public health leaders in the United States, England, Scotland, and Ireland during 1996 (see Case Study 2-A). The author conducted an hour-long conversation with each of these leaders to find out his or her view of the future role of public health agencies.

The public health leaders interviewed generally thought that they and business leaders have much in common. Good leadership is essential for the effectiveness of companies engaged in business and can increase the effectiveness of public health agencies as well. But although the leadership practices of business and public health leaders are similar, there are also important differences, which this book explores. For example, the social justice perspective that characterizes public health is more or less absent from the business world where a profit motive predominates. One of the leaders interviewed argued strongly that the social justice perspective is critical for public health but that public health leaders must be careful not to let this value interfere with the work that public health needs to do. One way of putting this is that social justice is only part of the leadership value system. Gardner[8] integrates that value with the values of freedom, social and ethnic equality, the worth and dignity of each individual, and the brotherhood of all human beings.

## Principle 1

The public health infrastructure and the system in which it is embedded must be strengthened by utilizing the core functions of public health and its essential services as a guide to the changes that should occur. The future of public health will be determined by the way in which core functions are carried out and essential services are provided. Public health leaders must evaluate the health status of the population, evaluate the capacity of the community to address its health priorities, and implement preventive measures to reduce the impact of or even avoid public health crises. Leaders must not rely on the current assurance models (service interventions) but need to implement new assurance models built on integrated and collaborative systems of service and program delivery. Leaders must also help to restructure the policies and laws that govern health and public health. Leaders must be policy makers who have a view of the future grounded in the realities of the present and built on the experiences of the past.

## Principle 2

The goal of public health is to improve the health of each person in the community. Public health leaders believe deeply that health promotion and disease prevention are possible. In fact, a focus on prevention is intrinsic to public health. In this regard, public health contrasts with the medical care system, which places an emphasis on treatment and rehabilitation. Every citizen needs to learn about the benefits of public health and how quality of life can be greatly improved if certain rules are followed.

A public health leader who truly believes in this principle will become a teacher and mentor for the community. Education will be the prevailing program model rather than medical care. The leader will reach out to schools, churches and synagogues, businesses, households, and health care providers and promote the vision of good health for all throughout life. The leader will also be concerned with the quality of care. If someone becomes ill, access to the best possible care is a community requirement. A visionary leader sees the total health system existing in the community and helps to ensure that the system is integrated and comprehensive, provides the services that are necessary, and does not contain duplicate services and programs, which are a waste of valuable resources.

A public health leader can play an important role in promoting a sense of community among community members. The leader might help define the values of the community and clarify the cultural aspects of the community life. Not all geographic areas have a cohesive cultural infrastructure. In an area that lacks such an infrastructure, the public health leader can help the community to define itself. (These issues will be addressed more completely in Chapters 4 and 6.)

## Principle 3

Community coalitions need to be built to address the community's public health needs. Public health is both a community responsibility and a population-based activity. This means that the mission of public health is to work with all groups in a community to improve the health of all members of the public.

All communities have assets and all sorts of community resources. Unfortunately, communities, like people in general, tend to be careless with their assets.[9] Consequently, each community needs to learn how to manage its assets if it doesn't know how to do that already. In short, it needs to take responsibility for its future. It may be too dependent on those who work in human services. Promoting good health is every citizen's responsibility. Public health leaders can play a critical role in helping the community move from a value system based on dependency to one based on shared responsibility. Public health leaders and their cousins in the human services field are thus the true servant leaders.[10]

Coalition building and other forms of collaboration require knowledge and creativity. First, coalitions made up only of managers are doomed to failure.[11] Coalitions need *leaders* to guide the process. Second, coalitions require trust among their members. If there is no trust, change will not occur. Third, there must be positions of power in a coalition. Key players must not be excluded or the process will fail. Expertise is also necessary so that informed decision making will occur. Fourth, the coalition must have credibility so that it will be taken seriously by others (both inside and outside the community) who can affect the implementation of the change agenda.

## Principle 4

Local and state public health leaders must work together to protect the health of all citizens regardless of gender, race, ethnicity, or socioeconomic status. Public health leaders firmly believe in the principle that all people are created equal. Several U.S. public health leaders interviewed by the author stated that the U.S. public health system must be understood within the context of the American political tradition and that it is impossible to be an effective public health leader without knowing about that tradition.

Access to service is sometimes affected by who you are. Women have found that the health care system does not always respond to their special medical needs. Public health leaders see that they have a responsibility to press for improvements in health care for women. They also have a responsibility to develop health promotion programs for women as well as men. For example, local health departments can take a leadership role in the development of breast examination programs for cancer prevention. Cultural and ethnic groups often have difficulty in accessing health programs because of color, language, or socioeconomic status. Diabetes-screening programs are often the first programs to go when funding cuts occur, despite the critical need for these programs in our communities. Public health leaders have important tasks to perform in protecting the rights of the unserved and underserved.

We live in a culturally diverse society. Our diversity is a strength as well as a weakness. Public health leaders must deal with their personal prejudices each day and consciously move beyond them to create a public health system that respects the needs of every citizen. State public health leaders must monitor the needs of all citizens as well as create the policies of inclusion that will lead to an improvement in the public's level of health. In addition, these leaders must make state legislators partners in this enterprise. The other critical partner is the *local* public health leader, who, in conjunction with the local board of health or county board of commissioners, is the gatekeeper for the community. What the state proclaims, the local leaders must adapt for local implementation. Local public health leaders must be extremely creative in the adaptation process. They must also speak loudly for the unique needs of their local community and take the local public health agenda to places where the state leaders do not tread.

## Principle 5

Rational community health planning requires collaboration between public health agency leaders, the local board of health (if such a board exists), other local and county boards, and other external community stakeholders. The relationship between the administrator of the local health department and the chair of the board of health needs to be a close one and based on a philosophy of equality and trust. The chair and the other members of the board of health do more than approve the health department budget and select the health administrator. The board members are residents of the community. They are the protectors of the community's interests and, with the administrator, serve an important gatekeeper function. Shared leadership and a shared vision are critical here. The health department and the board of health must be partners, not adversaries, which means they must work collaboratively to achieve agreed-upon outcomes. The exchange of information is an important part of the relationship, because relevant information is essential for the making of good public health decisions.

## Principle 6

Novice public health leaders must learn leadership techniques and practices from experienced public health leaders. Mentoring is a critical part of leadership. A mentor is a person who helps another person learn about the world and how it works.[12] Mentors also help people in their care choices. Mentors tend to be well-known individuals who help their proteges meet their major goals.[13]

Murray[14] discusses what she calls "facilitated mentoring," which is a process designed to develop effective mentoring relationships. It is also designed to guide the teaching of the person being mentored. If the mentoring experience is successful, there will be an impact on the mentor, the person mentored, and the agency promoting the mentoring experience.

Mentors are not threatened by the professional progress of their proteges. They personally feel good about the mentoring experience. All of the leaders interviewed by the author said that they had been mentored at various times in their public health careers. They thought that mentoring was important and that the need for mentoring does not stop with the attainment of a leadership position. Mentoring is beneficial to leaders throughout their careers. Furthermore, leaders who have been mentored have a responsibility to pass on the gift of learning they received.

## Principle 7

One issue of import is whether leaders are born or made. If leadership is innate, leaders wouldn't need to develop their skills, but if leaders are made, anyone has the potential to become a leader. The most defensible position is that leaders are both born and made—that some people are natural leaders with the talents necessary for successful leadership but nonetheless need to develop their leadership abilities.[15] That is the position taken in this book.

In fact, public health leaders must continuously work to develop their leadership skills. Leaders never stop learning. They are like detectives who pick up clue after clue in order to find the solution to a mystery. Leaders seek solutions to challenges rather than to mysteries, but the attainment of new knowledge is just as important for finding these types of solutions. Not only that, but each solution leads to new challenges and the need for additional learning.

Support for programs for lifelong learning is critical. There has been a tendency in recent years not to allocate funds for learning activities, partly based on the argument that the public does not want to pay for training programs. When the funds are available, they tend to be classified as discretionary and used for purposes other than training. Yet allowing leaders to improve their skills can lead to substantial benefits.[16] Very few public health practitioners have ever received major job-related training, to the detriment of the agencies they work for.

Over the past several years, a unique experiment has been underway, funded by the Centers for Disease Control and Prevention and state health departments. A national public health leadership institute and a number of state and regional leadership programs have been created to help state and local health department professionals, board of health members, local and state legislators, faculty members, and community leaders develop their leadership potential. The programs, which teach public health theory and practice, promote the education of public health professionals and, through them, the education of all citizens in a community. Public health leadership development, at its best, can create a partnership between public health leaders, the public health academic community, and the public health professional community in the public and private sectors. The main lesson learned from this experiment is that public health leadership development must build on the mission of public health but must orient itself to the future of public health. A second lesson is that these programs need to be experientially based and need to focus on projects that strengthen the infrastructure of the public health system. These programs also have the value-added result of increasing networking among the public health leaders who attend these programs.

## Principle 8

Leaders must be committed not only to lifelong learning but to their own personal growth. Self-esteem is a key factor in personal growth and is essential to the personal competence necessary to cope with life's challenges.[17] Further, the higher a leader's self-esteem, the more able the leader is to inspire others. Research on children has shown that children with high self-esteem are more willing to take risks and to assume leadership roles than children with low self-esteem.[18] Sethi has described the seven R's of self-esteem:[19]

1. *Respect.* It is necessary to respect and trust your employees.
2. *Responsibility and Resources.* Encouraging creativity among employees and delegating responsibility for tasks are essential.
3. *Risk Taking.* Only through risk taking can innovation occur.
4. *Rewards and Recognition.* People need to be recognized for their accomplishments.
5. *Relationships.* The quality and quantity of personal relationships have an impact on self-esteem.
6. *Role-modeling.* The work practices of an organization should be consistent with its values.
7. *Renewal.* It is critical to maintain a strong belief in lifelong learning.

Self-esteem is tied to each of the seven R's. Each factor affects the self-esteem of the leaders and their associates inside the agency and in the community. Building the self-esteem of leaders and associates is a prerequisite for the building of strong organizations.[20]

## Principle 9

The infrastructure of public health must be built on a foundation of health protection for all, democratic ideals and values, and respect for the social fabric of American society. The assumption underlying this principle is that physical, psychological, emotional, economic, and social health are all elements of the health of a community. By acting as role models for the community, public health leaders strengthen the infrastructure of public health in the community. This infrastructure is not just a physical building or an official agency called the department of public health; it comprises the entire community.

## Principle 10

Public health leaders should think globally but act locally. Although public health professionals practice their craft primarily at the community level, they should not ignore the rest of the world. Emerging viruses know no boundaries. Disease is carried not only on the wind but even in airplanes. Public health leaders need to be vigilant in looking for potential health problems. The Centers for Disease Control and Prevention has a national center for infectious disease that monitors emerging diseases globally, and public health professionals located throughout the world are investigating potential worldwide health problems such as the possibility of a pandemic influenza outbreak. Some multiregion crises have been documented in recent books, such as R. Preston's *The Hot Zone*,[21] L. Garrett's *The Coming Plague*,[22] and J. B. McCormick and S. Fisher-Hoch's *Level 4: Virus Hunters of the CDC*.[23] When a crisis hits, the international public health community must work together on the problem. Public health leaders thus have several overlapping communities to which they owe allegiance, and they must understand how to coordinate their multiple allegiances.

## Principle 11

Public health leaders need to be good managers. In the above mentioned interview study of public health leaders, the leaders pointed out that they, as heads of agencies, not only define their agencies' practice activities but also help to implement those activities. Managers do not have to be leaders, but tomorrow's leaders will need to possess both management and leadership skills (see Table 1-1). Reconciling these two sets of skills will not be easy, because they are based on two different ideological and talent perspectives. Managers are oriented toward ensuring that current systems are functioning smoothly. They tend to orient their activities to strengthening the public health agency in which they work. Leaders are change agents who are concerned with moving their agencies forward. Since change is unavoidable, today's managers will become obsolete if they cannot keep up with the ever-increasing pace of change. Leaders and dynamic managers will have to steer their organizations in new directions, and they will have to utilize cutting-edge leadership skills and managerial tools to do this.

**Table 1-1  A Comparison of the Characteristics and Responsibilities of Practitioners, Managers, and Leaders**

| Practitioners | Managers | Leaders |
|---|---|---|
| The practitioner implements. | The manager administers. | The leader innovates. |
| The practitioner follows. | The manager is a copy. | The leader is an original. |
| The practitioner synthesizes. | The manager maintains. | The leader develops. |
| The practitioner focuses on programs and services. | The manager focuses on systems and structures. | The leader focuses on people. |
| The practitioner relies on compliance and behavior change. | The manager relies on control. | The leader inspires trust. |
| The practitioner has a narrow view. | The manager has a short-range view. | The leader has a long-range view. |
| The practitioner asks who and where. | The manager asks how and when. | The leader asks what and why. |
| The practitioner's eye is on the client and the community. | The manager's eye is always on the bottom line. | The leader's eye is on the horizon. |
| The practitioner separates programs from services. | The manager imitates. | The leader originates. |
| The practitioner protects the status quo. | The manager accepts the status quo. | The leader challenges the status quo. |
| The practitioner is in the infantry. | The manager is the classic good soldier. | The leader is his or her own person. |
| The practitioner is a conflicted pessimist. | The manager is a pessimist. | The leader is an optimist. |
| The practitioner is a reflective thinker. | The manager is a linear thinker. | The leader is a systems thinker. |
| The practitioner follows the agency agenda. | The manager does things right. | The leader does the right things. |

*Source:* From *On Becoming a Leader* by Warren Bennis. Copyright © 1989, 1994 by Warren Bennis, Inc. Reprinted with permission of Perseus Books Publishers, a member of Perseus Books Group.

### Principle 12

Public health leaders need to walk the walk. They must not only define a vision but sell the vision and inspire others to accept it and try to realize it.[24,25] In his book on visionary leadership, Nanus[26] pointed out that there are four major types of leadership activity. First, a leader has to relate to the managers and other workers in the organization. The leader should be the guide to and motivator of action within the organization. Second, the leader has to relate to the environment or community outside the organization. A public health leader, for example, must carry the agency's vision and message into the community. Third, the leader has to influence all phases of the operation of the organization. Finally, the leader has to anticipate future events and move the organization forward in a manner that takes these events into account. If it is clear that managed care organizations will provide medical care for all members of a community, then the public health leaders of that community need to get the public health department out of the direct service business and into population-based health promotion and disease prevention.

### Principle 13

Public health leaders need to be proactive and not reactive. Up to the present, they have mostly tended to respond to public health crises as they occurred rather than focus on preventing crises. A reactive stance will probably always be part of the strategy of any state or local health department. However, reactivity tends to tarnish a health department's image. Public health agencies and professionals need to develop action plans to address the health needs of the citizens in their service area. Assessment activities will help to evaluate the health status of the community and give guidance for action. Action planning is more than planning for a crisis, which is an anticipatory activity that assumes a problem is on the horizon. Action planning is essentially preventive. Its goal is to create programs to prevent the occurrence of problems rather than create programs to deal with problems after they occur.

### Principle 14

Each level of the public health system has a need for leaders.[27] In fact, a leader does not need to have an official position to be a leader, and nonpositional power is likely to become more and more important. However, a defined leadership position does not hurt. Change will come from many different sources, and leaders will step forward to make sure the required tasks are accomplished. For example, if an environmental crisis occurs in a community, the environmental director from the health department, a community resident who is an engineer, a firefighter, a police officer, and others may form a leadership team to deal with the crisis. When the crisis has passed, the members of this ad hoc leadership team will then step back into their normal roles. Much has been written on this issue since the tragedy of September 11, 2001. The National Incident Management System is one example of this team effort to address a public health emergency.

Each level of an organization also has a need for leaders.[28] And like members of a community, members of an organization often share leadership tasks by forming a team to tackle issues. These critical shared leadership experiences are often ignored in the leadership literature.

## Principle 15

Public health leaders practice their craft in a community setting and must understand what a community is. A recent book stated that Americans are searching for a revitalized sense of community.[29] A community is more than a place; it consists of people living together who "participate in common practices; depend upon each other; make decisions together; identify themselves as part of something larger than the sum of their individual relationships; and commit themselves for the long term to their own, one another's and the group's well-being."[30(p.10)]

Human beings have a desire to be free and independent, but those who take independence as an absolute value risk becoming profoundly lonely by not including other people in their lives.[31] Being part of the community involves inclusivity, commitment, and consensus. It also can lead to a sense of realism, because communities, through the actions of individual members, contemplate and evaluate themselves. Finally, communities tend to be safe places, which is one reason Americans, with their increasingly well-founded fear of violence, have a renewed interest in the sense of community.

> **Leadership Tip**
>
> *Read your mail or answer e-mails when your energy level is low. Do important tasks when your energy levels tend to be high.*

In the now classic book *Habits of the Heart*,[32] Bellah and his collaborators argue that we Americans have become committed to the lexicon of individualism and have consequently lost our way morally. We are losing our sense of community and our commitment to improve society at large. Everyone from our politicians to our educators is pushing for a return to our moral roots, by which is meant a return to community.

Public health leaders have traditionally had a strong belief in community. Their focus, after all, is on improving the health of the communities they live and work in. Public health leaders also believe that they can strengthen their communities by working with community leaders to bring about change. If they are to be effective in bringing about change, they need to study and learn how their communities function. In particular, they need to know how to empower the members of their communities and get them to take their share of the responsibility for improving their own health.

## Principle 16

Public health leaders must practice what they preach. If they are promoting family values, they must live lives that are consistent with these values. If they are promoting good health and developing programs to get people to stop smoking, they should not smoke themselves.

This principle is not always easy to abide by. Some of our most successful leaders have personal lives that are in shambles. O'Neill called this the paradox of success.[33] Leaders often become prisoners of their official position and are unable to find a workable balance between their professional commitments and their private lives. Indeed, achieving a balance between work and home is becoming more difficult, as individuals are required to work harder due to such factors as downsizing. Decisions regarding the balance between work and home must be built into the culture of the places where we are employed,[34] especially as nowadays both spouses in a marriage usually work. The costs of not achieving a proper balance are high. Conflicting pressures and stresses can have serious health consequences.

I was running a leadership program and was planning for a six-month follow-up meeting to an initial program. All trainees from the first meeting were expected to come to the second meeting. One day before the second meeting was to occur, I received a telephone call from one of the trainees. She told me that her son was ill and that she was trying to find someone to take care of him. She was worried about missing the meeting. I asked her what she thought she needed to do. She said she felt she needed to stay with her son. I told her she had made the right choice. Balancing is making the right choice.

## Summary

The one thing that a review of the leadership literature makes clear is that leadership is a complex series of processes affected by many factors. These factors, for public leaders in particular, include the principles described above, which apply to leadership style, leadership practices, the public health system, the core functions and essential services of public health, and leadership tools (see Figure 1-1).

Leading is a multidimensional activity. Every leader uses leadership skills in his or her own way, which is to say that every leader has his or her own leadership style and unique set of personal talents. Every leader engages in a set of leadership practices and uses a unique set of tools. All these elements determine whether a leader is successful. Throughout this book, I will use a variety of examples, from public health case studies to a public health quiz for leaders. Public health quizzes will involve presenting several questions to a public health leader that grow out of one of the chapters in this book. The first quiz is with Dr. Virginia Caine, a former president of the American Public Health Association and the director of the Marion County Health Department in Indianapolis, Indiana.

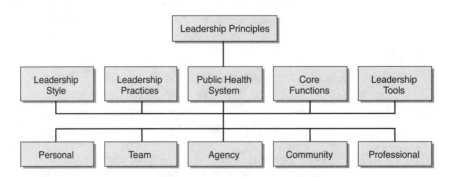

**FIGURE 1-1  Conceptual model of public health leadership**

---

## Case Study 1-A
## A Public Health Practice Quiz for Virginia Caine

### 1. How would you define leadership?

Leadership is

- Creating a vision others can see
- Promoting the capacity of other people to take action on that vision
- Taking a diverse group of people with different backgrounds and ideas, focusing the group on a common goal, and motivating the group to overcome obstacles and reach the goal

### 2. What do you think are the critical strengths needed to be a successful public health leader?

Successful public health leaders are those who are visionary, decisive, good communicators, change agents, and risk takers. They have the conviction of their values and are deeply committed to improving the health of everyone in this country.

These leaders are also politically astute, are able to listen and hear what people are really saying, are respectful of different cultures, have emotional intelligence, are resilient and future focused, and have a love for public health.

They understand that relationship building and collaboration are the cornerstones of public health work.

### 3. What will be the major challenges of public health in the next 10 years?

The major challenges for public health in the next 10 years include the following: the improvement of the health of everyone in the country; the strengthening of the public health infrastructure; the aging of the public health workforce; the changing demographic populations (age distribution, cultural diversity) and their impact on disparities; chronic diseases; lack of access to health care and the uninsured; global health; health promotion and behavior change; environmental hazards and global warming; and the integration of public health and traditional medical information systems.

Other challenges for public health include genomics and ethical issues, credentialing and accreditation, emerging infectious diseases and drug-resistant bacteria, and the ability to convene and collaborate with people across the political and opinion spectrum.

### 4. What needs to be done to develop a culturally diverse leadership workforce?

We need to encourage and promote diversity in our public health leadership training across the entire public health system, not just the public health departments. Also, public health agencies in collaboration with the education system, from preschool to the academic institutions, that is, colleges, need to create opportunities for students of all cultures to gain the knowledge and skills needed. Public health agencies need to promote more recruitment where it's robust and not passive of a culturally diverse workforce.

Some of these opportunities may include partnerships with diverse populations and organizations, providing scholarships, peer counseling, internships, and outreach educational endeavors for students of all cultures to gain the knowledge and skills needed to be 21st century public health leaders with appropriate incentives.

### 5. Is leadership in the private sector similar to leadership in the business sector?

Leadership is leadership no matter what system you are in.

> **Leadership Tip**
>
> *Think and act locally with*
>
> *global health issues involved*
>
> *in your activities.*

This chapter, besides offering an introduction to leadership, reviewed some of the main principles that public health leaders should be guided by. The next chapter presents various analyses of leadership styles and discusses essential leadership characteristics. Later chapters cover the three core functions of public health, associated public health practices, and important leadership tools and skills, among other topics. A major section of the book will examine the skills and competencies of public health leaders. This will be followed by an examination of leadership evaluation. The final section of the book will look at the future.

## Discussion Questions

1. What is your personal definition of leadership?
2. Who is a living person whom you define as a leader and why?
3. What, in your view, are the differences between business leaders and public health leaders?
4. How does creativity play a role in leadership activities?
5. How is collaboration related to leadership?
6. What role does social justice play in public health?
7. What are the main goals of public health?
8. What does it mean to say that public health leaders should think globally but act locally?
9. Is leadership different from management?

## Exercise 1-1:   Course Expectations

*Purpose:* to explore the expectations that students have at the beginning of a leadership course

*Key concepts:* expectations, leadership development, preconceptions

*Procedure:* Each student writes down initial thoughts or preconceptions about leadership and also writes down expectations for the course and for leadership training in general. The class then divides into groups of 5–10 members, and each group discusses the preconceptions and expectations. The students need to keep the lists they have created, for they will re-examine at the end of the course (in Exercise 18-1) what they thought at the start of the course. One way to make this a meaningful experience is to start a leadership journal in which your list becomes the first page of your journal.

## References

1. Institute of Medicine, *The Future of Public Health* (Washington, DC: National Academy Press, 1988).
2. Institute of Medicine, *The Future of the Public's Health* (Washington, DC: National Academy Press, 2003).
3. Institute of Medicine, *Training Physicians for Public Health Careers* (Washington, DC: National Academy Press, 2007).

4. J. P. Kotter, *Leading Change* (Boston: Harvard Business School Press, 1996).
5. S. E. Melendez, "An Outsider's View of Leadership," in *The Leader of the Future,* ed. F. Hesselbein et al. (San Francisco: Jossey-Bass, 1996).
6. Institute of Medicine, *Healthy Communities: New Partnerships for the Future of Public Health* (Washington, DC: National Academy Press, 1996).
7. S. M. Bornstein and A. F. Smith, "The Puzzles of Leadership," in *The Leader of the Future,* ed. F. Hesselbein et al. (San Francisco: Jossey-Bass, 1996).
8. J. W. Gardner, *Self-Renewal* (New York: W.W. Norton, 1981).
9. J. McKnight, *The Careless Society* (New York: Basic Books, 1995).
10. R. K. Greenleaf, *The Servant as Leader* (Indianapolis, IN: Greenleaf Center for Servant Leadership, 1970).
11. Kotter, *Leading Change.*
12. F. Wickman and T. Sjodin, *Mentoring* (Chicago: Irwin Professional Publishing, 1996).
13. L. Phillips-Jones, *The New Mentors and Proteges* (Grass Valley, CA: Coalition of Counseling Centers, 2001).
14. M. Murray, *Beyond the Myths and Magic of Mentoring,* rev. ed. (San Francisco: Jossey-Bass, 2001).
15. P. Hersey et al., *Management of Organizational Behavior,* 9th ed. (Upper Saddle River, NJ: Prentice Hall, 2007).
16. P. M. Senge et al., *The Fifth Discipline Handbook* (New York: Dell, 1994).
17. N. Brandon, "Self-esteem in the Information Age," in *The Organization of the Future,* ed. F. Hesselbein et al. (San Francisco: Jossey-Bass, 1997).
18. D. Baumrind, "An Exploratory Study of Socialization Effects on Black Children: Some Black-White Comparisons," *Child Development* 43 (1972): 261–267.
19. D. Sethi, "The Seven R's of Self-Esteem," in *The Organization of the Future,* ed. F. Hesselbein et al. (San Francisco: Jossey-Bass, 1997).
20. K. Blanchard and N. V. Peale, *The Power of Ethical Management* (New York: Fawcett Columbine, 1988).
21. R. Preston, *The Hot Zone* (New York: Random House, 1994).
22. L. Garrett, *The Coming Plague* (New York: Farrar, Straus & Giroux, 1994).
23. J. B. McCormick and S. Fisher-Hoch, *Level 4: Virus Hunters of the CDC* (Atlanta: Turner Publishing Co., 1996).
24. J. M. Kouzes and B. Z. Posner, *The Leadership Challenge,* 4th ed. (San Francisco: Jossey-Bass, 2007).
25. P. M. Senge, *The Fifth Discipline; The Art and Practice of the Learning Organization* (New York: Doubleday, 2006).
26. B. Nanus, *Visionary Leadership* (San Francisco: Jossey-Bass, 1992).
27. S. Helgesen, "Leading from the Grass Roots," in *The Leader of the Future,* ed. F. Hesselbein et al. (San Francisco: Jossey-Bass, 1996).
28. J. W. Gardner, *On Leadership* (New York: The Free Press, 1990).
29. C. R. Shaffer and K. Anundsen, *Creating Community Anywhere* (New York: Jeremy P. Tarcher and Perigee, 1993).
30. Shaffer and Anundsen, *Creating Community Anywhere.*
31. M. S. Peck, "The Fallacy of Rugged Individualism," in *In the Company of Others,* ed. C. Whitmyer (New York: Jeremy P. Tarcher and Perigree, 1993).
32. R. N. Bellah et al., *Habits of the Heart* (Berkeley, CA: University of California Press, 1985).
33. J. R. O'Neill, *The Paradox of Success* (New York: Jeremy P. Tarcher and Putnam, 1994).
34. J. Kofomidos, *The Balancing Act* (San Francisco: Jossey-Bass, 1993).

# CHAPTER 2

## LEADERSHIP STYLES AND PRACTICES

> But leadership in public health involves more than individual leaders or individuals in leadership positions. Public health is intimately involved in leadership as an agent of social change by identifying health problems and risks and stimulating actions toward their elimination.
>
> B. J. Turnock, *Public Health*

This chapter begins by examining several styles of leadership. Leadership style generally refers to the way a leader provides direction to his or her organization, how plans and programs get implemented, and how staff are motivated to do their work. The first model describes McGregor's distinction between two main leadership styles, referred to as Theory X and Theory Y. It then discusses another way of categorizing leadership styles, based on the Leadership Grid, and explores the view that a leader needs to use different styles in different situations. The next section of the chapter is devoted to an account of the characteristics that a leader must possess in order to lead effectively. The last section presents a discussion on the importance of talent as a critical component in leadership.

## Leadership Styles

### Theory X and Theory Y

In a classic study, McGregor discussed two leadership styles, Theory X and Theory Y, that are appropriate for different types of organizations.[1] Theory X is the more suitable for an organization in which the employees do not like their work situation and will avoid work whenever possible. In this case, the employees will have to be forced, controlled, or reprimanded in order for the organization to meet its goals and objectives. The employees are looking for control because they are not willing to guide the work process themselves. The thing they are most interested in is security.

McGregor noted that a situation in which employees are unhappy and need to be controlled will push leaders toward an autocratic style of leadership. Theory X represents a mainly negative approach to leadership. I had dinner with a local public health administrator at an American Public Health Association annual meeting several years ago. During the discussion, the question why this administrator did not send any of his staff to a leadership program was raised. His answer—that he was the leader and his staff did not need leadership development—exemplifies the Theory X style of leadership.

Theory Y is appropriate for an organization in which the employees like their jobs and feel that their work is natural and restful. Further, because they accept the goals and objectives of the organization, they tend to be self-directed and even to seek higher levels of responsibility. Finally, decision making occurs at all levels of the organization. Theory Y is essentially a democratic form of leadership. A public health administrator who had completed a state public health leadership program decided that he had benefited greatly from the training. Over the following five years, he sent most of his executive staff to the program to develop their leadership skills. Another 10 years have passed, and this director has begun to send his new staff through the same leadership development program. His actions exemplify the Theory Y style of leadership. Exercise 2-1 is intended to help elucidate the difference between Theory X and Theory Y.

## The Managerial Grid

Blake and Mouton adapted the Managerial Grid, a tool devised by Blake and his colleagues, to form the Leadership Grid (Figure 2-1).[2] There are 81 positions on the grid and five different leadership styles. The vertical axis represents concern for people and the horizontal axis represents concern for production (task-oriented behaviors). The location of each style on the grid is determined by where the style falls with respect to the two dimensions. For example, the *country club management* approach is characterized by a high level of concern for people and a low level of concern for production and is thus placed in the upper left-hand corner of the grid. This managerial approach creates a relaxed atmosphere and makes people happy to come to work in the morning.

If a leader is not seriously concerned about the well-being of the employees or about production, the result is *impoverished management*. In this style of leadership, the leader engages in the least amount of work necessary to solve a production problem.

The third approach is *team management*, in which the level of concern for employees and production is high. Strong trusting relationships develop, and all or most employees feel a commitment to accomplish the tasks at hand.

In the *authority-obedience approach*, the primary concern of the leader is to control the production process and increase productivity. The leader's concern for the employees' well-being is minimal.

*Organization man management* tries to balance the needs of the employees and the needs of production.

## Situational Leadership

Instead of using just one leadership style, leaders should use different styles for different situations, according to some authors.[3-6] The series of one-minute manager books, by Blanchard and others, tries to integrate the needs of organizations with the needs of both employees and customers. Blanchard and his coauthors designated their approach Situational Leadership II.[7,8] As with the Managerial Grid, leadership behavior is evaluated along two dimen-

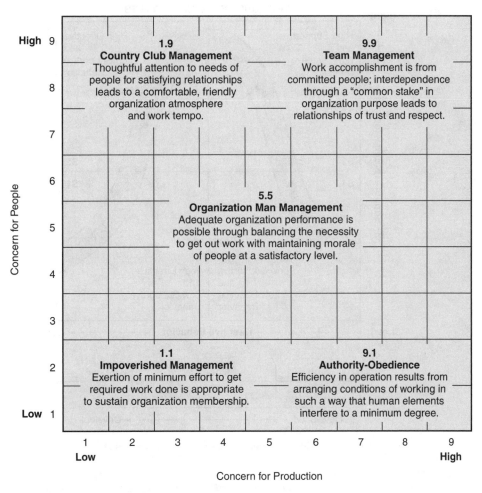

**FIGURE 2-1   The Leadership Grid®**
*Source:* Reproduced by permission. From Leadership Dilemmas—Grid Solutions copyright
© 1991 by Robert R. Blake and the Estate of Jane S. Mouton, Austin, Texas. Gulf Publishing
Company, Houston, Texas, 800-231-6275. All rights reserved.

sions: directiveness and supportiveness (Figure 2-2). The type of leadership
that is relatively nonsupportive and nondirective is termed a "delegating"
style of leadership. The type that is supportive but nondirective is termed a
"supporting" style of leadership. Leadership behavior that is highly supportive and highly directive constitutes "coaching," and leadership behavior that
is highly supportive and highly directive is called "directing."

The model is intentionally flexible. A leader will need to relate to an employee in a given situation using a specific leadership style, a style partly determined by the task and the employee's years in the organization. There are
certain assumptions here. First, there is the assumption that people want to
learn and develop their skills over time. Second, Blanchard pointed out that
there may be no guaranteed best leadership style to make this happen. In fact,
it may be that some people have a better capacity for learning than others do.

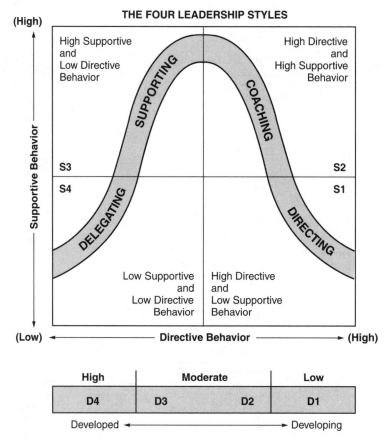

**FIGURE 2-2 Situational Leadership II**
*Source:* "The Four Leadership Styles"—from *Leadership and the One Minute Manager* by Kenneth Blanchard, Ph.D., Patricia Zigarmi, Ed.D. and Drea Zigarmi, Ed.D. Copyright © 1985 by Blanchard Management Corp. Reprinted by permission of HarperCollins Publishers, Inc.

There are clear overlaps between McGregor's analysis of leadership styles and Blanchard's. Theory X involves directing and some coaching. Theory Y involves some coaching, supporting, and delegating. However, the Situational Leadership II model is the more adaptive of the two. Hersey, Blanchard, and Johnson noted an overlap between McGregor's model and the Situational Leadership II model, but they thought that Theory X and Theory Y represented leaders' and managers' assumptions about leadership and that these assumptions often did not get translated into action.[9]

It is clear that leaders must use different strategies for different employees. Leadership occurs in a social context in which values and norms cannot help but influence the process of leading. One leadership approach will not work for every individual in an agency. Unfortunately, some public health leaders are inflexible and use one style predominantly. For instance, one local public health administrator believed it was necessary for him to use an authoritarian approach for managing his staff. Years later, he moved to a new public health agency that he discovered to be more democratic in form. He changed his leadership style but did not seem to learn that leadership style needs to be tied to the situation at hand and not to the agency.

## Other Analyses of Leadership Style

In a classic paper, Tannenbaum and Schmidt explored how a leader-manager might be democratic in some situations and autocratic in others.[10] As can be seen in Figure 2-3, both leadership styles are used to carry out the activities of the organization. In fact, most leadership practices fall between the two extremes. For example, the action of presenting ideas to subordinates and inviting questions from them involves the use of authority by the manager but also gives to the subordinates a degree of freedom or power. Tannenbaum and Schmidt's analysis is similar to the work of Lewin and his colleagues at the University of Iowa.[11,12] The Lewin group distinguished three leadership styles—autocratic, democratic, and laissez-faire. Their research showed that the democratic style seemed to be especially suitable for group process-oriented activities.

Bass and Stogdill found that leaders differ in the approach they take to leading their organizations, in part because of the variation in the issues they need to address.[13] Furthermore, they discovered that leadership behaviors generally fall on a continuum between task-oriented and relationship-oriented behaviors.

Fiedler explored the relationship between three factors that affect leadership effectiveness: personal relationships with work associates, the structure of the task to be performed by the work group, and the power associated with the leader's position in the organization.[14] These three factors can be combined in eight ways. According to Fiedler, leaders who are task oriented tend to be more effective in very favorable or very unfavorable situations than those who are relationship oriented. Leaders who are relationship oriented, on the other hand, perform better in situations that fall between the two extremes. Note that public health leaders must be both task and relationship

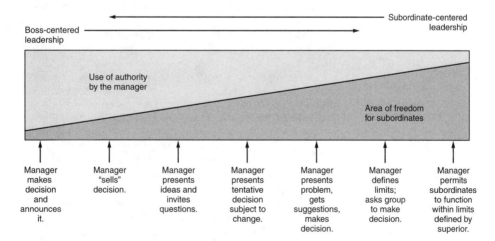

**FIGURE 2-3   Continuum of Leadership Behavior**
*Source:* Reprinted by permission of Harvard Business Review. From "How To Choose a Leadership Pattern" by R. Tannenbaum and W. H. Schmidt, May-June/1973. Copyright © 1973 by the President and Fellows of Harvard College; all rights reserved.

oriented, because public health programs demand good communication be-tween public health leaders and their constituents (see Chapter 11).

Hersey, Blanchard, and Johnson developed a typology of task- and relationship-oriented behavior: high-task and low-relationship behavior, high-task and high-relationship behavior, high-relationship and low-task behavior, and low-task and low-relationship behavior.[15] The authors added effectiveness-ineffectiveness as a third dimension (Table 2-1). As noted above, public health leaders need to exhibit high-task and high-relationship behavior.

In the 1940s, a series of studies was done by the Bureau of Business Research at Ohio State University.[16] The researchers defined leadership as the direction of group activities for the purpose of attaining a goal. Leadership, in their view, involved two types of behavior: initiating structure (task-oriented behavior) and showing consideration for the needs of employees (relationship-oriented behavior). The researchers hypothesized, on the basis of their data, that both types of leadership behavior are necessary, but they found little relationship between the two types of behavior.

Utilizing the Ohio State model elements, House formulated a path-goal model.[17] According to this model, a leader's task was to help followers attain their goals through appropriate direction and support. In other words, the leader points the way to the right path to enhance the ability of followers to reach their goals. In addition, House characterized leadership behaviors as either directive, supportive, participative, or achievement oriented.

**Table 2-1    How the Basic Leadership Styles May Be Seen by Others**

| Basic Style | Effective | Ineffective |
|---|---|---|
| High task and low relationship behavior | Seen as having well-defined methods for accomplishing goals that are helpful to the followers | Seen as imposing methods on others; sometimes seen as unpleasant and interested only in short-run output |
| High task and high relationship behavior | Seen as satisfying the needs of the group for setting goals and organizing work but also providing high levels of socioemotional support | Seen as initiating more structure than is needed by the group and often appears not to be genuine interpersonal relationships |
| High relationship and low task behavior | Seen as having implicit trust in people and as being primarily concerned with facilitating their goal accomplishment | Seen as primarily interested in harmony; sometimes seen as unwilling to accomplish a task if it risks disrupting a relationship or losing "good person" image |
| Low relationship and low task behavior | Seen as appropriately delegating to followers decisions about how the work should be done and providing little socioemotional support where little is needed by the group | Seen as providing little structure or socioemotional support when needed by members of the group |

*Source:* © 2006 Reprinted with permission of the Center for Leadership Studies, Inc. Escondido, CA 92025. www.situational.com. All Rights Reserved.

Researchers at the University of Michigan followed the Ohio State model by dividing leadership behaviors into those that were employee oriented (roughly equivalent to showing consideration for employees) and those that were production oriented (roughly equivalent to structure initiation activities).[18]

## Leadership Traits

Those who study leadership traits usually attempt to create an interface between the way leaders think and the ways they tie their thoughts into action on a daily basis. It is these traits that are reflected in the leadership styles of individuals. Traits seem to combine some innate qualities with qualities that seem to be learned. Bass and Stogdill reviewed studies of leadership traits and abilities done between 1948 and 1970.[19] Table 2-2 contains a list of all the traits

**Table 2-2    Factors Appearing in Three or More Studies of the 52 Surveyed**

| Factor | Number of Studies Found |
| --- | --- |
| Technical skills | 18 |
| Social nearness, friendliness | 18 |
| Task motivation and application | 17 |
| Supportive of the group task | 17 |
| Social and interpersonal skills | 16 |
| Emotional balance and control | 15 |
| Leadership effectiveness and achievement | 15 |
| Administrative skills | 12 |
| General impression (halo) | 12 |
| Intellectual skills | 11 |
| Ascendence, dominance, decisiveness | 11 |
| Willingness to assume responsibility | 10 |
| Ethical conduct, personal integrity | 10 |
| Maintaining a cohesive work group | 9 |
| Maintaining coordination and teamwork | 7 |
| Ability to communicate; articulativeness | 6 |
| Physical energy | 6 |
| Maintaining standards of performance | 5 |
| Creative, independent | 5 |
| Conforming | 5 |
| Courageous, daring | 4 |
| Experience and activity | 4 |
| Nurturant behavior | 4 |
| Maintaining informal control of the group | 4 |
| Mature, cultured | 3 |
| Aloof, distant | 3 |

*Source:* Adapted with the permission of The Free Press, a Division of Simon & Schuster, Inc. from *Bass & Stogdill's Handbook of Leadership: Theory, Research, and Management Applications*, Third Edition by Bernard M. Bass. Copyright © 1974, 1981, 1990 by The Free Press. All Rights Reserved.

and abilities reported in three or more of the studies. Leading the list are technical skills, social nearness and friendliness, task motivation and application, supportiveness toward group activities, social and interpersonal skills, emotional balance and control, and leadership effectiveness and achievement.

Kouzes and Posner compared the traits identified in 1987 and again in 2007 as the chief characteristics of admired leaders (Table 2-3).[20] The five most frequently mentioned leadership traits of the most admired leaders in 1987 were honesty, forward-lookingness, the ability to inspire, competence, and intelligence. In 2007, honesty still topped the list, followed by competent, forward-looking, intelligent, and fair-minded. Honesty was also reported as the number one trait in Canada, Australia, Malaysia, New Zealand (tied with forward-looking), and Mexico. Being forward-looking was reported as the number one trait of admired leaders in Denmark, Japan, Korea, Singapore, and Sweden.

A determination of the traits expected of leaders is used by the military in an effort to not only designate traits but also to use these traits as indicators

**Table 2-3    Characteristics of Admired Leaders**

| Characteristics | 2007 Respondents (Percentage of People Selecting) | 1987 Respondents (Percentage of People Selecting) |
|---|---|---|
| Honest | 89 | 83 |
| Forward-looking | 71 | 62 |
| Inspiring | 69 | 38 |
| Competent | 68 | 67 |
| Intelligent | 48 | 43 |
| Fair-minded | 39 | 40 |
| Straightforward | 36 | 34 |
| Broad-minded | 35 | 37 |
| Supportive | 35 | 32 |
| Dependable | 34 | 32 |
| Cooperative | 25 | 25 |
| Courageous | 25 | 27 |
| Determined | 25 | 20 |
| Caring | 22 | 26 |
| Imaginative | 17 | 34 |
| Mature | 15 | 23 |
| Ambitious | 16 | 21 |
| Loyal | 18 | 11 |
| Self-controlled | 10 | 13 |
| Independent | 4 | 10 |

*Note:* These percentages represent respondents from six continents: Africa, South America, North America, Asia, Europe, and Australia. The majority, however, are from the United States. Because the authors asked people to select seven characteristics, the total adds up to more than 100 percent.
*Source:* Reprinted with permission of John Wiley & Sons, Inc. From J. M. Kouzes and B. Z. Posner, *Leadership Challenge,* 4th ed. (San Francisco: Jossey-Bass, 2007).

of those that will reflect the values and culture of the military service and the country. For example, the Marine Corps lists 14 traits for people in the military who wish to become Marine leaders. Many, if not all of these traits may also reflect the expectation of a leader in public health. These 14 traits are:[21]

1. *Justice*, which is the practice of being fair and consistent;
2. *Judgment*, which is the ability to think clearly and in an orderly fashion for decision making;
3. *Dependability*, which reflects the ability to perform duties properly;
4. *Initiative*, which is taking action with or without orders;
5. *Decisiveness*, which is making good decision expeditiously;
6. *Tact*, which is dealing with people in a way that maintains good relations;
7. *Integrity*, which is honesty and truthfulness;
8. *Enthusiasm*, which is sincere involvement and enthusiasm in work;
9. *Bearing*, which is the way the leader conducts and carries him/herself;
10. *Unselfishness*, which is the avoidance of self comfort at the expense of the comfort of others;
11. *Courage*, which is calmness while recognizing fear;
12. *Knowledge*, which is acquiring the knowledge necessary to carry out one's work;
13. *Loyalty*, which is devotion to your country; and
14. *Endurance*, which is physical and mental stamina.

Leadership is dynamic, and there is probably no universal list of leadership traits that apply to all situations.[22] Nonetheless, whereas all the traits and abilities presented in Tables 2-2 and 2-3 are capable of enhancing the effectiveness of a leader, at least in certain circumstances, the 10 leadership abilities and practices described next have been singled out as especially important for successful leadership in the 21st century.

## Leadership Practices

First, leaders must be *knowledge synthesizers*. They must bring intelligence to the leadership enterprise. They need to know about past events, understand the realities of the present, and have a vision of the future. They must not only be experts in their chosen field but be familiar with many other areas as well. In public health, leaders need to understand the paradigm of core functions and essential services of public health as discussed in Part II of this book. Good leaders know how to use their knowledge to carve out a perspective and move their organization forward. Intelligence alone is not enough.[23] Self-awareness, self-control, self-confidence, commitment, integrity, the ability to foster change, and the ability to communicate with and influence others are all necessary.

Second, leaders need to be *creative*. They must not only manage large amounts of information but use it creatively to guide action. To do this successfully, they must ignore information that is not pertinent. It is hard to teach people to be creative, although most individuals tend to be creative in areas where they have high interest. When you have enthusiasm for what you are doing, there seems to be a natural flow to the process. It is possible for individuals to expand their creative abilities through practice, including through interacting with others in a social context.[24] Exercise 2-2 is designed to explore the creativity of the team members engaged in devising a solution to a public health problem.

Third, leaders need to be able to *create a vision* and get others to *share the vision* and demonstrate a *commitment to the vision* and the mission it represents. Creating a vision is not an easy thing to do, because it requires careful consideration of different scenarios that might occur if certain factors are present. Furthermore, creating a vision is next to pointless unless others can be convinced to share the vision. Pfeffer stated that a vision gets others to see beyond the obstacles of things to the important possibilities that can ensue in the future.[25] Long-term visions tend to allow people the opportunity to create many innovations, whereas short-term visions seem to be limited by the barriers that today's reality presents. Leaders also need to be flexible enough to modify the vision to better satisfy their partners in the visioning process. Finally, leaders need to fit the vision to a mission and devise an action plan to realize the vision.

Fourth, leaders need to foster and facilitate *collaboration*. No one in an organization exists in a vacuum, nor does anything get done in a vacuum. Turning a vision into reality requires the development of partnerships with external stakeholders and, in fact, the sharing of leadership. In shared leadership, each partner must respect the needs and wants of each of the other partners.

> **Leadership Tips**
>
> *Keep your knowledge and skills up to date. Be committed to lifelong learning.*

Fifth, leaders need to possess *entrepreneurial ability*. Traditional approaches to running companies and agencies no longer seem to be working. Leaders will increasingly need to explore alternate funding sources for their programs as well as learn how to use their resources in new ways.[26] This change in perspective will not only increase program efficiency but also program effectiveness. Perhaps surprisingly, leaders in the governmental public health sector need to learn these skills.

Sixth, successful leaders are *systems thinkers* who must also address the needs of complex environments. Acting as a change agent for an organization requires mastering the techniques of systems thinking as well as looking at the organization systemically.[27] Systems thinkers are consciously aware that everything is connected to everything else. The obvious problems plaguing an organization may be symptoms rather than root causes. A systems approach to change allows leaders to logically analyze the dimensions of the problems.

One way to put systems thinking into practice is to turn the organization into a learning organization—"an organization that is continually expanding its capacity to create its future."[28(p.14)] In a learning organization, the system becomes the guiding mechanism for change. This allows the organization to keep pace with the rapid rate of change in today's world, to function in a more interdependent manner, and to respond to the changing needs of society.[29] In a system, all the parts are interrelated, and activities that occur in one part affect all the others. The traditional linear approach to decision making is not appropriate for a true system. Systems thinkers see the big picture and are interested in the way organizations and individuals interrelate. They are students of change and the transformational patterns that affect change. Systems thinkers also think strategically. They try to determine strategies for facilitating change as they address the challenges of the system. These practices will be addressed more extensively in Chapter 4.

Seventh, leaders must *set priorities*. They have to determine what issues will be addressed within the organization. Because of the current focus on team development and community coalition building, leaders often set priorities in concert with team or community partners. Public health places a strong emphasis on the community assessment of health and disease, which helps in setting health priorities for a community. Because the health priorities are determined in concert with partners, subjective as well as objective factors tend to influence the priority-setting process. Decisions about priorities are often determined by political issues as well as community concerns.

Eighth, leaders need to *form coalitions and build teams*. They no longer practice the leader's craft in a vacuum, and they must be aware that their success depends on their being able to work with others. Because different individuals bring different expertise to the decision-making environment, teams are created to solve problems and make decisions. In teams, leadership is shared and different members move into the leadership position at different phases of the problem-solving process. Because of public health's strong community perspective, building coalitions to support the local public health agenda becomes critical. A community coalition is a team in which many community groups are represented, and it is a means of empowering the community to address its own problems.

Ninth, leaders, as pointed out previously, must not only bring a creative spark to the organization but also help put innovative ideas into practice. Therefore, they must become masters of the latest *management and leadership techniques*. This does not mean that they should adopt all the latest management fads. Rather, they should explore new techniques and integrate into their repertoire those techniques that will likely make the organization stronger, more productive, and more customer oriented.[30] The overall objective of managing is to guide the organization toward achievement of its vision. (Note that new management techniques will occasionally have to be adapted to the systems perspective, because even now many new techniques are linear in nature.)

Tenth, a successful leader acts as a *colleague, a friend, and a humanitarian* toward everyone in the organization. Leaders must be effective communicators and be able to empathize with colleagues, peers, and customers. They should protect the values of their organizations as well as the values of the communities in which they live. In fact, they will occasionally need to help define organizational and community values when necessary.

Most leaders of the 21st century, to be fully effective, will need to possess these 10 leadership abilities and characteristics. These abilities and characteristics provide a solid foundation for the activity of leading the process of developing a vision (and a mission) and bringing that vision to fruition. Each ability or characteristic will be revisited at appropriate places throughout this book.

## The Talent Issue

In the last several years, there has been an emergence of a new dimension of leadership that is tied to the relationship of talents of people and how these talents are reflected in the work of managers and leaders. Talent becomes a filter in which knowledge and skills get translated into action. Thus, it is more than a series of traits in that the combination of specific talents is unique in each individual. The following formula puts these new trends into perspective:

$$\frac{\text{Knowledge + Skills + Talent + Attitude + Personal Values}}{\text{Personal Strengths + Organizational Values}} = \text{Action}$$

The traditional view was that knowledge, attitudes, and skills led to action. Recent research shows that the process is more complicated.

In a number of books, the Gallup Organization has investigated the critical aspect of talent and how it impacts action.[31,32] What was discovered was that most organizations stressed the weaknesses of employees rather than their personal strengths. In order to address these weaknesses, individuals were often sent for training related to these weaknesses rather than training to make personal strengths stronger. In a study of 80,000 people in administrative positions, Buckingham and Coffman said that our orientation to weaknesses was incorrect.[33] Training does not substantially improve an individual's weaknesses. Our brains are wired to support our strengths rather than our weaknesses. This is the talent dimension. Thus, administrators have discovered that it is necessary to change our approaches to training and performance improvement. It is better to train people to use their personal talents more effectively.

The authors also pointed out that effective administrators have to become more expert at dealing with human capital issues. This means that they need to become more ready to hire people on the basis of their talents and not just on their technical knowledge and skills. It is in the day-to-day activities that an individual's talents are displayed. The administrator needs to let his direct reports define process on the basis of these personal talents. If this happens, then the administrator can concentrate on helping individuals determine outcomes and then measure performance on these outcomes. Thus, performance plays out on an individual's strengths rather than his or her weaknesses. The challenge then is to find the best fit for jobs on the basis of the combination of knowledge, skills, and talent.

In order to explore talent from the vantage point of strength. the Gallup Organization began an extensive research process to investigate what are the major talents of individuals. Buckingham and Clifton discussed this study of over two million people.[34] They reported that this research made the assumption that all individuals have a different combination of talents and strengths. Whereas using trait approaches tries to match individuals to the traits required for a job, talent research pointed out that each individual is different and it is important to create the best fit between these personal talents and strengths and the tasks to be performed. Because our brains are wired for our strengths, the combination of talents is unique to each of us. It is to our personal strengths that we need to move in our pursuit of knowledge and skills.

Out of the Gallup surveys was developed an instrument called Strength Finder, which is now in its second iteration.[35] This instrument measures 34 trait categories. The 34 talents are organized around four key themes, which are discussed by Coffman and Gonzalez-Molina.[36] First, there are themes involving relationships and how well we perform in these talents related to other people. The second theme involves our abilities to create impact in how we motivate people to act. Kouzes and Posner also listed enabling other people to act as a key leadership practice.[37] The third theme involves talents associated with our abilities to be action oriented. The final theme relates to our thinking talents. Table 2-4 lists the 34 talents related to the four themes.

An important lesson from this research is that an individual can become a strong performer within a particular job category and not be a strong performer in a higher level that requires a different set of talents that the individual may not have. The other part of the formula presented at the beginning of this section relates to the attitude that a person brings to his or her performance. Rath discusses how his grandfather Donald Clifton, who helped develop an instrument to measure strengths related to talent, also discussed the importance of positive thinking for managers and leaders.[38] The more positive reinforcement that the individual gets, the better the work performance becomes. The other numerator variable relates to the values that we bring to a job and to our other life activities. These values are also a guide to how we view our actions. The denominator of the formula on page X adds the way organizational values and our personal strengths filter the way we practice leadership and action. Our leadership style grows out of many of the factors listed in the formula, which affects the actions we take in problem solving and decision making. Experiment with the concepts in this section by doing Exercise 2-3.

**Table 2-4  Talent Categories of People**

| Relating Themes | Impacting Themes | Striving Themes | Thinking Themes |
| --- | --- | --- | --- |
| Communication | Command | Achiever | Analytical |
| Empathy | Competition | Activator | Arranger |
| Harmony | Developer | Adaptability | Connectedness |
| Includer* | Maximizer | Belief | Consistency[†] |
| Individualization | Positivity | Discipline | Context |
| Relator | Woo | Focus | Deliberative |
| Responsibility | | Restorative | Futuristic |
| | | Self-Assurance | Ideation |
| | | Significance | Input |
| | | | Intellection |
| | | | Learner |
| | | | Strategic |

* Previously "inclusiveness"
† Previously "fairness"
*Source:* From *Follow this Path* by Curt Coffman and Gabriel Gonzalez-Molina. Copyright © 2002 by the Gallup Organization. By permission of Grand Central Publishing.

## Summary

Traditional theories of leadership have tended to ignore situational factors that can influence which leadership style is best for a given set of circumstances. In addition, most of the leadership literature concerns leadership in the business sector, yet public agencies seem to work differently than for-profit companies. William Foege, a former director of the Centers for Disease Control and Prevention, has said on numerous occasions that social justice is the value that most motivates leaders in public health. Another way of saying this is that concern for people's well-being is primary. Case Study 2-A reviews some of the concerns and motivations of public health leaders.

---

**Case Study 2-A**
**Inner World to the Future: Leaders' Perspective on the Future**

*Louis Rowitz*

We are at a crossroads. Public health agencies appear to be under attack from multiple sources, including government entities, government superagencies, managed care organizations, the mass media, community groups, and disgruntled citizens. There is confusion about what the thing called "public health" is. There is concern about the involvement of public health agencies in direct medical service activities. Perhaps, some say, it is time for government to get out of the public health service business and spin off public health agency activities to the private sector.

To these concerns must be added a strong belief that leaders make a difference. Leaders bring hope and vision and have an ability to find solutions for the challenges that face the field of public health. It is to the training of public health professionals that the public health community looks as a possible way to strengthen the infrastructure of public health in this country and to clarify the vision of public health for the 21st century. There is a strong belief in the public health community that leadership skills can be taught. There is also a strong belief that a commitment to life-long learning is critical. For the last several years, national, regional, and state public health leadership programs have been developed. These programs have helped public health leaders increase their leadership skills and learn the latest techniques for improving and strengthening organizations. These programs have also trained public health leaders to work with communities to help define the role of public health at the community level. These programs have also stressed the importance of promoting the public health paradigm of core functions and essential public health services and of urging leaders to use their skills to build the public health system. These programs have developed unique approaches to training that promote an experiential application of all training materials back to the workplace and the community. The greatest challenge for these programs, other than the obvious one of financial sustainability, is the measurement of their long-term effect on the infrastructure of public health.

The combination of public health's challenges and the present-tense quality of our public health leadership programs, even when we talk about the future, raises an important series of issues related to where public health needs to go over the next several decades. The perspective is partly one of vision, but it is also one that goes to the very soul of the beliefs of public health leaders around the world. The experience of public health work changes us as professionals. Our inner world processes all our experiences and creates what the experimental psychologist Tolman called a cognitive map. Each experience changes the topography of our lives. This includes our personal experiences and our community living experiences as well as our professional experiences.

### Interviews with Public Health Leaders

During 1996, I began a personal odyssey to find out what public health leaders think about public health today and what they perceive will be public health's future. I traveled throughout the United States, England, Scotland, and Ireland conversing with public health leaders about the future of public health. I talked to more than 130 leaders in conversations that lasted about an hour. These conversations changed my cognitive map and my inner world by showing me the field of public health in ways that I had never perceived it. I talked to leaders at all levels of government. I talked to public health professionals at the federal, state, and local level in the United States as well as to academics. I talked to foundation professionals as well as professional trainers. I also talked to public health leaders who moved to the private sector. These leaders have given me insights about ways to strengthen our training programs in the future so that we can make public health more responsive to the needs of the public. They have also taught me what we do wrong and the importance of blending our strengths in solutions of our problems.

### Lessons Learned

Public health leaders live the reality of their chosen profession on a daily basis. They struggle with the crises of the day as well as with the concerns that public health faces as it progresses into the 21st century. Leaders in the United States face concerns with the impact of managed care on the public health field. Leaders in the United Kingdom and Ireland see public health within the context of a nationalized health service where managed care is a reality rather than a specter on the horizon. As I talked to U.S. leaders at the federal, state, and local levels as well as in both the public and private sectors, I found that all the leaders struggle with what that elusive field called public health is. The confusion extends to the issue of whether public health as a profession is different from public health as an organizational entity. U.S. public health is multidisciplinary as well as multisectorial in perspective. This means that we speak with many voices and do not always convey a unified message. Despite this multidisciplinary orientation, public health has a strong medical perspective and an increasingly economic one as well. One result is that the primary prevention goal of public health is sometimes lost as we pursue treatment and rehabilitation programs for underserved or unserved populations. Many leaders argue that the local public health agency must be a provider of last resort when there are limited medical services available for the people in local communities. As local public health agencies continue to act as direct service providers, leaders argue that managed care organizations' move into the local area of service is a threat to local health agencies that rely heavily on the service dollars received for direct service. However, public health needs to be seen as a partner in a total integrated health program in the community. Some leaders see public health agencies as playing the leading role in a comprehensive community-based health care system.

*(continues)*

**Case Study 2-A** *continued*

There is increasing acceptance of the core functions paradigm of assessment, policy development, and assurance, along with a lesser degree of acceptance of the essential public health services perspective. There is a concern that the core functions terminology is too abstract and confusing to people outside the public health field. U.S. leaders feel that we perform assessment activities fairly well, although we tend not to be conversant with the latest technology advances in informatics. Leaders at all government levels feel that they have a critical role in policy development but do not always exercise the policy opportunities that they have. Several leaders pointed out that public health leaders need to be students of the democratic process and understand how our political process works. The leaders are concerned that politicians and local board of health members or county board members have most of the control of the budget that drives the public health machine. They also believe that the relationship between the local health agency and its boards is often adversarial. Leaders argue that boards could become more of a voice for public health in the community than they currently are. In addition, these issues point to the question of how public health leaders can affect the decision-making process.

Most questions were raised about the assurance function and the difficulties in specifying completely our assurance role, because this is the role that underwent the most change during the last decade of the 20th century. There is agreement that public health needs to support a lifelong learning perspective and encourage and support continued educational and training opportunities for the public health workforce. However, training dollars are currently scarce.

Many leaders express concern about the future of public health in the United States and the increasing split between national public health concerns and state and local concerns. The agenda of each level of government is different and often not integrated with the issues of concern at other levels. In addition, we have not explored the possibilities of regional collaboration as a viable way to share programs across counties and other local entities and across states in different geographic areas. An added challenge concerns the absorption of public health into state human services umbrella agencies. However, some leaders feel that the umbrella agency model may increase the importance of public health agencies and leadership at the local level. Public health practice is really a local concern and needs to be protected. It must not become too parochial, because public health has a global perspective. State and local public health leaders need to think globally but act locally.

There are several other issues of concern to public health leaders. First, our assessment activities tend to ignore the important perspective of epidemiology, which provides methods for interpretation of data. Leaders often do not know how to use data for effective decision making. Second, public health needs to reclaim its primary prevention perspective and its key role in health promotion. Educational models should predominate in health promotion activities. Third, public health is developing academic and practice linkages, but not too many successful ones. Next, public health needs to do a better job in the areas of social marketing and health communications, because the public still does not know what public health is. Finally, public health needs to do a better job building community coalitions to address community public health needs. However, there is much to learn about the development of coalitions and how to keep up the interest of these coalitions over time.

In England, Scotland, and the Republic of Ireland, I saw national health systems in which public health often played a secondary role. In all three countries, public health is dominated by physicians. All other public health–related groups are in secondary support roles. Only physicians can head a public health program in a district. If other professionals want to move into a leadership role, they are often limited to roles in academic teaching settings. However, all public health physicians have received training in public health and have passed national credential examinations.

Purchasing of services becomes the primary role of the health service public health physicians. Primary prevention programs may exist in some areas, like immunization, but these programs are contracted out to local physicians or hospitals and clinics. A common complaint of the district physicians was their inability to use their public health knowledge in the health districts. They felt that a large amount of their professional energies were expended on conflicts with local managers, who are often not health trained. In England, public health physicians felt that public health is losing its foothold and becoming less visible. In the Republic of Ireland, public health offices were abolished for 20 years under the mistaken belief that all of the public health concerns of Irish society had been solved. Only in the past few years has public health been re-established in the districts. However, it is taking time for these offices to re-create public health programs. Scotland is an interesting case, in that community-based programs are being developed and supported within the Scottish office of the national health service.

The major lesson to be learned is that public health often has trouble surviving in a system in which all the citizens have access to services. However, primary prevention programs do not flourish in this environment without a vigorous struggle. Time pressure resulting from calendar overload becomes a problem. Bureaucracy and an overabundance of meetings at the local and national levels are the rule rather than the exception. In addition, each public health profession has its own organization, the agendas of these organizations conflict, and there is a consequent lack of agreement between these groups as to how to pursue a common public health agenda. However, these European countries are small, and most public health people know each other. This does offer opportunities for collaboration that are not often pursued.

**The Future**

Public health concerns never go away. Although it is possible to see variations in the ways public health is practiced, there will continue to be crises and issues of concern to the public health profession. There is growing anxiety about emerging infections and increasing resistance to the effects of antibiotics. Money available for health services is shrinking. Managed care organizations do not seem to hold all the answers for the health care needs of the American public.

The changing demographics of our population require public health interventions. The need for primary prevention activities and the development of health promotion and disease prevention initiatives remains critical. Ebbs and flows in the support for government-based public health programs will continue.

Public health leaders remain hopeful. They see growing support for leadership programs for the public health workforce. They project a growing influence of public health activities undertaken by local health departments. They are ambivalent about the movement to create superagencies at the state level, although they recognize that public health agencies need to work closely with other human services

*(continues)*

**Case Study 2-A** *continued*

agencies. Our technology knowledge will increase significantly over the next several decades. The Centers for Disease Control and Prevention will continue to be a major public health voice in this country. Public health will work more closely with its health care partners to develop more integrated systems of care. Some leaders see this collaboration as occurring from within an integrated health care system. Other leaders believe that public health agencies will remain part of the government system, because their oversight function must not be compromised. Closer linkages will evolve between academic institutions and public health agencies. Finally, public health's emphasis on core functions and essential services will lead to increased infrastructure strength in the future.

In summary, public health leaders bring a message of hope for the future. Public health will survive.

---

Given this fact of a people rather than a product orientation, the most balanced type of leadership in public health should probably be called, not organization man management (as it is designated in the Leadership Grid), but something like community collaboration leadership. A public health leader's concern for people encompasses many constituencies other than his or her work associates. Furthermore, production, in a public health setting, includes all sorts of programs and activities, from community assessment to the development of effective community interventions.

### Discussion Questions

1. What are the differences between the Theory X and Theory Y leadership styles?
2. What are the five leadership styles defined in the Leadership Grid?
3. What is an example of high-task, low-relationship leadership behavior?
4. How would you describe your dominant leadership style?
5. How flexible are you in modifying your dominant leadership style in situations that require a different style?
6. What are two examples of how you practice leadership?
7. What are five of the most cited traits of admired leaders?
8. What do you think are the most important traits a leader needs to possess?
9. Why do leaders of public organizations need entrepreneurial ability?
10. What are the similarities and differences between traits and talents?

### Exercise 2-1: Authoritarian and Democratic Leadership Styles

*Purpose:* to explore alternative approaches to decision making and to investigate how alternative leadership styles can influence program outcomes

*Key concepts:* authoritarian leadership style, democratic leadership style, decision making

*Procedure:* The class or training group should divide into two or more groups. Each group has the assignment to create a plan for developing a community's public health infrastructure using a given set of resources. The plan should address core infrastructure elements, including the local public health workforce, public health facilities and services, public health surveillance and information systems, and relationships with medical, social, community, government, and business organizations. To develop this plan, each team chooses a leader, who is given an envelope containing a note designating the leader as a supporter of the Theory X or the Theory Y leadership style. The leader guides the group through a planning process according to the characteristics of the leadership style assigned but does not inform the other team members which leadership style he or she is using. After half an hour, each team reports back to the class or training group as a whole, describing the exercise process, evaluating the leader, and describing the infrastructure plan chosen by the team and what its ramifications are.

### Exercise 2-2:   An Exercise in Creativity

*Purpose:* to generate solutions to a public health problem from several leadership perspectives and to learn how to use creativity to discover the best solution for a problem

*Key concepts:* community coalition, creativity, problem solving, team

*Procedure:* The class or training group should divide into small teams of five to eight people. Each member of each team should select a public health problem that concerns the particular member. The team then chooses one of the problems and tries to solve it from a personal perspective, a public health agency perspective, and a community coalition perspective. The exercise is repeated using the supposition that the mayor of the town or the governor of the state does not want public funds expended on the problem. The entire team should explore the advantages and limitations of the alternative solutions and the role that creativity plays in developing the solutions.

### Exercise 2-3:   Talent and Strength

*Purpose:* to become aware of when we make strong decisions and explore the underlying talents we have as leaders

*Key concepts:* talent, personal strengths, decision making

*Procedure:* Jot down in your journal or on a sheet of paper the last three decisions you made that demonstrate your effectiveness as a leader. Break down the class or training group into small teams of five to eight and discuss one example with your team where you showed your strength in making a decision. Looking at the list of talents in Table 2-4, determine what talents you displayed in your decision-making style.

## References

1. D. McGregor, *The Human Side of Enterprise* (New York: McGraw-Hill, 1985).
2. R. R. Blake et al., *The Leadership Grid* (Houston: Gulf Publishing Co., 1991).

3. K. Blanchard and S. Johnson, *The One Minute Manager* (New York: Morrow, 1982).

4. K. Blanchard and R. Lorber, *Putting the One Minute Manager to Work* (New York: Morrow, 1984).

5. K. Blanchard et al., *Leadership and the One Minute Manager* (New York: Morrow, 1985).

6. K. Blanchard et al., *The One Minute Manager Builds High Performing Teams* (New York: Morrow, 1990).

7. Blanchard et al., *Leadership and the One Minute Manager.*

8. Blanchard et al., *The One Minute Manager Builds High Performing Teams.*

9. P. Hersey et al., *Management of Organizational Behavior,* 9th ed. (Upper Saddle River, NJ: Prentice Hall, 2007).

10. R. Tannenbaum and W. H. Schmidt, "How to Choose a Leadership Pattern," *Harvard Business Review* (March–April 1958): 95–102.

11. K. Lewin and R. Lippitt, "An Experimental Approach to the Study of Autocracy and Democracy: A Preliminary Note," *Sociometry* 1 (1938): 292–300.

12. K. Lewin, "Field Theory and Experiment in Social Psychology," *American Journal of Sociology* 44 (1939): 868–896.

13. B. M. Bass, *Bass & Stogdill's Handbook of Leadership* (New York: The Free Press, 1990).

14. F. E. Fiedler, *A Theory of Leadership Effectiveness* (New York: McGraw-Hill, 1967).

15. Hersey et al., *Management of Organizational Behavior.*

16. R. M. Stogdill and A. E. Coons, eds., *Leader Behavior: Its Description and Measurement,* Research Monograph No. 88 (Columbus: Ohio State University, Bureau of Business Research, 1951).

17. R. J. House, "A Path-Goal Theory of Leadership," *Administrative Science Quarterly* 16 (1971): 321–338.

18. R. L. Kahn and D. Katz, "Leadership Practices in Relation to Productivity and Morale," in *Group Dynamics: Research and Theory,* eds. D. Cartwright and A. Zander (Evanston, IL: Peterson & Co., 1960).

19. Bass, *Bass & Stogdill's Handbook of Leadership.*

20. J. M. Kouzes and B. Z. Posner, *The Leadership Challenge,* 4th ed. (San Francisco: Jossey-Bass, 2007).

21. http://www.au.af.mil/au/awc/awcgate/usmc/leadership_traits.htm

22. Hersey et al., *Management of Organizational Behavior.*

23. D. Coleman, *Working with Emotional Intelligence* (New York: Bantam, 1998).

24. M. Csikszentmihalyi, *Creativity* (New York: HarperCollins, 1996).

25. J. Pfeffer, "No Excuses Leadership," *Leader to Leader,* 46 (Fall, 2007): 31–34.

26. D. Osborne and T. Gaebler, *Reinventing Government* (Reading, MA: Addison-Wesley, 1992).

27. D. L. Kauffman Jr., *Systems 1: An Introduction to Systems Thinking* (Minneapolis: Future Systems, Inc., 1980).

28. P. M. Senge, *The Fifth Discipline: The Art and Practice of the Learning Organization,* Revised and Updated (New York: Doubleday, 2006).

29. Senge, *The Fifth Discipline.*

30. S. P. Robbins and M. Coulter, *Management,* 8th ed. (Upper Saddle River, NJ: Prentice-Hall, 2005).

31. M. Buckingham and C. Coffman, *First Break All the Rules* (New York: Simon and Schuster, 1999).

32. M. Buckingham and D. O. Clifton, *Now, Discover Your Strengths* (New York: The Free Press, 2001).
33. Buckingham and Coffman, *First Break All the Rules.*
34. Buckingham and Clifton, *Now, Discover Your Strengths.*
35. T. Rath, *Strength Finder 2.0* (New York: Gallup Press, 2007).
36. C. Coffman and G. Gonzalez-Molina, *Follow This Path* (New York: Warner Books, 2002).
37. Kouzes and Posner, *Leadership Challenge,* 4th ed.
38. T. Rath and D. O. Clifton, *How Full Is Your Bucket?* (New York: Gallup Books, 2004).

# CHAPTER 3

---

# THE INTERFACE BETWEEN
# MANAGEMENT AND LEADERSHIP

---

> A manager is responsible for the application and performance of knowledge.
>
> Peter Drucker

There is an interesting training exercise called the Human Likert, which has a large group line up along a continuum.* The general instruction is to decide how each individual defines his or her professional life. On one side of the line are individuals who define themselves as public health practitioners with a major specialty such as an environmental health professional. In the middle of the line are those who define themselves as managers or administrators, and at the end of the line are those who define themselves as public health leaders. The facilitator then goes down the line asking people why they placed themselves as they did and whether they see themselves as moving along the line as they professionally advance in their chosen public health field. What this exercise does is demonstrate how people view their professional training, their personal definitions of management, and what they perceive as leadership. In a recent use of the Human Likert by me, one individual who defined himself as an environmental health professional said that he wanted to become an expert in his chosen field. He saw this as a demonstration of leadership without a specific designated leadership position in his organization. Those in the management position also saw that leadership could be demonstrated in a management position as well. Thus, it is possible to move horizontally as well as vertically in an organization. Horizontally, you advance by becoming the best public health practitioner that you can or the best manager or the best leader. If you want to move to a higher administrative position in your organization—a vertical move—it is necessary to move in the direction of your strengths rather than your weaknesses, as pointed out in Chapter 2.[1]

This chapter explores the connections between management and leadership. The following section examines the management issues and is followed by an example of matrix forms of organization that are being tried by the Centers for Disease Control and Prevention (CDC) through its goals management initiative. Next is a discussion of some of the connections between management and

---

*I learned this exercise from Dr. Magda Peck of the University of Nebraska Medical Center as she did this exercise before a maternal and child health leadership group.

leadership with a discussion of transactional and transformational leadership. A discussion of meta-leadership is then presented as one way to look at the interface between management and leadership. The final section of the chapter presents a road map that begins to demonstrate how these management and leadership functions interrelate.

## Managers and Management

As pointed out in Table 1-1, there are clear distinctions between managers and leaders. Managers are tied to the present and to the mission of the agencies that they serve. Leaders tend to be less bound by their home agencies or their positions although they need to be concerned about their vision for the agency and the support of the individuals who work in the agency to move the agency forward into the future. Leaders in public agencies allocate much of their time to building relationships with external stakeholders in the public health enterprise.[2] Although both managers and leaders tend to be tied to a specific agency position, the manager seems to be more locked into the requirements of the job than the leader does. Leaders are more oriented to their vision and the overall public health system, whereas the manager needs to concentrate on making the agency effective and efficient. The effective manager makes the dreams and visions of the leader real.

Another reality is that a specific individual may be hired into an administrative position (management) and be expected to carry out both management and leadership activities. This may not always be an easy task. People are different and they view the world in different ways. Browning has pointed out that people have different thinking attributes.[3] There are people who tend to be linear thinkers and are intrigued with rules, regulations, and protocols. They are structured in the way they do things. They tend to be organized and to resist change. These structured thinkers can be contrasted with people who tend to be analytical in their thinking. These are the problem solvers who are very logical and like abstract thinking. They like to put facts and numbers together. If we extend this structural and analytical thinking to the organizational level, we are probably talking about many governmental agencies that like process, analyze facts, follow rules and protocols, and tend to support a status quo perspective. Managers tend to fall into this classification of structural and analytical.

Browning stated that there are two other major thinking preferences. There are the conceptual thinkers who tend to want to view the big picture. They like change and tend to stir things up. For example, you think that you have the last draft of a technical report and the conceptual thinker will ask if you have thought about solution X. Conceptual people tend to be creative and look at new ways to achieve their visions and goals. The fourth thinking attribute is social. Those strong in this thinking preference tend to like to work in teams and show great concern for others. They tend to be empathic. Recent literature has pointed out that managers need to have strong people skills in today's environment.[4] Managers have to be able to fit people's talents into appropriate jobs that fit the needs of the organization.[5] The Browning Emergenetics Model can be seen graphically in Figure 3-1 where the analytical and structural half of the diagram represents left brain think-

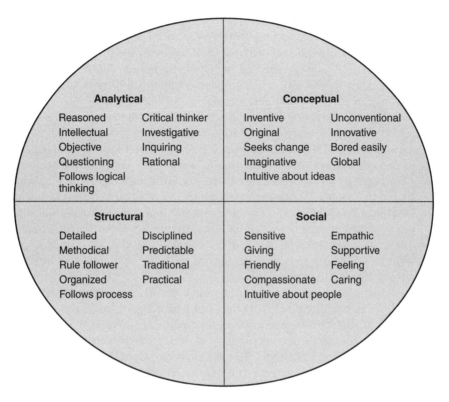

**FIGURE 3-1   Your Thinking Attributes**
*Source:* From G. Browning, *Emergenetics* (New York: Harper-Collins, 2006). With permission of the Author.

ing and the conceptual and social half represents right brain thinking.[6] Most people will show preference in more than one thinking attribute. All sorts of combinations are possible, from strong preference in one, two three, or four thinking attributes. However, the thinking preferences of an individual are filtered and affected by their behavioral attributes of expressiveness, assertiveness, and flexibility.

Management takes place within the context of an agency or an organization. In 1916, Fayol defined the five elements of management as prevoyance (planning), organizing, commanding, coordinating, and controlling.[7] Planning involves a series of actions to achieve organizational goals. Organizing involves the assignment of tasks to employees, fitting assignments into the existing hierarchical structure of the organization, and tying organizational goals to these work processes. Commanding is about leadership inside the organization. Some writers discuss the issues of employee productivity, turnover and absenteeism, job satisfaction, and other human capital issues for this function.[8] Wagner and Harter of the Gallup Organization strongly argue for following a 12-step model for engaging employees that will be the orientation of great managers.[9] Part of the motivation of employees involves the leaders in the organization sharing their vision with the managers. The coordinating and controlling elements involve the necessity for the manager to monitor activities of the agency and make corrections and realignments as necessary. Drucker defined the three tasks of management as determining the mission of the organization, creating a work environment that is productive and leads to worker achievement, and recognizing the social impact and social responsibility of the organization's activities.[10] It is interesting to note here that businesses as well as governmental public health agencies have a social impact and social responsibility dimension that for public health is related to the philosophy of social justice.

Fayol also developed a 14-principle guide for management that is as relevant today as it was when he formulated it early in the 20th century.[11] As can be seen in Table 3-1, the 14 principles cover all aspects of an organization's management, from a division of work to the creation of a positive environment in which people may work. A clarification regarding management needs to be made. Management activities will differ at different levels of the organization. Robbins and Coulter point out that technical skills will be necessary at the program level of the organization, with people skills becoming more important as you move up horizontally in the organization.[12] Conceptual skills become critical for the top managers and leaders in the organization. The leaders create change.

Administrators of state or local public health agencies or offices are generally appointed by elected officials or by local boards of health. New public health administrators tend to be seen as political appointees. These appointments to so-called leadership positions are in reality perceived to be high-level management positions. The job of these appointees is to manage the official public health agency. The new administrators face all types of organizational challenges during the early part of their tenure. As they accommodate to their new positions, demands from external community stakeholders need to be addressed. As community issues take precedence, the administrator may need to delegate managerial responsibilities to other people in the department.

**Table 3-1    Henri Fayol's 14 Principles of Management**

1. Division of Work (Specialization)
2. Authority
3. Discipline
4. Unity of Command (One Supervisor)
5. Unity of Direction
6. Subordination of Individual Interest
7. Remuneration
8. Centralization (or Decentralization)
9. Scalar Chain (Organizational Hierarchy)
10. Order
11. Equity
12. Stability of Tenure of Personnel
13. Initiative
14. Esprit de Corps

*Source:* From Fayol, *General and Industrial Management* (Paris: Dunod, 1916).

Working in government is not the same as working in business. It is not that the tools or skills necessary to work in these two sectors are very different, but rather that the public health leader needs to adapt these tools and skills to the public sector. There are at least four challenges for leaders who work in the public sector:[13]

(1) The public sector administrator has to work within the framework of laws, rules, regulations, and procedures defined by governmental entities. These laws, rules, regulations, and procedures put limits and restrictions on the public agency executive, which can affect mission, vision, performance, and progress at addressing public health issues.

(2) The performance of the agency is extremely visible to the outside world through legislative oversight and media scrutiny. Moore has stated that performance is affected by the challenge of creating public value for public sector issues.[14]

(3) The internal and external stakeholders that are affected by the work of public agencies are more numerous and representative of diverse value perspectives than in the business world. Each stakeholder has unique issues. There are multiple and diverse demands and levels of influence on the work of the agency.

(4) The realities of bureaucracy often impede or delay the ability of administrators to carry out the public's work in an effective, efficient, and timely manner.

Even though we live in a democratic society, people who work in government often seem to feel limited in their ability to move their agency agendas forward because of external scrutiny as well as political agendas.

It is incorrect to assume that all agencies are the same. Different agencies require different types of administrators to address these differences. There are at least four different organizational settings for the new administrator. Daly and Watkins define these settings as a start-up situation, turnaround, realignment or shift in priorities, and maintaining a successful organizational strategy.[15] Start-up and turnaround situations require that the new administrator needs to make changes quickly and does not

> **Leadership Tips**
>
> *Treat your board members as supporters and not enemies.*

have the leisure to learn about the organization and its staff as in realignment and success-sustaining organizations. Exercise 3-1 will allow the class or training group to experiment with Daly and Watkins's four organizational settings, utilizing a public health scenario.

During 2007, the National Association of County and City Health Officials (NACCHO) undertook a process of developing a plan for a new local health official orientation program. In concert with a NACCHO committee, the staff of the association began an interactive process of developing this program. The committee, NACCHO staff, and curriculum design consultants developed the curriculum.[16] It became clear early that the program needed to be strong on management issues because the committee composed of several seasoned health administrators strongly argued that new administrators need to spend time on management issues. Five specific competency expectations for new health officials were determined:[17]

(1) Clearly describe to their staff and variety of public audiences the roles and responsibilities of the new administrator within their local health departments (LHDs) and their LHD's roles and responsibilities within their local health system.

(2) Effectively engage elected officials, governing boards, and the state health department in carrying out the roles and responsibilities of their LHD.

(3) Effectively manage their LHD, including providing insight and direction of strategic planning and the agency's human, financial, and information resources.

(4) Effectively engage community partners in developing local public health systems for community health improvement and community preparedness initiatives.

(5) Rapidly access peer and coaching resources that may assist in developing leadership skills for addressing and resolving problems and issues that challenge local health officials.

Competency 3 clearly involves management competencies. Competencies 1 and 2 require both management and leadership activities. Competencies 4 and 5 are leadership competencies. What this means is that public health administrators have to do both management and leadership activities to carry out their jobs effectively. The cautionary consideration is that some people are great managers and some are great leaders. Bringing the two sets of talents and skills together may not always be possible.

It is clear that public health needs both excellent managers and excellent leaders. In order to address the management domain, the University of North Carolina School of Public Health and the Kenan-Flagler Business School have developed a model training program for managers. The Management Academy was created to develop teams of health professionals to address management challenges in community health.[18] The training curriculum helps individuals to improve their management skills, work in small groups on interactive management exercises, transfer new skills into action, build teams, create networks, and learn how to develop business plans. The curriculum includes information on managing people, business planning, human resources development, financial management, civic entrepreneurship, marketing, communication, partnerships, negotiation, program implementation, and team building. Steve Orton, the director of the Management Academy, answers the public health practice quiz in Case Study 3-A.

---

### Case Study 3-A
### A Public Health Practice Quiz for Steve Orton

**(1) What types of management training do public health professionals need?**
Public health professionals have widely varied skills and backgrounds, so individuals have different needs. Public health work does seem to present some specific challenges, though—and I believe that the current environment creates some challenges for managers across the board.

For public health, I think managers need training that builds skills in managing teams, because so much of the high-yield work they do involves convening teams, bridging differences, translating across disciplines and/or organizations, and sustaining effort (often without positional authority).

They need training in managing money, because so few of them have a background in finance. We have done pre-course assessments in the Management Academy for many years: too many public health managers have no confidence in their abilities to read a spreadsheet, create a budget, calculate a break-even point for a program, or understand the financial reports for the programs they manage. Few managers have taken finance in school, even those with MPH preparation. And few public health organizations have a culture of attending to finances, so managers don't have to learn money management to succeed. External pressures are building though—I think many managers now feel the need to develop finance skills.

Managers generally, not just in public health, need training that they can quickly translate into practice. I see a need for training in managing people effectively, so that they are engaged and committed and well-deployed.

Clearly, in each of these areas, it isn't sufficient to read the book or listen to the lecture about the topic: these are skills. It isn't even sufficient to have the individual ability, because in these areas the "competence" is in some sense collective: team-wide, organization-wide, even community-wide.

### (2)  How do we evaluate the effectiveness of this type of training?
Very carefully. I think that evaluating management training for professionals should make sure the process is working (and constantly improving), and should also seek measures of impact on behaviors and ultimately organizations, where management gets enacted. Training transfer to the workplace should always be the goal.

My own experience with this process convinces me that evaluation, and evaluators, should be integrated into design and quality improvement. Don't expect to determine effectiveness by hiring an evaluator after the program runs.

I say "very carefully" because I worry that some people have unrealistic expectations of what an educational intervention can accomplish, when so many forces act on organizations and communities. But I also worry that other people have such low expectations.

### (3)  How is management training different from leadership training?
Short answer: leadership training is big-picture; management training is nuts-and-bolts. At UNC, this is how we differentiate our leadership and management programs in executive education. For instance: leadership communication is about message mapping and media skills. Management communication is about communicating in a work team, writing e-mails, or crafting a good PowerPoint presentation.

### (4)  How do we create an interface between management and leadership training?
Education is not inoculation. Workforce development isn't a one-time shot; it's an individual and organizational commitment to keep learning. The best leaders, and the best organizations, are seeking out training continually, assessing themselves, strategizing, learning new skills, practicing, stretching, staying fresh. Personally, I think the individuals and organizations that get that are already doing a good job of integrating learning from lots of different sources.

The challenge for producers of training is to stay in touch with the needs of the audience to keep training relevant. The integration, ultimately, happens at the con-

*(continues)*

**Case Study 3-A** *continued*

sumer level—so those of us funding or implementing training programs need to stay tuned in.

**(5)  What is the next level of management training for public health professionals?** I think there is plenty of need for manager development at the current level! To me, the "next level" would be to have many more public health managers developing new skills. System-wide, we have plenty to do to make sure managers have reasons and resources to develop themselves in relevant areas.

## Matrix Organizations in Public Health

In recent years, there have been discussions about the difficulties of working in traditional hierarchical organizations. The concept of a silo has been used to reflect what goes on in vertical organizations when programmatic units become insulated from other programs within an organization or agency. There have also been discussions about changes in the way work is done in the public sector. Goldsmith and Eggers have discussed these issues within a governance by network model.[19] We are seeing the rise of third-party government where we contract with private firms and nonprofit organizations to do the work of government. There is also joined-up government activities where partnerships are created between two or more governmental entities to provide an integrated approach to delivering public programs. Changes in technology are also affecting our work relations in that it is possible to work on common projects from great distances using the Internet. Friedman described this process as evidence of a flattening world.[20] Goldsmith and Eggers also described consumer demand and the possibilities of customized service models in the future. Governmental employees involved in these new initiatives will find that the way they work will change. Instead of supervising employees in the agency, these new managers will find themselves managing portfolios of projects being done outside their home agency.

> **Leadership Tip**
>
> *Without trust, leaders often fail.*

With these changes possible, it becomes necessary to change our agencies as well. One model builds on the matrix form of management with the goal of leveling the organization to be more project or goal focused with techniques for coordinating activities across projects. Robbins and Coulter have defined a horizontal matrix structure as a form of organizational model involving program specialists from various functional units in an organization to work on a multidisciplinary team to carry out a project or goal-based program.[21] Figure 3-2 graphically shows a sample matrix structure model. The model labels each unit as a portfolio to reflect that the project or goal approach will allow the individual unit to manage all parts of a project or projects related to the unit program. The role of the steering committee is to be a group that includes a representative of each project or goal unit to supervise

**Overall Strategic Plan**

**FIGURE 3-2    Mapping the Horizontal in Matrix Structure: Overall Strategic Plan**

the whole project and to prioritize all the projects and goals of the organization.[22] The steering committee can also be the manager of the overall strategic plan of the organization.

On the positive side, this organizational model is flexible and allows for projects and goals to be added or subtracted as appropriate. This model also allows new projects to draw on the talents and strengths of people in the agency who will help benefit a specific project. Each unit staff also requires that both management and leadership processes happen. Creativity in the developing of new projects or sub-projects will also be encouraged.

There are also difficulties with the design. First, the matrix model is often superimposed on a traditional vertical organization. What this does is complicate the processes and work of the organization. On the one hand, the programmatic silos continue to exist at the same time as the matrix units are developed. The challenge then becomes how to have the silo teams buy into the matrix units' projects and goals. Marketing within the organization needs to be done to support the matrix structures.

There may also be control and communication difficulties with the model as well as resistance to the design by the established vertical organization. Some staff of the agency sometimes believe that they have two bosses and have to report to their silo supervisor as well as the team leader of the matrix unit. There is also the issue of power and the difficulty to share power. Credibility and trust issues also have to be addressed. There are possible methods for addressing some of these silo concerns. Lencioni has delineated a four-part model for this.[23] The model, if addressed early, may prevent some of the resistance to a project or goal-based horizontal matrix model. There needs to be a clear vision for the agency that is shared by all of the silo directors serving as a leadership team for the agency. Agency goals also need to be determined. These goals then are translated into clearly defined objectives or projects that can evolve into matrix units around these objectives or projects. These objectives then need to be aligned to standard operational requirements. Finally, there needs to be a methodology for measuring the results of the agency's activities and programs.

There are both management and leadership outputs from matrix structures. Table 3-2, which is adapted from the work of Paula Martin, shows these outputs.[24] The CDC provides us with an intriguing variation of the matrix model in its reorganization and goals development program. The next section will look at the CDC Health Protection Goals agenda as an example of the application of a modified matrix management program.

**Table 3-2  Management and Leadership Outputs**

Goals aligned with customers and partners
Processes aligned with customers
Capacity in line with the strategic plan
Resources deployed effectively
Performance improvement implemented as needed
Create standards and use common methodologies
Develop teams that produce results
Promote organizational learning
Collaborative leadership
Creation of an innovative portfolio
Shared leadership
High-performing teams
Working inside the organization and with external partners

*Source:* From P. Martin, *Quick Guide: The New Matrix Management* (Cincinnati: Martin Training Associates, 2005).

## CDC Futures Initiative[25]

Dr. Julie Gerberding, the director of the CDC, announced in June 2003 the start of a Futures Initiative to restructure CDC, prioritize its strategies for the 21st century, revamp its programs, and determine resources and needs. CDC professionals assigned to the Futures group collected information from CDC partners and customers. An extensive review was made of the agency's performance, organization, and operations. From all these deliberations, six strategic directions were formulated for the agency:

(1) Health Impact Focus
(2) Customer-centricity
(3) Public Health Research
(4) Leadership
(5) Global Health Impact
(6) Accountability

Dr. Gerberding and her leadership team said that it was necessary for the CDC to address the many new health and safety challenges for the 21st century within the United States and globally. These activities began with a project called the Futures Initiative. The major determination was to develop a management and strategic plan for the agency that would address many of these concerns. Gerberding had to sell the plan at a national level as well as at the agency level before many of the details of the initiative could be implemented.

There are two major changes that came about as a result of the Futures Initiative. The first was a major restructuring of the agency in April 2005 in an attempt to break down the silo model that had existed for a number of years and decrease the number of programs that reported directly to the CDC director. The second change involved the development of a number of health protection goals that would provide the direction for the CDC's work in the future. Ideally, these two changes would become integrated in a holistic manner. The new structure designated eight national centers:

(1) Environmental Health
(2) Injury Prevention
(3) Global Health
(4) Health Promotion
(5) Infectious Diseases
(6) Public Health Information, Health Marketing, and Health Statistics
(7) Terrorism Preparedness and Emergency Response
(8) Workplace Health and Safety

These national centers have a number of programmatic divisions with their own financial resources. These divisions have their own directors and tend to be resistant to many of the changes within the CDC. As can be seen in Figure 3-3, there are six coordinating centers and the National Institute for Occupational Safety and Health. The directors of these coordinating centers are supposed to work together to provide direction to the activities of the agency as well as provide mechanisms for the implementation of the CDC Health Protection Goals.

The Coordinating Center for Environmental Health and Injury Prevention includes the National Center for Environmental Health and the National Center for Injury Prevention and Control. The Coordinating Office for Global Health includes all global health initiatives. The Coordinating Center for Health Promotion includes the National Center on Birth Defects and Developmental Disabilities, the National Center for Chronic Disease Prevention and Health Promotion, and the Office of Genomics and Disease Prevention. The Coordinating Center for Infectious Diseases includes the National Center for HIV/AIDS, Viral Hepatitis, STD, and TB Prevention; the National Center for Immunization and Respiratory Diseases; the National Center for Zoonotic, Vector-Borne, and Enteric Diseases; and the National Center for Preparedness, Detection, and Control of Infectious Diseases. The Coordinating Center for Health Information and Service includes the National Center for Health Marketing, National Center for Health Statistics, and the National Center for Public Health Information. The Coordinating Office for Terrorism Preparedness and Emergency Response covers the preparedness initiatives for the CDC. The National Institute for Occupational Safety and Health covers the programs related to workplace safety and health. As pointed out, the national centers, with their individual directors and the divisions within centers, were to work horizontally with each other (modified matrix model) as well as vertically with their coordinating centers (a silo model). The National Centers have a leadership committee but not a steering committee, which is more traditional in matrix systems.

In addition to the coordinating centers, there are a number of offices tied to the director of the CDC. These offices include:

(1) Office of the Chief Science Officer
(2) Office of Chief of Public Health Practice
(3) Office of Chief Operating Officer
(4) CDC Washington Office
(5) Office of Strategy and Innovation
(6) Office of Workforce and Career Development
(7) Office of Enterprise Communication
(8) Office of Chief of Staff
(9) Office of Dispute Resolution and Equal Employment Opportunity

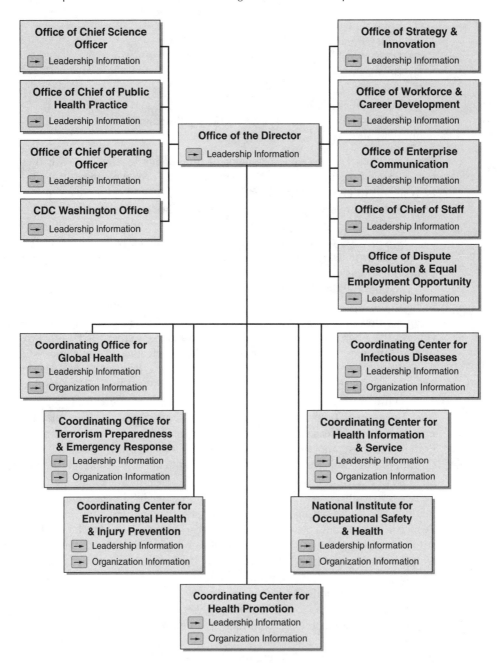

**FIGURE 3-3   CDC Organizational Chart (2007)**
*Source:* CDC Office for Enterprise Communications. Available at: www.cdc.gov/about/
organization/orgChart.htm. Accessed November 17, 2007.

The advantage of this new structural model is that it better programmatically represents the real program emphases of the agency as a whole. It also cuts down the number of direct reports to the CDC director.

Structurally, the new organization is extremely complex. It does not do away with silos. In fact, it creates silos within silos and several different matrices as well. It can become structurally hard to maintain over time. The leaders at the top do provide general management oversight to the agency as a whole, but communication throughout the new system is difficult in an agency oriented to both science and practice. The top leadership is insulated from the divisions in the national centers, which are embedded within the coordinating centers and which can affect morale and commitment to both the agency leadership and the goals and objectives of the agency programs. Each coordinating center and its national centers have the potential for creating all the negatives of a silo-based organization. Good management is definitely possible at the program level even though it is difficult for CDC leadership to get a grasp of all the activities in which the agency is engaged. Wagner and Harter stated that employees need to know what is expected of them at work.[26] The CDC structure limits communication to the front lines of the organization. There are now so many different organizational levels with managers at each level that many professionals feel removed from the decision-making activities of the agency. This can be observed by visiting and reading the entries on the blog site called CDC Chatter.[27] However, it becomes critical for meta-leadership techniques to be utilized in complex organizations that will help alleviate the frustrations tied to communication difficulties. Meta-leadership concepts will be introduced later in this chapter.

The second product of the CDC has been the development of health protection goals for the future. There are four major overarching goals for these now fourteen strategic goals. Table 3-3 lists the overarching and strategic goals. Two of the overarching goals became Strategic Goals 13 and 14. At an organization level, a determination was made to create a goals action team for each of the major goals. A matrix approach was taken. A goals team leader was recruited from other organizational units within the CDC and team members were also selected. Thus, another level of organization was created,

**Table 3-3   Centers for Disease Control and Prevention Health Protection and Strategic Goals**

Overarching Goal 1: Healthy people in every stage of life
    Strategic Goal 1: Start Strong (0–3 years)
    Strategic Goal 2: Grow Safe and Strong (4–11 years)
    Strategic Goal 3: Achieve Healthy Independence (12–19 years)
    Strategic Goal 4: Live a Healthy, Productive, and Satisfying Life (Adults, 20–49 years)
    Strategic Goal 5: Live Better Longer (Ages 50 and over)

Overarching Goal 2: Healthy people in healthy places
    Strategic Goal 6: Healthy Communities
    Strategic Goal 7: Healthy Homes
    Strategic Goal 8: Healthy Schools
    Strategic Goal 9: Healthy Workplaces
    Strategic Goal 10: Healthy Health Care Settings
    Strategic Goal 11: Healthy Institutions
    Strategic Goal 12: Healthy Travel and Recreation

Overarching Goal 3: People prepared for emerging health threats (Strategic Goal 13)

Overarching Goal 4: Healthy people in a healthy world (strategic Goal 14)

*Source:* From CDC Health Protection Goals and Strategic Goals.

which led to a second matrix structure within the agency. Each goals team leader and the team are responsible to a steering committee. Team members are responsible to the goals leader and the supervisor from the units in which they worked. Each goals team had the responsibility for the development of an action plan for its goal. These plans were reviewed from November 2007 into 2008. The alignment of the goals to budget will occur in 2008.

This CDC example represents the difficulty in changing a major governmental agency. Daly and Watkins would call this reorganization a turnaround model with the need for a strong leader who would need to utilize a command and control approach to create the changes necessary.[28] The director of the agency clearly had a vision for the future of the agency that is creative and innovative. She supported the organizational changes that she thought would do away with the silos of the past. She met with external stakeholders to explain the plan and gain their support. She assigned the new Office of Strategy and Innovation with the development of protocols to make the plan work. The reorganization was done, but new silos and several matrix structures came into being. The professional staff, including many researchers within divisions, resisted the changes and argued that the new organization did not reflect the work that needed to be done or the work in which they were engaged.

The new organizational structure was seen as overly complex with elements of traditional bureaucratic hierarchies still in place as well as matrix structures that were superimposed on the organization. Changes as those that have been made do not occur overnight. There is cultural change going on. Both leadership and management relationships need clarification. Different scenarios have to be tested. Exercise 3-2 will help you experiment with different options for change that might expedite the process. To aid you in the process, Case Study 3-B provides a public health quiz with Dr. Bradley Perkins, the director of the CDC Office of Strategy and Innovation.

---

**Case Study 3-B**
**Public Health Practice Quiz for Bradley Perkins**

**(1) How are the four Health Protection Goals reflective of the vision for the CDC over the next decade?**
The CDC's Vision for the 21st Century is Health Protection, Health Equity. The CDC is committed to achieving true improvements in people's lives by accelerating health impact and reducing health disparities. To achieve this vision, the CDC needed to change how it works and how it thinks as an organization.

Consequently, the CDC created a set of four overarching Health Protection Goals, which are supported by a number of strategic goals that help refine the scope of the goals and the annual Goal Action Plans and a set of 80 objectives that identify leading public health issues and that provide direction and focus for the CDC's work and collaborations.

**(2) How will the goals' action plans change programmatic emphases within the CDC?**
Having goal action plans will alter the way we view our programs and our planning at the CDC. Our planning now encompasses horizontal assessments of our programs and activities across the CDC to look for common areas of emphasis and focus and to increase efficiency and innovation in our approaches. For example, obesity cuts across multiple program areas, affects people of different ages, ties to numerous dis-

eases and conditions, and results from many risk factors. There cannot be a unilateral or isolated approach to the problems tied to obesity.

These plans will also help to shape the CDC's priorities and how we allocate resources. Programs that have health impact, that protect health, and that reduce disparities will be evaluated more favorably than those that do not.

### (3) How will the goals change the CDC's relationship with external partners?

There is going to be a process of aligning our priorities with our partners' priorities, but throughout the goals process, we have worked with our partners to develop our goals and to ensure that our partners had a say in developing the goals. Just as we evaluate our own programs, we have to look at the work our partners are doing, and again, those whose work leads to health impact, health protection, and reduced disparities will be evaluated accordingly.

Having Goal Action Plans will also provide external partners with high-level perspectives for achieving mutual goals and provide a baseline by noting the CDC's current response and key achievements within these areas.

### (4) How can goals be added or removed from the program?

The goals themselves will not be added or removed. Our four overarching Health Protection Goals set the direction and tone for the CDC's work. The strategic goals that describe ages, places, and other characteristics of the goals are also stable. But we will evaluate the objectives that support the goals annually, and we may modify these by refocusing them, removing them, or developing new objectives.

### (5) What are the management and leadership issues involved in the implementation of the goals matrix structure?

As with any new structure, there are management and leadership challenges. The CDC has been a traditional disease-focused organization and has been managed accordingly. Scientists are recruited for their expertise in particular diseases. However, as the CDC moves forward using goals as a framework, the focus of leadership and management has changed to more cross-cutting issues. Consequently, partnership and collaboration—both internally and externally—become critical.

For instance, we have 14 goal teams engaged in an annual planning process that spans the entire agency. The members of these teams are from across the agency, and following through with their recommendations and plans requires collaborative solutions. The management and leadership functions are no longer as direct as they were previously, but they must now be "matrixed" across divisions, centers, and coordinating centers. The Goals Steering Committee, which also comprises members from across the CDC, plays a critical oversight role, and continues to monitor the progress and challenges of the goals process. Changes to the structures are ongoing, based in large measure on input from a series of goals retreats.

---

## Transactional and Transformational Leadership

The CDC example above demonstrates how the line between what is leadership and what is management often becomes blurred. This relationship becomes even more complicated when we look at the issue of transactional leadership and transformational leadership where the management role seems to vanish altogether. Most discussions about leadership concern vision and change. Burns has pointed out that leadership is about reciprocity.[29] Through the development of relationships between partners with varying perspectives on values and motivation, the partners are often in conflict and competition in relation to the overarching goals, which should bring the leaders together to realize their goals and to work together to reach these goals. Moreover, these goals are influenced by the realities of the environment or communities in which these leaders come together.

Burns defined two critical types of leadership—transactional and transformational.[30] The transactional leader engages others in the reciprocal activity of exchanging one thing for another. Most management and leadership are related to the exchange of one thing for another. Transformational leadership examines and searches for the needs and motives of others while seeking a higher agenda of needs. Transformational relationships are intense and raise the participants to a higher level of mutuality and morality so that the interaction between leaders or between leaders and followers changes both parties. From these definitions, it can be argued that both transactional and transformational skills are important for leaders. They are complementary types of skill. Transformational leadership demands higher level negotiation activities and will lead to change at both the organization and systems level.

The attempt to put the concept of transactional leadership into action has led to a reinterpretation of this type of leadership to be a reconceptualization of management. The exchange of work for various types of rewards seems tied to the organization where there is an attempt to maintain the stability of the organization. Transformational leadership seems to be more about change. Table 3-4 demonstrates how these two leadership concepts are viewed today and also puts managers in the leadership camp.[31] In recognizing that public health leaders need to transform the public health system in which they work and also change the understanding and commitment to the work of public health with their internal and external partners, the National Public Health Leadership Development Network had to define the characteristics and competencies of a transformational leader.[32] The three major activities of the public health transformational leader involve the skills necessary to engage in the development of mission and vision as well as the development of skills related to monitoring and facilitating the process of change. The whole framework is discussed further in Chapter 17.

In order to begin to clarify distinctions between management and leadership, it is possible to begin this dialogue by creating a continuum from management to leadership. Figure 3-4 does this by putting management at the left side of the continuum and covering traditional management processes. Transactional leadership is at the center of the continuum and blends traditional management with the reciprocity concerns discussed by the Gallup Organization in its look at great managers. It is with transactional leadership that we can begin to see the interface between management and leadership. Transformational leadership and its change and vision agenda are on the extreme right side of the continuum. Most leaders need to have both transactional and transformational talents and skills.

## Meta-Leadership—A New Perspective

In 1990 in the last edition of the now classic textbook, Pickett and Hanlon pointed out that change is inevitable in public health.[33] Public health will have to work in new ways. This will require a flexibility that is often missing

**Table 3-4  Transactional vs. Transformational Leadership: Differences Between Managing and Leading**

|  | Transactional Leadership or Management Skills | Transformational Leadership or Leadership Skills |
|---|---|---|
| Performance: | Considered by leadership writers to produce ordinary performance | Considered by leadership writers to produce extraordinary performance |
| Goal: | To maintain the status quo by playing within the rules | To change the status quo by changing the rules |
| Goals arise out of: | Necessity, are reactive and respond to ideas. They are deeply imbedded in the organization's history and culture | Desires, they are active, shaping ideas, may be a departure from organization's history and culture |
| Emphasis: | Rationality and control, limits choices, focuses on solving problems | Innovation, creativity to develop fresh approaches to long-standing problems and open issues to new options |
| Attitudes toward goals: | Impersonal, if not passive attitudes | Personal and active attitude |
| Incentives: | Based on exchange of needs (i.e., "tit for tat") basis | Based on the greater good |
| Locus of reward: | Maximize personal benefits | Optimize systemic benefits |
| Requires: | Persistence, tough-mindedness, hard work, intelligence, analytical ability, and tolerance and goodwill | Genius and heroism |
| View work as: | Enabling processes, ideas, and people to establish strategies and make decisions | Creative, energizing, and emerging |
| Tactics employed: | Negotiate and bargain, use of rewards, punishment, and other forms of coercion | Inspire followers, create shared vision, motivate |
|  | Strive to convert win-lose into win-win situations as part of the process of reconciling differences among people and maintaining balances of power | Strive to create new situations and new directions without regard to reconciling groups or power |

*Source:* From T. D. Robertson, C. S. P. Fernandez, and J. E. Porter, "Leadership in Public Health," In L. E. Novick, C. B. Morrow, and G. P. Mays (eds.), *Public Health Administration,* 2nd ed. (Sudbury, MA: Jones and Bartlett, 2007).

in governmental organizations. This work will occur in a transorganizational environment where public health leaders will work with partners outside of their home agencies. In this new environment, leaders will have to understand the values that drive the different agendas of their partners. It will be

FIGURE 3-4   **Management & Leadership Continuum**

necessary to build coalitions and other forms of external alliances and part-nerships. Negotiation will be an important element in these new relationships. These transorganizational activities will demonstrate transformational lead-ership in action.

Meta-leadership is the new terminology for working across organiza-tions. Leaders need to move outside their organizational positions and utilize their talents, knowledge, and transactional and transformational skills to cre-ate new models for collaboration with partners. It requires a systems perspec-tive, an understanding of how values shape action, and risk-taking related to initiatives that may in part negatively impact their home organization. Henderson has defined the meta-leader as an individual who is able to con-nect the purposes, activities, and work of different agencies and organizations and their program components to achieve a greater good at the systems level.[34] Public health requires actions that cross agency boundaries. The meta-leader is able to align the core interests, motivations, and values of dif-ferent organizations into a new synergistic value orientation (meta-values) that will create an integrated vision and set of actions to create change. Marcus and his colleagues have used the word "connectivity" to refer to this process.[35]

The traditional leader gains power from the position that he or she holds in the organization that he or she represents. This power from their home organization can be called silo power. This power is closely allied to what we called transactional leadership. Meta-leaders need to gain trust, credibility, and power in their external collaborations as well as they demonstrate their trans-formational leadership skills. There are five dimensions to meta-leadership (Figure 3-5).[36] The meta-leadership model was developed to gain a better un-derstanding of how leaders function in crisis. Some event will impact how leaders will function. There may be challenges to defining the event from the vantage point of size and scope, scale, and the substance and understanding of what may have triggered it.

Some of the expected qualities of a leader in crisis include courage, cu-riosity, imagination, organizational sensibilities, persuasion, conflict manage-ment, crisis management, emotional intelligence, and persistence.[36] I have included in my discussions of crisis leaders such additional skills as systems and complexity thinking, collaboration skills, concerns for community safety, understanding of health law and ethics, understanding of risk and health communication, ability to determine tipping points and change strategies, and community-building.[37] Meta-leaders not only have to be masters of the ability to work within and between organizations, but they also have to be able to influence action inquiries and plans to make the results of the collaborations work in the real world. There may be a need to develop meta-managers as well as meta-leaders.

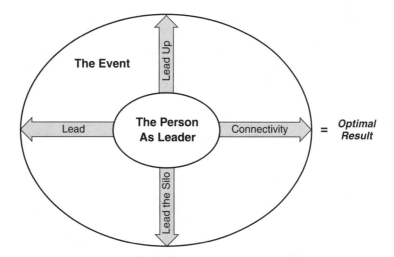

**FIGURE 3-5    The 5 Dimensions of Meta-leadership**
*Source:* From L. J. Marcus, B. C. Dorn, and J. M. Henderson, *Meta-Leadership and National Emergency Preparedness* (Cambridge MA: Harvard  Center for Public Leadership Working Papers, 2005). Reprinted with the permission of L. J. Marcus, I. Ashkenazi, B. Dorn, and J. Henderson.

Leading up has challenges. The meta-leader has to learn how to deal with boards, county commissioners, other elected officials, and subject matter specialists. As pointed out in Case Study 2-A, American public health leaders feel weakest in their policy development and advocacy roles. Henderson has pointed out that all crisis events in the United States are political.[38] In fact, almost all public health decisions also have political implications. When the leader is not successful in advocacy and other political relationships, it can impact the agency in a number of ways. Staff morale may be affected and the trust in the leader may decline as a result. The credibility of many local activities (scientific findings as well as agency decisions) may be questioned. This lack of credibility and trust may make it more difficult to resolve the conflict or crisis in a timely manner. Henderson recommends that meta-leaders manage up one level at a time.

Leading within the silo is important if followers are going to have trust in their leaders and believe in the vision and strategy formulated by the leader. Gaining input from all staff during the formulation of vision and strategy is important. External stakeholders from the political and nonpolitical realms need to be involved in this process as well. Good managers are needed in the silo to carry out the vision and strategy of the leader through agency operations and execution of strategy through action and through the connection of the strategy to activities of the agency as a whole. Henderson has pointed out that after leadership and management there needs to be a third phase to the process: evaluation. The evaluation phase involves the measurement of impact, monitoring change, measuring productivity and performance, and ensuring that all public health systems support a continuous quality improvement process.

It is in connectivity that meta-leaders shine. It is their work to connect the purposes and activities of the many organizations with whom they partner for the good of the public health agenda in their communities. Their curiosity and need to explore many creative avenues should affect the process of collaboration. They need to become expert in conflict leadership and how to resolve the differences in ideas that arise. The meta-leader is a risk-taker and needs to be able to address the consequences of his or her actions. Meta-leaders also need to be able to determine when their shared goals have been met.

## The Public Health Management and Leadership Road Map

Now it is necessary to put the management and leadership puzzle together. By adapting the Gallup Path to the governmental sector and adding the leadership dimension as well, it is possible to develop a public health management and leadership road map such as that in Figure 3-6.[39] Because public health has strong roots in the community, it is important to look at the context of public health as the starting point in our understanding of how the work of public health is accomplished. The public health agency becomes the coordinating organization from which to view the public health system as well as the specific activities of public health. The leader who is engaged is one who is able to work outside the agency with stakeholders from the political realm as well as from other sectors to improve the health of the public. This is meta-leadership in action. This high level of planning, negotiation, and action is tied to the role of the public health administrator leader within the transformational leadership role. The public health leader is often engaged in

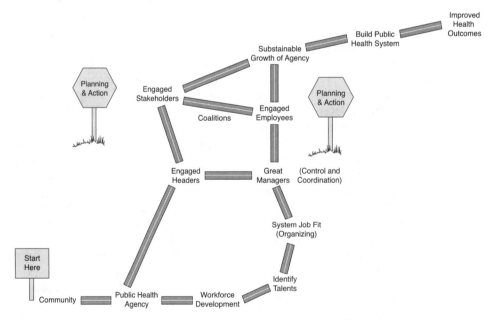

**FIGURE 3-6   Management & Leadership Roadmap in Public Health**
*Source:* Adapted from C. Coffman and G. Gonzalez-Molina, *Follow This Path* (New York: Warner Business Books, 2002).

these activities as a major part of the job of promoting the public's health. Because of the time-intensive nature of these activities, the leader often has to rely on engaged managers in the agency to carry out the day-to-day activities of the agency itself. In some instances and especially in smaller health departments, the leader may also have to carry out the activities of the manager as well.

The development of the public health workforce within the agency is often the responsibility of management. Following the work of the Gallup Organization on talents, the manager has to be able to identify the talents of workers and fit those talents within the system requirements of the agency and its programs.[40] In traditional management jargon, this involves the organizing function of management. The excellent and great managers also have control and coordination responsibilities. These managers also have to engage the agency employees in the work of the agency so that they understand the vision of the agency leadership. The management staff and the engaged employee have to interact on planning and action protocols as well because this is often a team effort.

As the leader continues to work with external stakeholders, engaged employees get to work with other staff of the engaged stakeholder groups in coalitions and other groups to carry out the specific tasks necessary to help the public improve its health status. If these leadership and management tasks are carried out well, there should be sustainable growth of both the public health agency and its community partners. With this growth, the infrastructure of public health and the public health system as a whole will be strengthened. The outcome of all these activities will be improved health outcomes in the community being served.

## Summary

This chapter has addressed the complex relationship between management and leadership. The functions of leaders and managers are clearly different even though it is necessary for leaders and managers to work together. In smaller jurisdictions, public health administrators will have to be both manager and leader. However, this marriage is not an easy one because the role of manager/leader requires two different sets of skills. The individual may have the talent to carry out one set of skills better than the other. It is important for the individual to understand his or her personal strengths and fit his or her talents to the needs of the organization in its current state of development. The next chapter addresses the critical concern of systems and complexity thinking, which impacts leadership in a significant way.

## Discussion Questions

1. What are the differences between management and leadership?
2. Do you think it is possible to be a great manager and a leader at the same time?
3. What are the differences between working in the governmental and the business sectors?

4. What are the relationships among traditional management, transactional leadership, and transformational leadership?
5. What is meta-leadership and why is it an important leadership approach?
6. What are organizational silos and how can communication between these silos be improved?
7. Give examples of how the Public Health Management and Leadership Road Map might work.

**Exercise 3-1:    Organizational Development and Strategic Health Priorities (Application of Daly and Watkins Model)**
Adapted from P. H. Daly and M. Watkins, The First 90 Days in Government (Cambridge, MA: Harvard Business School Publishing, 2006).

> *Purpose:* to see the relationship between the organizational structure of a public health agency and the way it then addresses local public health priorities.
>
> *Key concepts:* start-up, turnaround, realignment, sustaining-success perspective, health priorities
>
> *Procedure:* Scenario—The American County Health Department has been involved in carrying out a community health assessment in its county. American County has come up with four strategic health priorities:
>
> 1. Strengthen the public health workforce.
> 2. Address the needs of those who require public health services.
> 3. Improve health outcomes for cardiovascular diseases.
> 4. Create a broader sense of community connectedness.
>
> The class or training group will be divided into four groups of 8 to 10. One group will discuss the problem from the perspective of a start-up agency. The second group will address the problem from the perspective of an agency in a turnaround situation. Group 3 will discuss the scenario from the perspective of a realignment organization. The final group will discuss the priorities from the perspective of a sustaining-success organization. Your task as a leadership team for your county is to determine how to address these priorities when your agency is in one of the four organizational development phases discussed by Daly and Watkins. You have an hour to discuss these issues. Your team will then report to the class or training group as a whole on how you addressed these issues.

**Exercise 3-2:    Scenario-Building for the CDC**

> *Purpose:* to explore different approaches to organizational development and the CDC Health Protection Goals to increase the chance of success for the goals program
>
> *Key Concepts:* scenario-building, organizational restructuring, goals alignment, health protection goals, coordinating centers, silos, leadership, management
>
> *Procedure:* Utilizing the CDC example in this chapter, divide the training group or class into teams of 8 to 10. Each team is to develop two to three different scenarios for ways to integrate the Health Protection Goals into the CDC structure or to make proposals for the reorganization of the CDC in a more efficient and effective manner to make goals a part of the total CDC organization.

# References

1. M. Buckingham, *Go Put Your Strengths to Work* (New York: Free Press, 2007).
2. J. H. Fleming and J. Asplund, *Human Sigma* (New York: Gallup Press, 2007).
3. G. Browning, *Emergenetics* (New York: Harper-Collins, 2006).
4. C. Cherniss and D. Goleman, *The Emotionally Intelligent Workplace* (San Francisco: Jossey-Bass, 2001).
5. M. Buckingham and D. O. Clifton, *Now, Discover Your Strengths* (New York: Free Press, 2001).
6. Browning, *Emergenetics.*
7. H. Fayol, *General and Industrial Management* (London: Pittman Publishing, 1949).
8. S. P. Robbins and M. Coulter, *Management,* 8th ed. (Upper Saddle River, NJ: Prentice-Hall, 2005).
9. R. Wagner and J. K. Harter, *12: The Elements of Great Managing* (New York: Gallup Press, 2006).
10. P. F. Drucker, *The Essential Drucker* (New York: Harper Business, 2001).
11. Fayol, *General and Industrial Management.*
12. Robbins and Coulter, *Management,* 8th ed.
13. P. H. Daly and M. Watkins, *The First 90 Days in Government* (Cambridge, MA: Harvard Business School Publishing, 2006).
14. M. H. Moore, *Creating Public Value* (Cambridge, MA: Harvard University Press, 1995).
15. Daly and Watkins, *The First 90 Days in Government.*
16. B. J. Turnock and L. Rowitz, *NACCHO New Local Health Official Orientation Curriculum: Final Design* (Washington, DC: National Association of County and City Health Officials, 2007).
17. Turnock and Rowitz, *NACCHO New Local Health Official Orientation Curriculum.*
18. S. Orton, K. E. Umble, B. Rosen, J. McIver, and A. J. Menkens, "Management Academy for Public Health: Program Design and Critical Success Factors, *Journal of Public Health Management and Practice* 12, no. 5 (2006): 409–418.
19. S. Goldsmith and W. D. Eggers, *Governing by Network* (Washington, DC: Brookings Institution Press, 2004).
20. T. L. Friedman, *The World Is Flat* (New York: Farrar, Straus, and Giroux, 2006).
21. Robbins and Coulter, *Management,* 8th ed.
22. P. Martin, *Quick Guide: The New Matrix Management* (Carmel, NY: Martin Training Associates, 2005).
23. P. Lencioni, *Silos, Politics, and Turf Wars* (San Francisco: Jossey-Bass, 2006).
24. Martin, *Quick Guide: The New Matrix Management.*
25. http://www.cdc.gov
26. Wagner and Harter, *12: The Elements of Great Managing.*
27. http://cdcchatter.net
28. Daly and Watkins, *The First 90 Days in Government.*
29. J. MacGregor Burns, *Leadership* (New York: Harper and Row, 1978).
30. Burns, *Leadership.*
31. T. D. Robertson, C. S. P. Fernandez, and J. E. Porter, "Leadership in Public Health" in L. E. Novick, C. B. Morrow, and G. P. Mays (eds.), *Public Health Administration,* 2nd ed. (Sudbury, MA: Jones and Bartlett, 2007).

32. K.S. Wright, L. Rowitz, A. Merkle, et al., "Competency Development in Public Health Leadership," *American Journal of Public Health* 90 (August 2000): 1202–1207.

33. G. Pickett and J. J. Hanlon, *Public Health: Administration and Practice,* 9th ed. (St. Louis: Times Mirror/Mosby College Publishing, 1990).

34. J. M. Henderson, *Meta-Leadership and the Challenge for Public Health* (talk) (Raleigh: North Carolina State Health Director's Conference, 2007).

35. L. J. Marcus, B. C. Dorn, and J. M. Henderson, *Meta-Leadership and National Emergency Preparedness* (Cambridge MA: Harvard Center for Public Leadership Working Papers, 2005).

36. Henderson, *Meta-Leadership and the Challenge for Public Health.*

37. L. Rowitz, *Public Health in the 21st Century: The Prepared Leader* (Sudbury, MA: Jones and Bartlett, 2006).

38. Henderson, *Meta-Leadership and the Challenge for Public Health.*

39. C. Coffman and G. Gonzalez-Molina, *Follow This Path* (New York: Warner Business Books, 2002).

40. Buckingham and Clifton, *Now, Discover Your Strengths.*

# CHAPTER 4

# A SYSTEMS AND COMPLEXITY PERSPECTIVE

> Life was simple before World War II. After that, we had systems.
>
> G. Hopper

Public health is about the system. Medical care is more about management than leadership. Public health moves from a focus on the individual to a focus on all the people in a community. The change in focus requires a systems orientation with the need for public health leaders to understand systems and how they work. The 1998 Institute of Medicine report on public health defined the mission of public health from a systems perspective.[1] The mission involved the fact that society and thus the community has an investment in its population and this investment involves making sure that the health of the population is protected. This assurance activity includes the utilization of most current scientific and technical expertise available. All community stakeholders need to be involved in this process. The local public health agency will usually take a lead role in these activities. Thus, leadership within a systems perspective is critical.

Public health is a clear example of a complex adaptive system. Public health practice takes place within this complex adaptive system. Public health as a complex system has several properties:[2]

1. A focus on emergent patterns related to health outcomes of the population.
2. The health of the individual is affected by the body as a complex system in itself that interacts with many environmental factors.
3. Social networks and the interactions between people in many social situations adds an additional complexity issue to the occurrence of disease events.
4. Public health has a strong unpredictable political dimension that affects how public health issues are affected in communities.
5. Public health systems are affected by the array of health care programs in communities as well as the complex nature of insurance coverage.
6. Public health systems are affected by the education of the public health workforce as well as the location and size of the community, municipality, or county. Rural health jurisdictions are not the same as large urban ones.

In the next section, we will explore systems thinking and then discuss the issue of systems relative to management inside of an agency and working outside that agency. The following section will explore the issue of complexity and its impact on the work of public health leaders. Finally, a short note discusses some new systems possibilities.

## Systems and Systems Thinking

The modern emphasis on systems and systems thinking began to occur in the years after World War II but was impacted by the Macy Conferences from 1942 to 1951. These conferences involved many important thinkers of the time including anthropologists Margaret Mead and Gregory Bateson; the early computer scientist John von Neumann; the early leader on the issues of artificial intelligence Warren McCulloch; and Norbert Weiner, who founded the field of cybernetics.[3] In two influential books published in 1948 and 1950, Weiner discussed a new field called cybernetics and systems.[4,5] His perspective becomes clearer in his 1950 book on the human use of human beings. Cybernetics is the science of steering rather than rowing. Society can be mainly understood by the study of messages and the way these messages are communicated between man and machines. Cybernetics relates to the way that systems function regardless of whether the system is mechanical or social. Weiner also discussed the importance of feedback. Feedback is tied to performance and the importance of previous information and experience guiding present performance, especially when some unexpected event occurs. Both people and modern machines thus function in a similar way.

In the 1950s, the biologist von Bertalanffy pointed out that structure was a critical component in systems.[6] In fact, structure is more important than function. These principles can be applied to not only biology but to such diverse fields as sociology and electronics. In the 1960s, Forrester studied economic and social systems using computer simulation techniques.[7] The difficulty in understanding all aspects of the systems approach is that systems tend to be viewed from different perspectives by scientists and practitioners. Churchman viewed the systems approach from the perspective of the business community.[8] All approaches seem to see the system as a set of coordinated parts that pursue the accomplishment of a series of goals. Thus, an animal is a system, as is a community. The management scientist as well as the leader attempt to define the parameters of the system. The managers and leaders also define the environment in which the system will be viewed. This translates into the need to define goals, objectives, actions, resources, management requirements, and performance measurements as they impact on the parts of the system. According to Churchman, it is important to be aware that the systems approach is sometimes seen as too general for some management/ leadership professionals who feel that it eliminates the specificity of problems that need also to be addressed.

Senge expanded the issue of systems to the leadership and management area in the 1990s.[9] Systems thinking was seen as important for leaders. They need to see the big picture if they are to solve organizational and community problems. A systems perspective allows us to build learning organizations where people are able to systematically understand challenges to their organizations and communities as a methodology for getting the results that will help their organizations and communities to grow. In learning organizations, people expand their thinking and learning in a nurturing way.

Senge defined five disciplines to guide the work and understanding of learning organizations.[10] These five disciplines work together. The first discipline relates to personal mastery, which involves each person in a learning organization working to expand his or her knowledge and skills over time as well as building upon personal strengths. The second discipline involves the critical cultural dimension of mental models. Each individual has an outlook on the world based on personal values and experiences. It is important that the individual learn to understand these factors if he or she is going to work in organizations and communities to create change. Values clarification is an important component of learning organization activity. The third discipline is shared vision, which involves the buy-in of all people in an organization to the vision. Commitment to the leader's vision is a requirement for successful change strategies to come into being. The fourth discipline is team learning in which the members of a team, coalition, or partnership work together in a coordinated fashion. The fifth discipline is systems thinking in which all need to work together and view problems and challenges from the wide perspective of the total organization or the total community. Exercise 4-1 looks at the differences in solving a community health issue when the perspective is limited to public health and when it expands to the community as a whole. Other exercises on the five disciplines can be found in Rowitz.[11]

In recent years, Senge and his colleagues have been exploring the impact on the individual of working in learning organizations on systems issues. They have pointed out that the core capacity needed to look at the future collectively is called presence.[12] Systems thinking involves a change in perspective. It involves looking at the world in new ways. Status quo is no longer an option. Change is the reality. This new perspective means that our old ways of identifying ourselves and what we do must also undergo change. Our view must be forward-looking and not constantly on re-creating our past. These shifts in perspective mean that leaders will shift from a concentration on organizational hierarchies to an approach in which those leaders will work through shared social networks. This new view leads to a new model for this collective type of learning—Theory U.

Theory U is a new approach to integrating the five disciplines to these new approaches to collective learning and practice. Figure 4-1 shows the relationship between the five disciplines and the Theory U approach.[13] Working with others requires that the team inquire in depth as to the source and understanding of their mental models to see reality more clearly ("co-sensing"), find ways to increase the connections with the mission or purpose and the vision of the problem ("co-presencing"), and translate these visionary activities into feedback-based working action models ("co-realizing"). As can be seen in Figure 4-1, mental models, team learning, and systems thinking come into play in the processes of co-sensing and co-presencing. Co-presencing also shows the disciplines of personal vision and shared vision as happening. In the move from co-presencing to co-realizing, team learning and systems thinking play critical roles in the process.

Scharmer clarifies Theory U by defining five movements toward change as the U Process evolves.[14] He first adds the movement of "co-initiating,"

**FIGURE 4-1    The U Process and the Five Disciplines**
*Source:* P. M. Senge, *The Fifth Discipline,* Revised and Updated (New York: Double-day, 2006). Used by permission of Doubleday, a division of Random House, Inc.

which involves the process of engagement between people and environmental contexts with the importance of listening to others and what you perceive that you will need to do. This stage precedes "co-sensing" and starts the U Process. He then clarifies the movements after "co-presencing," when reflection and deep understanding need to occur. Then the movement of "co-creating" occurs when different strategies and scenarios for the future are explored. The final movement stage is "co-involving," when new models and innovations occur from the strong interrelationships between the people that are involved in the change process. This is the stage of transforming action that is shown in Figure 4-1 as "co-realizing." Scharmer points out that Theory U redefines leadership as a collective activity that will occur at all levels of the organization or community.

### Leadership in a Systems Environment

The importance of systems thinking for public health leaders became extremely visible as a result of the events of September 11, 2001. A number of training programs and modules related to crisis leadership have developed with this strong systems orientation. It is not that systems thinking has been absent from traditional leadership development programs; it just has become more critical in the training of crisis leaders who need to work in a public health preparedness environment. In the previous chapter, I explored some of the issues involved in better understanding the relationship between management and leadership. In this section, the relationship will be explored in the context of a systems-based world where there are connections across organizations (meta-leadership), across jurisdictions from local to state to national, and eventually around the globe.

The traditional management approach is linear in perspective. It involves rules, regulations, and procedures to make an organization work more effectively and efficiently. Leadership in today's knowledge, skills, talents, and practice world is more of a systems set of issues. Cabrera has developed a systems organizing model that is based on the four components of vision, structure, learning, and action (VSAL).[15] Figure 4-2 shows this model. These four components have a role in traditional linear and hierarchical organizations as well as in more systems-oriented or community-based organizations. Within each of the Cabrera quadrants, there is a continuum to demonstrate this move from traditional to systems orientations. The components are shown in a two-by-two contingency table format to show that all four parts are interactive with each other. Another important aspect to the model is that it builds on a theory, research, and action interrelationships, which for us is a demonstration of public health practice in action. The National Cancer Institute has used this model to show systems thinking in tobacco control initiatives.[16]

Starting with the quadrant-labeled vision, it is important to recognize that vision has generally been part of a consistent set of visioning tools tied to leadership in traditional as well as systems-oriented organizations. Vision is closely allied with the planning activities in an organization or agency. This will become clearer in the discussion of the leadership wheel in Chapter 5. For most organizations and agencies, the top administrator as leader has set the tone for the work of the organization through defining a vision, living the

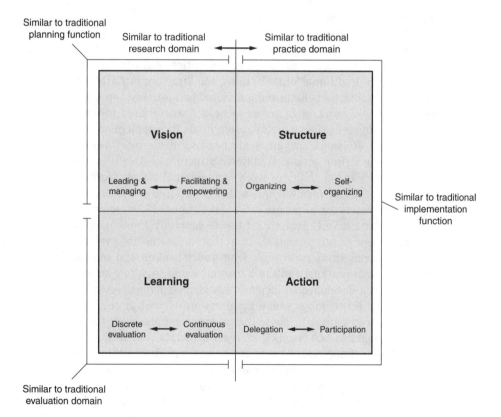

**FIGURE 4-2  Systems Organizing Model**
*Source:* Reprinted with the permission of Derek Cabrera. From Cabera, D. 2001. *Knowledge Age Operating System: Four Principles of Project Design. Version 1.0.* Loveland, CO: Project N Press.

vision, and inspiring others in the organization to support and take ownership of the vision.[17,18] The top administrator, as lead manager, and other
organization managers have the critical role of making the organization vision work in a practical way.

In a systems organizing perspective, vision becomes a collective activity
in which a leadership network approach defines a shared vision. Leadership
becomes more a demonstration of empowering others and facilitating the visioning process. Here, we see the use and development of many tools to help
in the process. For example, there is brainstorming where ideas get generated;[19] the six thinking hats framework for generating ideas and solving
problems;[20] the use of logic models to link planning and evaluation;[21] future
search techniques to define the future
and how to get there;[22] the Search
Conference, which is a participatory
model for visioning, creating strategic
goals, and developing action plans;[23]
facilitation to create participation, address conflict, make effective decisions,
manage meetings, and show how to use process tools for a group's work;[24]
and Communities of Practice where leaders from the community as well as
other stakeholders, including public health, meet face-to-face and virtually to
learn and share ideas for the possible development of resources to support
programs in a special area of interest.[25]

> **Leadership Tip**
> *Root your vision in reality.*

The second quadrant relates to structure, which involves the movement
from organizing people and activities by managers and leaders to the systems
orientation of self-organizing, which is a critical component in complexity
thinking.[26] In traditional organizations, the structure is fairly well-defined.
There are organization charts and individual performance appraisal processes,
and individuals' work often seems to be defined through inflexible job descriptions. This inflexible structure often limits the problem-solving possibilities and the decisions that are made because of the rules, regulations, and
protocols that define action. Traditional structure also defines who you can
talk to as well as the ability to work with external stakeholders.

The structure of the system is self-organizing and encourages leaders to
interact with all types of people and organizations. The structures that evolve
are tied to the networks that are created to support collaboration between the
partners. However, our present reality is that traditional and systems structures
coexist. Systems thinkers struggle with understanding and interpreting how
traditional organizations work in a systems world. A whole series of systems
tools has been developed to increase this understanding. Systems archetypes
are one such set of tools, where problems are viewed through a number of
graphic representations to show the underlying framework for success and
failure of programs and events.[27-29] These archetypes are used more in understanding why things are as they are rather than determining how to solve
these problems or events. Self-organizing systems do provide a different approach to these issues by creating an environment that allows for the structure to evolve as needed to address community and systems challenges.[30]

The third quadrant involves action. In traditional organizations, the leaders and managers tend to delegate work to their staff. How delegation occurs
is important. If we follow the recommendations of the Gallup Organization,
the great manager is one who fits the talents of each staff member to the tasks

that are to be done. People need incentives, rewards, and recognition for their work.[31] They are willing to do the work if it is tied to their talents, knowledge, and skills. As pointed out in the last chapter, these people skills are critical in today's organizations whether they are traditional in nature or more systems-based. The subtle but critical dimension here is for systems organizing leaders to work with their organizational colleagues to connect their work to the larger collective vision of the community or system as a whole. The philosophy is more than the original belief of thinking globally and acting locally. In systems, the philosophy now becomes acting locally for the benefit of the community and society as a whole. Local work has global consequences. It is at the local level that mission leads to the goals that bring vision into reality. Social entrepreneurs are leaders who use systems solutions to address global, national, and local social problems.[32]

The final quadrant involves the differences in learning in traditional organizations in contrast to systems organizations and communities. Best and his colleagues see learning within an evaluation context.[33] In traditional organizations, this evaluation learning is tied to the linear perspective related to planning, implementing, and carrying out programs. This type of evaluation is discrete and done as required by the project but tends not to be ongoing. Systems work that is ongoing is about creating learning organizations and learning collaboratively. Whereas the researcher or leader/manager defines activities for the organization, systems research is more participatory in nature. In systems, the needs of the researcher and the practitioner must be collaborative in nature.

In their simplest form, logic models involve the process of defining inputs, through-puts, and outcomes. They are oriented more toward traditional program structures and try to simplify discussions of cause and effect relationships and link them to process and outcome considerations. Best et al. see logic models as more traditional in nature and see systems dynamics with the important component of feedback as necessary to link the effects of programmatic actions as they influence factors such as those inputs in the logic model.[34] The effect of actions also affects the relationships between these actions and the outcomes that occur. The Centers for Disease Control and Prevention has developed a systems framework for evaluation. Figure 4-3 shows the elements of a systems approach to evaluation as a series of steps.[35] The inclusion of feedback opportunities at each step of the process would make this model even more acceptable to systems thinkers.

There are two interesting examples that will allow you to see the leadership issues in systems change. In November 2007, the Commonwealth Fund released a report outlining the issues necessary for the development of a high-performance health system for the United States.[36] First, it will not be possible to create such a system without a concern for public health issues. There will need to be an alignment between the health care system and the public health system in the areas of health promotion and disease prevention. Public policy and the political structure must find ways to promote healthy lifestyles. Without these public health dimensions, a reform of the American health system cannot occur. These public health concerns need to be aligned at a systems level with affordable coverage for all people with improvements in access to care and quality, efficiency, and cost control; aligned incentives and cost control through better information systems, payment

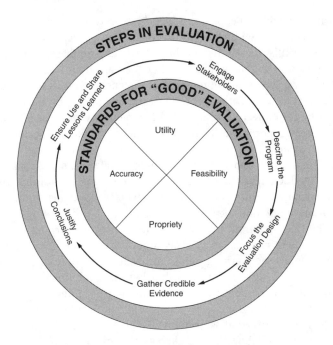

**FIGURE 4-3  Elements of Evaluation Framework for a System**
*Source:* Reprinted from Framework for Program Evaluation in Public Health, *Morbidity and Mortality Weekly Report,* Vol. 48, 1999, the Centers for Disease Control and Prevention.

reforms, better management of high-cost and chronic conditions, transparency through public reporting, improved administrative efficiencies, and elimination of unnecessary waste; accountable coordinated care; quality control and efficiency; and accountability among health leaders.

The second example, which illustrates the application of the systems-organizing VSAL model, is presented in Case Study 4-A. This study was developed by a team of public health professionals from Quebec who attended the Mid-America Regional Public Health Leadership Institute in 2002 and 2003 and undertook a study of ways to restructure the Quebec Public Health Program. The team also was concerned with the ways that leadership works in a system-wide program change.

---

## Case Study 4-A
### Leadership Issues Associated with the Development of the Quebec Public Health Program

*André Dontigny, Céline Farley, Isabelle Garon, Odette Laplante, Mariette LeBrun-Bohémier, Guy Poudrier, Jocelyne Sauvé, Lise Renaud*

**Once upon a time there was a program . . .**
In November 2002, Quebec's department of health and social services (*ministère de la Santé et des Services sociaux,* MSSS) made public its national public health program. This program defines the scope of public health action in Quebec and sets out the priorities and activities to be undertaken for the regional partners of public health departments (DSPs) and local partners (the local community service centers or CLSCs).

Our case study focuses on the challenges involved in developing this program and the leadership exercised by various stakeholders to meet these challenges. This document is an initial assessment resulting from consultation with several key stakeholders. It will serve as a basis for a discussion of the challenges with a group of Quebec's public health leaders. This discussion will allow us to gather ideas to help implement the program and prepare and implement the action plans resulting from it.

### Context and Stakeholders

Quebec's health and social services network, a deconcentrated system accessible to the whole population, is made up of several partners acting at different levels. At the provincial level, the MSSS funds this network and defines major orientations, policies, and programs, both curative and preventive. The 18 regional boards plan and coordinate services, allocate resources, monitor the budgets of the institutions in their region, and ensure that results are achieved for their region, whereas the institutions manage the care and services that they deliver. The regional boards also provide regional public health services through the mandate given to public health directors. The CLSCs provide curative and preventive services and are the local public health mandataries whereas the medical clinics deliver care and some preventive services. Finally, several community organizations provide preventive community services.

Over the last 12 years, the MSSS has produced about 20 documents addressed to public health stakeholders and other resources of the health and social services network. They are, for example, the Policy on Health and Well-Being (1990), the Framework for the Development of the Public Health Program, and the Organization of the Public Health Network (1992), a report focusing on the development of children, literally translated as "Quebec wild about its kids" (*Un Quebec fou de ses enfants*) (1993), Quebec Priorities in Public Health (1997), the Tobacco Act (1998), followed by the National Tobacco Control Program (*Programme national sur le tabac*) and the Public Health Act (2001). The most recent document is the Quebec Public Health Program (2002). To sum up, it seems that several documents have been introduced one after the other into the network in a short period of time and had to be absorbed, but they were not all associated with a plan to integrate these into practices.

The Quebec Public Health Program hoped to be different from the documents that preceded it. While striving to achieve the same high-quality document as its predecessors, it is intended to serve as a platform for mobilizing public health stakeholders and partners around the full scope of public health actions that are common to all of Quebec. The program, just like the Public Health Act, which was developed at the same time, was seen as a structuring measure to consolidate the public health infrastructure. It was an element in a vast project to strengthen and enhance the credibility of public health. The Quebec health and social services network has just undergone a period of major change, that is, a shift to ambulatory services in the context of budgetary pressure. This indirectly caused some disinterest from the authorities toward public health actions as the attention of the media and politicians, in Quebec and elsewhere, was once more focused on the overcrowding of emergency departments and the length of waiting lists.

*(continues)*

**Case Study 4-A** *continued*

The aim of the MSSS was to share a common vision of public health and to provide the conditions so that public health actions would be coherent, with a strong science base and carried out by all partners, that is, the health and social services network (the regional boards' public health departments and the CLSCs) as well as community organizations and partners in other sectors. It was hoped that the program would be the product of broad-based collaboration and participation of the entire network.

The key stakeholders who influenced this process were the Assistant Deputy Minister of Public Health and the Minister for Health and Social Services, who wished to strengthen the capacity of preventive health services; the National Public Health Director, who was particularly skillful at developing structuring measures, supported by a team of dynamic professionals; several public health directors; executive directors of CLSCs convinced of the advantages of working together; as well as the institute for public health (*Institut de santé publique* [INSPQ]), which could provide high quality expertise.

**Leadership Activities Linked to Policy Development**
The following activities linked to policy development have served as an analytical framework for this case study:

- Developing support, particularly by building coalitions, empowering other stakeholders, recognizing community assets and making representations on the health challenges targeted by the policy
- Clarifying values, creating a vision, linking that vision to the mission, using partners to establish the priorities on which this policy is to be based
- Organizing goals and translating them into action
- Organizing and seeking new resources, making organizational changes to better meet community needs
- Emphasizing innovation, delegating responsibilities for programming, supervising programs resulting from the policy

**Initial Challenges**
In the autumn of 2000, at the very beginning of the process of developing the Quebec Public Health Program, a number of challenges to be met were identified through interviews conducted with public health authorities at different levels. At the time, it was expected that the program would provide a way to strengthen the capacity of all public health teams to act effectively in partnership and to be recognized as such in the health and social service system and by other sectors. These challenges are as follows:

- The desire of the MSSS to increase the coherence and a more uniform access to public health services and interventions in Quebec's regions and local territories served by the CLSCs by defining the supply of public health services that are common to all regions and CLSC territories of Quebec
- The intention of the MSSS to use the program as a lever and a tool to mobilize all public health mandataries and support decisions on resource allocation
- The shared desire on the part of the MSSS, DSPs, and CLSCs for the program to give public health a greater role in the political space of the health and social services network and to confirm the importance of promotion and prevention, particularly in CLSCs

- The desire to conserve a degree of regional and local flexibility
- The recognition of CLSCs as public health mandataries in their own right, which is in keeping with the spirit of the public health bill being developed at the time and the need for them to assert themselves as such
- The fear on the part of a number of public health departments and CLSCs that a program would be too constraining and that it would stifle innovation and not take into account regional or local characteristics
- The choice of all public health mandataries to establish a participatory process to define the program, one in which all public health organizations would be involved under the leadership of the MSSS

Another major issue underlying the process was to reach an agreement on the content of the program, since the first attempt 10 years earlier had been transformed into seven "national priorities" in public health, because an agreement could not be reached on the content of an entire program.

On the whole, the idea of developing a national public health program, which was provided for under the act respecting health services and social services since 1993,[1] but never written, originated from the MSSS. It mainly reflected the search for coherence in public health activities, which often varied from one region and one CLSC to the next, and did not address some major health challenges. This desire also reflected a recognition of the need to make more room for public health within the health and social services system.

Although several public health departments shared this vision, others feared that their regional flexibility would be reduced because the act respecting health services and social services defined their responsibilities but not the explicit link with the central level, except in the event of a health threat. For their part, the CLSCs appeared to be happy to participate in the process but had to assert themselves as a new stakeholder in the planning of public health activities. On the other hand, they had to figure out how to restore the importance of activities that deal with the cause of health and social problems, because they had to increase their ambulatory care activities during periods of budgetary pressure, therefore often at the expense of prevention.

While the program was being written, the Public Health Act,[2] which was being developed at the same time, was used as another opportunity to provide the legal foundation on which to build the public health program and to confirm and specify the role and responsibility (and accountability) of the stakeholders in the program and its implementation.

### Clarifying Its Foundations, Orientations, and Values

The task of specifying the foundations, clarifying the vision as well as the orientations and values to be conveyed by the program, was a challenge in itself because there was no consensus on vision and content. Although the values were, to a certain extent, shared and supported by professionals at all levels, several schools of thought had to be reconciled in terms of boundaries of the public health domain, philosophies, and intervention practices. The entire process of drafting the program, which took more than two years, was used in part to do this conciliation.

At the time, there was no program model from elsewhere that could simply be copied. The program was therefore written with a view to innovating and reconciling knowledge on practices that have been proven to be effective. Fairly early on in the process, the writing team, supported by the advisory committee, suggested that

*(continues)*

**Case Study 4-A** *continued*

interventions be grouped under main areas or domains, which required that, as much as possible, actions be carried out with common partners and be based on common determinants. Although several times during the writing process doubts were raised about this "perspective," it served as the basis throughout the construction of the program.

### Organizing the Process

The work structure to be used in developing the program was defined in the spring of 2000, based on a central idea, that is, a participatory process in which all levels of the public health organization would be involved[3] (MSSS, the INSPQ, DSPs, CLSCs) to ensure the highest quality product and support for the program by organizations with a public health mandate, even though the legal framework allowed the MSSS to establish the program on its own.

Partners from within[4] the health and social services sector joined these representatives to form an advisory committee with the responsibility of providing an opinion on the content of the program. For its part, the main working committee was made up of managers and professionals from different levels of the public health organizations (the MSSS, the INSPQ, public health departments). The working groups responsible for developing the contents of the program were mainly made up of public health professionals and resources at the regional and national as well as the local levels. Finally, a team of MSSS professionals supported the process and led the working groups. Partners from other sectors and community organizations were invited to participate in developing the program only on a few occasions.

The choice of this structure demonstrates the wish of the public health mandataries to, on the one hand, assess the situation "among themselves" in order to plan public health activities and, on the other hand, to promote the maximum participation of the public health mandataries without weighing down the process by broadening it to other sectors. It was agreed that the trans-sectoral partners and community organizations would be asked to participate later, during consultations on the draft program. However, the choice of this work structure was not neutral; rather, it reflected the need of public health mandataries to plan public health activities together before turning to outside partners. The stage of recognizing community assets was carried out by professionals who made up the working groups, who brought with them the concerns of their communities (based on needs assessments previously conducted by the CLSCs and DSPs), and then validated by the CLSCs; the program's authors took for granted that these assets existed without describing or examining them.

### Agreeing on "What"

A crucial stage was defining the conceptual framework (see Figure 4-4), which represented the will to clearly define the scope of public health action by the functions exercised, to structure public health activities according to intervention areas or domains,[5] and to guide these activities based on health and social objectives aimed at enhancing health and well-being as well as reducing the major health problems through interventions known to be effective. This was done in the autumn of 2000.

Moreover, the proposal of an ethical framework and the choice of action strategies, also in the autumn of 2000, helped to identify the set of fundamental values on which the program would be based. Through this process, it was possible to identify consensus on the values that would constitute guideposts to support the ethical consideration on the choice of interventions to be carried out and to guide the in-

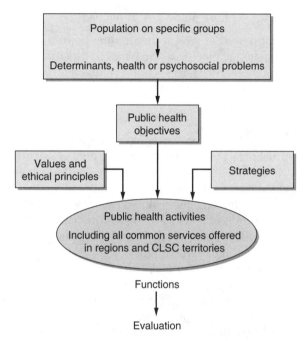

**FIGURE 4-4   Components of the Quebec Public Health Program**

terventions themselves. The key values are the public interest; beneficence and non-maleficence; respect for confidentiality and private life; responsibility; solidarity; recognition of the potential of individuals and communities and the necessary protection of individuals, groups, and communities that are at risk; and justice.

Another crucial stage was determining the program's actions and activities, which mainly involved identifying main health and psychosocial problems as well as determining effective interventions to act on the problems and their determinants. This process was carried out in sub-groups by more than 200 public health professionals. It involved considerable work carried out intensively over four months (during the winter of 2001) and then continued for nearly a year, until January 2002. This process was supervised by the program's main working committee and the professional team of the MSSS. The latter was also responsible for determining whether the material met the criteria of inclusion of activities in the program. During this stage, the professionals attempted to influence the program content through their work and expertise (but also through representations).

The sometimes poor adherence to the criteria of inclusion in the program, particularly regarding whether or not the activities belonged to the field of public health or were effective; the speed with which discussions took place between the professionals who had developed the content and the ministerial team (a speed that prevented the professionals from having the decisions validated by their working groups); the difficulty in uniformly applying the criteria of inclusion of activities; the lack of clarity about how the priorities could be determined; and the fear of seeing certain areas of expertise being left out of the program are all elements that gave rise

*(continues)*

**Case Study 4-A** *continued*

to tensions during that period. It was at that turning point that a professional suggested conducting a strategic analysis of the issues in order to clarify the issues, expectations, fears, conditions for success, and pitfalls, and beginning to focus on "how" to manage change rather than focusing only on "what" the content of the program should be.

### Which Priorities?

Furthermore, the program's advisory committee and the public health authorities met a few times to validate the proposed contents and to establish priorities. The lack of consensus on the need to use duly established criteria to determine the priorities as well as on the relative importance of the proposed activities made this operation difficult. However, an exception should be noted, that is, a meeting held at the end of the development process, in which the criteria of feasibility and opportunity made it possible to determine, on the basis of consensus, the activities to be conducted during the first stage of the program.

In general, despite efforts and good will, some deficiencies were observed in the transmission of information throughout the process of development of contents and establishment of priorities. Indeed, information was perceived to have been insufficiently communicated or was communicated too late between the different groups (MSSS-DSPs-INSPQ-CLSCs, between the authorities and the professionals or other resources), and even within the same group. Apart from a newsletter that was disseminated by the MSSS a few times and on an irregular basis and the information transmitted to the national roundtables on public health (which include the regional and central public health organizations, except for CLSCs) and to the management committee of the MSSS's General Department of Public Health (*Direction générale de santé publique*), few mechanisms had been specified and established to communicate information between members of the advisory committee and the organizations where they came from and between the authorities and professionals or other resources, except for a periodic and widely disseminated information letter and consultation meetings' reports.

The speed of the process involved in this stage and the lack of time to disseminate information by the drafting team account, but only partly, for the unsteady flow of the information transmitted, and especially received, during the program's development. The lack of information received only partly explains the tensions observed during this stage and the lack of synergy between the organizations and the different levels of the same organization during this stage of program development. Much of this perception of lack of information may have reflected the expectations of the professionals, in particular those who had been involved in the working groups, that they would participate in all stages of decision making and drafting the program.

### The Writing and Consultation Stage

The writing of the program's consultation draft (first full draft of the text) began in July 2002 following an advisory committee meeting in which the majority of members agreed with the comments made. This consultation, which had been postponed for a few months in relation to the initial schedule, was to last from eight to ten weeks. However, this process was upset by the ministers' agenda. Although the consultation was to be launched during the Annual Public Health Days (*Journées annuelles de santé publique*) in November 2002, the ministers wished that the program be disseminated during this event instead. The consultation draft therefore had to be finished sooner than expected and the consultation period was thus limited to around 12 days. It was intended for the public health organizations only, except for the principal intersectoral ministerial partners concerned by the program. Thus it was deemed unfeasible and inappropriate to consult the national groups of community organizations during such a short time, because the latter would not have enough time to consult their members.

Within this context, it was clear that the program could not be appropriated during such a brief consultation process, in particular by the CLSCs and the trans-sectoral partners, and an appropriation stage was to be planned for later. However, the matter of the minister missing the opportunity to launch the program was considered to be worse, given the risk of missing a key opportunity for appropriation by the minister and decision makers in the health and social service network. The assistant deputy minister thus decided to put his cards on the table during a teleconference with the regional and local public health partners.

Despite these difficult conditions, the responses to the consultation were most generous. Indeed, nearly all the organizations consulted sent their comments to the MSSS within the prescribed time. Moreover, the comments made were excellent and most were rapidly integrated. The regional and local public health leaders also seemed to agree that the opportunity provided by the ministers to rapidly disseminate the program should be grasped while the long-awaited synergy was present.

**The Home Stretch . . .**

The final draft of the program was thus written (including all the comments, many of which involved major rewriting), formatted, and printed in record time (4 weeks).

The program was launched as planned on the Annual Public Health Days by the Minister for Health, Social Services, Youth Protection and Prevention, a rallying assistant deputy minister, and before representatives of all public health levels who seemed to enthusiastically welcome the first Quebec public health program.

**What Comes Next . . .**

The development of regional action plans followed by that of local action plans are crucial stages during which public health directors and executive directors of CLSCs will have to exercise strong leadership at their respective level in order to formulate their action plans for implementing the program in their respective territory. Moreover, these stages are critical for program appropriation by professionals in the DSPs and workers in CLSCs as well as their partners. The development of regional and local action plans will also be a key moment to involve the community organizations and other trans-sectoral partners in the development of action plans and to seek their support for the program and the action plans.

The program's implementation has begun. The Follow-up Committee of the Quebec Public Health Program, which includes representatives of all public health organizations (MSSS, INSPQ, DSPs, CLSCs) has held it first meeting. Its members accepted the mandate to jointly follow up the program's implementation as well as its evolution based on the population's health needs and the organizational and financial contexts. This committee will be required to play a key role in supporting the program's implementation. Lastly, training activities and evaluation activities, which will make use of the services of all public health stakeholders, are essential to the successful implementation of the program.

Although the program's publication is the end of a decisive stage, other issues in the implementation of the program are just as crucial:

*(continues)*

**Case Study 4-A** *continued*

- Changes in practice to be reconciled, supported, and facilitated
- Changes at the organizational level to facilitate changes in practice
- Professional and management leadership at all levels to promote implementation and a dynamic evolution
- Coherent actions of public health teams that are based on effective or promising interventions relying on community assets, and foster innovation
- Mechanisms for reconciling different perspectives with partners as well as within and between public health teams
- Obtaining funding to support implementation

### Conclusion

**Building alliances.** Special efforts were made to ensure the development of a program that fosters a broad consensus, both within the public health network and with key partners in its implementation. However, the appropriation exercise must continue, in particular in the development of regional and local action plans because the network's people were not all closely involved in the process, particularly at the local level, but also in the regional and national organizations. Training and appropriation activities will be critical for the effective implementation of the program.

**Clarifying values.** The program clearly raises the ethical issues associated with public health action and makes a solid synthesis of evolving concepts and practices in public health, taking account both of the importance of public policies and the empowerment of communities, while proposing actions that are most likely to have an impact on avoidable morbidity, injuries, and mortality. In brief, this is a visionary program that will require time and sustained concerted efforts for appropriation and implementation.

**Organizing goals.** The prioritization of activities must nevertheless be continued in collaboration with the regional and local partners and will be reflected in the regional and local action plans, taking advantage of the strengths and minimizing the weaknesses due to the fact that the program is vast, not having reduced the the proposed interventions enough through prioritization.

Additional effort will be needed to quantify certain goals and promote evaluation in order to measure and follow the degree of achievement, which could not be finalized before the release of the program. Evaluation is nevertheless a major issue of the program. The aim of improving the operation of the evaluation parameters will be to facilitate the follow-up of the program's implementation as well as the capacity to report on the degree of achievement of goals. Lastly, the periodic evaluation can also be instrumental in supporting the program's visibility and implementation.

**Seeking new resources.** The program's adoption seems to have further contributed to the government's intention to increase funding for prevention. A first commitment to increase existing funding for public health actions by 25% was made by the government in March 2003. Another major issue relates to the network's capacity to promote the transition from intention to action and to invest in activities considered to be priority activities in terms of their potential impact on the health of the population.

**Emphasizing innovation.** By the very nature of its content and mission, the program leaves necessary room for innovative approaches while promoting its implementation. In brief, through the development of the program and the resulting activities, a context that is conducive to its implementation at the political level (associated with funding) seems to be emerging. Local, regional, and national organizations can take advantage of this context to intensify their collaboration, in particular by providing the conditions that are conducive to the program's implementation (achievement of the action plan). This increased collaboration should be accompanied by the identification of other means to foster stronger public health leadership and infrastructure in this new context.

### Notes

1. The act respecting health services and social services stipulated that the minister "establish the public health program, take the measures that are best suited to ensure the protection of public health, and ensure national and inter-regional coordination" (R.S.Q., c. S-4.2, s. 341.9).
2. Adopted in December 2001, the Public Health Act sets out four basic functions of public health: surveillance and monitoring, prevention, promotion, and health protection. It replaces the Public Health Protection Act, which dated back 25 years. It also defines the components of the program, the regional and local action plans, and the responsibilities of the mandatories.
3. The fact that people who were "committed" rather than "representatives" had been chosen to create a product that was based on the best expertise available rather than on the interests of the parties resulted in situations of quid pro quo, in terms of the information and the involvement of stakeholders from participating organizations at several stages of the process.
4. The advisory committee included a member of each of the following organizations: College of Physicians, Professional Association of Nurses, and several others.
5. The intervention areas are (a) development, adjustment, and social integration, (b) lifestyles and chronic diseases, (c) unintentional injuries, (d) infectious diseases, (e) environmental health, and (f) occupational health.

---

*Note: Special thanks to Marthe Hamel, coordinator of program development, to the DSP, the MSSS, for the text's history and basis.*

---

## The Paradox of Inside/Outside: A Complexity Concern

In traditional public health organizations and agencies, the walls of the building that house the public health entity serve as virtual boundaries from the outside community. Within the agency, programmatic silos also become isolated from the total mission and vision of the public health enterprise. When the administrator works with the community, the other staff of the agency often remain far removed from the administrative leader's work with the community. With the increasing complexity of public health as a community system, the leader struggles with these issues. Traditional agencies and organizations are like machines. These entities tend to concentrate on the individual people, parts, programs, and silos rather than on the whole organization or agency. When a part breaks, it is necessary to fix it or the whole will suffer. These organizations tend to be hierarchical in structure with generally a command and control type of leader. The status quo tends to be the governing principle. The mission of the organization often does not align well with the activities of the organization.[37] You do not get aligned thinking or action until the vision of the leader drives the action.[38]

This machine view tends to limit the effectiveness of the work of public health. This machine view creates a world that is delimited by boundaries.[39] Wheatley believes that this machine model is extremely limiting and does not deal with organizations and communities as living systems. Systems often function in a chaotic manner and not according to the logic of the more linear mechanistic model. Systems are about chaos and change. Systems thinkers need to get away from the study of an organization or community as a machine and concentrate on the human relationships that drive the system. Wheatley and Kellner-Rogers pointed out that a system is holistic in that it is not really a sum of its parts.[40] There are no separable parts. A system is basically about relationships between people. Exercise 4-2 will give you the opportunity to explore the differences between organizational and community collaborative skills.

The complexity model of systems is clearly an innovative approach that builds on the following premises:[41]

(1) The universe is a living system that is creative in nature and exists at all levels from the microbe level to the cosmos.
(2) Life's energy is oriented toward organization. Life becomes more and more complex as it develops diversity and requirement for sustainability.
(3) Life is oriented toward defining a self and is organized to create an identity.
(4) Life self-organizes at all levels of complexity as networks, patterns, and structures emerge without external pressures.
(5) People do not like to be controlled. If left alone, they will use their intelligence, talents, creativity, and ability to adapt, and they will search for meaning and organize themselves in appropriate ways.
(6) Organizations are also living systems that follow all of the above premises.

In several books, Wheatley defines this new complexity paradigm in terms of the following dimensions:[42-45]

(1) Focus on relationships and not facts, positions, and structure
(2) Concentration on the importance of interconnectedness, which creates a web of relationships
(3) Constantly evolving
(4) Concentration of process rather than only on outcomes
(5) Systems are different in different places
(6) The agenda is always on order out of chaos and the process is always messy
(7) Life seeks organization and use messes to get there

At the organization level then, it is process and not structure that drives action. Structure needs to come out of the process. As soon as a group is brought to together to address a public health issue—tobacco control, for example—a structure will evolve to address the issue. In Figure 4-5, Rogers shows graphically that the phenomenon of organizations starts with the interrelationship between structures and systems organized around the processes needed to carry out action.

From organizations and their processes of change, the individual and especially the leader develop identity through the organizing process, from the information collected and from the relationships as they develop to how this affects action. Rogers adds the important level of meaning, action, and trust because these activities create the capacity for change and evolving organizations. To gain clarification on Rogers, who is an international consultant on complexity in organizations, a Public Health Quiz appears in Case Study 4-B. Exercise 4-3 shows how groups change as a result of new members entering the discussion.

**FIGURE 4-5    Complexity and Organizations**
*Source:* Reprinted with the permission of Myron E. Rogers.

---

## Case Study 4-B
### A Public Health Practice Quiz for Myron Rogers

**1. How do systems thinking and complexity thinking differ?**

Complexity theory is a subset of systems theory. When thinking about organizational life, it's most useful to consider living systems theory, as opposed to cybernetics, which is fundamentally about machines as systems. Systems thinking is a way of understanding the phenomenon of life as an interrelated, interconnected, dynamic whole. Life is a pattern of relationships, and more precisely a network of patterns of relationships. The old mechanistic view of the world was answering the question "What is a thing made of?" Systems thinking seeks to answer the question "How is a thing made?" This is a shift in thinking from things to processes; from parts to the

*(continues)*

**Case Study 4-B** *continued*

whole; from linear, predictable steps to nonlinear, unpredictable outcomes; from analysis of substance to seeing patterns; from neat and nested hierarchies to messy and dynamic networks; from matter to relationships; from control to order.

If systems theory explores the process nature of wholes, complexity theory seeks to understand how patterns emerge from networks, and how order emerges in a system. Scientists have long noted that over time, the evolution of a living system and its environment produces more complex patterns, relationships, and networks. This creates the ability of a system to respond to complexity in its environment in a way that preserves the system, even as the system changes itself to preserve itself. The basic question in complexity theory is "What are the simple rules that allow a system to continually self-organize into higher levels of complexity, capable of better response to an unpredictable environment over time?"

An understanding of complexity theory allows us to see how the dynamic patterns of a system come into being. I would say that complexity theory is actually a theory about simplicity. We seek to understand the simple rules which, when freely iterated over time, produce the ability to respond to complex environments and adapt successfully. The understanding of adaptation—how a system learns, grows, and thrives—is a central feature of complexity theory.

Consider for a moment the difference in applying either the mechanistic view of the world or the complexity view of the world. A mechanistic approach seeks to control the parts of the system. In organizational life, this translates into the imposition of rules, regulations, policies, procedures, micro-measurement, and micro-management. The outcome over time is complex bureaucracies with little ability to respond quickly to new information or new events in the environment. In the complexity view, the focus is on adaptation and learning, and therefore focuses on some simple rules or conditions that, iterated over time, create greater access and system-wide intelligence and enable coherent responses. In a mechanistic approach, you could look at the policy manual of an organization as the history of mistakes people have made, and each time a mistake was made, a rule was created to make sure no one else ever makes the same mistake. In a complex adaptive systems view, the essential need is to foster open networks of relationships, based on a shared sense of who we really are and what we are trying to do, and allow immediate response to whatever arises, then distributing the learning, as feedback, across the network, creating greater capacity for responsiveness in the future.

**2. Why is relationship building so critical to organizational change?**
It is the quality of the relationship within and across the system that determines the systems' access to information, its ability to respond coherently to the challenges it faces, and its ability to learn, grow, and develop.

I worked with the U.S. Army back in the 1990s. A challenge for the Army is how to create the capacity for rapid decision making and action in local units in response to immediate conditions, while still serving the objectives of the whole. The Army recognized that traditional command and control would not serve it in a time of confusion and complexity in the battle theater—it's too slow and cumbersome and relies on limited intelligence (that of a small group of leaders). How do you create this capacity for rapid response from which emerges coordinated, system-wide action? The answer lies in the development of a coherent identity, built on a shared view of what is significant, what really matters, and how we should act. But this identity cannot be imposed. Meaning is constructed, not dictated. Individual soldiers have a local experience and make sense of it based on their own interpretation. So, we might have a shared experience in an event, but we don't make sense of it in a way that will create shared meaning of its significance. This results in fragmented learning, and therefore fragmented, incoherent action over time, and ultimately, a fragmented identity, based on where you sit.

In any experience, each person holds a different and unique view of what transpired. And each person is wrong in the sense that his or her view is incomplete. We need to tap into the range of experience people have, and construct a shared view of the event, in order to tap into the intelligence that is everywhere in the system. Our ability to tap into this intelligence is a function of the quality of our relationships. If we believe that information has a hierarchy, that the captain's experience is of greater value than the private's, we'll lose information that is critical to our learning, and therefore our ability to adapt to changing circumstances. Creating a quality of relationship that invites people's experience without judgment, evaluation, or blame is essential to creating a learning organization. When evaluation is present, learning is absent.

It is the quality of our relationships across hierarchies, roles, and divisions that determines our access to information that is within the system. Access to the information and intelligence in the system determines our ability to learn and to create the freedom to act in response to what really matters. This is the key capacity of high-performing organizations.

**3. What factors cause governmental agencies to change from traditional mechanistic organizations to systems-based organizations?**

One clarification here: governmental agencies are systems and operate following the dynamics of life, whether we chose to acknowledge it or not. When we are operating mechanistically, we are working against these dynamics. The dynamics of life—self-organizing, self-generating, emergent networks of relationships, fed by information—are unstoppable. When we work mechanistically, we only predictably create unintended consequences. We then spend our energy trying to fix what showed up that we did not intend, and we become focused on the unintended, rather than on what we need and what to be.

So, what would cause a governmental agency to shift its view of how to get the results it wants from a mechanistic to a systems approach? I think there are many possible answers to this question, but the one I most frequently hear from my clients, who are leaders of complex organizations, is their awareness that more is possible. That no matter how well they've done, they haven't really tapped into the potential of their people. They are seeking a better way, a simpler way, a way that results in greater service to all their stakeholders. They set off on a path of inquiry, willing to explore new possibilities and new ideas, and have a willingness to experiment.

Of course, sometimes what creates this shift is crisis or failure in the system. As the organization becomes more rule bound, over time it reaches a kind of inertia, unable to act reliably and rapidly to sudden shifts in the environment. People have two common reactions at this point—do what we've been doing with more force (use a bigger hammer), or consider what the source of problem is. Once you go beyond trying to manage and control the phenomena and ask the question "What is the source of this problem," new options for organizing become possible.

**4. Do leaders need special knowledge, talents, and skills to work in a complexity environment?**

Well, yes and no. I would say leaders everywhere need to focus on certain talents and skills that they've neglected if they've been leading mechanistically, through

*(continues)*

**Case Study 4-B** *continued*

command and control. And, they need to let go of some qualities they've been rewarded for inappropriately.

I believe most importantly that certain qualities of character are essential for leading in these times. One is humility. Another is compassion. A leader in public education once defined these for me in the most compelling way:

> *Compassion is when I realize you don't have the whole picture.*
> *Humility is when I realize I don't either.*

This sense that we need each other, that we each possess a piece of the picture, that none of us knows it all creates a willingness to be curious and engage people everywhere in finding a shared understanding of what matters and why. I think great leaders possess these qualities in their DNA. They've shed the heroic ideals of leaders having all the answers and saving people. This heroic, mechanistic model leads to robbing people of their own competence. Many leaders trap themselves and limit their people by moving every problem up the hierarchy, to be solved above and far away from the problem, and then impose the solution in linear steps. Leaders who create true organizational capacity hold their people in the problem long enough and well enough for them to find their own solution, and regain their own competence. They see their role as nurturing relationships, connecting people to each other around questions and work that matters, and thereby connecting the system to more of itself.

Of course, this can require some special skills. Some knowledge of high-engagement, high participation processes that bring the whole system into the room is useful. Some self-mastery that allows the leader to hold people in the space of exploration and chaos longer than they are comfortable being there, long enough for new ideas and insights to develop, is helpful. And finally a willingness to hold the organization in new processes and ways of working together long enough for people to regain their sense of competence is essential.

I'd add to this a good dose of curiosity. Curiosity drives the desire to truly explore the source of a problem or challenge, and motivates the leader to seek answers everywhere in the system. This act alone is a powerful impetus for change.

### 5. Why are the three levels of change in your phenomena of organizational change so important?

This model of change helps people understand how change works and why it doesn't. It is a powerful tool for understanding the source of an issue or problem.

At the phenomenal level, we're dealing with the material form of organization—the stuff we can see and touch. Our mechanistic heritage says that this is where change should be made. For instance, if the organization isn't working right, it must be because the structure is wrong. So, we move chairs, create new and more or less complicated arrangements, in an attempt to align the parts of the system. If we do this right, the parts will add up to a whole that is what we want.

But is this anyone's experience? Structural, materialistic change has been the route for 50 years or more, and the pace of this kind of change is accelerating. Yet, when we examine what happens with structural change, the only predictable outcome is unintended consequences. What is the source of the unintended consequences we experience?

I suggest that the source of the unintended consequences is how a new structure is taken up by the "dynamics of organizing" in the next level of the model. When we change a structure, we are not just changing where people sit and who they report to—we are challenging their identity. What I've come to see as important, how I've learned to be contribute, and what I've been valued for is now disrupted. The network of relationships I've built that helps me do work that matters is shattered, and now information that is essential is lost. This usually results in resistance. The source of the resistance is my sense of my identity being threatened or rejected. Now, I'm seen as a resistor, and additional pressure is applied to me. Leadership chants a mantra: "People resist change." But this is not so. People resist *being* changed.

If we are working with the dynamics of organizing, then we are seeking to engage everyone in developing a shared view of what matters and why, what works, and what doesn't. As our collective sense of what is truly significant grows, our ability to take right action in the moment expands. This shifts the work of leadership to connecting the system to more of itself. The work is about nurturing the network of relationships, accessing the intelligence and information in the system, and generating a shared sense of identity. It's about deciding how we belong together. The ability to make meaning that is coherent across the system grows, liberating intelligent action everywhere in the system. Learning thrives; adaptation is possible without command and control.

This model provides a good map for understanding what is really happening in the organization, and why. It can be a path into the source of intelligence or the cause of stupidity in our collective actions. Just work with it from where you are. Start anywhere, but follow it everywhere.

---

## A Short Note on the Flattening World

Collaborations are changing on a daily basis. Technology is changing the ways that we expand our collective capabilities and creativity to create change, innovations, growth, and new measures of success. With the growing concern on the spread of infectious diseases around the world and the potential impact of the spread of these diseases in the United States, public health leaders have become concerned about the global nature of public health and its eventual impact on public health at the local level. It is thanks to technology and specifically the ability to collectively share information through the Internet that many of our discussions on systems and complexity are evolving to a new level of development. Friedman has discussed 10 forces that he believes are affecting our perspective on all the work done in the business and the governmental sector.[46] The first force relates to the fall of the Berlin Wall and the closely timed event of the personal computer and the Windows 3.0 operating system. These two events in 1989 changed the world as we know it. Communication between the peoples of the world changed. Thus by 1995, the World Wide Web expanded the connections of people in ways unknown before (flattener 2). The other flatteners included work flow and community-developed software, uploading, outsourcing, offshoring, supply-chaining, insourcing, informing, and all other types of technological development. One of my colleagues has developed an online course. Students sign up for the course and do all the work of the course online. My colleague can respond to the students on a regular basis from anywhere in the world, including a French café.

As the world shrinks, public health professionals are beginning to track diseases around the world on the Internet and with public health colleagues worldwide. The concept of "Wikinomics" was coined to demonstrate how mass collaborations are possible and how these new forms of collaboration in a complex world are affecting leadership in public health.[47] In fact, the computer now allows anyone to participate in the activities of the world in ways he or she never could before. In discussing Wikinomics, Tapscott and Williams use the term "peer production" to refer to the new possibilities for people joining together on the Web and addressing any issue of concern.[48] The online encyclopedia Wikipedia allows anyone to add or delete information from a specific entry. YouTube can be used to post videos on various subjects. Second Life allows you to test new ideas in a second-life world where you can be whoever you want to be. Many other examples can be given to demonstrate that all our institutions and organizations will be affected by these changes in technology. Leadership in a complex world will be different.

## Summary

The world as we know it has changed significantly since this book was first published in 2001. This chapter has looked at traditional organizations and the shifts that are occurring in public health as we move to a community- and systems-based view of the work that we do. Our systems perspectives are also being affected by an increasing understanding of the role of chaos and complexity in our lives. Edward de Bono argues caution as these changes occur.[49] The decisions that we make need to be simple even in a complex world. People have trouble understanding complex and convoluted decisions. It is important that we strive for simple explanations without much jargon if we are to be successful leaders.

## Discussion Questions

1. Explain public health in the context of a complex adaptive system.
2. What is a learning organization, and what is the role of a leader in it?
3. What are the five disciplines of the learning organization?
4. What is "Presence" and "Theory U"?
5. Describe the differences between traditional linear organizations and systems-based organizations.
6. What is complexity thinking and how does it relate to systems thinking?
7. Explain the four components of the systems-organizing model of vision, structure, learning and action.
8. What are social entrepreneurs?
9. How are systems thinking, complexity thinking, and leadership affected by a flattening world?

## Exercise 4-1:   Childhood Obesity and Systems Thinking

*Purpose:* to examine the difference in solving a public health issue from a public health perspective and from a community systems perspective

*Key concepts:* traditional linear thinking, systems thinking, meta-leadership

*Procedure:* Childhood obesity is becoming an epidemic in the United States. Your county has seen a 20% increase in childhood obesity cases in the last five years. Your local health department decides to create a public health intervention to address the problem. Internal staff meet to come up with a program plan for the project. Professor McDavid from the local university feels that the proposed initiative of the local health department is too narrow and that childhood obesity needs to be seen as a systems problem that needs county-wide attention with many different stakeholders involved.

1. Divide the class or training group into teams of 8 to 10. Half the teams will develop a program from only a public health agency perspective and half the teams from a systems perspective working across agencies.
2. Spend an hour devising the strategy and plan for your team.
3. Present the plan to the group as a whole.
4. Discuss the differences in the two types of plans.

### Exercise 4-2: Organizational and Community Collaborative Skills

*Purpose:* to explore the different types of management and leadership skills to work inside a public health agency and the skills necessary to work collaboratively with external stakeholders

*Key concepts:* management, leadership, meta-leadership, collaboration, talents, linear thinking, systems thinking

*Procedure:* Divide the training or class into small groups of 6–8 people. Each group will get a large piece of flip chart paper and a colored marker. Half the groups will create a list of the talents and skills necessary to be a manager/leader inside a public health agency. Half the groups will create a similar list for leaders working collaboratively with external stakeholders. Groups will present their list to the group or class as a whole. Comparisons of the lists will then be made.

### Exercise 4-3: Complexity Through Rotation

*Purpose:* to examine how the rotation of people in a group changes its internal dynamics

*Key concepts:* complexity, relationships, self-organizing systems

*Procedure:* All people need to be organized into groups of 8–10. Start your work on this exercise by discussing the following question: How are these times of stress affecting you personally? After 10 to 15 minutes, have one of the people in your group move to another group and someone from another group move into your group. The next question is "How difficult is it to work across departments in this agency (or students can answer this question by talking about difficulties in working in different groups in different classes) and what can we do about it?" After 10 to 15 minutes, the rotation is done again and the next questions are "Do we work in ways that support interconnectedness rather than separateness? How can we break down our silos?" After another 15 minutes, rotate again and answer the question "If public health is a system, how does our agency reflect the systems needs of our state?" After 10 to 15 minutes, there is a final rotation with the question "How do we improve our relationships with our community partners?" Debrief the exercise after the 15-minute discussion.

## References

1. Institute of Medicine, *The Future of Public Health* (Washington, DC: National Academy of Press, 1988).
2. G. H. Eoyang, "Public Health and Human Systems Dynamics: What Can We Learn from Each Other?" *Complexity Science in Practice: Understanding and Acting to Improve Health and Healthcare* (Allentown, PA: Plexus Institute, 2003).
3. J. O'Connor and I. McDermott, *The Art of Systems Thinking* (London: Thorsons, 1997).
4. N. Weiner, *Cybernetics* (Cambridge, MA: MIT Press, 1948).
5. N. Weiner, *The Human Use of Human Beings* (Boston: Houghton Mifflin, 1950).
6. L. von Bertalanffy, *General Systems Theory* (New York: Braziller, 1968).
7. J. Forrester, *Industrial Dynamics* (London: Productivity Press (Taylor and Francis), 1961).
8. C. W. Churchman, *The Systems Approach* (New York: Laurel Books, 1970).
9. P. M. Senge, *The Fifth Discipline* (New York: Doubleday, 2006).
10. Senge, *The Fifth Discipline.*
11. L. Rowitz, *Public Health in the 21st Century: The Prepared Leader* (Sudbury, MA: Jones and Bartlett, 2006).
12. P. Senge, C. O. Scharmer, J. Jaworski, and B. S. Flowers, *Presence* (Cambridge, MA: Society for Organizational Learning, 2004).
13. Senge, *The Fifth Discipline.*
14. C. O. Scharmer, *Theory U* (Cambridge, MA: Society for Organizational Learning, 2007).
15. D. Cabrera, *Knowledge Age Operating System: Four Principles of Project Design, Version 1.0 Workbook* (Loveland, CO: Project N Press, 2001).
16. A. Best, P. I. Clark, S. J. Leischow, and W. M. K. Trochim, *Greater Than the Sum: Systems Thinking in Tobacco Control* (Washington, DC: National Cancer Institute, Tobacco Control Monograph Series, 18).
17. J. M. Kouzes and B. Z. Posner, *The Leadership Challenge,* 4th ed. (San Francisco: Jossey-Bass, 2007).
18. M. Lipton, *Guided Growth* (Boston: Harvard Business School Press, 2003).
19. A. F. Osborn, *Your Creative Power: How to Use Imagination* (New York: Charles Scribner, 1948).
20. E. De Bono, *Six Thinking Hats* (New York: Little, Brown and Co., 1999).
21. W. K. Kellogg Foundation, *Logic Model Development Guide* (Battle Creek, MI: W. K. Kellogg Foundation).
22. M. R. Weisbord and S. Janoff, *Future Search* (San Francisco: Barrett-Kohler, 1995).
23. M. Emery and R. E. Purser, *The Search Conference* (San Francisco: Jossey-Bass, 1996).
24. I. Bens, *Facilitating with Ease* (New York: John Wiley & Sons, 2000).
25. E. Wenger, R. Mcdermott, and W. M. Synder, *Cultivating Communities of Practice* (Boston: Harvard Business School Press, 2002).

26. Best et al., *Greater Than the Sum: Systems Thinking in Tobacco Control.*
27. Senge, *The Fifth Discipline.*
28. D. H. Kim and V. Anderson, *Systems Archetype Basics* (Watham, MA: Pegasus Communications, 2007).
29. Rowitz, *Public Health in the 21st Century: The Prepared Leader.*
30. M. J. Wheatley, *Leadership and the New Science* (San Francisco: Berrett-Kohler, 1999).
31. R. Wagner and J. K. Harter, *12: The Elements of Great Managing* (New York: Gallup Press, 2006).
32. D. Bornstein, *How to Change the World: Social Entrepreneurs and the Power of New Ideas* (New York: Oxford University Press, 2007).
33. Best et al., *Greater Than the Sum: Systems Thinking in Tobacco Control.*
34. Best et al., *Greater Than the Sum: Systems Thinking in Tobacco Control.*
35. Centers for Disease Control and Prevention, "Framework for Program Evaluation in Public Health," *Morbididty and Mortality Weekly Report Recommendations and Reports, 48, RR11,* 1–40.
36. The Commonwealth Fund Commission on a High Performance Health System, *A High Performance Health System for the United States* (Washington, DC: The Commonwealth Fund, November 2007).
37. S. Goldsmith and W. D. Eggers, *Governing by Network* (Washington, DC: Brookings Institution Press, 2004).
38. J. Steffen, *Aligned Thinking* (San Francisco: Berrett-Kohler, 2006).
39. Wheatley, *Leadership and the New Science.*
40. M. J. Wheatley and M. Kellner-Rogers, *A Simpler Way* (San Francisco: Berrett-Kohler, 1996).
41. Wheatley and Kellner-Rogers, *A Simpler Way.*
42. Wheatley, *Leadership and the New Science.*
43. Wheatley and Kellner-Rogers, *A Simpler Way.*
44. M. J. Wheatley, *Turning to One Another* (San Francisco: Berrett-Kohler, 2002).
45. M. J. Wheatley, *Finding Our Way* (San Francisco: Berrett-Kohler, 2005).
46. T. L. Friedman, *The World Is Flat* (New York: Farrar, Straus, and Giroux, 2006).
47. D. Tapscott and A. D. Williams, *Wikinomics* (New York: Portfolio, 2006).
48. Tapscott and Williams, *Wikinomics.*
49. E. De Bono, *Simplicity* (London: Penguin Books, 1999).

# CHAPTER 5

# THE LEADERSHIP WHEEL AND ORGANIZATIONAL CHANGE

Devote yourself to loving others, devote yourself to the
community around you, and devote yourself to creating
something that gives you purpose and meaning.
                              Morris Schwartz, *Morrie: In His Own Words*

Good leadership depends on systems thinking. This type of thinking focuses on ways to implement, in the short and long term, system components necessary for meeting identified needs. To ensure that systems thinking is effective, public health agency leaders must support the systems perspective and make certain staff understand what is involved in a systems approach to change. Communication must be frequent enough to allow the staff to help manage the implementation of strategic policies. The leader is responsible for guiding the implementation activities and presenting to the community the steps being taken by the agency in response to local public health issues.

Team building is a critical part of leading a public health agency (see Chapter 6). The leader creates teams inside the agency and coalitions outside to address the programmatic needs of the agency. Once the members are appointed, the teams need to clarify the values that will guide their activities. Community coalitions and partnerships have basic similarities to teams, and their development resembles team development.

Public health leaders must:

- think systemically and act strategically
- create a learning organization
- coordinate knowledge management activities
- promote and support the change process
- support the values of the agency and the community
- understand the relationship between system inputs, program interventions, and outputs
- monitor and evaluate the effects of change
- practice systems thinking at the five levels of leadership (see Chapter 6)

The remainder of this chapter covers the main stages in the systems approach to organizational change as represented by a leadership wheel (Figure 5-1). Strong leaders with a high level of commitment must serve as the conveners and inspirational voices for the process. These stages include values clarification, construction or revision of the agency's mission and vision,

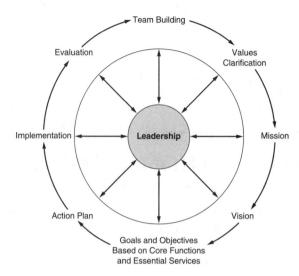

**FIGURE 5-1** **Systems Approach to Organizational Change**

identification of goals and objectives, development of an action plan, implementation of the action plan, and assessment of the effects of the implementation. As a systems-based working model, the leadership wheel sees the integration of planning and action. An important consideration in this whole process is the need to understand the assumptions that provide a foundation for all the activities that occur as part of the systems perspective for both internal and external stakeholders.[1] In actuality, we often do not have all the knowledge necessary to the understanding of a public health or programmatic need before we start to work on it. The assumptions we make will depend on whether we take a linear perspective on an issue or we take a systems perspective. This assumption approach is tied to what Churchman has called an inquiry system.[2] An inquiry system involves the process of creating a system of interrelated parts or components that provide a holistic perspective on the appropriate knowledge to address a problem or challenge.

## Values Clarification

Blanchard and O'Connor make a distinction between the Fortune 500 and the Fortunate 500.[3] The latter are businesses in which management by values occurs. In the management-by-values process, which can take three years to complete, an agency goes through three stages. The first stage involves clarification of the agency's mission, values, and vision. The second stage involves communicating the agency's newly clarified mission, values, and vision to others. The final stage, which is the most complex, involves aligning the leadership and management practices of the agency with its stated values. In the case of public health leadership, the alignment of practices and values applies to the individual, team, agency, community, and professional level.

An agency's culture is made up, in part, of the values and beliefs that the members of the agency have in common.[4] These values and beliefs guide the members' individual and collective behavior. Also part of the agency's culture are the rituals and myths that have grown out of the agency's history. For example, a myth might be created about a former administrator, who, as an avid promoter of public health in the community, might be idealized as a public health hero. Treating the administrator as a hero has its benefits, because it reaffirms the importance of health promotion. Yet it can also have a downside. For one thing, it may lead to organizational stasis, for the myth suggests that everything the administrator did, every policy decision made, is above question, and thus the current members of the agency may be more reluctant to make necessary changes than if they viewed the administrator as praiseworthy but fallible.

Agency rituals might include a special public health award given to a community organization each year at an annual luncheon. If this award is named after the former administrator, the ritual supports the myth. A new public health administrator with new ideas and a new vision for the agency will need to work with the agency staff to redefine its values, and thus the current myths and rituals—and even the agency's physical layout, which is a component of organizational culture—may need to be changed.

A value, according to Rokeach, is "an enduring belief that a specific mode of conduct or end-state of existence is personally or socially preferable to an opposite or converse mode of conduct or end-state of existence."[5(p.5)] Each community has a unique configuration and a unique set of values, and the local public health agency is a reflection of these values. Societies that are geographically and politically separated from each other tend to develop different community approaches to dealing with their particular problems.[6] For example, a county with a mostly rural population will have different public health priorities than a county with a mostly urban population. Rural health leaders often have to do more with less. They have less money, fewer staff than large urban health departments, sometimes geographic isolation, limited technical resources, lower salaries for staff, and often fewer external partners.[7] Case Study 5-A examines some of these issues as well as leadership wheel issues in a local public health response to a potential smallpox outbreak in a rural county.

---

### Case Study 5-A
### Pustules Proliferate in Dairyair County—A Local Public Health Response to a Smallpox Outbreak: A Case Study in Assurance
### Mid-America Regional Public Health Leadership Institute, April 2003

*Sue Becker, Kurt Eggebrecht, Sherry Gehl, Sue Kunferman, Jody Langfeldt, Cheryl Mazmanian, Lora Taylor*

**Opening/Introduction**
The risk of smallpox being used by terrorists as a bio-weapon is becoming a viable threat to citizens of the United States. In the event of a smallpox outbreak, health care providers, emergency service personnel, and state and local governments are

*(continues)*

**Case Study 5-A** *continued*

going to be working in a crisis mode to not only treat the victims, but to contain the outbreak and begin mass vaccination. Communities and especially individual neighborhoods may be initially left to fend for themselves during the onset of the crisis.

Ensuring that the health needs of the citizens of Dairyair County are met is the responsibility of Jo Jersey, the director/health officer of the Dairyair County Health Department. Jo is a member of Dairyair County's community response team and has been trained in the Incident Command System.

Dairyair County is located in north central Wisconsin. It has a population of 100,000 people. Farming is the main industry of the county, with eight migrant farms supplying the majority of the workforce. A number of smaller factories are located in the county, the largest of which is the Cow Pie Factory, employing 3,000 workers. The median annual income in this county is $29,000. The largest municipality in this county is the small urban center Lodge City (40,000 population), with other surrounding rural communities making up the rest of the population. A rural newspaper, the *Dairyair Daily*, provides a daily newspaper to most of the residents of Lodge City, with limited circulation to the rest of Dairyair County. Two local radio stations, WSPOX and WPUS, are both linked to the county emergency broadcast system.

**Case Body**

The county executive, Wanda Windbag, has just been notified of a $400,000 Community Preparedness Grant that has been awarded to the county to be used for bioterrorism preparedness. She is soliciting input from community leaders on how these dollars should be spent to prepare the county to respond to a bioterrorist attack. The perception of a bioterrorism event occurring in Dairyair County is believed to be so remote that most residents and local officials gave little weight to the warnings and preparations going on about them. For example, Fire Chief Blaze Arson was skeptical of the likelihood of a biological attack. He is convinced, and is working to influence county supervisors to agree, that the county's limited resources should be devoted to personal protective equipment and training for firefighters. Sheriff Sly Straightshooter believes, as a result of the training he received from the Federal Bureau of Investigation, that the likely scenario will be a car bomb at the Dairyair administration building. He is advocating for security badges for all county employees and that bomb reduction film be placed on the windows of the administration building. The executive of General Hospital, Mavis Moneypenny, has contacted the governor expressing concerns regarding the hospital's lack of sufficient decontamination equipment and negative pressure rooms and is advocating for funding to improve the situation. Although supportive of the local health department's planning effort, the hospital's lack of resources makes it incapable of fulfilling its role. Cricket Copyright, the aggressive reporter of the *Dairyair Daily*, is pressuring County Executive Windbag to disclose how these limited resources will be used.

Jo Jersey, aware of the real risk to the community in the event of a bioterrorism event, particularly a smallpox outbreak, had been working closely with the state and the Centers for Disease Control and Prevention (CDC) on educating and vaccinating her staff. Plans were being developed to educate the other members of the Incident Command Team and the political leaders regarding the unique issues the community would face in a biological emergency. Tommy Tabletop, the Dairyair county director of emergency management, has not embraced the recommendations of Jo Jersey to sponsor a biological incident exercise due to his limited knowledge and lack of understanding regarding bioterrorism issues.

As the discussion and political wrangling continued, on January 1, 2003, a woman from Lodge City walked into the local emergency department (ED) with a four-day history of fever, malaise, headache, and severe backache. She currently is exhibiting a pustule type rash covering most of her extremities and face. As usual for a holiday, the ED was very busy, with at least 45 people present. Two days following the woman's presentation in the ED, a family of four, mom, dad, and two children, walked into the local health clinic exhibiting the same symptoms. The clinic was busy with 28 people in the waiting room and a staff of 10. After much testing and significantly more exposure, the tentative diagnosis was variola major, better known as smallpox. During the next 48 hours, 10 more people in Dairyair County were tentatively diagnosed with smallpox. The suspect smallpox patients were either quarantined at home, or for those requiring hospitalization, placed in an isolation area in the local hospital.

The unexpected had occurred. Local health officials began working on a plan to vaccinate all the citizens of Dairyair County. The CDC had released the vaccine. With more and more cases of smallpox presenting every day, it was imperative that the entire population be vaccinated. Never had the community faced this type of emergency, a biological one.

Within 48 hours and the diagnosis of 20 cases of smallpox, the community was in a panic. Clinic and hospital staff were afraid to go to work. The school superintendent, following a recommendation from Jo Jersey, closed all schools. Absenteeism in all workplaces was at an all-time high. People were isolating themselves and their families. The shelves in the stores were emptying fast. Following the advice of Jo Jersey, Tommy Tabletop activated the Incident Command Center and delegated the leadership role to Jo Jersey. Under Jo's leadership, it became clear that this was a public health emergency that would require a nontraditional approach by the community emergency response team in Dairyair County.

Utilizing the state and the CDC mass vaccination protocols, clinics were established throughout Dairyair County. Jo assigned Tommy Tabletop the task of recruiting and organizing medical and nonmedical volunteers to assist with these clinics. Sheriff Straightshooter was assigned the role of public information officer. A community moratorium was ordered on public events. An emergency communications network was established. The CDC Web site was recommended as the source for information on smallpox. In addition, working with the media partners, municipal leaders assured the community that sufficient vaccine had been acquired to immunize all of the citizens of Dairyair County and it would be made available to residents at multiple immunization clinics throughout the county. Chief Arson was assigned to work with the coroner's office and the hospitals to ensure the appropriate handling of the deceased.

Seventy-two hours after the first case of smallpox was diagnosed, the first of many vaccination clinics occurred. Clinics were set up on a daily basis at numerous sites around the county. An exhaustive public awareness campaign on the need to be vaccinated was launched throughout the county. After a 10-day vaccination effort, with no additional residents presenting for vaccination, it was determined that only 75,000 smallpox vaccinations were provided, leaving 25,000 citizens unprotected and unreached by the vaccination efforts.

---

Some general truths about values are worth noting. First, certain values are universal, whereas others occur only in specific locales. There is a clear recognition that there are some values that are universally held. These universal values tend to be heterogeneous in content with some tied to our human nature and some tied to living in cultural groups. Brown has tied the study of universal value systems to both human biology and evolutionary psychology.[8] Second, values tend to be organized into value systems. Third, people generally have the values they do because of the socialization they have undergone. Fourth, values are present in every social situation.

The increasing diversification within many communities has led to changes in value systems and in some cases to a confusing diversity of values. To ensure that a system of shared values evolves, a community must undertake a process of value clarification. This type of process respects diversity but is aimed at elucidating the dominant values of the community. A vision cannot be realized unless it is built on an infrastructure of shared core values.

With an awareness of universal values, 24 leaders from around the world and from various professions were asked to address this.[9] They reached a consensus that the following values were universal: love, truthfulness, fairness, freedom, unity, tolerance, responsibility, and respect for life. Some widely shared values were nonetheless not universally shared, but these were listed as well: courage, wisdom, hospitality, obedience, peace, stability, racial harmony, respect for women's place in society, and protection of the environment. In the case of American culture, two other widely shared values should be added to the group: health protection and quality of life. Americans, among others, are concerned about the effect that disease can have on quality of life. Public health leaders promote a public health agenda oriented toward improving the quality of life of people in their service communities.

Americans are also concerned about having a choice.[10] In the health reform debate in the early 1990s, the potential for the loss of choice of medical provider (and loss of power over other aspects of medical care) was a critical factor in the defeat of the Clinton plan. It almost became more important than the potential benefits of universal health care. (To partially fill out the list of American cultural values, Americans are preoccupied with the biggest and newest consumer products, pursue dreams even when the chance of success is slight, are impatient, and tend to improvise in the making of changes. All these need to be taken into account in designing public health policies.) It is interesting to examine the Commonwealth Fund report on the future of the American health care system discussed in Chapter 4 because many of the issues discussed in the Clinton health plan are being reexamined today.

Shared values play an important role in any reform of the public health system. Exercise 5-1 is intended to illuminate the relationships among personal, professional, organizational, and community values.

Public health leaders, as protectors of the values of the agency and the community, must emphasize the importance of maintaining high ethical standards inside the agency and in the community. One necessary task is to do an ethics check. Are the procedures used in the agency and the community legal? And even if legal, are they consistent with the values of the agency and the community? Leaders also need to examine the relationship between the science of public health, the facts that guide public health practice, and the explicit knowledge that comes from our formal learning.[11] As can be seen in Figure 5-2, which evolved from my discussion with Dr. Patrick Lenihan, who was the 2003 president of the National Association of County and City

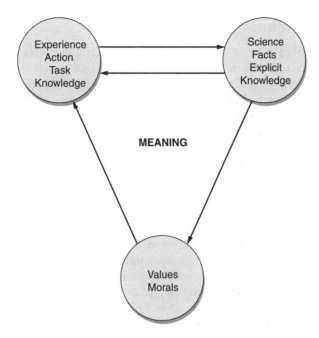

**FIGURE 5-2    Leadership & Meaning**

Health Officials, the science and explicit knowledge dimension of a public health system needs to be understood in relationship to the experiences, action activities, and tacit knowledge that grows out of practice and internal agency learning and operations. Tacit knowledge is difficult to communicate because it involves the internal understandings of people to the experiences they have filtered through their personal values and beliefs. The science and experience dimensions are quite interactive but derive meaning after being screened by our values positions. It is not knowledge, experience, or values alone that are important; it is the meaning that is attached to these activities that is the important dimension. Leaders and managers have the critical role of translating tacit knowledge into explicit knowledge so that there is meaning in these events for internal and external stakeholders. This translation helps the organization address similar problems in the future.

Public health leaders, besides identifying values, must consider how these values will affect the implementation of programs. They should be aware that the process of values clarification can simplify the solution of many local public health issues. Following is a list of strategies for clarifying values and promoting them in the agency and community:

- Learn which values are universal (or nearly universal) and promulgate them in the community.
- Learn which additional values prevail in the community and in the agency.
- In conjunction with agency members and community partners, integrate universal, community, and agency values.
- Evaluate prevailing values and revise those that need to be changed.
- Develop a shared values statement.

## Mission and Vision

Leaders need to be oriented toward the future and help create the vision that guides the activities of the agency. They must also inspire their colleagues to share the vision and use it to guide their activities. Therefore, the next task after values clarification is to evaluate both the agency's mission and the current vision for the agency (or create a new one).

An agency's mission and the vision must reflect each other. A vision is a picture of what, according to its leaders, the agency's future should be like. The agency's mission is the role it sees itself playing in the community. If the vision and mission truly reflect each other, then the agency, in fulfilling its mission, will help realize its vision (i.e., help bring about the kind of future it desires).

In addition, public health, like other areas of society, is changing rapidly, and an agency's vision and mission must change in concert. For example, disaster preparedness and response, public-private partnerships, emerging infections, drug resistance, mental health, and community violence are issues, some newer than others, that public health must address. A public health agency's mission statement must be revised periodically to take into account new problems or other developments that have occurred in the public health arena.

An organization's mission defines its purpose—its reason for existing.[12] A standard mission for a public health agency is the promotion of health and the prevention of disease. If an agency views itself as having this mission, then it should not be primarily involved in providing direct services with a strong medical orientation.

A mission statement can be short or long. It can be a statement of the agency's general purpose or it can detail the agency's role in several areas. According to Wall and colleagues, a mission statement needs to answer four questions:[13]

1. What is the purpose of public health?
2. How does the public health agency intend to coordinate its values and actions?
3. Who makes up the constituencies of the agency?
4. How does the agency link the present with the future?

Pearce and David claim that a mission statement should address such things as the customer market (community), service-related issues, geographic concerns (global, national, state, or local), the level of technology, the requirements of agency survival, the personal concerns of the agency's leaders, the agency's philosophy, and the image of the agency in the community.[14] Albrecht recommended addressing the environment of competitors, economic concerns, political concerns, legal concerns, and social issues.[15] Wilson cautioned that a mission statement may leave out critical organizational activities, which sometimes shrivel financially and programmatically if not included in the mission.[16]

A mission statement should be inspiring, for the public health agency's workforce needs to embrace the mission.[17] Getting the staff members to do this could be difficult, because many of them have a minimal background in public health. Many will have been hired to perform clinical functions rather than engage in community-oriented preventive activities.

The mission is an important determinant of the agency's goals and objectives and should be closely tied to the agency's action plan. Therefore, the agency leaders must communicate the mission to community partners and constituents as well as to the agency workforce.[18] One strategy is to ask partners and constituents to read the mission statement in order to evaluate its clarity.

There is a question whether the mission or vision should be developed first. Typically, a public health agency has a clear idea of its mission but an undeveloped vision of its future. In a case like this, the mission is virtually given and the vision is what must be worked on. Sometimes an organization's mission and vision are both treated in a single statement that covers the present and the future. For example, the public health mission enunciated in *Healthy People in Healthy Communities* can also be viewed as a vision of the future.[19]

As pointed out earlier, managers are focused on protecting the integrity of their organization, whereas leaders are visionary and committed to change. Therefore, leaders can often benefit from developing their visioning skills. A vision can be likened to a blank canvas on which the leader sketches a possible future. Although a vision statement is about the future, it is often written in the present tense, which is one method of expressing the strong connection between the "now" and the "then."

Two cautionary notes: First, leaders are responsible for more than creating a vision. They need to motivate others and to play a major role in the development of action plans. Second, leaders may need to give up power in order to bring the vision into reality.[20] For example, they may be required to make changes in the organizational chart.

Following is a brief description of one method for developing a vision statement. First, the visioning team lays out the values and principles that will guide the visioning process. Second, the team develops a glossary of terms to go along with the shared mission statement. Third, it includes key constituents in the visioning process. Fourth, it describes the functions of a vision statement and how the vision statement to be created will be used. Fifth, the visioning team discusses the future and where it wants public health activities to go. (The team should consider scenarios likely to occur if the agency moves in certain directions. Scenario building is an important step in the visioning process.) Next, the team redefines terms and relates them to concepts in the glossary. Then it devises a vision statement based on the work it has done. The construction is followed by general editing, which occurs in smaller teams. The final step is to reach a consensus on the vision statement. Of course, once the vision statement is agreed upon, it is necessary to audit progress toward the implementation of the vision.

Following is a summary of the steps public health leaders need to take in order to develop a mission and vision for their agencies:

- Use a mission statement to guide the daily activities of the public health agency.
- Create a vision statement to guide the activities of the agency as it moves forward in time.

- Use visioning skills to create the vision.
- Involve colleagues and community partners in the development of a shared mission and vision.
- Develop a glossary of public health terms for colleagues and community partners.
- Review the mission and vision statements yearly.

Mission and vision are also affected by whether the leader is a traditional thinker who defines public health in a narrow sense as tied to the programmatic activities of the governmental public health agency or more systemically from the perspective of the community as a whole. Because leaders often work from the inside of their agency to the outside and also recognize the possibilities and concerns of external stakeholders as an outside to inside approach, the practice of action inquiry needs to occur.[21] Action inquiry is a systems activity of transformational leaders that should lead to mutual approaches to addressing public health challenges. It is through action inquiry that knowledge and action will come together.

## Goals and Objectives

The next task in the systems approach to organizational change is to translate the mission and the vision into measurable goals and objectives. The mission statement is framed in general terms and does not contain the details of how the mission is to be fulfilled. Nor does the vision statement lay out how the vision is to be realized. Goals are more specific than either the mission or vision, and objectives are more specific still. They are, so to speak, the individual steps on the way to fulfilling the mission and realizing the vision.

Goals can be classified in several ways. One distinction is between organizational goals, which the activities of the organization are intended to achieve, and order goals, which are pursued as a means of preventing certain events from happening.[22] Organizational goals can be further divided into the stated goals of an organization and the actual, sometimes hidden, goals of the organization. Creating a fit between organizational goals and systems goals is an important leadership activity. Goals can also be classified in terms of the areas of human activity to which they pertain, as seen in the division between economic, cultural, social, and political goals.

Objectives are the quantitatively and qualitatively measurable steps needed to achieve the goals of the organization. Along with the goals, they are used to guide the managerial processes for which public health agency leaders are responsible. The goals and objectives also need to reflect the vision of the agency and community or the vision or goals need to be revised. Specifically the leader then has the responsibility for:

- translating the agency's mission and vision into programmatic goals and objectives
- discovering any hidden goals that may sabotage activities (action inquiry)
- considering the budgetary requirements necessary to realize the goals and objectives
- examining goals to determine if they are translatable into action

Exercise 5-2 explores the relationship between an organization's mission, vision, and goals and objectives.

## The Action Plan

The next step is to develop an action plan for achieving the goals and objectives identified in the preceding stage. The action plan consists of operational steps that, if performed, will lead to the attainment of the stated goals and objectives. In this step, the agency leaders are required to be especially creative, because the action plan will almost certainly demand innovative approaches to achieving the goals and objectives. Creativity is called for by the structural tension that exists between the vision and the current reality. A creative leader looks for ways of resolving the tension in order to move the organization forward.[23]

Brainstorming is frequently used at this stage, because it is an effective way of discovering worthwhile ideas. In addition, the leaders, in creating an action plan, must take into account the environment (the agency and its community) and the resources needed to carry out the plan.[24] Another set of techniques involves scenario planning, which is the development of stories to examine variations in eventual outcomes in bringing vision into reality. Scenario planning uses many tools including forecasting, forces for change, tabletop exercises, computer simulations, environmental changes, politics, and systems tools and techniques.[25]

> **Leadership Tip**
>
> *Public health is about adapting to change. There is really no status quo.*

The creative process can be divided into three stages.[26] First comes the germination phase, in which the leader uses personal excitement to address the problems that need to be dealt with. In the second stage, the organization and its employees begin to adapt to the leader's agenda. In stage 3, the process is completed. At the end of stage 3, the leader often starts the process over again.

Some management experts suggest that devising strategies for goal attainment is more effective than an action plan. Mintzberg, for example, argued that the action plan approach is too narrow.[27] For one thing, it separates strategic thinking from the goal-attainment process, and the separation prevents leaders from responding creatively to the changing environment. In Mintzberg's view, planning is an incremental process and is not something that can be done all at once. One way of proceeding is to create an action plan that addresses only a few important areas. If the plan is too complex, failure may result.[28] Note that if the strategic approach is used, the strategies chosen may in fact replace goals in the minds of the various constituencies.

One way of looking at an action plan is as a process of learning through action. Constant feedback is a necessary part of the process. If progress toward the goals is not occurring, revisions in the plan will need to be made. The leaders may have to go back to previous stages and repeat them. Feedback in systems is in actuality quite complex as can be seen in Figure

5-3.[29] This diagram demonstrates that a critical aspect of action is to close the gap between a designated goal or set of goals and a series of action steps. Part of the reason for this gap is that there may be hidden goals in the system that come to the forefront when specific action steps are implemented. As actions steps are implemented, unexpected occurrences may also happen that change the system. This fits the Wheatley argument that change is messy and chaotic.[30]

One point to mention here is that government agencies tend to be highly bureaucratic because of the legislative need for oversight and accountability. As may be expected, civil service requirements often work against organizational change, and networks are often difficult to form in bureaucratic organizations. Yet, an interesting phenomenon is occurring that may help in overcoming some of the barriers caused by bureaucratization. Over half of the states have an in-state or regional public health leadership institute, and such institutes are facilitating the development of leadership networks. Web sites, forums, chat rooms, and other forms of electronic communication are making networking easier.

The structure of any organization is multilayered, and those devising an action plan need to take account of the hidden parts of the organization's structure.[31] Furthermore, they need to keep in mind that any stage in the implementation of the plan will be affected by all the previous stages. They also must pay attention to authority issues and the impact that the implementation of the plan will have on the workforce, because major changes can alter a staff member's sense of identity.

A number of strategies, including the following four, can be used to reduce the problems likely to arise from a major change. First, resulting changes in roles and relationships should be determined as the action plan is being created. Staff will worry about no longer having a job when the process

**FIGURE 5-3   Feedback Loops in a System Dynamics Model**
*Source:* A. Best, P. I. Clark, S. J. Leischow, and W. M. Trochim, *Greater Than the Sum: Systems Thinking in Tobacco Control* (Washington, DC: National Cancer Institute Tobacco Control Monograph Series, 2007).

is completed—and in fact jobs may vanish as a result of the implementation. Second, the human resources office may have to be reorganized or its practices reformed in light of the proposed change. Third, an information system capable of monitoring the implementation process may have to be created. Finally, the financial management of the organization may have to be altered.

One way to measure the effectiveness of an action plan is to use the balanced scorecard model developed by Kaplan and Norton.[32] This model evaluates the degree of success from the financial, internal organization process, customer, and learning and growth perspectives. What the balanced scorecard demonstrates is that action planning needs to be aware of the many different dimensions to action planning activities. We need to be careful to include all the dimensions in our action activities. Oversimplification can be as much of a problem as can too much complexity. For an action plan to work, according to the authors, the leaders of the organization must communicate the mission and vision, the goals and objectives, and the action plan to all the relevant constituencies. Second, the leaders must understand and be able to explain to these constituencies the linkage between the action plan goals and the rewards associated with good performance—what might be called "encouraging the heart."[33] Third, the process of developing the plan must include target setting. Fourth, the action plan must include feedback and learning components.

An action plan can usher in a new era for the organization or be its death knell. It is more likely to benefit the organization if it is created by means of a well-thought-out method and is implemented using the strategies mentioned above. Following is a list of guidelines that public health leaders should follow when engaged in action planning:

- Develop an action plan tied to the agency's mission, vision, and goals and objectives.
- Use strategic planning techniques for action planning (see Chapter 13).
- Formulate operational steps or strategies for each goal and objective.
- Know the resources that are needed and the resources that available to implement the action plan.
- Explore existing barriers to successful action planning.

- Use the balanced scorecard model to measure the effectiveness of the action plan.

## Implementation

The implementation of an action plan for the purpose of achieving goals and objectives and thereby realizing the agency's vision *is* the practice of public health, or at least part of it. During implementation, the leaders of the agency have the task of communicating the mission, vision, and goals and objectives of the agency to the staff and community constituents and doing this within the governing paradigm of the public health core functions of assessment, policy development, and assurance. In short, the leaders must become a bridge between the agency and the community.

Very little has been written about the implementation of action plans in the field of public health. Yet it is clear that implementation of an action plan can involve many of the same activities public health leaders normally engage in as part of their responsibilities. These include:

- identifying community leaders and other external stakeholders
- delegating tasks to staff members and community partners
- establishing relationships with constituents
- communicating health information to the community
- working with the legislature
- working with the county board or local board of health

In a survey of California public health officers and executives, the respondents stated that their work encompassed budgeting, programming, disease control, staffing, environmental issues, health issues related to foreign nationals, and issues arising from undocumented care.[34] The researchers examined the lessons that the public health leaders had learned from their daily activities. These lessons included the importance of accuracy of information, flexibility, the total involvement of all stakeholders, action based on vision, patience, and providing information to the public.

## Evaluation

After an action plan is implemented, the results of the implementation need to be evaluated. The object of the evaluation is to determine to what degree the goals and objectives were achieved. Although the leaders of a public health agency will not be directly involved in gathering and analyzing the evaluation data, they will use the conclusions of the evaluation to determine what steps to take next to realize the agency's vision.

Leaders of an agency need data to foster a culture of evidence-based practice within the agency and among community constituents. For one thing, public health leaders are seen as sources of knowledge about community public health issues, and ensuring that evaluation data are gathered and publicized in some form confirms the legitimacy of their role as knowledge providers. In addition, the data will show the effects of the agency's activities on the residents of the community and, assuming they are mostly positive, will confirm the legitimacy of the agency's role as a protector of the community's health.

The evaluation process has been analyzed as consisting of six separate steps:[35]

1. posing questions about the program
2. setting effectiveness standards
3. designing the evaluation
4. collecting the data
5. analyzing the data
6. reporting the results

Not part of the evaluation process itself but an essential step nonetheless is the use of the results to determine further changes that need to be made.

Evaluation seems to frighten American health professionals, who tend to think evaluation data will jeopardize their jobs. In Great Britain, on the other hand, public health leaders seem convinced that evaluation helps strengthen programs.

## Summary

This chapter describes the main stages in the systems approach to organizational change. The first step is for the organization to clarify its values. Once it does that, it can more easily construct a mission for itself and create a vision of its own future. The next task is to determine which goals and objectives, if achieved, will lead to the fulfilling of the organization's mission and the realization of its vision. Then comes the development of an action plan designed to accomplish the goals and objectives. The action plan needs to be implemented, which constitutes the fifth step. The last step, of course, is to do an evaluation to determine whether the goals and objectives were accomplished and whether their accomplishment led to the realization of the organization's vision. Usually the evaluation uncovers changes that need to be made if the vision is to be realized.

### Discussion Questions

1. What are the similarities and differences between systems thinking and strategic thinking?
2. What are the values that characterize public health in the United States or in your home country?
3. How do an organization's mission and its vision differ and how are they similar?
4. What is the relationship between goals and objectives and vision?
5. What is an action plan and what is the typical purpose of such a plan?
6. What are four strategies for reducing the seriousness of problems resulting from major changes?
7. What are the six steps in the evaluation process?
8. What is the role of leaders in the change system defined by the leadership wheel?

### Exercise 5-1:   Shared Values Team Assignment

*Purpose:* to elucidate the relationships among personal values, community values, organizational values, and professional values

*Key concepts:* community coalition, community values, organizational values, personal values, professional values, value alignment, meaning

*Procedure:* The class should divide into teams of four or five members each. Each team pretends to be a community coalition charged with creating a shared values position statement intended to guide the coalition as it addresses the community's public health needs. The statement should integrate personal, organizational, community, and professional values—the values that guide our personal lives, the organization we work in, the community we live in, and the profession we are members of. Each team will perform the following steps:

1. Each team member writes down on a Post-it one of his or her personal values. The member acting as "mayor" (facilitator) collects the Post-its and sticks them on a poster board in a column. The team reviews the values to see if a pattern emerges.

2. Each team member writes down on a differently colored Post-it (one of another color than the Post-its used in step 1) a community value (the team members should choose from among the values held by the community in which they live). The mayor collects the Post-its and puts them on the poster board in a column next to the personal value Post-its. The team reviews the community values and compares them with the personal values.

3. Each team member writes down on a differently colored Post-it a professional value held by public health practitioners. The mayor collects the Post-its and puts them on the poster board in a third column. The team reviews these values and discusses the ways in which they are consistent or inconsistent with the values previously listed.

4. Each team member writes down on a differently colored Post-it an organizational value held by the organization in which he or she works. The mayor collects the Post-its and puts them on the poster board in a fourth column. The team reviews the values listed and discusses their relationship to the other sets of values.

5. The team reviews all the values listed and creates a values list that reflects the shared interests of all the team members (remember, the team members are pretending to be representatives of the organizations in a community coalition).

6. Each team presents its list of values to the whole group.

### Exercise 5-2: The Vision Thing

*Purpose:* to elucidate the initial steps in the systems approach to organizational change; the role of a public health agency's mission, vision, and goals and objectives; and the connections between these

*Key concepts:* goals and objectives, mission, vision

*Procedure:* The class should divide into agency work teams of five to ten members each. The first task is for each team to act as an ad hoc committee assigned the job of drafting a mission statement for a public health agency. If a glossary of terms is necessary, one should be drafted. After the mission statements are completed, the teams present them to the class as a whole, which then develops a shared mission statement.

In the second task, each team acts as a committee that has been assigned the job of developing a vision statement utilizing the shared mission statement created in the first task. Some team members should be designated as senior staff and others as front-line staff. After the vision statements are completed, the teams present them to the class as a whole, which then develops a shared vision statement.

In the third and final task, each team develops goals and objectives statements that indicate what actions must be achieved in order to implement the agency's mission and vision.

## References

1. I. I. Mitroff and H. A. Linstone, *The Unbounded Mind* (New York: Oxford University Press, 1993).
2. C. W. Churchman, *The Design of Inquiring Systems* (New York: Basic Books, 1971).
3. K. Blanchard and M. O'Connor, *Managing by Values* (San Francisco: Berrett-Koehler, 1997).
4. P. Hersey et al., *Management of Organizational Behavior,* 9th ed. (Upper Saddle River, NJ: Prentice Hall, 2007).
5. M. Rokeach, *The Nature of Human Values* (New York: The Free Press, 1973).
6. R. M. Williams Jr., *American Society: A Sociological Interpretation,* 3rd ed. (New York: Knopf, 1970).
7. Center for Rural Public Health Practice, *Bridging the Health Divide: The Rural Public Health Research Agenda* (Pittsburgh: University of Pittsburgh, 2004).
8. D. E. Brown, *Human Universals* (Boston: McGraw-Hill, 1991).
9. R. M. Kidder, "Universal Human Values: Findings on Ethical Common Ground," *Futurist* 28, no. 2 (1994): 8–13.
10. J. Hammond and J. Morrison, *The Stuff Americans Are Made Of* (New York: MacMillan, 1996).
11. H. Mintzberg, B. Ahlstrand, and J. Lampel, *Stategy Safari* (New York: Free Press, 1998).
12. S. P. Robbins and M. Coulter, *Management,* 8th ed. (Upper Saddle River, NJ: Prentice Hall, 2004).
13. B. Wall et al., *The Visionary Leader* (Rocklin, CA: Prima Publishing & Communication, 1992).
14. J. A. Pearce Jr. and P. R. David, "Corporate Mission Statements: The Bottom Line," *Academy of Management Executives* (May 1992): 109–116.
15. K. Albrecht, *The Northbound Train* (New York: American Management Association, 1994).
16. J. Q. Wilson, *Bureaucracy* (New York: Basic Books, 1989).
17. N. M. Tichy, *The Leadership Engine* (New York: Harper Business, 1997).
18. E. Marzalek-Gaucher and R. J. Coffey, *Transforming Healthcare Organizations* (San Francisco: Jossey-Bass, 1990).
19. T. Norris and L. Howell, *Healthy People in Healthy Communities: A Dialogue Guide* (Chicago: Coalition for Healthy Cities and Communities, 1998).
20. Wall et al., *The Visionary Leader.*
21. B. Torbert and Associates, *Action Inquiry* (San Francisco: Berrett-Kohler, 2004).
22. A. Etzioni, *A Comparative Analysis of Complex Organizations* (New York: The Free Press, 1971).
23. R. Fritz, *The Path of Least Resistance for Managers* (San Francisco: Berrett-Kohler, 1999).
24. E. E. Bobrow, *Ten Minute Guide to Planning* (New York: Macmillan, Spectrum, and Alpha Books, 1998).

25. G. Ringland, *Scenario Planning: Managing for the Future* (New York: John Wiley and Sons, 1998).

26. R. Fritz, *The Path of Least Resistance* (New York: Fawcett, 1984).

27. H. Mintzberg, *Mintzberg on Management* (New York: The Free Press, 1989).

28. Albrecht, *The Northbound Train.*

29. A. Best, P. I. Clark, S. J. Leischow, and W. M. Trochim, *Greater Than the Sum: Systems Thinking in Tobacco Control* (Washington, DC: National Cancer Institute Tobacco Control Monograph Series, 2007).

30. M. J. Wheatley, *Leadership and the New Science,* 2nd ed. (San Francisco: Berrett-Kohler, 1999).

31. P. M. Senge et al., *The Fifth Discipline Fieldbook* (New York: Bantam, 1994).

32. R. S. Kaplan and D. P. Norton, *The Balanced Scorecard* (Boston: Harvard Business School Press, 1996).

33. J. M. Kouzes and B. Z. Posner, *The Leadership Challenge,* 4th ed. (San Francisco: Jossey-Bass, 2007).

34. J. C. Lammers and V. Pandita, "Applying Systems Thinking to Public Health Leadership," *Journal of Public Health Management and Practice* 3, no. 4 (1997): 39–49.

35. A. Fink, *Evaluation Fundamentals* (Newbury Park, CA: Sage Publications, 1993).

# CHAPTER 6

# THE FIVE LEVELS OF LEADERSHIP

> Effective leaders are capable of reframing the thinking of those
> whom they guide.
>
> D. R. Conner, *Managing at the Speed of Change*

A leader is a person who inspires others to action and guides their undertakings. These others can be members of a team, employees of an agency, or heads of groups that have formed a coalition, an alliance, or a partnership, for example. In other words, leaders in public health, as in other arenas, operate on different levels. The major difficulty in conceptualizing what leadership is relates to the fact that we live in an ever-changing world that demands that leaders adapt to these changes in a continuous way. Each day leaders face new technical challenges for which solutions need to be found. These challenges require more than the usual solutions tied to an authoritative position or to the standard operating procedures of an organization or community. All we need to do is look at the events of September 11, 2001, to see that the world has changed. Heifetz and Linsky pointed out that these adaptive challenges require solutions that are innovative, perhaps experimental, and create new forms of adjustment.[1] Adaptive change may require a change in attitude, values, and behavior, or a new interpretation of events.

Sometimes this new perspective may involve trying to see the situation from the perspective of others. I have suggested to students that simply changing their seats from one class session to another will give them a new perspective of me as teacher. I recently saw this effect in a management training program. The trainees were asked to develop a new public health program during the first six months of the training. During the second six months, the trainees' task was to develop a business plan for their new program. They reported that the business plan project gave them a whole new perspective on their project and the feasibility of making the project work. Heifetz and Linsky have added a variation on this technique, which they named the balcony exercise. If you are at a dance, you tend to concentrate on dancing with your partner. If you go to the balcony between dances, you get a different view of the proceedings.

It is also important to understand what entices people into leadership roles. Over the last 20 years, there has been a strong belief that leadership can be taught. Many public health leadership programs have come into being with the goal of training public health professionals to be better leaders with the belief that leadership is one of the key dimensions in building a stronger public health system. Parks has stated that there are important explanations of why people want to be leaders.[2] She calls these explanations "hungers" and discusses five of them as follows:

1. hunger to contribute and make society better
2. hunger to be in an authority position
3. hunger to implement and explore systems issues
4. hunger to show others how to adapt to change
5. hunger to demonstrate moral courage in behalf of the "common good"

This chapter first discusses the abilities that public health leaders need at any level, including the personal level (i.e., when dealing with another individual one on one), then goes on to consider the particular abilities and strategies that they put to use in heading a team, heading an agency, working within a community collaboration activity, or guiding their profession toward improvement. As we proceed, it is important to remember that each of the five levels of leadership provides a foundation for the next level of leadership. It is almost like going up a flight of stairs on which we need to go up the first stair before going to the second stair. Skipping a stair might trip us up.

## Personal Leadership Development

This section considers some of the prerequisites for being an effective public health leader at any level. These prerequisites include a commitment to social justice, an understanding of democracy, an understanding of the political process, communication skills, mentoring skills, decision-making skills, and the ability to balance work and life outside work.

### Values

Public health leaders, to be fully effective, must be committed to the values that characterize public health, especially social justice. However, they need to be careful not to let the social justice agenda prevent them from doing the tasks that need to be done. Furthermore, social justice is a broad concept and encompasses a range of different issues. The predominant social justice issue of concern to almost all public health leaders is equity in access to care. On the other hand, no consensus exists that, for instance, there should be a radical redistribution of wealth in the society at large.

A commitment to a value such as equity in access to care entails a willingness to challenge the political status quo and act as an advocate for the public health agenda. Leaders are supporters of organizational and community values and should be on the front lines in attempts to make public health practices and policies conform to these values.

### Politics and Governance

Public health leaders need to understand the political system of the location in which their activities take place. In this country, they need to understand how the American version of democracy works at the local, state, and national levels and how to influence the political process. As an example, the author, on a visit to the office of a public health professional in a state health department, noticed *The Federalist Papers* and de Tocqueville's *Democracy in America* on the shelf. The public health leader said that he often referred to these books for guidance in making decisions.

One question that arises is whether there is a difference between government (or governance, the activity of governing) and politics. Governance, in large part, consists of administering programs and adjusting them to fit policies developed as part of the political process.[3] Unfortunately, these policies sometimes are not founded on the best available evidence but instead reflect the personal concerns (including the desire to get reelected) of the politicians who vote them into existence. Several years ago, I talked to a state legislator about having a school of public health supply data on specific health issues of interest to the legislator. He refused the offer, because, according to him, he did not need data to make his decisions. (As someone has pointed out, politicians have spin doctors whereas government agencies have spokespeople.[4] That says something about the difference between politics and government.)

Public health agencies are government agencies, and public health leaders are implementers of policies set by politicians. This creates interesting possibilities for a partnership between the political and governmental sectors. Leadership theories often focus exclusively on organizational tasks, such as setting organizational policies and motivating the workforce, but public health leaders need to develop the skills necessary for working with elected officials. Their role is to use the values, mission, vision, and goals and objectives of their agency to clarify public health issues and ensure that the policies created to deal with these issues will have a good chance of being effective.

## Communication and Empowerment

The AIM Leadership Model is based on the idea that leaders have to learn to take *a*ction, learn how to *i*nfluence the field, and be *m*otivated by the process.[5] According to the model, the five building blocks of effective personal leadership are communication, the empowerment of followers, a focus on key issues, linkage to others, and life balance. Each of these building blocks is affected by leadership style and practices as well as the systems approach to organizational change.

Good communication skills are critical. Effective communication has several aspects, including slowing the thought processes, increasing understanding, testing conclusions, listening constructively, getting to the essence of things, and exploring areas of disagreement.[6] In addition, gender differences, racial or ethnic differences, and age differences can affect whether messages are received as intended.[7] Leaders need to understand all the factors that influence communication so they can synthesize public health information into effective messages (see Chapter 11).

Leaders, in trying to empower work and community associates, often act as their mentors. Interaction between leaders and constituents is critical,[8] and leaders need to empower "followers" in ways that give them the chance to be more effective as well as to develop their own leadership skills. Followers are themselves people with exceptional talents, and, according to one study, 80% of the effectiveness of a project is due to the followers and only 20% to the leadership.[9]

## Leading and Following

Also, followers in one situation become leaders in another, and many public health practitioners see themselves in both leadership and follower roles. Public health practitioners who work for public health agencies see themselves as professionals first and even leaders in their profession, but those who are part of a traditional public bureaucracy are frequently expected to be less leaders than followers, which can create a contentious work environment.

Members of a board of health often see themselves as powerful individuals and therefore as natural leaders. Health administrators also see themselves as leaders rather than followers. This may lead to conflict. For example, a health administrator addressing a group of public health professionals in a leadership program said that it was his job to protect board members from gossip and controversies. A local board of health president who was in the training program said that if the health administrator kept information hidden from board members, someone in the community would give them the information instead. Board members need information and lose trust in health administrators who hold back information.

Another board of health president pointed out that the administrator of the health department was his employee, because he could fire the administrator and recommend cutting the local health department budget. This shows how important it is for the board of health members and the public health administrator to develop an understanding that they are partners. In this regard, governance has an important role to play.[10] A governance public health framework should include mechanisms for organizing values, carrying out the public health mission, formulating goals and objectives, developing realistic action plans, resolving conflicting agendas, determining the need for structural change, improving the relationship between the board and the health department, and developing mechanisms to share governance with the appropriate governmental body. As one public health leader stated:

> To create effective governing boards, we must examine our values and determine why our boards need to exist. Once we discover our common purpose, we can develop skills and processes to improve our effectiveness. Boards and administrators need a shared vision, commitment, and leadership to make goals a reality. As public health leaders, it is our job to develop boards that are a part of our leadership teams and join us in creating healthy communities.[11(p.11)]

## Agenda Setting

Public health leaders should learn about and use the systems approach to organizational change (see Chapter 5) and the public health core functions model (discussed in detail in Part II) to ensure that their agencies' agendas are tied to the core functions of public health. In addition, they need to master the art and science of public health. Leaders are the grand integrators of science and practice, and part of their job is to explain public health issues to health professional associates and community partners.

Leaders should acquire agenda-setting skills. An organization needs to prioritize the problems that it is facing and create action plans that deal with the largest problems first.[12] Figure 6-1 presents a model for agenda setting that includes the creation of a media agenda, a public agenda, and a policy

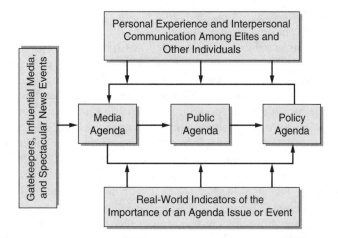

**FIGURE 6-1   Three Main Components of the Agenda-Setting Process: The Media Agenda, Public Agenda, and Policy Agenda**
*Source:* From Rogers and Dearing, Agency-Setting Research: Where Has It Been? Where Is It Going? in *Communication Yearbook,* Vol. 11, J. A. Anderson, ed., p. 5, © 1988 by Sage Publications, Inc. Reprinted by permission of Sage Publications, Inc.

agenda. The fact that public health leadership practice takes place in a government setting means that community realities affect the agenda-setting process. Also influencing the process are gatekeepers, the media, and spectacular news stories (e.g., a story about children becoming ill after eating in a fast-food restaurant).

## Barriers to Effectiveness

In 1988, the Institute of Medicine issued a report stating that the public health system in the United States was in disarray.[13] The report listed a number of barriers that reduce the ability of public health leaders to be effective, including the following:

- a lack of a consensus on the content of the public health mission
- inadequate capacity to carry out the essential public health functions of assessment, policy development, and assurance of services
- disjointed decision making uninformed by the necessary data and knowledge
- inequities in the distribution of services and the benefits of public health
- disharmony between the technical and political aspects of decisions
- rapid turnover of leaders
- an inadequate relationship between public health and the medical profession
- organizational fragmentation
- problems in relationships between layers of government
- an inadequate development of necessary knowledge across the full array of public health needs
- a poor public image of public health, inhibiting necessary support
- special problems that unduly limit the financial resources available to public health

Without question, the public health system in the United States needs to become more effective, and public health leaders will be at the forefront of attempts at reform.[14] One problem is that public health agencies are dealing with more complex problems today than previously, and the complexity of problems in the areas of infectious diseases and chronic diseases will probably continue to increase. Therefore, organizational stability may not be possible to achieve. In addition, public health professionals come from different disciplines with different approaches to problem solving, which leads to professional disagreements.[15] It will only be through collaboration that effective problem solving and decision making will occur.

In a speech before the Illinois Public Health Leadership Institute in 1992, George Pickett said that public health leaders need to increase their skills transorganizationally; that is, they need to be able to understand and communicate with others in community sectors with values and priorities different from theirs. Public health leaders are often deficient in collaboration skills,[16] and consequently they are sometimes prevented from cooperating effectively with leaders from important sectors, such as the business community and the religious community. Fortunately, obstacles to cooperation are becoming less frequent. The discussion on meta-leadership in Chapter 3 presents theses issues of working across organizational silos as presenting leaders with important new skills.

It should be noted that, in general, leaders who are extremely effective tend to be key players in rather than reactors to the change going on around them.[17] Effective leaders, when confronted with a problem, typically consider a wide range of options and seem to know how to select the important factors first. They also think in terms of win-win and try to arrange it so all parties are winners in a dispute. They are good listeners who try to understand others and their perspectives before trying to make themselves understood. They are excellent synthesizers who try to foster cooperation and collaboration. Finally, they constantly *renew* themselves through training, education, exercise, values clarification, and so on.

## Leadership Style

Public health leaders need to develop an appropriate leadership style (see Chapter 2). Autocratic and directive styles work best when the leader structures the tasks and the workers are willing to do what the leader asks. In public health, the democratic style seems to work better.[18] Participative forms of leadership, in which staff members are involved in the problem-solving process, facilitate the building of a consensus and the acceptance by the staff of the decisions arrived at. Collaboration should be viewed as a creative process whose goal is to discover new approaches and new solutions for old problems.[19]

## Dealing with Diversity

Professional diversity in public health brings its own set of problems.[20] Practitioners from different professions view public health differently. Public health leaders need to look at public health in its totality and develop strategies for integrating the different approaches. Exercise 6-1 provides an opportunity to consider the issue of professional diversity and its impact on public health strategies.

Public health leaders need to confront not only professional diversity but gender, race, ethnic, and age diversity. For example, the so-called glass ceiling for women still exists,[21] and therefore public health leaders must conscientiously promote gender equality. The first step is to gather the data necessary to determine whether gender inequalities exist and, if so, where they exist. The next step is to hire a consultant to evaluate the agency's environment and its receptiveness to gender equality. The third step is to use a benchmarking process (comparing the agency with the best agencies not the average ones) to identify best practices for achieving gender equality and taking full advantage of the skills that women bring into the workplace. The final step, so to speak, is to prepare oneself for a backlash. Case Study 6-A is an interview with Dr. Joyce Lashof, who has held a number of public health leadership posts over the last 40 years. The interview explores some of the gender issues that public health leaders typically confront.

Diversity encompasses gender, age, race, ethnicity, sexual orientation, work and family issues, education, work experiences, tenure within the agency or organization, personality, risk tolerance, geographic region, and religion.[22] A unified diversity enhancement program for public health professionals and clients may be difficult to construct because of the different issues that are prominent in each diversity category.

---

### Case Study 6-A
### A Leadership Interview with Joyce C. Lashof, MD

*Shirley F. Randolph*

*Joyce C. Lashof, MD, is dean emeritus, School of Public Health, University of California at Berkeley. Her most recent previous positions include president of the American Public Health Association; dean, School of Public Health, University of California at Berkeley; president, Association of Schools of Public Health; assistant director, Office of Technology Assessment, U.S. Congress; senior scholar in residence, Institute of Medicine, National Academy of Sciences; deputy assistant secretary for Health Programs and deputy assistant secretary for Population Affairs, U.S. Department of Health, Education, and Welfare; and director, Illinois Department of Public Health.*

The first name that comes to mind when one thinks of women leaders in the field of public health is Joyce C. Lashof, MD. Dr. Lashof has done it all. After four decades in public health leadership positions, she is, quite simply, the quintessential public health leader.

And she did it all while successfully integrating her workplace duties with her responsibilities as the wife of a university professor (her husband, Richard, is a well-known mathematician) and the mother of one son and two daughters—two of whom have made Joyce and Richard grandparents, and all of whom are growing as young professionals in their chosen fields. Her insights into leadership issues, particularly as they apply to women, are perceptive and fascinating.

*(continues)*

**Case Study 6-A** *continued*

One of the first areas Dr. Lashof and I explored during an interview several years ago dealt with the challenge women often experience when faced with men as "gatekeepers" to upward mobility.

**What have been your greatest challenges when confronting the male monopoly on power and men as gatekeepers on the upward path to leadership?**
There was definitely a problem early in my career. Moving up depended a good deal on having a mentor who paved the way. At the beginning of my career, after I received my MD from Woman's Medical College of Pennsylvania and completed my residency in medicine at Montefiore Hospital in New York, I went to the University of Chicago first as a physician at the Student Health Services and then as an assistant professor in the Department of Medicine.

I served year to year on a one-year appointment for three years and then asked for a regular three-year appointment. I was told by the chairman of the Department of Medicine that he would never give a married woman a tenured track appointment because she would leave and go where her husband's career took him. Needless to say, I was unhappy about the situation and told him "thanks, but no thanks" to another one-year appointment. That was in 1960. At that time, of course, there were no laws about discrimination and affirmative action.

Luckily, colleagues referred me to Dr. Mark Lepper at the University of Illinois, College of Medicine, and Presbyterian-St. Luke's Hospital, Chicago. Mark offered me a faculty appointment in the Department of Preventive Medicine at the University of Illinois and arranged an appointment as assistant attending physician at Presbyterian-St. Luke's Hospital. This led to a series of succeeding appointments and long-term collaboration.

In many ways, Mark was a mentor who opened doors for me. Most specifically, he appointed me research director of a study of health needs of poverty populations funded by the Office of Equal Opportunity (OEO). It was this study that led to recommendations that health centers to serve the disadvantaged be opened in Chicago. The study was well received by the OEO and resulted in the further development of a proposal to open a health center on Chicago's West Side. The West Side's Mile Square organization approached Presbyterian-St. Luke's about developing such a health center. We put together a proposal for an OEO-funded Mile Square health center. The proposal was successful and Mile Square Health Center was the second OEO-funded health center in the country. I served as its director for five years.

During this same period of time, I was promoted to attending physician and director, Section of Community Medicine, at Presbyterian-St. Luke's Hospital. As the only woman to head up a section, during staff meetings I was the lone woman sitting around the table with all the men. They were more or less accepting of me, but I could sense that in their eyes I was not quite an equal. I walked a thin line between asserting myself and not being too assertive.

When Dan Walker became Illinois's government in 1973, he said he was going to appoint women to his cabinet. He did and I became the first woman to be named the director of a state public health department. I think I ought to thank the women's movement!

**What changes in the male monopoly are occurring as we move into a new era with a new vision about women as leaders and managers?**
Things are certainly changing. Obviously there are now laws against overt discrimination against women. But just as important as the legal ramifications of discrimi-

nating against women (or anyone else), the fact is that women have proved themselves capable and are accepted as leaders and managers. In addition, women are networking more. Not being the only woman sitting around a table with a group of men makes a real difference in relationships with colleagues. And the younger generation of men are much more accepting of women in peer relationships. Men who are not comfortable with women as leaders and managers and who do not accept them as colleagues are a dying breed.

**How did you counteract the obstacle of discrimination in the workplace because you are a woman? Was discrimination more or less a problem as you moved from mid-level management to top leadership roles?**
Of course the way I counteracted the first obstacle at the University of Chicago was by leaving. Beyond that, I think I just did the best job I knew how to do. I worked hard to be sure that I met *every* expectation and did not give anyone any excuses to criticize me because of my gender.

Then again, sometimes I just ignored the problems and sometimes I took a little action. For example, at Presbyterian-St. Luke's, we would sit around the table and select interns and residents. We would come to a woman applicant and the men would make comments like "Let's take her . . . she is really attractive." I would wait until we came to a likely male applicant and then I would say, "Yes, I think we should take him . . . he's quite a handsome fellow."

Problems related to discrimination because of my gender became less and less as I moved up. It was easier working with younger men and women. But, some of the "old-timers," both in terms of age and length of service in an agency, were still a problem that had to be faced.

**Is it your sense that leadership opportunities are increasing or decreasing for top leadership positions for women?**
In many ways top leadership opportunities for women are increasing. For instance, more women are serving as directors of state health departments, as deans of schools of public health, and in high-level leadership positions at all levels of government. On the other hand, I look at medical school professorships and I'm not sure that the number of women professors has increased. I think people are looking for women to fill leadership roles, but it is still a problem when you look at the top jobs.

**Are the opportunities for women to fill leadership positions greater or lesser in the field of public health?**
There are greater opportunities for women in public health. I think one reason for this is the more liberal nature of the public health field, the result being more opportunities and less discrimination. Public health professionals have a commitment to equality, social justice, women's rights, minority rights, etc. In addition, a career in public health often gives a woman the opportunity to be a leader in politics and in government by virtue of the position she holds.

**Are the attributes and characteristics of successful women leaders different than they are for successful men leaders?**
Women's leadership styles tend to be different from men's to some degree. Whether those differences are the things that account for success is the question. Are women more successful as leaders because they have different values and styles? This is a research question and an issue that is currently being studied. In my experience,

*(continues)*

**Case Study 6-A** *continued*

especially earlier on in my career, I found women to be more sympathetic, compassionate, much less aggressive, less domineering, and more inclusive . . . all very valuable traits when one looks at leadership. We know now that research studies regarding capable leadership indicate that those who have an inclusive leadership style are more effective. Obviously, there are always exceptions to this rule. Taken as a whole, the inclusive leadership approach is lower key; it is more sharing and more "motherly." One of the best compliments I received as assistant director of the Office of Technology Assessment was that I was good at "mothering" them, but I could also kick their rears when I needed to!

**In addition to being a successful public health leader in a variety of forums, you are also a wife, mother, and grandmother. How did you integrate the workplace with your private life responsibilities and "juggle" the complexities that resulted from your various roles?**
It has been a real juggling act! Of course, things got easier as my three children grew up, but at times it was wild! One of the very conscious decisions I made early on in my career was to move toward public health and research in the medical care area because it was less competitive and would result in a less intensive demand on my time, which gave me more time to be with my family. Before I made this decision, I had been working in infectious diseases. I observed how competitive this field was and felt that with three young children at home it wasn't what I wanted to do. I wanted to be home with my husband and children at night and on the weekends, holidays, etc. When the children were all in school and busy with their individual activities, the balancing act became easier. Also, I was very fortunate in having the same full-time housekeeper for over 20 years.

My need to spend time with my family was one of the main reasons why I decided to go into public health and medical care research. It was really serendipity . . . opportunity knocked through Mark Lepper's mentoring and I was there.

**The present job market is very competitive for public health practitioners regardless of gender. What leadership skills are most important for women to cultivate who are presently at the lower and middle levels of a public health organization?**
First and foremost, one needs to know one's field. One has to be looked at as one who is a good problem solver. My advice is to learn how to be objective and analytical and how to be fair. Other important leadership skills include developing an inclusive leadership style, learning how to be a good listener and to reflect on what you hear. One leadership skill that is absolutely essential is knowing how to relate well to other people and to be honest in those relationships.

**As public health redefines its role within a new health care delivery system that is likely to emerge as the result of some form of health care reform, will there be different or "new" opportunities for women in public health leadership positions?**
If the whole health care system becomes more and more competitive through a corporate approach, some women will be able to fit into that structure as leaders. If we move into a system that is accountable for populations (core functions included), opportunities for women to attain top leadership positions certainly should increase. As public health grows and strengthens its positions as an integral part of the health care delivery system, there will be increasing leadership opportunities for both women and men.

One way for public health leaders to deal with diversity issues is to empower staff so that they become advocates for themselves. It is important to understand how human beings in our society act and what needs they have. In his classic work *Motivation and Personality,* Maslow defined a hierarchy of needs.[23] At the most basic level, individuals want their physiological needs met. Second in order of importance are their safety needs. In other words, issues of job security and amount of income are critical for most people. Next come social needs, including the need for recognition by colleagues. One level up, people want to experience a sense of self-esteem. They want to take pride in their work and hence want to be empowered to do a good job. A professional who works well and without the need of much direction will usually be allowed the freedom to design his or her own activities, an almost sure way of increasing self-esteem. Finally, people have a need for self-actualization—the ability to make personal dreams become reality.

## Balancing Work and Play

Work has a tendency to take up most of a leader's waking hours, and family life can suffer as a result. O'Neil called this dilemma the paradox of success.[24] In his view, the myth of success is that success offers complete fulfillment, that success is tied to how much money is made, and that success increases freedom. In fact, success causes a constant craving for more success and hence can lead to a kind of bondage. Factors that can help a leader keep a balance between work life and private life include self-knowledge, managing conflicting pressures, and maintaining a concern for how others feel.[25]

Women seem to be very proficient at balancing personal and professional interests. For working women with a family, work and home are full-time jobs that they typically seem to handle equally well. At work, women, by redesigning their positions and demanding employee training and development, are helping to break traditional organizational molds.[26] They are also helping to break down the barriers between home and work by pushing for flex time, child care, and family leave.

This section raised and discussed many issues related to personal leadership development. Following is a list of leadership strategies that can be used to increase one's leadership skills and abilities:

- Be a value role model. Live the values that the community espouses.
- Understand the democratic process and how it affects the public health system.
- Translate political policy into action.
- Improve communication skills.
- Be a mentor to others.
- Learn to follow when appropriate.
- Be partners with the agency's governing board.
- Learn agenda-setting skills.
- Address barriers to effective public health practice.
- Explore community partnerships.
- Be creative in finding new funding sources.
- Balance work and family.
- Increase leadership opportunities for others.

## Leadership at the Team Level

Public health leaders do not work alone. Public health practice is a group activity. Therefore, among the most important skills a leader can possess are those that are necessary for building and maintaining teams and increasing their effectiveness.

A team is a group of people who come together to pursue a common purpose.[27] The results of the team's activities are often greater than the sum total of the results that would have occurred had each team member been acting alone.

Each team member should be viewed as leader although one person will generally become the official leader. The team leader will share information in an equitable manner with other team members.[28] The leader will build trust in the team process and share authority and power with other members. The leader will also intervene when necessary to move the team forward. The expectation is that all members will be involved in the performance of the team tasks.

Team members who are also members of the public health agency may need to act as a link between the team and the agency and community constituents. These team members, in particular, will need to learn the skills of conflict resolution and negotiation (see Chapter 14). When a skilled leader guides the team process, creativity and innovation are the result.

### Reasons for Creating Teams

The reasons for creating teams include the following: First, a team allows an organization to use the leadership skills and talents and the multidisciplinary backgrounds of its staff. For example, multidisciplinary team that includes nurses, social workers, and environmental health specialists, among others, might be assembled to address the low level of prenatal care in the community. Second, creating a team allows the members time to get to know each other and to develop a sense of togetherness in the context of shared leadership. In general, team members find they can communicate with each other better even once they have left the team or the team has been disbanded. In addition, they learn how to cooperate and collaborate, and cooperation and collaboration increase productivity.[29] Finally, team decision making produces decisions that are supported by the majority of the team's members.

Teams that are created to lighten a supervisor's workload are often doomed to failure.[30] Teams are not a replacement for training and not a way for leaders to observe the opinions and working style of the staff. Teams do not necessarily increase the personal productivity of their members. They need leaders to clarify issues and set the parameters of their activities.[31] One of the strengths of teams is that they are flexible and can reorient themselves as roadblocks occur. Yet the freedom teams are given can be a weakness as well. Teams sometimes fail because they lack discipline and a sense of responsibility for achieving the desired outcomes. When team members realize that they will be completely in charge of their activities and will have the power to make decisions, they sometimes abuse this power, with negative results for the agency. This risk can be reduced if the agency leaders make clear to each team how they expect it to proceed and what results they expect it to achieve.

Leadership teams work differently than management teams. Management teams carry out the instructions of a supervisor. Their tasks are circumscribed, and there is very little room for creativity or innovation. Leadership teams share leadership with the public health administrator, who openly delegates decision-making power to them. In some leadership teams, the health administrator becomes a team member. If given the trust of the agency administrator, leadership team members become committed to the agency and lose their fear of reprisal. They feel that they are respected for their expertise and ability to innovate. They also know that their recommendations will be seriously considered.

## Facts about Teams

Katzenbach and Smith studied teams in 30 organizations, including businesses, schools, and social agencies.[32] They found that teams were critical for building quality organizations and improving customer service. The authors came up with 10 findings about teams in general.

The first finding is that teams are created to address a performance challenge, and indeed a leadership team must have a purpose (mission) if it is to succeed. The second finding is that the team's composition and its purpose need to be thought through. Not every leadership team should be of the same size or professional composition. Third, leaders need to promote team performance opportunities. As the leaders view the organization, they will find these opportunities exist throughout. Fourth, many teams composed primarily of people at the top fail because of the other demands made on these individuals' time and energy. Fifth, organizations and their leaders find it easier to work with individuals than with teams. Everything, including the hiring of people, the determination of salary, the construction of career paths, and the monitoring of performance, is oriented toward the individual. Teamwork seems to go against the structure of individual responsibility.

The sixth finding is that organizations committed to high performance standards are more likely to use teams than organizations with lower performance standards. Seventh, very few high-performance teams exist. High-performance teams can be either leadership or management teams. However, leadership teams are generally clearer on the purpose for which they were created. They take control of their activities and promote the development of relationships between their members. They build team activities upon good communication. The leaders maintain their flexibility, work productively together, and recognize the accomplishments of their leader colleagues. Leadership teams also seem to have high morale. (High-performance teams can be created using the PERFORM model, propounded by Blanchard and colleagues.[33] The acronym stands for *p*urpose, *e*mpowerment, *r*elationships and communication, *f*lexibility, *o*ptimal productivity, *r*ecognition and appreciation, and *m*orale.)

The eighth finding is that teams do not replace organizational hierarchies. Instead, teams enhance these hierarchies, partly because they are able to cross over structural boundaries. Because of the strong community orientation of public health agencies, leadership teams can be used to address community concerns. These teams may include community partners among their membership.

The ninth finding is that teams are small learning organizations that integrate performance and learning. Typically a team will do research on a subject related to its purpose. Team members also learn team-building and leadership skills. They often learn that each member is a leader or potential leader. The conjoining of performance and learning in teams is generally a plus, since their conjunction throughout an organization is often a prerequisite for the organization to increase it effectiveness. This applies to public health agencies as well.

The final finding is that teams are effective in addressing new issues as well as old issues. In the case of old issues or problems, they often discover new solutions. One reason teams are good at discovering solutions to problems is that they view the problems from a systems perspective rather than using the traditional cause and effect approach.[34] They are also experts at sharing information and coordinating actions, and members of one team frequently tie their activities to the activities of other teams working on different though related issues.

The important question is why so many teams fail when their importance to the work of public health is so important. Lencioni has pointed to five major dysfunctions that affect the success of team-based activities.[35] First, teams fail when there is a lack of trust either in their organization or in their leadership. This includes the implicit leadership of the team as well. Second, team members fear conflict and contesting the decisions of other team members. Conflict is not necessarily a personal issue, but rather is often an issue related to the challenge that the group must address. The third dysfunction relates to the level or lack of commitment of team members to the process. The Leadership Wheel presented in Chapter 5 pointed to the important dimension of values clarification and the need to get all team members to commit to the team activities or project. If there is a lack of commitment, then the fourth dysfunction occurs. The lack of accountability will often affect the effectiveness of team activities. The fifth dysfunction relates to the problem of ignoring the results of the teamwork regardless of the reasons. If the boss had the team do busywork or did not allow the team any involvement in the decision-making process, all the dysfunctions come into play. There will be no trust, no conflict on the surface, no commitment to the process, no accountability, and obviously no attention to the results.

Teams build social capital, which brings people together in a way that individuals alone cannot do. Building social capital helps to develop trust, allows for shared leadership and creativity, expands social networks for the team members, develops shared purpose in team activities, levels the playing field for the members in terms of equity, increases collaboration and commitment, enhances knowledge-sharing, and fits different talents of individuals into a comprehensive whole.[36] At the individual level, teamwork provides many benefits to the individual as well and creates satisfaction and sometimes personal rewards in the accomplishments of the team.

## Team Classification

Many writers have attempted to classify teams. One helpful classification is as follows:[37] Natural work teams are made up primarily of individuals who work together as part of their regular activities. These teams, which can be either management or leadership teams, are usually given a set of designated activities to perform. Cross-functional teams, the second type, include members who have different functions within the organization. They are primarily leadership teams. Corrective action teams are management teams assigned to work on the solutions to problems that are already determined. Finally, hybrid teams address issues not addressed elsewhere in the organization. They may be either management or leadership teams, and they utilize the techniques associated with all the other types. Local public health departments use all four types of teams.

### The Importance of Empowerment

Teams and their members need to be empowered by administrators to take active decision-making roles.[38] Empowerment, which gives team members the freedom to use their knowledge, experience, and skills to address important issues,[39] tends to increase their commitment to the agency and the level of their performance as well. Empowerment must come from the agency leader, and there appears to be a direct relationship between the amount of responsibility staff are given and the degree of their empowerment.[40]

The transfer of power to a team must be real and not merely nominal. A public health leadership team from a state public health leadership institute worked with a local health department to develop a lead-screening program for children. The administrator allowed the team to work on the creation of this new program because she had been told by the state to develop the program. However, the administrator viewed the team members as outsiders, and, though she told them that she had respect for them and would seriously review any recommendations they made, she used the team merely to show the state that she was complying with its request and had no intention of implementing the team's recommendations. This is an example of team activity subverted by a hidden agenda. The power to have an impact on the development of a program through recommendations was implied but was in fact an illusion.

As Figure 6-2 shows, empowerment is related to organizational values, leadership activities, human resource systems, and the structure and activities of the organization. Empowerment is often used as a tool for the improvement of programs and services.

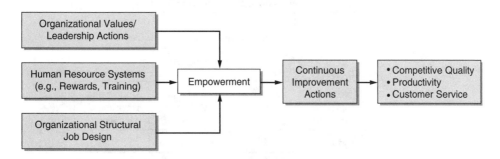

**FIGURE 6-2  Empowerment in Contemporary Organizations**
*Source:* Reprinted with permission from R. S. Wellins, W. C. Byham, and J. M. Wilson, Empowered Teams, p. 23, © 1991, Jossey-Bass Inc., Publishers.

## Teams and Leadership Style

In Chapter 2, the situational leadership model was briefly discussed. The model identifies four leadership styles: directing, coaching, supporting, and delegating. This same classification can be applied to team-based activities (Figure 6-3).[41] When a team is first created, the leader is involved in formulating the team's purpose and determining the activities to be performed. The leader, in other words, is using a directive style. During the next phase, the leader, acting as a coach, clarifies the team's activities. The leader then begins to involve team members in decision making, a process that falls into the category of providing support. In the final phase, the leader empowers the team members, and empowerment, as pointed out above, is closely related to the delegation of responsibility.

It is also important to concentrate on the leadership activities associated with working on teams. LaFasto and Larson discussed the six tasks of team leadership.[42] First, leaders clearly need to focus and pay attention to the goals

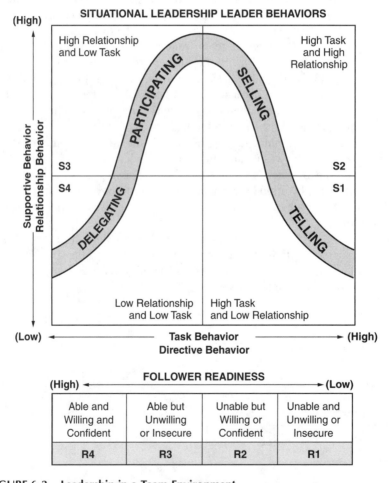

**FIGURE 6-3    Leadership in a Team Environment**
*Source:* © Copyright 2006. Reprinted with permission of the Center for Leadership Studies, Inc., Escondido, CA 92025. All rights reserved.

of the project that will occur during the teamwork. Second, the critical nature of collaboration within the team to get the work done is an important leadership activity. Third, team members like to think and feel that the team process builds their confidence in the way the work is progressing. Team members want to see short-term and long-term results in the work. Team leaders need to help build this confidence and need to be willing to keep team members knowledgeable about external events that affect the work of the team. Secrets defeat teamwork. The fourth leadership activity involves leaders demonstrating technical knowledge and abilities. This activity also means the leader will ask for help or technical assistance when necessary. The fifth leadership activity involves keeping the team on track by setting priorities. It is important to keep the team on task and prevent distractions if possible. When priorities change, leaders must make note of this to the team. The sixth and final task relates to the necessity of managing performance, giving feedback through the group process, and rewarding results.

## Team Preparedness

Of course, teams are at different places in their involvement in and commitment to the tasks they have been assigned, and leaders need to monitor team readiness, which ranges from unable and unwilling to carry out the team assignment to able and willing and confident (Figure 6-3). In some cases, leaders may have to utilize planning strategies for key team members as well as for the team as a whole.

One useful team technique, based on the so-called skunkworks model, is to send a team to a neutral place away from the organization to work on issues related to the team's activities.[43] The "skunkworks" is a subteam composed of experts on the topic that is the focus of the team activities. These team members tend to be transformational leaders who will move the organization forward.

## Team Members

Mallory studied the characteristics of various types of team members.[44] Some members tried to take control of the activities of the team, and these he labeled *dominant* members. These individuals do well in structured situations with a well-defined purpose. The *influencers* tend to be creative and extremely talented in interpersonal relationships. They also tend to be optimistic and try to keep the team together. The *balancers* look at the big picture in an objective manner and try to reconcile the differences between the team members. The *loyalists* are committed to the status quo. Each actual team member, although mainly of one type, has at least a little of every personality characteristic associated with any of the four types. Exercise 6-2 is based on this personality typology. It is intended to get you to reflect on the type of team member you are likely to be.

Team members benefit in several ways from working on a team. First, they gain experience in working together with colleagues on a project.[45] They also learn problem-solving skills, interpersonal relationship skills, and new technological information. In addition, they learn about accountability from a personal perspective as well as a team perspective and become more committed to the team's goals and objectives.

**The Life Cycle of Teams**

Teams have a life cycle that is similar to the life cycle of human beings.[46] A team starts out as an infant and disbands as it ages and finishes its tasks. Organizational leaders must develop the ability to function as team leaders at each stage of the team life cycle. This is especially true in the public health field, where so many leadership activities occur in a team setting.

Following are guidelines that organizational leaders should use when creating and working with teams:

- Develop teams to address agency or community public health problems.
- Choose multidisciplinary team members for their expertise and leadership qualities.
- Allow teams to make decisions and recommendations for change. Share power and control.
- Share information.
- Intervene in the team process when necessary.
- Do not create teams to alleviate your workload.
- Use the skunkworks technique for dealing with team issues.
- Tie team development to performance standards.
- Put a time limit on the activities of the team.

## Leadership at the Agency Level

In a recent book on management in the health field, the authors claimed that nowadays managers have to integrate clinical practice skills and management skills.[47] The view propounded here is that public health leaders have to integrate public health practitioner skills and management and leadership skills (see Table 1-1 and Chapter 3).

Currently, public health agencies typically have a management orientation. In the 21st century they will need to become consumer and community driven.[48] The leadership expertise of agency staff will need to be increased if the agencies are to keep up with the speed of change. Figure 6-4 shows the relationships among management theories, the health care environment, clinical expertise, and consumer health care expectations. Most of the items listed are relevant to public health as well as medical care. Two missing items that pertain particularly to public health are building community coalitions and health promotion and disease prevention.

Public health agencies, along with other types of organizations, are undergoing many reforms but need to change further. For one thing, they have not fully incorporated the lessons of business. They are still run as traditional bureaucracies, although community groups are trying to take a role in the making of decisions about public health issues.

In a bureaucracy, the managers and leaders are often far removed from the daily activities of the staff,[49] yet they feel the need to control these activities. Perhaps this is one reason that Peters and Austin urged the importance of "managing by wandering around."[50] Of course it is true that leaders need to monitor operations, but they also need to delegate authority to managers and staff members.[51] By doing this, they can help make the profession-

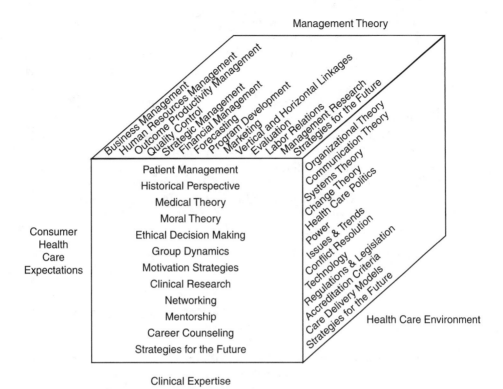

**FIGURE 6-4  Characteristics of the Health Care Management Role**
*Source:* J. G. Liebler and C. R. McConnell, *Management Principles for Health Professionals,*
4th ed. (Sudbury, MA: Jones and Bartlett, 2004).

als in their organization excited about coming to work in the morning.
Leaders need to remember that associates are customers too.

In the late 1950s, Drucker noted that traditional bureaucratic organizations were gradually becoming knowledge-based organizations.[52] Public
health agencies have always been knowledge based, and in fact the business
community can learn much from the public health leaders about knowledge-
based organizations and how they work. However, the models for knowledge
management are more developed on the business side. For example, Tiwana
has examined the four phases of knowledge management strategies for
knowledge-based organizations.[53] First, it is necessary to evaluate the present structure for dealing with knowledge in an agency (an infrastructure
issue). Second, it is important to develop the system related to knowledge in
terms of the analysis dimension, the design of the system, and how it is developed. Third, the issue of deployment and how to use the results of the system become critical. Finally, it is necessary to determine the return on
investment for the system, the performance evaluation of the system, and
making refinement as necessary. Public health leaders have an important role
in knowledge management. It will be important for leaders to apply these
phases to public health and to modify the models to better reflect the knowledge management aspects of public health practice.

Public health leaders, in order to thrive in the ever-changing environment, need to make a commitment to change and to focus on increasing customer satisfaction, fostering innovation, empowering staff, and instituting appropriate structural reforms.[54] Leadership is not just a matter of charisma; it is hard work.[55]

Nanus identified four main leadership roles (Figure 6-5).[56] First, public health leaders (to keep to the focus of this discussion) are spokespeople who present the contemporary public health issues to the community. Second, they are "direction setters" and involve community leaders in prevention activities and in the search for ways to increase the level of health in the community. Third, they act as coaches or mentors for agency associates as a means of improving the agency's effectiveness. Finally, they act as organizational change agents.

## Looking into the Future

If public health leaders are oriented to change and want to become catalysts for change, they need to develop program scenarios for possible futures. This means that they should look for societal trends to guide agenda setting for the agency. They need to be students of change, in other words, and look closely at the predictions of futurists.

The social scientist Alvin Toffler tried to make sense of the changes that are occurring now by looking at past periods of vast social change.[57,58] Toffler identified three waves of societal and organizational change. The first wave was the agricultural revolution, the second was the industrial revolution, and the third, which is occurring now, is the information revolution.

**External Environment**

| Present | Spokesperson | Direction Setter | Future |
| | Coach | Change Agent | |

**Internal Environment**

**FIGURE 6-5  Leadership Roles**
*Source:* Reprinted with permission from B. Nanus, *Visionary Leadership,* p. 13, © 1992, Jossey-Bass Inc., Publishers.

Toffler developed what he called social wavefront analysis, by means of which a scientist can supposedly analyze the leading edge of a wave to predict its future. In *Creating a New Civilization,* he and Heidi Toffler examined the effects of the shift from the second wave to the third wave.[59] Political tensions have arisen between those whose thinking was formed during the industrial period and the new leaders of the information age. An interesting question can be framed regarding the present structure of government in this country. If government reflects its era, does this mean that the old governmental organizational structures, created prior to the industrial age but refashioned during that era, are now obsolete and need to be reworked to fit the information age?

If Alvin Toffler is correct, then public health will undergo major reforms in the 21st century. Even if he isn't, it is unimaginable that public health will remain perfectly static. The developments and trends likely to drive changes in public health agencies in the 21st century include the following:

*New models of public health.* The direct service activities of local public health departments will continue to decline in the next 20 years.[60] New program and service models will emerge, and community-based public health activities will increase.

*Team-based problem solving.* More multidisciplinary teams, both ad hoc and permanent, will be created to address public health concerns. Use of the team approach will lead to the structural leveling of organizations. Team success will empower the public health workforce and increase the self-esteem of individual health professionals.

*Community health coalitions based on partnership.* Public health activities take place in a community setting. Consequently, community partners as well as staff members need to be empowered. Also, partners need to have their expectations met and even exceeded.[61] If their expectations are exceeded, they will become "raving fans" of the agency.

*Privatization of assurance activities.* Privatization of service provision and program development will become a reality in the future. One local health department struggled with running a mental health program in its county. It also owned the building where mental health services were provided. The program was being operated at a loss, and the health department decided to contract out the delivery of mental health services. A contract was signed (although the department kept oversight responsibility), the building was sold, and the deficit vanished.

*Decentralization of responsibilities.* Community partners can do some of the work. If they become involved in public health, all sorts of activities will occur. Empowered communities address community issues.[62] Financial issues become less important because community volunteers will find a way to get things done even when the money is not there. Power must be shared to be effective.

*Community-wide governance.* Governance will need to be incorporated into the activities of the agency and the activities of the community partnerships.

*Revision of values.* Public health leaders not only will be protectors of the community's values but will help create new or revised value statements that reflect societal and cultural changes. It is interesting to note that politicians defend the status quo while organizational leaders support the generation of new values. Nonetheless, there seems to be a lag between the development of new values in the society and their adoption at the agency level.

*New political structures.* There appears to be a trend on the horizon that may affect the future activities of agencies in the public sector. A number of states and local jurisdictions have combined public health departments and human services departments into superagencies. These mergers have caused some public health professionals to wonder whether public health has a future. However, my study of public health leaders indicated that these leaders are generally very hopeful about public health. Public health problems will not go away and will still have to be addressed by agencies headed by public health leaders.

*Third-wave leaders.* The leaders of the new age are breaking down barriers to collaboration. These leaders know how to build their agencies using self-directed teams with high performance standards. Third-wave leaders also are expert at community building and empowerment. The goals of the agency become integrated with community goals. Third-wave leaders are innovative, creative, flexible, and adaptable to change.

*Integration of individual and community goals.* Public health leaders must articulate the relevance of public health initiatives to the personal life of individual citizens. In an interview, one public health leader talked about an initiative designed to respond to the nationwide increase in tuberculosis cases. The leader, who worked for a congressional representative, pointed out that tuberculosis would need to be present in the representative's jurisdiction for him to be concerned about the problem. The unfortunate fact is that the societal perspective of public health practitioners—the attitude that protection of the public's health is a matter of social justice—has yet to be accepted by our elected officials.

*Complete community empowerment.* Citizens as well as public health professionals need to be empowered to carry out public health activities. Empowerment leads to shared responsibility for addressing the public health needs of the local jurisdiction.

*Universal access to services.* The service system of the future will be comprehensive. Programs will be integrated across agencies, and community coalitions will work together to address health needs. Leadership will be shared.

Due to the terrorist events of September 11, 2001, preparedness will take center stage in the activities of public health with new skills required of public health leaders in this new environment. Although public health will still be local in practice, it will be global in perspective and orientation.[63]

## Public Health Functions

From the 1840s to the 1940s, six basic local health agency functions evolved: the collection and interpretation of vital statistics, sanitation, communicable disease control, the provision of maternal and child health programs, health education, and the provision of laboratory services.[64] In the period between 1940 and 1980, other functions were added, including the provision of environmental health services, the development and provision of personal health services, the coordination of community health services, the operation of medical care and public health facilities, area-wide planning, and the assessment of the adequacy of health services. The year 1988 saw the release of the Institute of Medicine report on public health. This report promoted the use of core functions to organize the activities of public health at the community level.[65]

Public health leaders have changed as public health has changed. They have adapted to new developments and devised innovative approaches to performing the standard public health functions. Although somewhat dated, Table 6-1 presents a comparison of the activities of a local health department in 1947 and 1995.[66] Since 1995, local health departments have continued to change. Many direct service activities have been outsourced. Local health departments have reoriented some of their activities to emergency preparedness and response activities.[67]

Not all states have local public health agencies. In states that do not, the state health department operates like a local agency. In states with local agencies, the activities of the state health department leaders are separate from the activities of the agency leaders. For example, state health departments have tended to stay away from the provision of direct services, especially in the case of services being provided by local public health agencies.[68] A state health department may provide special services that the local agencies do not offer. It also is likely to be engaged in overseeing and coordinating public health activities in the state.

State health department functions include communicable disease control, tuberculosis control, venereal disease control, acquired immune deficiency syndrome monitoring, sanitation, industrial hygiene, dental health, laboratory services provision, public health nursing, case management, maternal and child health program provision, public health education, technical assistance, public health workforce training, development of new local health departments, epidemiologic surveillance, regulation of health care facilities, licensure, inspection, cancer screening, and many more. The state health department also serves as the repository for state health data. Since 2001, the activities related to emergency preparedness and response have been added to the list. There clearly is still a need for inclusion of emergency mitigation and recovery dimensions for public health work as well.

State health department leaders are responsible for organizing the state public health system to reflect its mission, vision, and goals and objectives. They need courage to carry out their action plans in the face of community opposition and must know how to reform the state public health system without overstepping the boundaries of the state political system, for, among other reasons, the state is the conduit for funding for local public health agency programs.

## Responsibilities of Public Health Leaders

Leaders of local public health agencies have the responsibility to promote their agencies. They make sure the agencies are viewed as repositories of public health information as well as providers of high-quality programs and services. They develop relationships with the leaders of public health agencies throughout their state and also develop partnerships with community health providers.

Funding, of course, is critical for strengthening the public health system, and there is currently intense competition in the entire health industry for additional money.[69] Public health leaders need to be involved both in the allocation of public health funds and in the funding for related health service programs. They will need to make strong arguments for public revenues.

**Table 6-1    Comparison of Public Health Practice Performance Measures Used in 1947 and 1995**

*Examples of Performance Measures from Evaluation Schedule (1947)*

Hospital beds: percentage in approved hospitals

Practicing physicians: population per physician

Practicing dentists: population per dentist

Water: percentage of population in communities over 2,500 served with approved water

Sewerage: percentage of population in communities over 2,500 served with approved sewerage systems

Water: percentage of rural school children served with approved water supplies

Excreta disposal: percentage of rural school children served with approved means of excreta disposal

Food: percentage of food handlers reached by group instruction program

Food: percentage of restaurants and lunch counters with satisfactory facilities

Milk: percentage of bottled milk pasteurized

Diphtheria: percentage of children under 2 years given immunizing agent

Smallpox: percentage of children under 2 years given immunizing agent

Whooping cough: percentage of children under 2 years given immunizing agent

Tuberculosis: newly reported cases per death, 5-year period

Tuberculosis: deaths per 100,000 population, 5-year period

*Consolidated Panel of Core Function-Related Performance Measures (1995)*

Assessment

For the jurisdiction served by your local health department, is there a community needs assessment process that systematically describes the prevailing health status in the community?

In the past three years in your jurisdiction, has the local public health agency surveyed the population for behavioral risk factors?

For the jurisdiction served by your local health agency, are timely investigations of adverse health events, including communicable disease outbreaks and environmental health hazards, conducted on an ongoing basis?

Are the necessary laboratory services available to the local public health agency to support investigations of adverse health events and meet routine diagnostic and surveillance needs?

For the jurisdiction served by your local public health agency, has an analysis been completed of the determinants and contributing factors of priority health needs, adequacy of existing health resources, and the population groups most affected?

In the past three years in your jurisdiction, has the local public health agency conducted an analysis of age-specific participation in preventive and screening services?

Policy Development

For the jurisdiction served by your local public health agency, is there a network of support and communication relationships that includes health-related organizations, the media, and the general public?

In the past year in your jurisdiction, has there been a formal attempt by the local public health agency at informing elected officials about the potential public health impact of decisions under their consideration?

For the jurisdiction served by your local public health agency, has there been a prioritization of the community health needs that have been identified from a community needs assessment?

*(continues)*

**Table 6-1**  *(continued)*

In the past three years in your jurisdiction, has the local public health agency implemented community health initiatives consistent with established priorities?

For the jurisdiction served by your local public health agency, has a community health action plan been developed with community participation to address priority community health needs?

*Examples of Performance Measures from Evaluation Schedule (1947)*

Tuberculosis: percentage of cases reported by death certificate

Syphilis: percentage of cases reported in primary, secondary, and early latent stage

Syphilis: percentage of reported contacts examined

Maternal: puerperal deaths per 1,000 total births, 5-year rate

Maternal: percentage of antepartum cases under medical supervision seen before sixth month

Maternal: percentage of women delivered at home under postpartum nursing supervision

Maternal: percentage of births in hospital

Infant: deaths under 1 year of age per 1,000 live births, 5-year rate

Infant: deaths from diarrhea and enteritis under 1 year per 1,000 live births, 2-year rate

Infant: percentage of infants under nursing supervision before 1 month

School: percentage of elementary children with dental work neglected

Accidents: deaths from motor accidents per 100,000 population, 5-year rate

Health department budget: cents per capita spent by health department

*Consolidated Panel of Core Function-Related Performance Measures (1995)*

During the past three years in your jurisdiction, has the local public health agency developed plans to allocate resources in a manner consistent with the community health action plan?

*Assurance*

For the jurisdiction served by your local public health agency, have resources been deployed as necessary to address the priority health needs identified in the community health needs assessment?

In the past three years in your jurisdiction, has the local public health agency conducted an organizational self-assessment?

For the jurisdiction served by your local public health agency, are age-specific priority health needs effectively addressed through the provision of or linkage to appropriate services?

In the past three years in your jurisdiction, has there been an instance in which the local public health agency has failed to implement a mandated program or service?

For the jurisdiction served by your local public health agency, have there been regular evaluations of the effect that public health services have on community health status?

In the past three years in your jurisdiction, has the local public health agency used professionally recognized process and outcome measures to monitor programs and to redirect resources as appropriate?

For the jurisdiction served by your local public health agency, is the public regularly provided with information about current health status, health care needs, positive health behaviors, and health care policy issues?

In the past year in your jurisdiction, has the local public health agency provided reports to the media on a regular basis?

*Source:* With permission, from the *Annual Review of Public Health,* Volume 18. © 1997 by Annual Reviews, http://www.AnnualReviews.org.

Public health leaders have become more entrepreneurial since the 1990s. They received grants from and developed contracts with public and private funding organizations to supplement their base budgets. Fund-raising needs to be tied to the mission and vision of the public health agency.

Public health leaders are concerned with excellence in public health. They act as role models for emerging public health leaders. They develop benchmarks for best practices. In their oversight role, they motivate community providers to improve their performance. They work with the leaders of other organizations to develop a comprehensive, integrative approach to improving public health in the community. Public health agencies do not want to duplicate programs or services adequately provided by others, although they might offer competing services if the quality of a community provider's services is open to question.

Public health agency leaders have important responsibilities toward agency staff. They must honestly monitor and evaluate job performance and job satisfaction.[70] If job evaluations are done fairly and regularly, staff will be able to learn their full job responsibilities and meet them more effectively. In addition, public health leaders must be enthusiastic about the task of protecting public health and be able to motivate their colleagues to be enthusiastic as well, by fostering collaboration and sharing power with them, for example.[71] They also should cheer colleagues and their progress. Einstein's formula $e = mc^2$ has been reinterpreted as enthusiasm equals mission times cash and congratulations. People have to be cheered and they also have to be paid for their efforts.

As noted already, leaders need to empower agency staff. Empowerment must occur at the team level, the agency level, and the community level. Table 6-2 presents a list of principles of empowerment.[72]

In summation, at the agency level public health leaders have the responsibility to:

- understand how the agency functions
- delegate authority whenever possible

**Table 6-2    Ten Principles of Empowerment**

1. Tell people what their responsibilities are.
2. Give them authority equal to the responsibilities assigned to them.
3. Set standards for excellence.
4. Provide them with training that will enable them to meet the standards.
5. Give them knowledge and information.
6. Provide them with feedback on their performance.
7. Recognize them for their achievements.
8. Trust them.
9. Give them permission to fail.
10. Treat them with dignity and respect.

*Source:* "Ten Principles of Empowering People" from *10 Steps to Empowerment* by Diane Tracey. Copyright © 1990 by Diane Tracey. Reprinted by permission of HarperCollins Publishers, Inc.

- monitor client satisfaction
- make structural changes in the agency to accommodate new or emerging public health issues
- encourage knowledge management systems development
- explore alternate futures for the agency
- apply the core functions model to agency activities (see Chapter 7)
- empower the agency staff and the community residents

## Leadership at the Community Level

Leadership at the community level requires more systems-based skills than are utilized at the team and agency levels. At this level, public health leaders work to increase the visibility of the public health agency. In interviews with 100 American public health leaders, the author found consistent agreement that the public lacked in-depth knowledge about public health. Thus, public health leaders have a duty to provide public health information to the business community, the medical and health industry community, social agencies, and the general public. Public health leaders need to develop skills in community building in order to work with community groups to create an environment for positive social change.

Figure 6-6 shows the dimensions of public health leadership. Public health leaders build on the core functions model, which are discussed in detail in Part II of this book, regardless of the level of leadership, while taking into account the political and social realities that affect the agency and the community. Public health agencies must take into consideration social and political issues if they are to survive. For one thing, they are mandated by funding sources to provide certain basic services and programs. (This raises the issue of the proper balance between mandated services and community-based services and programs not included in the mandated services protocol.)

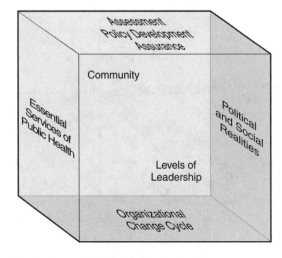

**FIGURE 6-6    Dimensions of Public Health Leadership**

## The Nature of Community

Over the last couple of decades, business discovered community.[73] Business leaders now see that community involvement needs to be part of the practice of business. Public health agencies, by their nature, serve communities, but serving a group of citizens who live in a specified geographic area does not mean that community issues are being addressed. My study of public health leaders found that their efforts at developing community coalitions have been uneven at best. Almost all of the respondents stated that public health agencies have not been successful in getting the public to understand public health.

Community is more than bricks and mortar. It is more than a place to live. It is the place in which our dreams and aspirations are or are not fulfilled. When we talk about improvement in our quality of life, community is part of the improvement process. Community is the place where values are put into action. Community is a complex system made up of individuals, families, politicians, health organizations, human services agencies, churches, schools, businesses, business organizations, and so on (Figure 6-7). It is a system that accepts challenges, and to develop the resources to deal with them it needs to be built on the strengths of its constituent parts, not on their weaknesses.[74]

One view currently prevalent is that we need to rediscover civility.[75] Civility requires that community leaders be open to the opinions of other people and other organizations. Further, public health leaders must transfer the leadership skills they use at the team and organizational levels to the community level. Leaders build communities in all their leadership activities.

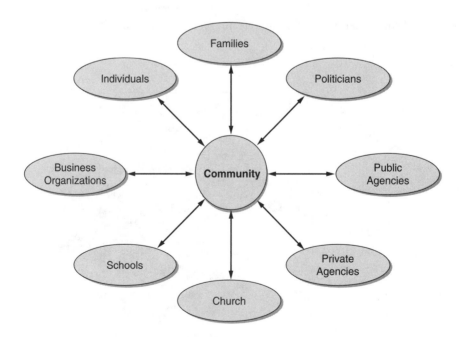

**FIGURE 6-7   Community Constituents**

It should be noted that public health concerns are part of almost every crisis that confronts a community. Exercise 6-3 is intended to explore what is likely to occur when a community experiences a natural disaster.

## Advocacy Through the Media

Media advocacy is an important way to promote public health programs and services.[76] Public health leaders should learn how to use the media to create support for agency goals. For example, they should consider sending letters on a regular basis to newspapers and other sources to increase the visibility of public health.

Think of the importance of using the media in the following situation: a public health leader in a conservative, middle-class community discovers that five cases of human immunodeficiency virus infection have recently been discovered. A statistic like this can hit the nerve center of a community. It is the public health leader who will have the skills to defuse the crisis and get community constituents to become partners in dealing with the problem.

One of the most important responsibilities of public health leaders is to promote prevention at the community level.[77] Our knowledge of health and disease is constantly growing, and new technologies and community-based prevention strategies are continually being developed to address public health concerns. The public needs to be convinced of the importance of using these technologies and strategies. It is the job of public health leaders to make the case.

## Linking Programs

There is a good argument that public health programs should be linked together where possible.[78] The Centers for Disease Control and Prevention has helped create Prevention Research Centers in a number of universities. Many, if not all, of these centers rely on community support to carry out their activities. Public health leaders, who see the future of their agencies as tied to primary prevention rather than direct services, know that linkage to academic programs will strengthen the infrastructure of public health in their communities.

## Community Building

Community building is a complex process that does not occur overnight. Peck analyzed it into four stages.[79] In the first stage, various community representatives who have formed a coalition pretend to have the community's interests at heart in order to gain acceptance for their own agendas. Peck called this the pseudocommunity stage. The second stage, which begins when the coalition realizes that community concerns are not being addressed, is one of chaos. Next comes the stage of emptiness, in which the leaders have to empty themselves of all their preconceived notions about the community and its concerns. It is extremely difficult for the leaders to leave their agendas at the door. The fourth stage is when true community comes into being.

Organizations involved in building a community need leaders.[80] These leaders must be students of the community and its culture and be able to involve individuals with different power bases in community change. Because each community resident has an agenda to which he or she is committed, leaders have to find ways to reconcile the differing agendas.

Community coalitions ideally should be learning organizations.[81] The members of a coalition need to examine their predispositions and how these predispositions affect the community-building process. In addition, the scientific perspective needs to be incorporated into the group's deliberations.

Community building is best achieved through the use of collaborative leadership.[82] Following are 10 factors that can contribute to the success of collaboration and community building:

1. good timing and a clear need
2. strong stakeholder groups
3. broad-based involvement
4. credibility and openness of process
5. commitment and/or involvement of high-level leaders
6. support or acquiescence of "established" authorities or powers
7. overcoming mistrust and skepticism
8. strong leadership of the process
9. interim successes
10. a shift to broader concerns[83]

## Coalition Building

Coalition building is an important part of empowering communities. Public health agencies can no longer work in isolation. Community leaders need to be involved in addressing public health issues. The major advantage of a coalition is that all voices are heard and programs can be developed that better reflect the health needs of the community. The major disadvantage is that being part of a coalition is time consuming.

Cohen and colleagues developed an eight-step model for developing community coalitions (Table 6-3).[84] The model is based on the experience of the Contra Costa County (California) Health Services Department Prevention Programs. The authors define a coalition as a group of interested parties (individuals and organizations) that want to influence the attempt to solve a critical problem. The coalition members need to develop strategies for each of the eight steps and know when to move to the next step.

**Table 6-3   Eight Steps to Building an Effective Coalition**

Step 1: Analyze the program's objectives and determine whether to form a coalition.

Step 2: Recruit the right people.

Step 3: Devise a set of preliminary objectives and activities.

Step 4: Convene the coalition.

Step 5: Anticipate the necessary resources.

Step 6: Define elements of a successful coalition structure.

Step 7: Maintain coalition vitality.

Step 8: Make improvements through evaluation.

*Source:* Reprinted with permission of Contra Costa Health Services, *Developing Effective Coalitions: An Eight Step Guide.* © 1994, Contra Costa County Health Services Department Prevention Programs.

A coalition can have many advantages. It can help to save resources. It can influence a large number of people in a community through its diversified membership. It can create an agenda that is more comprehensive than the agenda of any single community organization. It can create a network for the sharing of information, a network that could be used beneficially by the local public health agency for purposes of marketing and fostering change in the community. In addition, coalition members gain satisfaction when they see positive things happen, and a coalition can influence emerging grassroots organizations as they explore their roles in the community.

Building community through coalitions that are responsible and credible is an important goal of public health leaders. A report from the Centers for Disease Control and Prevention stated that public health should use a process called community engagement.[85] Community engagement involves collaboration between people who are in the same geographic area, share special interests, or are in similar situations. A mixture of social science and art, community engagement integrates the ideas of culture, community, coalition building, and collaboration. The report reviewed the literature for examples of successful engagement and presented a list of the principles of community engagement (Table 6-4).

Partnerships are collaborative relationships that involve more than minimal cooperation. They tend to evolve through the same steps outlined in the systems model of organizational change (see Chapter 5). Partnerships have a

**Table 6-4   Characteristics of Successful Community Engagement**

- Community engagement efforts should address multiple levels of the social environment, rather than only individual behaviors, to bring about desired changes.

- Health behaviors are influenced by culture. To ensure that engagement efforts are culturally and linguistically appropriate, they must be developed from a knowledge and respect for the targeted community's culture.

- People participate when they feel a sense of community, see their involvement and the issues as relevant and worth their time, and view the process and organizational climate of participation as open and supportive of their right to have a voice in the process.

- Although it cannot be externally imposed on a community, a sense of empowerment—the ability to take action, influence, and make decisions on critical issues—is crucial to successful engagement efforts.

- Community mobilization and self-determination frequently need nurturing. Before individuals and organizations can gain control and influence and become players and partners in community health decision making and action, they may need additional knowledge, skills, and resources.

- Coalitions, when adequately supported, can be useful vehicles for mobilizing and using community assets for health decision making and action.

- Participation is influenced by whether community members believe that the benefits of participation outweigh the costs. Community leaders can use their understanding of perceived costs to develop appropriate incentives for participation.

*Source:* Reprinted from Public Health Practice Program Office, *Principles of Community Engagement,* 1997, Agency for Toxic Substances and Disease Registry, the Centers for Disease Control and Prevention.

vision and a mission, they have goals and objectives, and they develop and implement action plans and evaluate their degree of success. The late Reverend Everett Hageman, who was one of the founders of the National Association of Local Boards of Health (NALBOH), was a major supporter of leadership development in public health, and I spent many hours talking to him about the importance of partnership. After Hageman's death, I put together a list of principles based on discussions with him. The principles that pertain to partnerships follow:

- Leave time to get to know your community partners on a personal level.
- Partnership is part of the human condition.
- Working together is better than fighting.
- Learn by listening to your partners.
- True partnership is the gourmet approach to organization.

Each community coalition needs to be revitalized on a regular basis. A community coalition often seems to work better when a community crisis is occurring.[86] When the crisis is over, people tend to move away from the coalition back to their own personal agendas. Thus, public health leaders need to be aware of this fact and make an extra effort to keep community coalitions alive after crises are resolved.

### National and International Communities

Thus far the discussion has been on leadership in local communities, but there are also national and international communities that offer an arena for action by public health leaders. National leaders, like local leaders, act as advocates for public health. They keep the public informed about health issues. They work on the construction of a national mission and vision as well as public health goals for the future. They collaborate with leaders at the state level on the creation of a coordinated nationwide approach to public health. They collaborate with national elected officials to ad-

---

**Leadership Tip**

*When you are given another committee assignment, ask the following questions:*

*(a) Why me?*

*(b) I am willing to be on this committee for the next 3 months, then I will come back and discuss whether I should continue on this committee.*

*(c) Tell committee chair that you do not want to be on another committee for life. You want the group to decide on how long the committee will remain in existence. If more time is needed, you want to determine whether you will continue to serve.*

dress key public health concerns, including the training of the public health workforce.

On the international level, public health leaders implement public health programs in countries where public health is not a priority. These leaders need to develop skills to enhance their ability to improve the quality of life of people in these countries. Rather than reinvent public health, these leaders develop networks with public health leaders throughout the world to share model program methods for addressing specific public health problems. As already stated, public health leaders need to think globally about public health concerns while acting locally (to protect community residents from potential health crises). Building healthy communities is partially a matter of applying knowledge gained from all parts of the world to local conditions. The importance of the 2005 International Health Regulations (IHR) cannot be overestimated. These rules and regulations were agreed upon by 193 countries. These countries believe that these international rules and procedures will help to make the world safe from potential threats to global health. The IHR were approved by the World Health Organization in the summer of 2005.[87] These rules will affect every community in the world.

Most of the strategies and techniques discussed in this chapter have universal application. Following is a list of guidelines of special pertinence for public health leaders working at the community level:

- Build trust.
- Form coalitions.
- Develop partnerships.
- Teach community groups about the core public health functions.
- Do community building with partners.
- See the community as a system.
- Encourage coalitions or partnerships to continue after a public health crisis has been resolved.
- Use the media to promote best practices in public health.
- Push a prevention agenda.
- Understand the connections between public health at a global level and public health at a local community level and their connections.

## Leadership at the Professional Level

Despite the multidisciplinary nature of public health, its leaders need to speak with a unified voice. Public health as a profession takes precedence over the particular educational backgrounds of the public health workforce. The following situation occurs much too often. A physician with almost no background in public health was appointed the administrator of a large county health department. He made decisions from a medical viewpoint and felt that physicians were the only ones who were qualified to do the department's work. He ran the department using a direct medical service approach and totally ignored the population-based approach to public health.

Public health practitioners tend not to travel to professional meetings or for professional development. Many local health departments have a small staff and are reluctant to let employees go to meetings. Funds for professional development are generally minimal, and paying for professional development is typically considered by taxpayers to be a waste of money. Yet public health leaders know that it is important to communicate with other public health professionals. Some of these leaders go to the annual meetings held by the various public health associations and even take a leadership role in these associations. They help to create public health policy that will trickle down to the local public health programs. Leadership development training seems to be a factor here. For example, most of the presidents over the last 15 years of the Illinois Public Health Association were either faculty members or fellows of the Mid-America Regional Public Health Leadership Institute (Illinois, Indiana, Wisconsin, and Michigan).

Public health leaders need to become active participants of the American Public Health Association (APHA). This association represents all segments of the professional public health workforce. It is at the annual meetings of the APHA that national public health policy tends to be made. The National Association of County and City Health Officials (NACCHO) is a key national organization for local health leaders. The Association of State and Territorial Health Officials (ASTHO) is a similar national organization for state health leaders. Leaders should also consider taking key roles in the various associations for state and county public health directors. Board of health leaders can also become involved in a national organization for boards (NALBOH). Following is a list of guidelines for leaders who wish to make a mark in the profession of public health:

- Promote public health as a profession.
- Encourage staff to become involved in state and national public health associations.
- Be active in state and national public health associations.
- Run for office in these associations.

## Summary

Leaders need to operate on five different levels. On the most basic level, they need to know how to exert their influence as leaders on other individuals person to person. To do this, they need a whole range of skills and abilities, from communication skills to the ability to balance work and private life. Regardless of the level at which the leader works, commitment and passion for the work are critical. Leaders strongly believe in what they do. Bolman and Deal believe that there is a spiritual quality to leadership that is difficult to explain or study.[88] However, it can be seen in the work and the dedication of leaders. Thus, leadership is not only about money; it is also about all the things that make us wake up in the morning with anticipation for the job we have to do today. Leadership at the personal level is about our passion in action.

Leaders also must be capable of functioning in teams, either as team leaders or as ordinary team members. Some of the leadership skills needed for teamwork are also needed on the personal level, but some are different. It is on teams that we see the mission of our work in action.[89] It is at the team level that we also see the emotional aspects of working together and creating networks of collaboration and friendship.

Public health leaders are often the heads of public health departments or agencies and thus need agency-level leadership skills as well. Their duties as agency heads include such things as mission and vision statement development, fund-raising, job performance evaluation, and role modeling. At the agency level, leaders also see systems thinking in action. It is the big picture that guides our work.

Public health is obviously community oriented, and so public health leaders need to be able to play a major role in the community, by acting as advocates on public health issues and building coalitions to deal with such issues. They thus need advocacy skills and coalition-building skills, among others. At the community level, we can see the passion and commitment of our partners.

Finally, public health leaders, like other public health practitioners, have an obligation to try to improve the field of public health, by becoming involved, for instance, in professional organizations such as the APHA, NACCHO, ASTHO, and NALBOH. Many leaders have told me that the networking that occurs at the national level is important and helps leaders to sustain their strong beliefs that public health can make a difference. Fighting our battles legislatively becomes easier when we work with our public health colleagues. Professional friendships often become lifelong.

## Discussion Questions

1. What is the difference between politics and governance?
2. What is the relationship between communication and empowerment?
3. What are several of the main barriers preventing public health leaders from being as effective as they could be?
4. What is one way public health leaders can deal with the increasing cultural diversity in the public health workforce?
5. What are some of the main reasons for creating and using teams?
6. What are the main agency-related responsibilities of public health leaders?
7. What are the main community-related responsibilities of public health leaders?
8. How do partnerships differ from other types of collaborative relationships?
9. How can public health leaders further the interests of the public health profession?

## Exercise 6-1:  The Drawbacks and Benefits of Professional Diversity

*Purpose:* to explore how professional diversity affects public health decision making

*Key concepts:* decision making, diversity, professionalism

*Procedure:* There has been an increase in teen gang violence in Midcity over the last 10 years. The mayor and the city council have asked the Midcity Department of Health to develop a plan to address this public health problem. The class should divide into teams to discuss the problem. Each team will have a designated leader from a different profession (e.g., physician, nurse, social scientist, environmental health specialist, or business expert). In addition to discussing the issue at hand, which should be done for half an hour, each team should reserve 5 to 10 minutes to examine how the professional background of the leader influenced the process and the outcome of the discussion. Each team will then report its conclusions and observations to the class as a whole.

### Exercise 6-2:   Leadership and Team Building

*Purpose:* to explore leadership behavior in team situations

*Key concepts:* team building, leadership in teams, leadership style

*Procedure:* Using the Mallory personality typology, each group member, using the worksheet, should classify him- or herself as one personality type or as a combination of types and analyze the degree to which he or she possesses the characteristics associated with all four types. The group should then break into teams and discuss the results of the self-evaluations, focusing on issues that are critical to team development, such as team communication, discussion facilitation, consensus development, priority setting, and conflict resolution.

**Table 6-5   Worksheet for Team Building**

Utilizing the personality typology for leaders, classify yourself relative to the percentage of each type that you may have. Fill out the worksheet and discuss it with your team. The discussion will help you see issues that are critical to team development.

1. Name

| 2. Personality Type | % of this type |
| --- | --- |
| Dominant | |
| Influencer | |
| Balancer | |
| Loyalist | |

3. Previous outstanding achievements in team activity, if applicable
4. Previous problems in team activity, if applicable
5. Outstanding achievements in overall job performance
6. Problems in job performance
7. How you act under pressure
8. How you react to a lack of structure
9. Ability to get along with others
10. Potential future position in agency
11. Current extracurricular activities requiring teamwork

*Source:* Reprinted with permission from E. Mallory, *Team-Building*, pp. 17–18. © 1991, National Press Publications.

### Exercise 6-3:   A Community in Crisis

*Purpose:* to explore the role public health leaders play in dealing with a natural disaster

*Key concepts:* collaboration, community crisis, strategic planning

*Procedure:* In February, California is hit by storm after storm. The town of Crisona is flooded for a two-week period, the entire town is evacuated, and eventually mudslides begin to occur in the surrounding hills.

The class should divide into teams of 6 to 10 members. In each team, half the members are assigned to play the role of Crisona City Council members, including the role of the mayor and of the head of the Crisona Department of Public Health. The remaining team members are to act as community leaders. These leaders and the head of the Department of Public Health testify about the disaster and offer suggestions for addressing it. The city council listens to the testimony and then works with the community leaders to develop a strategy for dealing with the crisis. The whole team should develop a one-page consensus statement outlining a strategy for responding to the crisis.

## References

1. R. A. Heifetz and M. Linsky, *Leadership on the Line* (Boston: Harvard Business School Press, 2002).
2. S. D. Parks, *Leadership Can Be Taught* (Boston: Harvard Business School Press, 2005).
3. P. M. Senge et al., *The Dance of Change* (New York: Bantam, 1999).
4. A. Delaney, *Politics for Dummies* (Foster City, CA: IDG Books, 1995).
5. P. Capezio and D. Morehouse, *Secrets of Breakthrough Leadership* (Franklin Lakes, NJ: Career Press, 1997).
6. E. Tosca, *Communication Skills Profile* (San Francisco: Jossey-Bass, 1997).
7. D. Tannen, *You Just Don't Understand: Women and Men in Conversation* (New York: Morrow, 1990).
8. J. W. Gardner, *On Leadership* (New York: The Free Press, 1990).
9. R. Kelley, *The Power of Followership* (New York: Doubleday, 1992).
10. J. Carver, *Boards That Make a Difference,* 2nd ed. (San Francisco: Jossey-Bass, 1997).
11. V. Mamlin-Upshaw, "Creating Effective Boards," *Leadership* 2, no. 3 (1993): 1, 11.
12. J. W. Dearing and E. M. Rogers, "Agenda-setting," *Communication Concepts* 6 (1992): 1–98.
13. Institute of Medicine, *The Future of Public Health* (Washington, DC: National Academy Press, 1988).
14. B. J. Turnock, *Public Health: What It Is and How It Works,* 4th ed. (Sudbury, MA: Jones and Bartlett, 2008).
15. Turnock, *Public Health.*
16. Turnock, *Public Health.*
17. S. R. Covey, *The Seven Habits of Highly Effective People* (New York: Simon & Schuster, 1989).
18. M. M. Chemers, "Contemporary Leadership Theory," in *The Leader's Companion,* ed. J. T. Wren (New York: The Free Press, 1995).
19. R. Hargrove, *Mastering the Art of Creative Collaboration* (New York: McGraw-Hill Business Week Books, 1998).
20. Turnock, *Public Health.*
21. S. Wellington, "Breaking the Glass Ceiling," *Leader to Leader* 6 (1997): 37–42.
22. R. R. Thomas Jr., "Diversity and Organizations of the Future," in *The Organization of the Future,* ed. P. Hesselbein et al. (San Francisco: Jossey-Bass, 1997).

23. A. H. Maslow, *Motivation and Personality* (New York: Harper & Row, 1954).
24. J. R. O'Neil, *The Paradox of Success* (New York: Jeremy P. Tarcher and Putnam, 1993).
25. Capezio and Morehouse, *Secrets of Breakthrough Leadership.*
26. S. Helgesen, "Women and the New Economy," *Leader to Leader* 4 (1997): 34–39.
27. C. Mallory, *Team-Building* (Shawnee Mission, KS: National Press Publications, 1991).
28. S. P. Robbins and M. Coulter, *Management,* 8th ed. (Upper Saddle River, NJ: Prentice Hall, 2005).
29. Mallory, *Team-Building.*
30. Mallory, *Team-Building.*
31. P. F. Drucker, *Management: Tasks, Responsibilities, Practices* (New York: Harper & Row, 1985).
32. J. R. Katzenbach and D. K. Smith, *The Wisdom of Teams* (Boston: Harvard Business School Press, 1993).
33. K. Blanchard et al., *The One Minute Manager Builds High Performance Teams* (New York: Morrow, 1990).
34. P. M. Senge, *The Fifth Discipline Fieldbook* (New York: Doubleday, 1999).
35. P. Lencioni, *The Five Dysfunctions of a Team* (San Francisco: Jossey-Bass, 2002).
36. D. Cohen and L. Prusek, *In Good Company: How Social Capital Makes Organizations Work* (Boston: Harvard Business School Press, 2001).
37. P. Capezio, *Supreme Teams: How to Make Teams Really Work* (Shawnee Mission, KS: National Press Publications, 1996).
38. Wellins et al., *Empowered Teams* (San Francisco: Jossey-Bass, 1991).
39. K. Blanchard et al., *The Three Keys to Empowerment* (San Francisco: Berrett-Koehler, 1999).
40. Wellins et al., *Empowered Teams.*
41. P. Hersey, K. H. Blanchard, and D. E. Johnson, *Management of Organizational Behavior,* 9th ed. (Upper Saddle River, NJ: Prentice-Hall, 2007).
42. F. Lafasto and C. Larson, *When Teams Work Best* (Thousand Oaks, CA: Sage Publications, 2001).
43. T. Peters and N. Austin, *A Passion for Excellence* (New York: Random House, 1985).
44. Mallory, *Team-Building.*
45. J. R. Katzenbach and D. K. Smith, *The Wisdom of Teams* (Boston: Harvard Business School Press, 1993).
46. Capezio, *Supreme Teams.*
47. J. G. Liebler and C. R. McConnell, *Management Principles for Health Professionals,* 4th ed. (Sudbury, MA: Jones and Bartlett, 2004).
48. Liebler and McConnell, *Management Principles for Health Professionals.*
49. J. Q. Wilson, *Bureaucracy* (New York: Basic Books, 1989).
50. Peters and Austin, *A Passion for Excellence.*
51. K. Blanchard and S. Bowles, *Gung Ho* (New York: Morrow, 1998).
52. P. F. Drucker, *Landmarks of Tomorrow* (New York: Harper & Row, 1957).
53. A. Tiwana, *The Knowledge Management Toolkit,* 2nd ed. (Upper Saddle River, NJ: Prentice-Hall, 2002).
54. T. Peters, *Thriving on Chaos* (New York: Knopf, 1987).
55. P. F. Drucker, *Managing for the Future* (New York: Truman, Talley Books, and Dutton, 1992).
56. B. Nanus, *Visionary Leadership* (San Francisco: Jossey-Bass, 1992).
57. A. Toffler, *The Third Wave* (New York: Bantam, 1980).
58. A. Toffler and H. Toffler, *Creating a New Civilization* (Atlanta: Turner Publishing Co., 1994).

59. Toffler and Toffler, *Creating a New Civilization.*
60. P. K. Halverson et al., *Managed Care and Public Health* (Gaithersburg, MD: Aspen Publishers, 1998).
61. K. Blanchard and S. Bowles, *Raving Fans* (New York: Morrow, 1993).
62. M. DePree, *Leading Without Power* (San Francisco: Jossey-Bass, 1997).
63. L. Rowitz, *Public Health in the 21st Century: The Prepared Leader* (Sudbury, MA: Jones and Bartlett, 2006).
64. W. Shonick, *Government and Health Services* (New York: Oxford University Press, 1995).
65. Institute of Medicine, *The Future of Public Health.*
66. Shonick, *Government and Health Services.*
67. Rowitz, *Public Health in the 21st Century: The Prepared Leader.*
68. Shonick, *Government and Health Services.*
69. Turnock, *Public Health.*
70. D. J. Breckon, *Managing Health Promotion Programs* (Gaithersburg, MD: Aspen Publishers, 1997).
71. J. M. Kouzes and B. Z. Posner, *The Leadership Challenge,* 4th ed. (San Francisco: Jossey-Bass, 2007).
72. D. Tracy, *10 Steps to Empowerment* (New York: Harper-Collins, 1992).
73. F. Hesselbein et al., eds., *The Community of the Future* (San Francisco: Jossey-Bass, 1998).
74. J. P. Kretzman and J. L. McKnight, *Building Communities from the Inside Out* (Evanston, IL: Northwestern University Center for Urban Affairs, 1993).
75. M. S. Peck, *A World Waiting to Be Born* (New York: Bantam Books, 1993).
76. L. Wallack and L. Dorfman, "Media Advocacy: A Strategy for Advancing Policy and Promoting Health," *Health Education Quarterly* 23, no. 3 (1996): 293–317.
77. R. C. Brownson and E. A. Baker, "Prevention in the Community: Taking Stock," *Journal of Public Health Management and Practice* 4, no. 2 (1998): vi–vii.
78. R. C. Brownson et al., "Demonstration Projects in Community-based Prevention," *Journal of Public Health Management and Practice* 4, no. 2 (1998): 66–77.
79. M. S. Peck, *The Different Drum* (New York: Simon & Schuster, 1987).
80. R. H. Rosen, *Leading People* (New York: Viking, 1996).
81. P. M. Senge, "Creating Quality Communities," in *Community-building,* ed. K. Gozdz (San Francisco: New Leaders Press, 1995).
82. D. O. Chrislip and C. E. Larson, *Collaborative Leadership* (San Francisco: Jossey-Bass, 1994).
83. Chrislip and Larson, *Collaborative Leadership.*
84. L. Cohen et al., *Developing Effective Coalitions: An Eight Step Guide* (Pleasant Hill, CA: Contra Costa County Health Services Department Prevention Programs, 1994).
85. Centers for Disease Control and Prevention, Agency for Toxic Substances and Disease Registry, *Principles of Community Engagement* (Atlanta: CDC Public Health Practice Program Office, 1997).
86. Peck, *A World Waiting to Be Born.*
87. Medical News Today, "International Health Regulations Enter Into Force," *Medical News Today,* June 16, 2007.
88. L. G. Bolman and T. E. Deal, *Leading with Soul,* 2nd ed. (San Francisco: Jossey-Bass, 2001).
89. R. Wagner and J. K. Harter, *12: The Elements of Great Managing* (New York: Gallup Books, 2006).

# Leadership Applications in Public Health

# CHAPTER 7

# INTRODUCTION TO THE CORE FUNCTIONS OF PUBLIC HEALTH

> The underlying premise of Healthy People 2010 is that the health of the individual is almost inseparable from the larger community and that the health of every community in every state and territory determines the overall health status of the Nation.
>
> *Healthy People 2010*

Part II focuses on the core functions of public health—assessment, policy development, and assurance—and the role of leadership in ensuring that these functions are carried out effectively by public health organizations. This chapter introduces the core functions, and the next three chapters each discuss one of the core functions in detail.

The overall mission of public health, as noted already, is to fulfill "society's interest in assuring the conditions in which people can be healthy."[1(p.4)] What this means, of course, needs to be spelled out, and one way of doing this is to divide the mission into its main parts, or core functions. There are various sets of core functions one might choose, but the trio mentioned above is certainly among the most defensible. Protecting and improving the general health of people in the community (the mission of public health) must begin with an evaluation of the current level of health and the current threats to health in the community (assessment). Following the assessment comes the step of developing policies to address the health threats or problems. Then the policies are implemented to improve the public's health (assurance). This step can be viewed as the last in a three-step process, but it must be followed by an evaluation of the effectiveness of the implementation, which will start the whole process over again, for the evaluation will undoubtedly uncover further problems or show that the implementation was only partially successful, leading to further policy development and implementation (Figure 7-1). This latter point demonstrates again the importance of feedback as a mechanism for making change.

## Core Functions of Public Health

Many human service fields struggle with the issue of credibility. Part of the lack of credibility is due to the fact that the public often does not understand

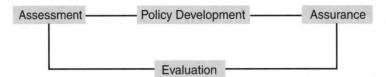

**FIGURE 7-1 The Government Role in Health**
*Source:* Reprinted with permission from Institute of Medicine, *The Future of Public Health,* p. 43, © 1988, National Academy Press.

the nature of the services being provided. Developing a paradigm can help to increase public understanding. A paradigm of public health, for example, can define the structure and parameters of public health work. The core functions model of public health is such a paradigm.

A paradigm is a map with boundaries that elucidates a major area of endeavor.[2] Public health leaders, to an extent, see the world in terms of core functions (or, in other words, a core functions paradigm). They also see it in terms of a leadership paradigm and a management paradigm. Sometimes leaders will substantially revise a paradigm or replace it with another. This is called a paradigm shift.[3] A paradigm shift, which usually takes a long time to be completed, creates a new set of rules, procedures, and perspectives.

*The Future of Public Health* first described the core functions paradigm.[4] The functions of assessment, policy development, and assurance are tied to the phases of public health practice. Assessment involves the identification of health problems, policy development involves the identification of possible solutions, and assurance involves the implementation of the supposed solutions (usually in the form of programs and services). Public health leaders have major responsibilities associated with each core function. It can be argued that these core functions are a universal model for understanding how human services programs work. At a clinical level, this model may also make sense. For example, an individual comes to a physician complaining of certain symptoms. The physician *assesses* the situation and the symptoms. The physician then puts the symptoms together according to the general rules and protocols of the medical profession and makes a diagnosis. This grows out of medical *policy* and procedures. The physician then defines the intervention, which is *assurance* in action. Thus the core functions operate at both an individual (clinical) and a population-based level.

Policy development is seen as linking assessment to assurance. In reality, policy development is often an afterthought in the American public health system—that is, assurance activities sometimes occur before policies are developed. Many public health leaders with whom I have spoken nevertheless have pointed out that leaders need to be effective in the policy development area if they are to create a comprehensive public health system.

One limitation of the original core functions model is that it does not show the interaction between the functions. A second limitation is that "the concepts of assessment, policy development, and assurance, while useful in the public health community itself, have been difficult to translate into effective messages for key stakeholders, including elected officials and community groups. These concepts need to be translated into non-technical language that these groups understand."[5(p.50)]

It is worth viewing the core functions model as an interactive system rather than as linear. Figure 7-2 presents the core function model as a system, with the added element of governance. Governance and public health practice are the glue that makes the entire interactive system cohere and function as it should. It is therefore a central concern for leadership at all levels of the public health system.[6] Governance in public health is a community responsibility, which means that the community needs to be empowered to become more involved in policy development. If all people involved in public health become empowered, then governance as demonstrated through sound and effective public health practice will be part of the infrastructure of the entire public health system.

Figure 7-3 combines the core functions model and the leadership wheel systems model of organizational change (see Figure 5-1). The assessment of need in a community starts the system cycle, allowing leaders to think and act strategically as well as tactically. Leaders then decide on the best strategies for improving health and engage in action planning, which is oriented toward developing tactics for meeting the responsibilities of public health through the practice of the public health core functions. Public health leaders also need to monitor public health activities to ensure they are effective. This important systems view can clearly be seen in Case Study 7-A, which was written by a group of academics and public health practitioners as part of their leadership development experience. This case on a natural disaster was developed from the perspective of the assurance function but clearly demonstrates the other two functions as well.

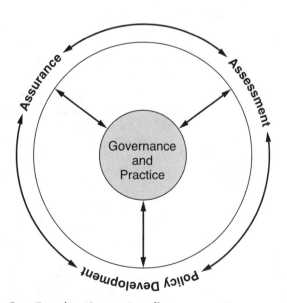

**FIGURE 7-2   Core Functions System Paradigm**

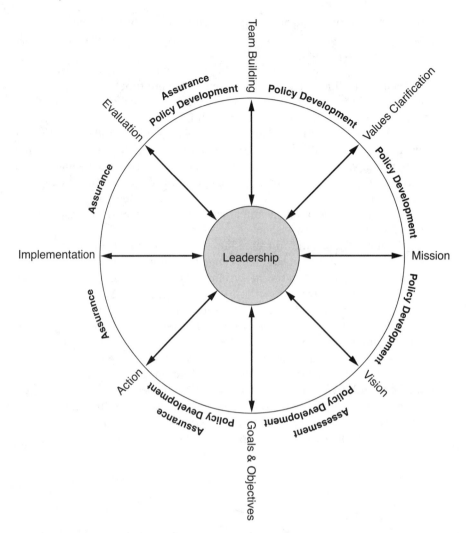

**FIGURE 7-3    A System Approach to Public Health Leadership Including the Core Functions**

---

### Case Study 7-A
### The Flood

*A Case Study in Assurance and Leadership, Mid-America Regional Leadership Institute Year 15 Fellows: Barb MacGregor, Rashmi Ganesan, Dina Kurz, Lisa Stefanovsky, Donovan Thomas, and Lynne Doyle.*

The city of Robinson is located along the picturesque Muddy River. This big, beautiful river has a history of winter ice jams causing flooding of some of the adjacent low lying areas. Two neighborhoods in Robinson, Atlantis Drive and Sunken Boulevard, which until a few years ago had been predominately summer cottages, have been affected by the floodwaters many times. These communities are constructed within the 100-year floodplain. Waterfront property in this area has been increasing in value, and it is considered a very desirable place to live. Therefore, many of the property owners in these neighborhoods have chosen to live in these homes year-round.

The Robinson City Health Department (RCHD), Environmental Health Section, has two sanitarians that have been with the department for 20 years and had an environmental health director who retired in late 2004 after 38 years of service. In early 2005, the RCHD hired a new health officer (Mr. Ivan) who was formerly a KGB agent, and a new environmental health director who had tremendous experience in mortuary science (Ms. Rigormortis). This new team had ideas for significant departmental change and immediately began declaring its authority by reorganizing. This met with resistance from staff, who had a long history of effectively carrying out the goal of the RCHD Environmental Health Division: to provide protection from environmental threats through education, collaboration, and enforcement of laws and regulations that assure a safe and healthy future for Robinson residents.

In the first week of January 2006, a large ice dam formed on the Muddy River, causing the worst flood in 40 years. Sunken Boulevard and Atlantis Drive were the areas most severely affected. Most homes had about four feet of standing water in their main floor, and many cars were underwater. Drinking water wellheads were completely submerged and the residential septic systems saturated.

The Sunken Boulevard and Atlantis Drive neighborhoods consisted of approximately 60 homes and cottages that were built in the 1940s and 1950s. The structures were built prior to public health regulations for well and septic systems and before city/township building regulations had been developed. Neither well nor septic systems met modern public health code standards for floodplain areas. However, it is important to note that the local health department's environmental health section had been routinely inspecting and passing the well and septic systems in these neighborhoods for years. The neighborhoods had been informally "grandfathered" through the system due to the extreme cost and difficulty of completely updating the well and septic systems to current standards. In some cases, costs of updates would have forced some residents to sell their properties.

Residents in the Sunken Boulevard and Atlantis Drive neighborhoods evacuated their homes voluntarily during the 2006 flood. These residents were forced to find alternative housing with family or friends or at local hotels, or they accepted emergency housing assistance from the Red Cross. These families were also expected to continue to pay their mortgages on homes that were underwater and uninhabitable.

From an environmental health standpoint, the following public health issues were identified by the RCHD for the homes and property within the flooded areas:

1. The drinking water supply was threatened and exposed to surface water contamination from the Muddy River, and potentially from raw sewage from the flooded septic systems.
2. Septic systems were saturated and nonfunctioning, which meant the systems were either backing up into the homes or spilling over into the groundwater and surface water.
3. The conditions of the homes themselves were compromised due to the standing water and ice, the future drying process, and subsequent potential mold problems.
4. Structural foundations were compromised due to ice flows and the heavy forces of water.

*(continues)*

**Case Study 7-A** *continued*

In addition, electric power had been cut off to the neighborhoods during the flooding due to safety concerns.

Approximately one week after the flooding forced residents from their homes, a town hall meeting was held at a local elementary school as many residents began to ask what they would need to do to move back into their homes. Ivan the health officer, representatives from law enforcement, and city officials met with residents to discuss the problems caused by the flood. Ivan the health officer chose to steadfastly uphold his interpretation of the public health code and told residents at the town hall meeting that they would not be able to move back into their homes until their wells and septic systems were brought up to the current health code. This message was delivered as an autocratic directive with little compassion for the situations the residents faced. This set the stage for the residents to become very angry and distrustful of the RCHD.

This situation presented a great number of problems for the citizens affected by the flooding, as well as challenges for the public health staff who had to contend with its aftermath. Certainly, this event offered an opportunity for the Health Department's key decision makers to exercise leadership and demonstrate good decision making while ensuring the health and safety of the community.

The environmental health team had the responsibility in this situation to investigate the impact the flooding had on private water and sewer systems; monitor the health of the citizens affected; inform and educate the public regarding health issues the flooding caused; collaborate with community partners to help identify and provide solutions for immediate and future problems; and uphold laws and regulations to protect the community's health. All tasks would have to be completed while working under public pressure in a challenging environment. The need for leadership was clear to ensure that necessary services were maintained and community needs addressed.

In the early stages of the flood, multiple agencies were involved to address the situation, including the health department, city authorities, utility companies, the county emergency services director, city police, the fire department, the Federal Emergency Management Agency (FEMA), and the State Department of Environmental Quality. Despite some very qualified individuals, no agency or individual took charge of the situation or helped residents understand how they could get back into their homes. One resident of the area was quoted in the local paper, "We just want some honest answers. I thought the government was supposed to help us. Why do we pay taxes?"

It was two to three months before the ice dam melted and the floodwaters completely receded. Many residents claimed financial burden and difficulties due to the flood.

As the floodwaters slowly withdrew, Ivan the health officer declared that the septic systems had failed and therefore could not operate again. In a department meeting Ivan said, "I don't care what it costs to fix them; nobody moves in without our approval—NOBODY." Ms. Rigormortis agreed, stating, "Although I don't really know how a septic system works, I know this isn't good."

In March 2006, in his attempt to ensure compliance with the public health code, Ivan the health officer assembled the environmental health staff to "discuss" the options for rebuilding the affected septic systems. Ivan directed that residents would have to install new systems that met current code before they could return to their homes. Options approved by Ivan the health officer included:

1. Building individual sewage holding tanks on stilts. These tanks (about $5,000 per tank to install) must be pumped out every two weeks at a cost of $200 to $300 per pump.
2. Constructing 6-foot elevated septic mounds to meet flood-level elevation requirements, which would cost each residence approximately $10,000.
3. The residents could build a community sewer system at the cost of over $1,000,000 (roughly $20,000 per residence).
4. All drinking water wells would have to be tested and replaced if not installed to current sanitary code (many were shallow wells with no construction record, and therefore did not meet current requirements).

At the same time, the City Planning and Grants Department was working with FEMA to apply for a grant that would buy the flooded homes. This option failed because the governor refused to declare a state of emergency, stating that the emergency was not large enough. Another federal grant was pursued that would buy the properties at 75% of appraised value, and the purchased properties would be deeded to Robinson City (approximately one-third of the homeowners later elected to enter into this agreement). Finally, the State Department of Transportation became involved and announced that it was interested in buying four properties in the neighborhood as part of a future highway expansion.

Unfortunately, the residents viewed this activity as a forced government land acquisition. A resident was quoted, "They don't care about us; they just want our land. I don't trust any of them."

Investigation of these options stalled progress for approximately two to three months (May–June 2006) after the water had receded. The residents were still unable to move back into their homes, and many were running out of resources and temporary housing. It was suspected that a few residents had returned to their homes illegally.

After months of heated debate, mistrust, anger, and inaction, a major change in the situation came when Ivan the health officer and Ms. Rigormortis resigned together to leave the stress of local government and start an alpaca farm. Ivan was heard saying as he left, "This is the most dysfunctional city government I have ever seen. Llamas are smarter than these people." Ms. Rigormortis agreed, stating, "Although I don't really know much about llamas, I know this isn't good."

For the first time in the six months since the flood began there was an opportunity for alternate opinions and direction. Critical partners in the situation began to think "outside of the box" and considered potential alternatives to the interpretation of the sanitary codes that would allow residents to move back into their homes safely. The city administrator, the new health officer, the new environmental health director, and other subject matter experts met and proposed the following criteria for resettlement:

1. Wells needed to be disinfected and water samples needed to pass inspection.
2. Wells needed to be physically protected from future flood exposure by either elevating casings or using a "snorkel" system.
3. Septic tanks needed to be pumped by certified haulers and receive a certificate of inspection.

*(continues)*

4. Contingencies were put in place so when the owners went to sell the homes, the well and septic systems would need to be brought up to code, which included installing holding tanks.
5. Homeowners would need to move out of their homes if the area flooded again. The affected water and septic systems would have to be reevaluated prior to resettlement.

Homeowners were offered these options as well as the buyout option at a second town hall meeting held in late June 2006. The goal of this meeting was to get information to the homeowners so they could make informed decisions about their properties and futures. A very different approach to assurance was used at this town hall meeting. The focus was on answering questions, listening to the concerns of the residents, problem solving, and working collaboratively with other agencies. One resident said, "They finally sent someone to listen to us and fix the problem."

The Health Department continued to hold public meetings monthly as residents considered the various options and slowly returned back to their homes. Meanwhile, residents who had returned to their homes prior to the cleanup called the RCHD and local health facilities complaining of hay fever–type symptoms, running noses, itchy red eyes, and skin rashes. As these calls poured in, it was evident that there was no policy to mitigate other health hazards, such as mold. There was disconnect between environmental health functions and personal health functions to address such issues. Previous leadership had frowned upon interdepartment collaboration between both divisions and had created animosity and a lack of communication within the organization.

The new health officer and new environmental health director worked with the Health Education Division to create educational fact sheets related to mold exposure. Additionally, a 1-800 hotline number was established in collaboration with the Information Services Department to educate the community about possible mold exposure. The health officer worked with the city administrator to provide options for hiring private companies to remediate the mold problems. The cleanup and recovery phase continued over the course of several months.

There are many different styles of leadership. A good leader must remain flexible because different issues often require different strategies. Leadership is dynamic, and there is no universal list of leadership traits that apply to all situations. During this event, it was important for the public health leader to support and enable the public health staff to act, because this situation required not only leadership but more leaders. By empowering others to act, leadership responsibilities could be shared. Communication was also a key issue; it was important to communicate and build trust with the citizens affected. A good leader is able to take complex information and simplify it so it has meaning to a broad audience. Likewise, the ability to communicate difficult information while leading others forward is vital to success. In addition, it was equally important for the leader to cultivate collaboration with community partners. This situation could not be handled solely by the Health Department.

Natural disasters can cause events that lead to public health emergencies. Assurance and policy development play crucial roles in mitigating disasters. Although sheltering is not a basic function of public health, enforcing laws and regulations that protect and ensure safety is an essential public health service. This includes meeting both the environmental and personal health needs of the community. In developing solutions to community problems, a local health department must engage residents and essential community partners in a form of collaborative leadership. This leads to connectivity and creative solutions.

Connectivity also spans across other agencies to create forms of meta-leadership that link public health, law enforcement, city, and county government. The new health officer assessed the emotional and cultural intelligence of the community, presented them with options, educated residents on potential hazards, and effectively managed the public health emergency. Meta-leaders exercise good active forms of leadership in an organization and cross organizational boundaries to protect the health and welfare of community residents.

Policy development plays a role throughout the process of protecting and improving the public's health. First, mission and vision development is a form of policy development. Second, whenever an evaluation is conducted, whether of a team, a community coalition, a program, or a service, the information gathered may suggest that policy revisions or entire new policies may need to be instituted. Obviously, though, assessment and policy development activities are pointless unless the policies chosen are implemented.

## Core Organizational Practices

Efforts have been made since the late 1980s to further define the role of government within the U.S. public health system. In 1989, the Public Health Practice Program Office of the Centers for Disease Control and Prevention initiated a process to identify the core organizational practices necessary for governmental agencies to carry out the mission of public health.[7] Representatives from government public health agencies and related associations identified 10 organizational practices that help illuminate the three core functions, which are obviously more general in nature. The major criticism of this model, which is unfortunately not utilized today, is that it tends to be somewhat narrow in perspective and more about the public health organization than the public health system. However, this model begins the process of seeing that the public health organization needs to look outward to its community and its external stakeholders. The public health agency is part of the local public health system and needs to define the organizational practices that will make the organization an effective partner in the local system. There are still leadership activities associated with this model that are required if the local public health system is to be strengthened. Table 7-1 does demonstrate that these 10 organizational practices begin to provide an operational definition of a functional local public health department.

### Assessment Practices

There are three organizational practices tied to the core function of assessment. The first, which concerns the health needs of the community, involves establishing a systematic needs assessment process that is coordinated by the

**Table 7-1   Leadership and the Organizational Practices**

| Core Functions | Organization Practices | Leadership Activities |
| --- | --- | --- |
| Assessment | 1. Assess the health needs of the community. | Lead the community assessment process. |
| | 2. Investigate the occurrence of health effects and health hazards in the community. | Collect and utilize information to enhance the investigation. |
| | 3. Analyze the determinants of identified health needs. | Integrate data with decision making. |
| Policy development | 4. Advocate for public health, build constituencies, and identify resources in the community. | Build coalitions; empower others; engage in public health advocacy; recognize community assets. |
| | 5. Set priorities among health needs. | Clarify values; create a vision; tie vision to mission; use partners to set priorities. |
| | 6. Develop plans and policies to address priority health needs. | Organize goals and objectives; translate goals into action. |
| Assurance | 7. Manage resources and develop organizational structure. | Search for new resources; make organizational changes to better address community needs. |
| | 8. Implement programs. | Stress innovation; delegate programmatic responsibility to others; oversee programs. |
| | 9. Evaluate programs and provide quality assurance. | Support program evaluation; evaluate data collected; monitor performance. |
| | 10. Inform and educate the public. | Use mentoring and training to educate workforce; use social marketing and health communication to educate public. |

*Source:* Adapted from W. W. Dyal, *Public Health Infrastructure and Organizational Practice Definitions,* 1991, Public Health Practice Program Office, the Centers for Disease Control and Prevention.

local health department and its leadership team and directed toward gathering data on the health status and health needs of the community. Although public health leaders initiate the process, community participation in the process is essential.

The second practice involves the investigation of health hazards in the community, especially timely epidemiological research to identify the magnitude of the health problems, their duration and location, health trends, and populations at risk. As obvious as the importance of epidemiological research is, it is not routinely done. A significant challenge for smaller health departments is doing investigations without an epidemiologist or behavioral scientist on the staff. Another significant challenge is finding the necessary funds.

Public health leaders need to understand how data are collected and used to monitor health status and uncover health hazards.

The third practice is the analysis of identified etiologic and contributing factors that place certain segments of the population at risk for adverse health outcomes. The data generated by the assessment process are used as raw material for this type of analysis. Public health leaders need to understand how to analyze data and how to use data for decision making.

## Policy Development Practices

There are three organizational practices identified for the policy development core function. The first involves the following activities: acting as an advocate for public health, building community constituencies, and identifying resources in the community. These activities are important because they help generate supportive and collaborative relationships with public and private agencies as well as with potential community partners and thereby create organizational mechanisms for the effective planning, implementation, and management of public health programs and services. These activities are also essential for developing action plans in cooperation with community partners.

> **Leadership Tip**
>
> *All leadership decisions are framed by the core functions and essential public health services.*

The fifth practice is the setting of priorities. Criteria used in ranking health problems include the size and seriousness of the problems, the acceptability of the problems, the economic feasibility of solving them, and the effectiveness of the interventions developed to address them. Priority setting is not a completely objective process. For example, a concern about personal safety may exist even without a high community crime rate. If the community groups or politicians push hard enough, the community coalition in concert with the public health agency leader may designate violence as a key issue despite a lack of statistical validation. Public health leaders, in determining health priorities for the community, use value clarification skills, visioning skills, and partnership skills.

The sixth practice is the development of plans and policies to address the prioritized health needs of the community. The development process involves establishing goals and objectives to be accomplished by means of a systematic plan that focuses on local community health needs and the equitable distribution of financial and nonfinancial community resources. This practice requires the participation of the community stakeholders and representatives from other related agencies. Public health leaders will guide the development of goals and objectives and help translate them into action steps.

## Assurance Practices

The final four organizational practices are associated with the assurance core function. The seventh involves managing resources and developing an organizational infrastructure to carry out the public health agenda. Critical leadership and management skills are necessary for the acquisition, allocation, and control of human, physical, cultural, and fiscal resources. Managing resources also encompasses maximizing the operational functioning of the local health system through the coordination of community agencies' efforts and the avoidance of the duplication of services. The issue of duplication is complicated by the professional protection of programs and resistance to the abolition of duplicative services. The seventh practice is unique in that it applies organizational considerations to the issue of public health agency operations. Public health leaders will search for new resources and alter their organizations to better reflect changing health priorities in the community.

The eighth organizational practice involves action plan implementation, which often involves the creation of services and programs. Plan implementation demands creativity and sound leadership, because legislative mandates must be interpreted and statutory responsibilities must be translated into programs. Public health agencies and health departments are usually given the task of providing population-based services, whereas personal services are seen as the responsibility of the medical care system. Public health leaders stress innovation in program development, delegate programmatic responsibility to others, and take an oversight role in monitoring program performance.

> **Leadership Tip**
>
> *Schedule your reading time, phone call time, and all other activities in your calendar. When an emergency meeting occurs or if your supervisor calls, immediately reschedule activities that are being displaced.*

The ninth practice involves the evaluation of program activities. First, there is the issue of quality assurance—whether the program activities are being performed in accordance with professional and regulatory standards. Second, there is the issue of effectiveness—whether the program is achieving the intended goals and objectives. Third, there is the question of revision—whether the program needs to be reformed or resources need to be redirected. Given all the discussion in recent times on reinventing government, it makes sense for public health leaders to use evaluation data for purposes of reorganization. Leaders will need to support program evaluation, evaluate the data collected, and support performance monitoring.

The last assurance practice involves the provision of public health information to the community. Public health agencies have a responsibility to educate the residents of the community on ways to improve personal health—a responsibility they have not always fulfilled. They need to develop health education initiatives in order to increase health knowledge, change attitudes about unhealthy behaviors, and foster healthy habits. To meet their educational responsibility, public health leaders need to learn health communication skills, translate research intervention results into practice, and create linkages to academic institutions in order to develop health education strategies. They also need to use social marketing and health communication strategies to reach community residents and to use mentoring and training to educate the public health workforce. The goal is to get the entire public to view public health issues as important. People must be made to realize that public health hazards put everyone at risk, not just the poor.

As can be seen from the discussion of the 10 practices, the public health model is extremely complex and needs a committed leadership to make it work. Turnock and colleagues, who have studied the core functions and organizational practices, claimed in an article that the 10 organizational practices have been applied in the local health department system as a way to build capacity.[8] It appears that public health leaders and other public health professionals understand the model and feel that it is applicable to their work.

In a follow-up article, Turnock and colleagues reported on current use of the 10 practices.[9] In a study of health departments, 50% of 208 respondents stated that they employed the 10 practices. Use was higher for the practices associated with the policy development core function, and it was also higher for departments serving a population of 50,000 or more and for smaller local health departments organized at the city or city-county level.

In a 1995 study, Turnock, Handler, and Miller investigated the relationship between the application of the core functions paradigm and the effectiveness of public health practice activities using a random sample of local health departments stratified by population size and type of jurisdiction.[10] They found that the U.S. public health system did not reach the proposed national health objectives for the year 2000 to a significant degree. In addition, the goal of having 90% of the population served by a local health department utilizing the core public health functions was not achieved. The researchers found that there was only 54% compliance on implementation of the core functions and organizational practices, about 4% higher than in the previous survey.

Voices had been raised that the core functions model is too abstract, and it was replaced with a model that includes an emphasis on research activities in local public health systems. There seems to be general agreement about what public health does and little agreement about what public health is. The essential public health services model approach to public health, which is discussed next, can be viewed as the systems perspective step toward a better understanding of what public health practitioners do in communities and how they do it. Public health is at a crossroads because of all the changes and proposed reforms in the health system.[11] Yet it must be kept in mind that public health, because it is population based and community oriented, is importantly different than other health professions, whether at the local, state, regional, or federal level.

## Essential Public Health Services

The public health system will be affected by the implementation of any proposals for a national health system (Figure 7-4) or indeed by any substantial changes in the medical care system. Yet what the effects will be is largely a mystery, especially because the core functions paradigm is still confusing to

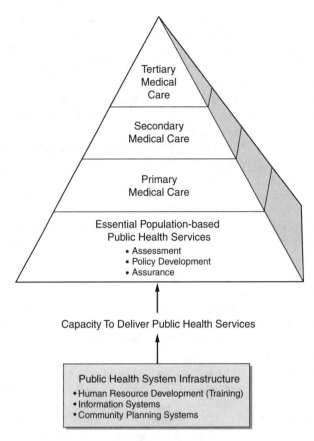

**FIGURE 7-4  Public Health: The Foundation of a National Health System**
*Source:* Reprinted from E. L. Baker, et al., Health Reform and the Health of the Public, *Journal of the American Medical Association,* Vol. 272, No. 18, pp. 1278–1282, 1994, American Medical Association.

policy makers and citizens, although the identification of organizational practices associated with the core functions helps to elucidate the paradigm. To offer further help, Baker and colleagues presented a list of essential public health services that are community based rather than organization based. This list, unlike the models of public health discussed thus far, includes research, enforcement of laws and regulations, and the assurance of a competent health services workforce.

Table 7-2 lists not only essential services but also related leadership activities, and Table 7-3 gives a brief description of each of the 10 services.[12] Leaders have key roles in the delivery of all of the essential services. There is a significant overlap in the leadership activities associated with the organizational practices approach and the essential services approach. The new leadership activities are associated with the three essential services not specifically covered in the organizational practices approach. With regard to enforcement of laws, public health leaders enforce laws and regulations that protect the health of the community. With regard to development of a com-

**Table 7-2    Leadership and the Essential Public Health Services**

| Essential Public Health Services | Leadership Activities |
|---|---|
| Monitor health status to identify community problems. | Use data for decision making. |
| Diagnose and investigate health problems and health hazards in the community. | Use data for decision making. |
| Inform and educate people about health issues and empower them to deal with the issues. | Engage in mentoring and training, social marketing, and health communication activities; empower others. |
| Mobilize community partnerships to identify and solve health problems. | Build partnerships; share power; create workable action plans. |
| Develop policies and plans that support individual and community health efforts. | Clarify values; develop mission; create a vision; develop goals and objectives. |
| Enforce laws and regulations that protect health and ensure safety. | Protect laws and regulations; monitor adherence to laws. |
| Link people to needed personal health services and ensure the provision of health care when otherwise unavailable. | Stress innovation; delegate programmatic responsibility to others; oversee programs. |
| Ensure a competent public health and personal health care workforce. | Build a learning organization; encourage training; mentor associates. |
| Evaluate effectiveness, accessibility, and quality of personal and population-based health services. | Support program evaluation; evaluate data collected; monitor performance. |
| Do research for new insights and innovative solutions to health problems. | Utilize research findings to guide program development. |

*Source:* Adapted from J. Harrell and E. Baker, *The Essential Services of Public Health,* 1997, American Public Health Association.

petent workforce, they build learning organizations based on systems thinking and support continuing education opportunities for the public health workforce. With regard to research, they utilize research findings to guide program development. Figure 7-5, which was originally designed by the Health Resources and Services Administration, shows the relationship between the core functions and the 10 essential public health services.[13] It is presented as a circle to demonstrate that public health works in a system. Essential Service 10 is seen as research for systems management and greater understanding of how the public health system carries out its activities.

If we think of the three core functions as the trunk of a tree, organizational practices constitute one branch that led to a dead end, and the essential public health services constitute another branch that has continued to grow. The two approaches (organizational practices and Essential Public Health Services) do have much in common, and because the essential services approach has predominated, it has been modified to include the organizational practices that are not now part of it (i.e., setting priorities among

**Table 7-3 Essential Public Health Services**

*Monitor health status to identify and solve community health problems:* This service includes accurate diagnosis of the community's health status; identification of threats to health and assessment of health service needs; timely collection, analysis, and publication of information on access, utilization, costs, and outcomes of personal health services; attention to the vital statistics and health status of specific groups that are at higher risk than the total population; and collaboration to manage integrated information systems with private providers and health benefit plans.

*Diagnose and investigate health problems and health hazards in the community:* This service includes epidemiologic identification of emerging health threats; public health laboratory capability using modern technology to conduct rapid screening and high-volume testing; active infectious disease epidemiology programs; and technical capacity for epidemiologic investigation of disease outbreaks and patterns of chronic disease and injury.

*Inform, educate, and empower people about health issues:* This service involves social marketing and targeted media public communication; providing accessible health information resources at community levels; active collaboration with personal health care providers to reinforce health promotion messages and programs; and joint health education programs with schools, churches, and worksites.

*Mobilize community partnerships and action to identify and solve health problems:* This service involves convening and facilitating community groups and associations, including those not typically considered to be health related, in undertaking defined preventive, screening, rehabilitation, and support programs; and skilled coalition-building ability in order to draw upon the full range of potential human and material resources in the cause of community health.

*Develop policies and plans that support individual and community health efforts:* This service requires leadership development at all levels of public health; systematic community-level and state-level planning for health improvement in all jurisdictions; development and tracking of measurable health objectives as a part of continuous quality improvement strategies; joint evaluation with the medical health care system to define consistent policy regarding prevention and treatment services; and development of codes, regulations, and legislation to guide the practice of public health.

*Enforce laws and regulations that protect health and ensure safety:* This service involves full enforcement of sanitary codes, especially in the food industry; full protection of drinking water supplies; enforcement of clean air standards; timely follow-up of hazards, preventable injuries, and exposure-related diseases identified in occupational and community settings; monitoring quality of medical services (e.g., laboratory, nursing homes, and home health care); and timely review of new drug, biologic, and medical device applications.

*Link people to needed personal health services and ensure the provision of health care when otherwise unavailable:* This service (often referred to as "outreach" or "enabling" services) includes ensuring effective entry for socially disadvantaged people into a coordinated system of clinical care; culturally and linguistically appropriate materials and staff to ensure linkage to services to special population groups; ongoing "care management"; transportation services; targeted health information to high-risk population groups; and technical assistance for effective worksite health promotion/disease prevention programs.

*Ensure a competent public and personal health care workforce:* This service includes education and training for personnel to meet the needs for public and personal health service; efficient processes for licensure of professionals and certification of facilities with regular verification and inspection follow-up; adoption of continuous quality improvement and lifelong learning within all licensure and certification programs; active partnerships with professional training programs to ensure community-relevant learning experiences for all students; and continuing education in management and leadership development programs for those charged with administrative/executive roles.

*Evaluate effectiveness, accessibility, and quality of personal and population-based health services:* This service calls for ongoing evaluation of health programs, based on analysis of health status and service utilization data, to assess program effectiveness and to provide information necessary for allocating resources and reshaping programs.

*Research for new insights and innovative solutions to health problems:* This service includes continuous linkage with appropriate institutions of higher learning and research and an internal capacity to mount timely epidemiologic and economic analyses and conduct needed health services research.

*Source:* Adapted from J. Harrell and E. Baker, *The Essential Services of Public Health,* 1997, American Public Health Association.

**FIGURE 7-5   Core Functions and Ten Essential Services of Public Health**
*Source:* DHHS. www.health.gov/phfunctions/images/pubh_wh2.gif, accessed October 14, 2003.

health needs, managing resources, and developing organizational structure). The National Association of County and City Health Officials (NACCHO) put the pieces together and came up with an operational definition of a functional local public health department. NACCHO was clearly aware that local health departments take many forms, but they need to support the core functions and 10 essential public health services within a public health systems approach.[14] The local public health department represents the governmental public health presence at the local level. The way they will do this is to follow a set of standards as is noted in Table 7-4. The residents of a community will hold their local public health responsible for adhering to these standards.

Following is a list of leadership activities related to the core functions paradigm:

- Put the core functions model into practice.
- Develop leadership skills to carry out the essential public health services approach.
- Increase commitment to the model by the public health workforce and by community partners.
- Utilize a systems perspective in implementing the essential public health services

**Table 7-4   Standards for a Functional Local Health Department**

Understands the specific health issues confronting the community, and how physical, behavioral, environmental, social, and economic conditions affect them.

Investigates health problems and health threats.

Prevents, minimizes, and contains adverse health effects from communicable diseases, disease outbreaks from unsafe food and water, chronic diseases, environmental hazards, injuries, and risky health behaviors.

Leads planning and response activities for public health emergencies.

Collaborates with other local responders and with state and federal agencies to intervene in other emergencies with public health significance (e.g., natural disasters).

Implements health promotion programs.

Engages the community to address public health issues.

Develops partnerships with public and private health care providers and institutions, community-based organizations, and other government agencies (e.g., housing authority, criminal justice, education) engaged in services that affect health to collectively identify, alleviate, and act on the sources of public health problems.

Coordinates the public health system's efforts in an intentional, noncompetitive, and nonduplicative manner.

Addresses health disparities.

Serves as an essential resource for local governing bodies and policy makers on up-to-date public health laws and policies.

Provides science-based, timely, and culturally competent health information and health alerts to the media and to the community.

Provides its expertise to others who treat or address issues of public health significance.

Ensures compliance with public health laws and ordinances, using enforcement authority when appropriate.

Employs well-trained staff members who have the necessary resources to implement best practices and evidence-based programs and interventions.

Facilitates research efforts, when approached by researchers, that benefit the community.

Uses and contributes to the evidence base of public health.

Strategically plans its services and activities, evaluates performance and outcomes, and makes adjustments as needed to continually improve its effectiveness, enhance the community's health status, and meet the community's expectations.

*Source:* National Association of County and City Health Officials, *Operational Definition of a Functional Local Health Department* (Washington, DC: NACCHO, 2005).

Exercise 7-1 is intended to help the readers explore the core functions paradigm and learn how the core functions are related to organizational practices, essential services, and strong public health leadership.

## Summary

This chapter introduced the core functions of assessment, policy development, and assurance as a paradigm for the practice of public health. Public health leaders have roles and responsibilities related to each of the functions. As a way of illuminating the three functions, the chapter described the early 10 organizational practices model associated with the three functions and the systems-based essential public health services model that predominates today. With this move from an agency-focused view of public health to a systems-based approach, an innovative operational definition of a functional local public health department has been developed by NACCHO and will become an important cornerstone in the development of a national accreditation program for local health departments. The idea of accreditation will be expanded to state health departments as well.

### Discussion Questions

1. What are the three core functions of public health?
2. What is a paradigm and what is a paradigm shift?
3. What are the similarities and differences between the organizational practices and the essential services of public health?
4. What leadership activities are required for priority setting?
5. What is one of the main criticisms of the core functions model of public health?
6. What are the reasons for creating an operational definition of a functional state and local health department?

### Exercise 7-1:   The Core Functions Debate

*Purpose:* to explore the core functions of public health and their relationship to organizational practices and essential public health services

*Key concepts:* assessment, assurance, core functions, essential public health services, organizational practices, policy development

*Procedure:* The class should divide into teams of 5 to 10 members. Each team is assigned a core function and the task of constructing an argument that purports to show why this function is the most important of the three core functions. In constructing the argument, the team should use the organizational practices and the essential services associated with the core function to clarify the nature of the function. It should also discuss the leadership issues involved. One team should be given the task of preparing an argument favoring a model in which all three core functions are treated as equally important. Each team selects a spokesperson to present its argument, and then all the teams vote on the arguments to determine which is most persuasive.

## References

1. Institute of Medicine, *The Future of Public Health* (Washington, DC: National Academy Press, 1988).
2. S. R. Covey, *The Seven Habits of Highly Effective People* (New York: Simon & Schuster, 1989).
3. J. A. Barker, *Paradigm* (New York: Harper Business, 1992).
4. Institute of Medicine, *The Future of Public Health*.
5. M. A. Stoto et al., eds., *Healthy Communities: New Partnerships for the Future of Public Health* (Washington, DC: National Academy Press, 1996).
6. P. Block, *The Empowered Manager* (San Francisco: Jossey-Bass, 1987).

7. W. W. Dyal, *Public Health Infrastructure and Organizational Practice Definitions* (Atlanta: Centers for Disease Control and Prevention, Division of Public Health Systems, Public Health Practice Program Office, 1991).

8. B. Turnock et al., "Implementing and Assessing Organizational Practice in Public Health," *Public Health Reports* 109, no. 4 (1994): 478–484.

9. B. J. Turnock et al., "Local Health Department Effectiveness in Addressing the Core Functions of Public Health," *Public Health Reports* 109, no. 5 (1994): 653–658.

10. B. J. Turnock et al., "Core Function-Related Local Public Health Practice Effectiveness," *Journal of Public Health Management and Practice* 4, no. 5 (1998): 27–32.

11. E. L. Baker et al., "Health Reform and the Health of the Public," *JAMA* 272, no. 18 (1994): 1278–1282.

12. J. Harrell and E. Baker, *The Essential Services of Public Health* (Washington, DC: American Public Health Association, 1997).

13. www.health.gov/phfunctions/images/pubh_wh2.gif, accessed October 14, 2003.

14. National Association of County and City Health Officials, *Operational Definition of a Functional Local Health Department* (Washington, DC: NACCHO, 2005).

# CHAPTER 8

# LEADERSHIP AND ASSESSMENT

[Assessment] involves identifying and studying important data sources.

G. Pickett and J. J. Hanlon, *Public Health*

Assessment brings public health agencies and communities together as partners. Ideally, the leaders of a public health agency should work with a number of community groups to determine the health needs and health priorities of the community. Over the last century, public health has developed a number of methodologic approaches to studying the health status of a community. One important lesson is that the determination of community health needs and strategies for dealing with these needs must take into account community boundaries, community resources, and the local culture. Otherwise, intervention strategies risk being rejected by community residents and will then wind up being largely ineffective. Another important lesson is that public health agencies must not ignore community groups and individuals in determining the community's public health priorities. The tendency of all types of human service organizations to ignore community input may have contributed to making communities overly dependent on outside help.[1]

Public health agencies have long used epidemiological methods and demographic and social science techniques to obtain an objective picture of community needs. The difficulty with this approach is that it is based on the assumption that problems exist. According to McKnight, human service organizations need to use an anti-diagnostic approach that focuses on evaluating the capacities and strengths of the community and the flexibility of community leaders.[2] In short, these organizations should first do an assets assessment. Once the strengths of the community are determined, the problems of the community can be addressed from a positive perspective.

## The Assessment Process

Local health departments often view a complete community needs assessment as a burden rather than a tool for guiding their activities. The solution is for them to treat assessment as an ongoing dynamic process. If health department leaders incorporate assessment activities into everyday activities, assessment won't appear as a monumental task, because assessment data will be gathered as a matter of course.

Despite awareness on the part of public health professionals that assessment is a critical activity, they are often confused about the nature of assessment. Probably the best way to approach assessment is to focus on its basic component, which is problem identification.[3] It is with regard to this component that community research activities become especially important. Exercise 8-1 explores the issue of developing assessment strategies for an emerging gang problem in a small city.

The first step in the assessment process is to design a durable integrated public health information system.[4] The accomplishment of this step calls for a true partnership, based on public health leadership principles, among local and state health departments, national health-related agencies (including the Centers for Disease Control and Prevention [CDC]), and citizen groups and other agencies. The data systems must be designed to allow growth and the incorporation of new technologies and new databases as they become available.[5]

The second step is to identify community resources and evaluate their effectiveness.[6] Public health leaders need to be students of the community in which they work. They must examine the community health resources, such as health facilities, health professionals, available medicines and vaccines, and emergency medical transportation systems. They must also look at other community resources, such as sanitation programs, education programs, disaster response plans, and mental health and other counseling programs, to determine their availability and effectiveness. Their availability should be analyzed in terms of proximity, accessibility, affordability, acceptability, and appropriateness. The effectiveness measures should include such factors as population size relative to need, proportion of the population in need reached by existing community services, program effectiveness, program costs, and the cost to cover the population not covered. Finally, alternative program approaches should be evaluated.

The third step is to utilize the data that are collected.[7] These data need to be transformed into information that public health leaders can use for effective decision making. Indeed, assessment activities should lead directly to the policy development activities discussed in the next chapter. Public health leaders often fail to express information clearly, and they lose credibility with policy makers as a result. They should present the data simply and straightforwardly, not in a convoluted fashion. They should also orient the presentation to the specific audience receiving the information. The presentation should answer questions that have been posed. Public health leaders need to learn the art of presentation so that the recipients are educated by being given the information.

Case Study 8-A, which describes the leadership activities of a disease surveillance group, explores obstacles that can prevent an assessment from being successful and ways of overcoming these obstacles.

---

### Case Study 8-A
### Removing Obstacles for Assessment: the MSDH Disease Surveillance System

*Kate Wright, Mahree Fuller Skala, Ronald Gribbons, and Adelaide Merkle*

The following case study reviews a selection of problems faced by many disease-oriented or risk factor-oriented public health surveillance systems. Some surveillance systems may not be comprehensive or may contain fragmented disease registries, holding large quantities of surveillance data not utilized to their full potential. This ultimately affects not only local public health and well-being but also state, regional, and national efforts to identify public health problems and implement interventions to control and prevent them.

### Middle State Health Department

*Surveillance System Problems*
Surveillance for communicable diseases has been one of the most visible and critical assessment functions of the Middle State Department of Health (MSDH). Like other state health departments, MSDH reacted to the need for assessment of communicable diseases by designating for itself which diseases were necessary to track.

The department developed its own requirements for collecting data on both individual and outbreak cases and added them to the federal report list. Various reporting procedures were developed by six different MSDH programs responsible for surveillance of various reportable diseases. Program-specific procedural differences resulted in the development of different report forms, several targeted reporting sources, and six separate surveillance databases.

Required information was provided to MSDH by various health providers, who could report directly to their local health departments or to MSDH. Most reports were forwarded by local agencies intending to maintain control over "local" surveillance functions. Even if accurate data were forwarded by some local authorities in an efficient manner, this did not create a "real-time" data system available to MSDH for critical decision support when needed. The largest cities in the state were exempted from state reporting requirements, which resulted in additional complications, including the existence of different local ordinances, report forms, and procedures.

As a result of the lack of system-wide tools and procedures and policies, the problem of underreporting of communicable diseases became increasingly apparent during the late 1980s and early 1990s. Depending on the seriousness and rarity of the disease and the accessibility of the reporting system, a range of from 10% to 90% of diagnosed disease cases were reported, annually. Many factors were blamed for the underreporting of communicable disease surveillance data. These included misunderstandings by providers regarding reporting requirements and confidentiality and the inconvenience of compliance given the wide range of reporting procedures and forms. Analysis of surveillance data did not present complete or accurate conclusions regarding disease trends, with the result that policy development and prevention and control measures to reduce public health risks were less than optimal.

*History and Background Information*
Historically, the public health system in Middle State was based on cooperation between autonomous local health departments and the state health department. The relationship was formalized through contractual arrangements that provided state general revenue funds to the local jurisdictions for core public health activities, including disease surveillance. Most local health departments received the majority of their funding from local taxes, Medicaid charges, and federal funding for nutritional and other services for mothers and children. These departments reported to local governing boards and set their priorities based on local constituent demands and funding source requirements.

*(continues)*

Local health departments in cities with less than 75,000 residents were governed by MSDH administrative rules regarding the list of and procedures for reporting disease and health conditions. Larger cities were exempted from these rules by law but were required to establish their own reportable disease lists and submit surveillance data to MSDH. In practice, most cities used the state list along with their own versions of the report form and the processes and procedures. Over time, additional diseases were added to the state report list but rarely were any diseases deleted. The criteria for adding a reportable disease included disease severity, the number of individuals affected by it, and the availability of public health measures to prevent or control it. In 1994, there were 49 diseases and conditions listed in the CDC list of nationally reportable diseases, of which most were included in the MSDH list of designated diseases.

The location where a disease case entered the surveillance system depended on the disease, the patient's residence, and the initial recipient of the information. State administrative rules defined those responsible for reporting requirements, although there were no penalties for failure to comply. The list included physicians, laboratories, school nurses, day-care providers, and nursing homes. Hospitals were not included on the list, although they often completed reporting requirements for physicians. In practice, laboratories were the chief source for disease reporting, followed by hospitals and physicians.

Both local and state jurisdictions were responsible for disease control activities, and the locus of responsibility depended on the disease. Local health authorities were responsible for investigating and controlling most reportable diseases, but state authorities would step in when local control was not assumed. MSDH policy specified the need for cooperation with local authorities in cases requiring state involvement. In fact, many smaller local health departments did not have full-time disease control personnel, and these often requested MSDH to assist with surveillance and follow-up activities.

The complexity of the MSDH surveillance system grew over time. Within the Division of Epidemiology, six of the seven programs maintained their own disease registries. Three of these programs (sexually transmitted disease (STD)/acquired immune deficiency syndrome (AIDS), tuberculosis (TB), and Immunization) received most of their funding from categorical federal grants. Program managers and supervisory staff were CDC employees assigned to MSDH as advisors; the CDC determined most aspects of their operations, including the diseases tracked, the data reported to the CDC, and even the computer database programs and record format used. Local and district data were transmitted weekly, through computer-modem transmission, to the Miscellaneous Diseases Program Office, where they were aggregated and sent to the appropriate registries, including national reportable data, which were also transmitted to the CDC.

The largest of the division's registries, the STD database, received 18,500 case reports in 1994. The TB registry added approximately 10,000 tuberculosis infections and 270 cases per year. The Immunization database added fewer than a hundred cases per year to several hundred per year, varying with the occurrence of outbreaks. The Miscellaneous Diseases and Zoonotic Diseases programs, supported by meager state general revenue funds, shared one centralized disease registry, which in 1994 received approximately 9,000 case reports. The Environmental Health program had two established registries, one for occupational fatalities and one for blood lead-screening results. Each used specialized methods and database formats mandated by federal funding agencies and entered and analyzed data in the program office. About 160 occupational fatalities and 30,000 blood lead-levels were annually recorded.

MSDH distributed specialized case report forms for STDs, TB infection, TB disease, miscellaneous diseases (also used by Zoonotic Diseases and Immunization), miscellaneous diseases reported by laboratories (used by several programs), human immunodeficiency virus (HIV) infection, AIDS, occupational fatalities, and lead screening. In 1994, a new set of specialized forms was being developed by the Environmental Health program for additional reportable conditions. The major metropolitan health departments developed their own case report forms for most of the reportable diseases. A few MSDH forms were universally accepted, most notably for HIV and AIDS. As a result of the variances in report form acceptance and use, physicians, pediatricians, internists, and emergency department physicians, who initially diagnosed most reportable diseases, used at least 10 different report forms to meet surveillance obligations. In addition, each reportable disease had requirements regarding whether it should be reported immediately, by telephone or by mail, and whether the form should be sent to the local health department, district office, or directly to MSDH.

The division's largely decentralized system had positive and negative attributes. Local control allowed physicians and other sources to report to their city or county health department, which helped minimize delays in local case investigation and implementation of control measures. Each large urban and suburban health department and each MSDH district office had access to its own database to track workloads, complete investigations, analyze for local assessment and planning purposes, such as determining trends, identifying high-risk populations, and generating report source feedback reports to local agencies. Localized data entry also reduced the workload burden for MSDH disease registry clerical staff. Although local authorities with investigation resources preferred to maintain control, local control resulted in variations in local policies, procedures, and report forms. These variations affected the quality and accuracy of surveillance procedures, data analyses, report transmissions, and timely disease investigations and follow-up.

### The Challenge
In July 1994, three opportunities for change created visibility for those wanting to address problems and begin reinventing the surveillance system. First, MSDH's capacity in the area of environmental epidemiology was expanded. This created an opportunity for allocation of new resources to expand the surveillance system to include environmental and occupational conditions that were not previously reported and increase the accuracy of and number of reporting sources for surveillance data. The division director, Mr. Jenkins, realized the importance of not dedicating new resources to perpetuate and further complicate the existing system. Other individuals supporting the need for change included the state epidemiologist and the program chiefs of the following programs: STDs/HIV/AIDS, TB, Immunization, Zoonotic Diseases, Environmental Epidemiology, and Miscellaneous Diseases. At the local level, the Communicable Disease directors from West City, East City, Suburban East City, and Southwest City, the largest cities in the state, expressed similar concerns.

While these needs were surfacing, the Middle State agency for licensing of physicians offered its newsletter as a forum for informing physicians about disease surveillance reporting obligations. They asked the division to provide their newsletter staff with a precise and succinct description of the state's system and reporting

*(continues)*

**Case Study 8-A** *continued*

requirements. During the same period, the MSDH director's office identified population health measurement as a priority and created an initiative to assist local health departments in developing community assessment and strategic-planning activities. Local support for this initiative was based on increasing demand for consumable and accurate data on the health status and needs of local populations. Local departments wishing to access all data for community assessment had to request surveillance data from each MSDH program.

As a result of these developments, Mr. Jenkins became more aware of the complexity of the disease-reporting system in Middle State and identified a pressing need to expand surveillance for environmentally induced conditions, teach physicians how to use the reporting system, and make local disease data accessible for local community assessment projects. His challenge, as a leader, was to simplify the system in order to improve its efficiency, accuracy, sensitivity, and ability to have an impact on the continuous improvement of disease-preventing investigation and follow-up policies and procedures. In general, the challenges confronting the division were complicated by:

- the variety of division programs involved
- different categorical funding sources
- different federal requirements due to ties to the CDC, including different data criteria for each program
- lack of a centralized database
- the obligation of various report sources to submit disease reports, complicated by different disease-specific requirements and report forms
- the involvement of different levels of the public health system in surveillance data management and response

**Postscript: Taking Action**

In October 1994, Mr. Jenkins called a meeting of the program chiefs to discuss possible solutions to the problems facing the division. The following suggestions were made:

*Develop a generic report form.* This was supported by Immunization, Miscellaneous Diseases, and Environmental Health but rejected by STD/AIDS and TB. The program chiefs believed that specific, detailed information about clinical history and treatment was essential to determine the appropriate follow-up procedures for each case.

*Utilize electronic disease-reporting methods.* The Miscellaneous Diseases program advocated the use of fax and computer bulletin board technology to make reporting easier. This would require development of a simple generic form that could be faxed and scanned.

*Centralize the reporting locus or "target."* Some of the larger, well-funded programs advocated centralization of reporting requirements. They requested that all reports be sent directly to MSDH. Others warned that additional (unavailable) resources would be required to handle the increased workload and that centralized reporting could delay local response and investigation. There were additional concerns that transmission of all reports to MSDH would erode communication lines between local health providers and public health departments.

Next, Mr. Jenkins contacted the local communicable disease directors to solicit their input. They were supportive of the concept of a generic report form; West City and Suburban East City already had generic forms in local use and would continue to use them regardless of any changes MSDH implemented. All local directors insisted that local disease reports should be sent directly to them to prevent unacceptable delays in investigation and creation of a negative impact on local reporting relationships. Opinions on fax reporting were divided; some sites were already receiving most of their reports by fax.

A division disease surveillance work group was established that included members from each of the disease control programs, the four city communicable disease directors, and three other members from local health agencies involved in surveillance and follow-up. The committee chose simplification of reporting requirements as its first priority. Its tasks included:

- updating the disease report list
- reducing the report categories to two
- eliminating outdated report requirements
- expanding the categories of sources required to submit disease reports (it added hospitals to the list) and defining group practice requirements
- developing a generic disease report form

The committee accomplished these objectives during the spring of 1995 and received board approval the following August. In October 1995, these policy changes were published in the Middle State Register for public comment. It was expected that policies recommended by the committee would go into effect by April 1996.

All jurisdictions involved were in agreement over the use of the new generic report form as well as other policy-simplifying report requirements. These changes represented a major shift in collaboration at all levels to ensure meeting public health needs. However, the remaining challenges were formidable. The fundamental problem regarding the locus of responsibility for reports entering the system and local jurisdiction over local disease surveillance continued to raise concerns. Providers remained unclear as to where reports should be sent. The issue of managing disease surveillance data from customer source to an electronic system that could transmit information to the appropriate locus and ensure disease investigation and follow-up also remained a challenge. As of 2008, this system is still in operation.

## Essential Services Associated with Assessment

As noted in the previous chapter, two essential services are associated with the core function of assessment. The first involves monitoring health status to assess the health needs of the community. The researchers who defined the 10 organizational practices also gave performance indicators for each practice. These performance indicators have been adapted to the essential services paradigm. It is important to note that the performance indicators are transferable from the organizational practice paradigm to the essential public health services paradigm, but the systems perspective of the essential services paradigm takes the activities and uses them in a total community context. In addition, the performance indicators serve as a guide to the public health agency in the community assessment process. The five organizational practice indicators show whether the essential service is actually in place:[8]

1. A community health needs assessment planning process is in place.
2. Needs assessment includes community input.
3. Morbidity and mortality data are obtained from vital records.

4. Morbidity and mortality data are obtained from other sources.
5. Behavioral risk factors are included in the community needs assessment.

The second essential service involves diagnosing and investigating the occurrence of adverse health events and health hazards in the community. This essential service has six performance indicators (also adapted from the organizational practices):

6. Epidemiological surveillance systems are functioning.
7. No preventable mortality or morbidity occurs as a result of delays in surveillance
8. Health needs identified by the needs assessment are analyzed.
9. Determinants and contributing factors are identified.
10. Health needs of population groups are analyzed.
11. Existing health resources are analyzed.

The remainder of this chapter discusses the various approaches to needs assessment that have been developed in recent years. Public health has begun to use the community assets model in the Mobilizing for Action through Planning and Partnerships (MAPP) assessment process discussed below. As soon as needs assessment becomes a leadership partnership activity, assessment and policy development move closer together, and it is out of the marriage of these two core functions that assurance activities come into being.

## Assessment Methodologies

This section presents four methodologic approaches to community and organizational assessment. Each of these approaches, despite being analyzable into a set of operational steps, requires leaders to be creative in their supervision of assessment activities. The leaders, of course, must delegate many of the activities to managers and other professional staff.

## APEX*PH*

In 1987, the Assessment Protocol for Excellence in Public Health (APEX*PH*) project was started under a cooperative agreement between the American Public Health Association (APHA), the Association of State and Territorial Health Officials, the CDC, the National Association of County and City Health Officials (NACCHO), and the National Association of County Health Officials.[9] Two major groups were established, a steering committee and an APEX*PH* working group. What eventually developed was a voluntary process for organizational and community self-assessment, a process for planned improvements, and methods for continuing evaluation and reassessment. The critical component is a set of procedures that local health departments can use to assess public health concerns. The final report and the manual created by the two working groups pointed to the differences between their approach and other approaches, some of which are indicated by the following outline of APEX*PH*:

1. APEX*PH* is a true self-assessment protocol that can be used by an agency to meet its needs and those of the community.

2. APEX*PH* leads to a practice-based plan of action.
3. APEX*PH* concentrates on a local health department's administrative and leadership capacity, the basic structure and organization of the local health department and its place in the community, and the community's actual and perceived problems instead of technical performance compliance with programmatic objectives by specific public health programs.
4. APEX*PH* offers opportunities for the local health department to assess its relationship with other local government agencies, with the community as a whole, and with state and federal agencies. The protocol can give guidance on ways to strengthen partnership relationships and obtain needed support.
5. APEX*PH* offers an approach by which the health department and its leadership will become accepted by the community as major players in the public health arena. It includes a community assessment process, health priority setting, policy development, and activities to ensure that the health needs of the public are being met.
6. APEX*PH* is adaptable to different local situations and different arrays of resources.

By following APEX*PH*, public health leaders fulfill the responsibility of the local agency to perform a community assessment. They will also increase their and the agency's credibility within the community and foster strong partnerships with community groups. The principles of APEX*PH* include these:

1. Because government has a primary responsibility to ensure the health of the public, health departments need to provide direction for their communities in assessing health problems, developing policies, and addressing community health problems.
2. Because leadership and accountability go together, health departments must establish and meet competency and practice standards that are seen by their communities as appropriate to health protection and health promotion.
3. Because public health practitioners are often placed in difficult situations in which hard choices need to be made, health department leaders have to be risk takers who shape their programs to the communities that they serve in ways that the communities will find acceptable.
4. Because public health problems demand a strong, coordinated, authoritative response, state and local health departments need to discover techniques for working in partnership with each other so as to strengthen each other's resources and authority.
5. In order to set health priorities utilizing scientific knowledge, health department leaders must become health information experts. They must routinely provide information to their communities and aid their communities in the development of community-based health plans.
6. Owing to the multidimensional nature of public health problems, health departments have to find creative approaches to solving local health problems using a wide variety of community resources.
7. With a strong belief that improvements in the health of the public require active community ownership and commitment, health

departments need to develop and maintain partnerships with community agencies, community leaders, interest groups, and representatives of high-risk population groups.

APEX*PH* is a three-part process. Part I is an organizational capacity assessment—an eight-step internal review of the health department itself (Figure 8-1). The object is to evaluate the health department's administrative structure and its capacity to undertake a community assessment (Part II of APEX*PH*). The internal review is performed by the health department director and a team of key staff members. As Figure 8-1 shows, the review in-

**Step 1**
Prepare for Organizational
Capacity Assessment

**Step 2**
Score Indicators for
Importance and Current Status

**Step 3**
Identify Strengths
and Weaknesses

**Step 4**
Analyze and Report
Strengths

**Step 5**
Analyze Weaknesses

**Step 6**
Rank Problems In
Order of Priority

**Step 7**
Develop and Implement
Action Plans

**Step 8**
Institutionalize the
Assessment Process

**FIGURE 8-1    Flowchart of Steps in Assessing Organizational Capacity**
*Source:* Reprinted from *Assessment Protocol for Excellence in Public Health,* 1991, the Centers for Disease Control and Prevention, National Association of County and City Health Officials.

cludes preparing for further steps, scoring indicators in regard to importance and current status, identifying strengths and weaknesses, analyzing and reporting agency strengths, analyzing weaknesses, ranking problems, developing and implementing action plans, and institutionalizing the assessment process.

Part II of APEX*PH* is a community assessment. Public health leaders need to reach out and involve the community in the assessment process. The process involves evaluating the health of the community as well as identifying community strengths and the potential role of the health department in addressing health problems. (How community strengths are to be determined is not clearly laid out.) Part II also provides for the utilization of objective health data and the community's perceptions of community health problems. Those responsible for the community assessment gather demographic data, socioeconomic data, environmental data, and data on years of potential life lost, access to primary health care, other health indices, perinatal indicators, the leading causes of mortality, the estimated prevalence of disease, and the leading causes of hospitalization. They then construct a community health problem summary, rank the top 10 contributors to years of productive life lost, and develop a community health plan.

The final part of the APEX*PH* process is called "completing the cycle." In this part, public health leaders integrate the plans developed previously into the ongoing activities of the health department and the community it serves. This part involves policy development, assurance, monitoring, and evaluation of plans developed in Parts I and II. As a result of the total APEX*PH* process, the leaders make recommendations for changes in current services or the development of new services. They also usually find ways of improving the functioning of the local health department (capacity building). The protocol guidelines are quite comprehensive and allow for assessment to be an ongoing agency process.

Beginning in the late 1990s, NACCHO, in partnership with the CDC, engaged in a revision of APEX*PH*. The new protocol, called MAPP, ties assessment to essential public health services as well as to the National Public Health Performance Standards (set by the CDC). It stresses the importance of community partnerships in the public health enterprise and the importance of measuring the outcomes of public health programs. Leadership is necessary at all levels of the assessment process.

## MAPP[10]

With the MAPP process, there was a shift from the agency-based community assessment process to a process that was systems based. Although some local health departments still choose the APEX*PH* approach to assessment, many health departments are moving to the MAPP model. The series of tools that were developed began a process of seeing strategic planning as a set of activities tied to the community health improvement process. MAPP was developed in a partnership between NACCHO and the Public Health Practice Program Office of the CDC. Between 1997 and 2000, a work group was established to develop this new approach by community representatives, CDC representatives, and academicians. The vision for MAPP is "communities achieving improved health and quality by mobilizing partnerships and taking strategic action."

Seven principles were designated to serve as the foundation for MAPP and to aid implementers in the understanding of the reasons behind the MAPP innovations. The seven principles are:

1. Systems thinking
2. Dialogue
3. Shared vision
4. Data to inform the process
5. Partnerships and collaboration
6. Strategic thinking
7. Celebration of successes

It is important to note that these seven principles support the activities of public health leaders discussed in Part I of this book.

MAPP was designed by the work group to include the following elements:

1. Community-driven and community-owned approach
2. Builds on previous experiences and lessons learned
3. Utilizes traditional strategic planning concepts at a community level
4. Creates and strengthens the local public health system
5. Creates governmental public health leadership opportunities
6. Uses essential public health services to define public health and its work
7. Brings four community assessments together to provide a comprehensive strategic plan

With the seven principles and the seven elements in mind, NACCHO compared the APEX*PH* process with the new MAPP process, which can be seen in Table 8-1.

**Table 8-1 Comparison Between APEX*PH* and MAPP**

| APEX*PH* | MAPP |
|---|---|
| • Build local health department (LHD) leadership | • Build LHD leadership, but also promote community responsibility for the health of the public |
| • Assess LHD capacity for delivering public health services | • Assess capacity of entire local public health system |
| • Operational planning | • Strategic planning |
| • Focus on health status | • Focus on health status, community perceptions, forces of change, and local public health system capacities |
| • Develop plans to address needs | • Strategically match needs, resources, ideas, and actions |

*Source:* NACCHO, "MAPP," http://mapp.naccho.org/FullTextIntroduction.asp. Accessed December 11, 2007.

As can be seen in Figure 8-2, there are four integrated assessments that occur as a local public health system engages in the MAPP process:

1. *Community themes and strengths assessment.* Themes that engage community groups and residents as well as perceptions about quality-of-life issues. Community assests are also explored.
2. *Local public health system assessment.* Capacity of the local public health system to carry out the 10 essential public health services, which include performance standards tied to the essential services.
3. *Community health status assessment.* Analyzes data about health status of residents, quality-of-life issues, and potential risk factors.
4. *Forces of change assessment.* Forces at a local, regional, national, or international level that will affect the community and the health of the public.

As can be seen in Figure 8-2, the MAPP process involves partnership development, visioning, the assessments themselves that need to be done on an ongoing basis, identification of strategic issues, the formulation of goals and objectives, and evaluation and implementation of the results of the process.

There is also an assessment strategy tied to environmental health. PACE-EH is an assessment protocol for determining community excellence in environmental health.[11] The strategy uses a systems framework and is strongly

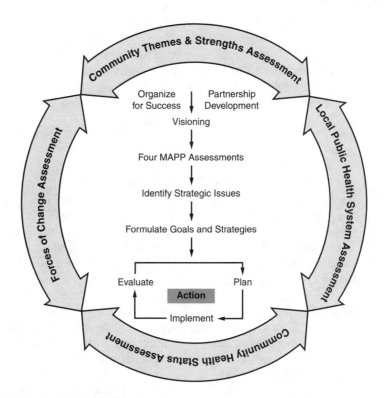

**FIGURE 8-2    MAPP Model**
*Source:* NACCHO, "MAPP". http://mapp.naccho.org/FullTextIntroduction.asp. Accessed December 11, 2007.

committed to community engagement. The protocol assumes the involvement of local public health agencies that organize and facilitate the process. PACE-EH has four goals:

1. Evaluate environmental health conditions
2. Target populations at risk
3. Set priorities
4. Support health equity and social justice

A major limitation of the assessment protocol is that it does not utilize the 10 essential public health services paradigm per se although it can be used to operationalize these 10 services for environmental health. There is a leadership challenge in that environmental health needs to play a key role in the public health agency and in the public health system by showing other leaders how public health and environmental health need to be integrated.

# PATCH

The CDC was one of the partners in the development of another assessment protocol, the Planned Approach to Community Health (PATCH). Other participants included state and local health departments and community groups. The protocol was designed in the mid-1980s to strengthen the capacity of state and local health departments to plan, implement, and evaluate community-level health promotion activities targeted at priority health problems.[12] It was developed in response to a shift in federal policy regarding categorical grants to states. Although PATCH includes strong assessment components, it has strong policy development and assurance components as well. It can be used to link local, state, and federal public health agencies, yet it is oriented toward local public health initiatives. Consumers are also essential partners in the PATCH process.

PATCH, like APEX*PH* and MAPP, has a methodology communities can use for planning, conducting, and evaluating health promotion and disease prevention programs.[13] The methodology includes procedures for establishing a health promotion team, collecting and using local data, setting health priorities, planning and implementing programs, and evaluating the results. The promotion of PATCH was tied to the *Healthy People 2000* health objectives, and although some health departments still utilize the PATCH process, the number is shrinking.

The object of PATCH is to inculcate behaviors that are conducive to health. The process uses educational techniques, public health policy, and environmental strategies to encourage community residents to choose healthy lifestyles. Each community, in conjunction with its public health leaders, needs to do its own community assessment, set its own health priorities, formulate solutions, and take ownership of its programs.

The main principles of the PATCH process include the following:[14]

1. Community members must participate in the process.
2. Data should guide program development.
3. A comprehensive health promotion strategy must be developed.

4. The evaluation of programs should emphasize ways of improving them.

The PATCH procedures can be adapted to various health problems and communities. The whole process can be analyzed into five phases, which are summarized below.

## Phase I: Mobilizing the Community

Public health leaders must use their coalition-building skills to involve the community in the PATCH process. They first need to complete a demographic profile of the community so as to identify the best community leaders and organizations to recruit. During this phase, the public health leaders must also work at informing the community about the PATCH process.

## Phase II: Collecting and Organizing Data

The community work group, which includes community leaders, obtains and analyzes data on mortality and morbidity and their causes. It also collects behavioral data. Community groups may identify other sources of data that might be useful. The data are then analyzed in order to determine the leading health problems in the community.

The community work group should collect extensive data on the community and compare its community's statistics with state and national statistics. The addition of data from multiple sources will aid the group in other phases of the PATCH process. The assessment should include data on the causes of death and disability and identify ways of preventing premature death and disability (Table 8-2).

Both quantitative and qualitative data are collected. Among the quantitative data are mortality and morbidity data gathered from state and local health departments, state and local social service departments, the state department of highway safety, state and local police departments, boards of education, voluntary agencies, hospitals, major employers or the chamber of commerce, and colleges and universities. Among the qualitative data are community opinion data. In order to get this type of information, it is necessary to identify community leaders, develop a series of survey questions, train interviewers, conduct interviews, collate and analyze data, and prepare a report of the results. The survey results will allow problems to be ranked according to the number of times they were mentioned. Public health leaders need to discuss the survey results report with community groups.

## Phase III: Choosing Health Priorities and Target Groups

Behavioral data as well as other relevant data are presented to the community work group, which then analyzes the behavioral, social, economic, political, and environmental factors that affect behaviors and thereby put community residents at risk for disease, death, and injury. After reviewing all the behavioral data, the community group sets health priorities and appropriate community objectives and decides which priorities are to be addressed initially.

**Table 8-2   Contributors to the Leading Causes of Death**

| | Heart Disease | Cancers | Stroke | Injuries (nonvehicular) | Influenza Pneumonia | Injuries (vehicular) | Diabetes | Cirrhosis | Suicide | Homicide |
|---|---|---|---|---|---|---|---|---|---|---|
| *Behavioral risk factor* | | | | | | | | | | |
| Tobacco use | • | • | • | • | • | | | | | |
| High blood pressure | • | | • | | | | | | | |
| High blood cholesterol | • | | P | | | | | | | |
| Diet | • | | P | | | | | | | |
| Obesity | • | • | | | | | | | | |
| Lack of exercise | • | • | • | | | | | | | |
| Stress | P | | P | • | | • | | | | |
| Alcohol abuse | • | • | • | • | | • | | • | • | • |
| Drug misuse | P | • | P | • | | • | | • | • | • |
| Seatbelt nonuse | | | | | | • | | | | |
| Handgun possession | | | | • | | | | | • | • |
| *Nonbehavioral risk factor* | | | | | | | | | | |
| Biological factors | • | • | • | | • | | | • | • | |
| Radiation | | • | | | | | | | | |
| Workplace hazards | | • | | • | | • | | | | |
| Environmental | | • | | | | | | | | |
| Infectious agents | P | • | | | • | | | | | |
| Home hazards | | | | • | | • | | | | |
| Auto/road design | | | | | | • | | | | |
| Speed limits | | | | | | • | | | | |
| Health care access | • | • | • | • | • | • | | • | • | • |

P = possible

*Source:* Reprinted from *PATCH: Planned Approach to Community Health*, 1994, the Centers for Disease Control and Prevention.

## Phase IV: Developing a Comprehensive Intervention Strategy

In this phase, interventions are chosen, designed, and eventually implemented. Existing health resources, policies, environmental supports, and programs need to be identified before new programs are created so that duplication of services can be avoided. The work group begins to explore the assurance function of public health and develops a comprehensive health promotion intervention plan, including strategies, a timetable, and a schedule for completing tasks.

## Phase V: Evaluating PATCH

In this phase, an evaluation work group is set up by the public health leaders. The work group's job is to evaluate progress, including improvements in the health of community residents, through the use of standard evaluation methods. The purpose of the evaluation is to provide feedback to program participants and public health leaders so they can enhance the effectiveness of the interventions.

Steckler and colleagues evaluated 27 PATCH sites that had been functioning in 13 states for one to three years.[15] Figure 8-3 shows a presumptive PATCH model containing the steps that 72% of the sites had completed. All 25 sites had completed a behavioral risk factor survey, which is discussed later in this chapter. Of the 18 sites that had completed the six CDC training workshops, 55.6% had completed most of the PATCH processes. The researchers found that PATCH was well liked by the participants. Funding for the process, however, tended to be a problem. Finally, PATCH was perceived to be effective as a community organization process by almost half of all state and local coordinators as well as by community leaders.

## Model Standards

A third major assessment methodology is based on model standards.[16] The model standards project, developed under the auspices of the APHA, was an attempt to bring together the various approaches to community assessment and apply the tools of assessment to the *Healthy People 2000* health objectives as a way of determining how and to what extent the objectives were being achieved. It was assumed that communities would adapt the national health objectives to local needs, in particular by a process in which community leaders and agencies, under the guidance of public health leaders, would set health priorities. Eventually, plans would need to be developed for programs designed to achieve the local health objectives.

The following principles are intended to guide the use of model standards:[17]

1. The health objectives should be measurable and reality based.
2. Plans should be flexible, and community coalitions should quantify their objectives and develop local strategies for addressing problems.
3. Community-wide partnerships that focus on the community as a whole should be fostered.
4. Government is the "residual guarantor" of health services, which means that a government agency provides the services directly or ensures their delivery by a public or private community-based organization.

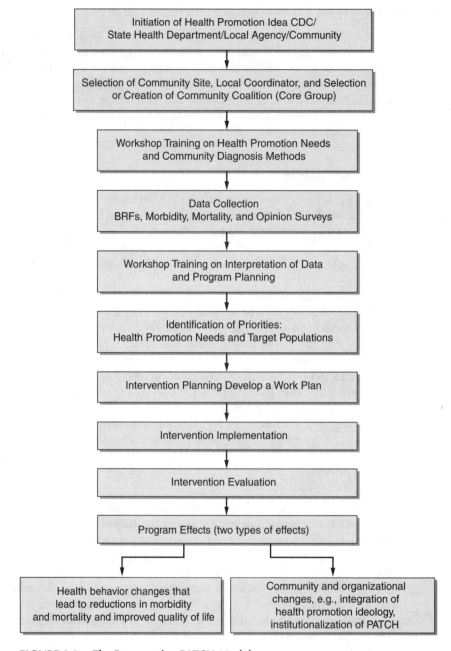

**FIGURE 8-3 The Presumptive PATCH Model**
*Source:* Reprinted from *PATCH: Planned Approach to Community Health,* 1994, the Centers for Disease Control and Prevention.

5. Negotiation is the secret to relationships between agencies.
6. The use of the term "standards" implies that the objectives are uniform (in the interests of equity and social justice), and the use of "guide-lines" suggests the existence of local decision-making discretion.
7. Assurance and accessibility to services are requirements of model standards.

8. Program development is emphasized rather than professional practice considerations.

In August 1990, a meeting was held at the CDC headquarters in Atlanta. The meeting, attended by representatives from the major U.S. public health organizations, focused on how local communities could best use planning methods in order to meet the objectives for the nation for the year 2000. Out of the discussion came the 11 steps of the model standards process:[18,19]

1. Determine and assess the role of one's health agency.
2. Assess the lead health agency's organizational capacity.
3. Develop an agency plan to build the necessary organizational capacity.
4. Assess the community's organizational and power structures.
5. Organize the community to build a stronger constituency for public health and establish a partnership for public health.
6. Assess the health needs of the community and its available resources.
7. Determine local priorities.
8. Select outcome and process objectives that are compatible with local priorities and the *Healthy People 2000* objectives.
9. Develop community-wide intervention strategies.
10. Develop and implement a plan of action.
11. Monitor and evaluate the effort on a continuing basis.

The model standards methodology can be used in conjunction with other assessment methodologies, such as APEX*PH*, PATCH, and MAPP. In *The Guide to Implemented Model Standards,* it was argued that APEX*PH* improves the public health infrastructure in the community by enhancing the community's capacity to perform the core functions of assessment, policy development, and assurance.[20] PATCH was seen more as a generic planning and implementation tool geared toward chronic diseases prevention and health promotion programs. The guide recommended that a community choose either APEX*PH* or PATCH but not both, although there are overlaps and connections between the two methodologies. Today, the advice would be to use MAPP. The model standards process is oriented toward the health priorities for the nation, and model standards are organized into four categories within each of the 22 priority areas of *Healthy People 2000:* health status, risk reduction, services and protection, and community surveillance. In essence, the model standards approach creates a blueprint (with extensive fill-in-the-blank forms) for addressing the health priorities at the local level. The integration of APEX*PH*, MAPP, or PATCH with the model standards approach would provide a comprehensive tool for discovering what a community needs to reach its goals.

An interesting extension of the model standards approach was presented in a report by Randolph and Ford.[21] A model standards work group worked with the model standards project staff to design and review community strategies for public health. The strategies were developed for the purpose of training staff to involve the community in the model standards process. A series of steps for "putting it all together" was also constructed. The first step is to choose the head of a lead agency to serve as coordinator of activities and meetings, collector and disseminator of data and information, and overall moderator and reporter for each of the various activities. The local health department head should take on this leadership role if possible. The role will allow the health department head to help improve public health in the community by:

- aiding the community in the assessment of local health problems by using health education methods
- establishing appropriate laws, regulations, and policies to protect the health of the public
- establishing and maintaining practice standards that encourage public confidence
- involving community residents in the planning of community-wide programs
- developing partnerships through linkage with the state health department and other local government agencies also involved in activities related to public health
- developing community resources to address problems
- acting as a trustee and guarantor (leadership roles) that the health needs of the public are being addressed
- encouraging flexibility in the development, adaptation, and elimination of programs based on the health needs of the community
- following the 11 steps for implementing the model standards[22]

The model standards project attempts to integrate the various assessment procedures. All three assessment methodologies are oriented toward collecting health status information about the residents of a community. They all require public health leaders to implement the assessment process. They just do it in different ways. The role of public health leaders in any kind of assessment is to:

- lead the community assessment process
- use health information data in decision making
- carry out the assessment using one of the assessment methodologies
- communicate the assessment results to the community

The major limitation of model standards is that it was not updated for the 21st century. This is not to say that the protocol could not be adapted for MAPP and other new assessment approaches. As new strategies develop, there is a tendency to ignore the strengths of previous approaches.

## Other Assessment Approaches

Assessment is one of the major responsibilities of public health. The public health system is organized to provide needed programs and services, and public health leaders therefore constantly look for innovative assessment techniques that can help gauge community health status. This section discusses several assessment techniques that can be used in conjunction with the methodologies described above.

Since the mid-1980s, telephone surveys have been conducted in the United States as a means of estimating the prevalence of specific behaviors associated with health problems.[23] For example, telephone survey data have been collected on cigarette smoking, dietary fat intake, level of physical activity and exercise, seatbelt use, and screening tests for early detection of disease. The information obtained has then been used by states to develop state and local health interventions.[24,25]

For instance, a San Francisco study used the behavior risk factor survey to evaluate differences between Latino and non-Latino white adults.[26] Telephone interviews were done with 652 Latinos and 584 non-Latino whites selected by random digit dialing. The researchers found that Latino men and women were less likely to consume alcoholic beverages and consumed fewer drinks per week than non-Latinos. The Latinos were more likely to be sedentary. Latino women were less likely to smoke and to have had a Pap smear or a clinical breast examination than their non-Latino counterparts. The researchers argued that the data showed that health programs targeted at Latinos would be beneficial. They also stressed the importance of providing information in Spanish.

In recent years, the value of community health report cards that provide an overall picture of community health status has been debated. Their advantages are clear. Community health report cards can help public health leaders monitor the overall health of the community in a straightforward way, and if they are written in easy-to-understand language, they provide a means of informing the community of its health status over time.

One type of report card can be created using Comprehensive Assessment for Tracking Community Health (CATCH), a system developed at the University of South Florida School of Public Health.[27] CATCH was used to produce a ranking of community health problems in 11 Florida counties by combining information on more than 200 indicators that was drawn from multiple data sources. The system allows public health agencies to compare their health indicator scores with those of other agencies.

> **Leadership Tip**
>
> *Use the essential public health services model to drive action.*

Trends over time can be identified so that an agency can check its progress in improving community health.

The report card approach has been explored by managed care systems. Both managed care and public health use population-based approaches to health.[28] Both are concerned with the cost of health care. Managed care organizations (MCOs) use population-based assessments of their membership groups to deliver the most cost-effective quality care at the lowest price. Public health professionals are taking leadership roles in the managed care sector, for they have long supported a population-based approach to community health improvement.

The survival of MCOs depends on their evaluating the health needs of their membership. The Health Care Financing Administration and private health care systems use Health Plan Employer Data and Information Set (HEDIS) to compare the quality of care delivered by health maintenance organizations. HEDIS, which monitors the effectiveness of care provided, is essentially an assessment tool. Some MCOs use a life care plan model oriented toward helping members increase their health potential by stressing prevention, wellness, better management of chronic conditions, and increased personal responsibility for health.[29] MCOs also conduct market research to determine whether their services are perceived to be of high quality, and they assess their programs to see if the programs reflect their mission.

MCOs and public health agencies both engage in some of the same monitoring and assessment activities.[30] They both do health risk assessments, community health assessments, health policy assessments, health systems assessments, and comparative analyses of populations and systems; they also both monitor adherence to quality standards, health outcomes, planning effectiveness, and cost-effectiveness. Leadership is critical in all of these activities. Leaders from the public and private sectors need to develop partnerships to create integrated systems of assessment and care in communities.

Attempts have been made to build leadership activities directly into the assessment process. The Healthy Communities approach is an example. The goal is to foster healthy lifestyle choices by community residents from birth to death and to share the responsibility for community health among residents, public health practitioners, and community leaders.[31] The community as a whole explores health issues in detail, and the dialogues between community residents and public health practitioners are part of an overall community assessment. Communities that have implemented the Health Communities approach may use any of the assessment techniques discussed previously.

In assessing the health status of a community, public health leaders:

- use national databases when appropriate
- coordinate the use of assessment techniques in the public and private health care sectors
- explore the pluses and minuses of regularly released community report cards
- explain community health report cards to the community
- work to integrate HEDIS with public health assessment techniques so as to better identify the needs of the community

## Public Health Informatics

Assessment depends on data collection and the use of information system techniques, and therefore public health leaders need to know how to design data collection activities, employ the latest information technologies, interpret data, translate data into useful information, and build data systems that utilize an evidence-based approach. Public health informatics is a new specialty designed to give leaders the necessary knowledge to perform these tasks.[32]

Public health informatics uses analytical tools such as meta-analysis, risk assessment, economic evaluation, public health surveillance, expert panels, and consensus conferences. It also uses new tools associated with geographic information systems (GISs). GISs are user-friendly data representations (in the form of spatial maps) that provide leaders with information on health risks, underlying causes of disease transmission, and the effectiveness of public health interventions and can demonstrate needed structural changes in the health system at the community level.[33]

Data are the raw facts of public health. Collected according to objective criteria, they tend to be quantitative in nature, although there is increasing support for collecting qualitative information, which can sometimes provide especially deep insights into public health issues. Information is processed data.[34] The translation of usable quantitative data into useful information involves computer-related information technology.[35] Qualitative information may also be computer analyzed, but such information often takes the form of stories, focus group findings, or anthropologic field materials. Public health leaders use information to inform and educate the public, make decisions, develop policy, and implement appropriate public health interventions.

Following are six principles that pertain to the use of information systems by public health leaders:[36]

- Public health leaders need to use data from two different data systems. One data system reports on the delivery of direct services and on program encounters (e.g., a case management meeting or a home visit). The second system collects population-based data.
- Public health leaders need to remember that people are complex, integrated beings but that programs are fragmentary (i.e., each program focuses on just one part of the whole person).
- Leaders need to advocate for information that integrates different types of data so that they can better understand the health concerns of community residents.
- Public health consumers must get something back from data collectors. They need to know why data are being collected and must be given feedback.
- Data systems need to be flexible and should be designed to meet the needs of local health leaders as they monitor the health of community residents.
- Information systems need to be compatible so that leaders can access different data sources using just one computer. (The Internet is becoming a very useful data source for public health leaders because all the data on Web sites are accessible by anyone with Internet software.)
- Public health leaders need to respect confidentiality. The public wants to be assured that personal information will be kept private.

Because public health draws data from multiple sources, including sources from different disciplines, public health leaders need to understand the different perspectives of the various professions and learn how to synthesize data from different sources. Information science, computer science, and computer technology are advancing, and public health leaders need to keep up with the changes. Leaders may not be personally responsible for data collection, but they must be able to define the data they need to make effective policy decisions. They must also be involved in the development and design of the information system.

An interesting example of cooperative sharing of information is the community health status indicators project supported by NACCHO, the Association of State and Territorial Health Officials, and the Public Health Foundation. The goal of the project has been to regularly provide community-specific public health data reports to local public health leaders in counties across the United States. The reports have included information on actual causes of death, risk factors for premature death, access to care, preventive services use, and county demographics. They also summarize health measures and compare data from counties with similar demographics. The profiles were removed from the Health Resources and Services Administration Web site in October 2002, but are available from the Public Health Foundation. Plans are underway to revive the project.[37]

Another example was the CDC's Information Network for Public Health Officials (INPHO). INPHO had several goals, including improving communication among public health leaders throughout the United States, increasing the accessibility of information, and utilizing information technology to expedite the exchange of information.[38] INPHO was tied to a vision of using telecommunication technology to help build public health infrastructure through increased connectivity, increased access to information, and data exchange.[39] The CDC funded several INPHO projects to create networks and investigate the barriers to access within present data systems. During the first decade of the 21st century, partially as a reaction to the events of September 11, 2001, INPHO was replaced by the Public Health Information Network (PHIN) with the redefined mission of being a national network facilitated by the CDC to improve the capacity of the national public health network to use and exchange information electronically. PHIN has standards and technical requirements for information systems based on best practice.[40]

Illinois is one state that has struggled with the issue of how to create useful and integrated information systems. Case Study 8-B, a review of the early history of the development of the Illinois Cornerstone project, describes the development of an integrated system for providing information on maternal and child health (MCH) to health professionals. Public health leaders need information if they are to positively affect the communities that they serve. To ensure they receive the necessary information, they should:

- take training courses in informatics
- learn techniques for the collection of health status indicators
- learn how to interpret data and turn them into useful information
- learn how to access information on the Internet
- explore different analytical tools for better understanding data
- utilize quantitative and qualitative information
- become involved in the development of information systems
- integrate conflicting data systems

---

### Case Study 8-B
### Cornerstone: Illinois's Approach to Service Integration

*James R. Nelson*

**Background**
As federal and state governmental agencies became more involved in community health services, funding was increasingly offered through grants for specific diseases and other public health issues. Over a 20-year period, this funding approach resulted in numerous discreet, single-purpose programs, each with its own reporting requirements and information system. Unintended consequences of this phenomenon were fragmented, episodic, and incomplete service delivery; repetitive registration processes; redundant data collection and reporting; nonstandard assessments; incomplete understanding of clients' service history; and inconsistent documentation of

services. Fundamentally, the core functions of public health—assessment, policy development, and assurance—were undermined by the continued proliferation of discreet and separate services.

Recognizing the significance and extent of discreet service delivery, the Illinois Department of Public Health, and now the Illinois Department of Human Services, moved to integrate the services of several health programs. At the heart of the issue was the need for a mechanism that would facilitate and encourage service integration and, ultimately, improve the health outcomes of Illinois residents. After considerable research and development, as well as the active participation of a diverse group of health care and human service providers, the department implemented a package of tools that redesigned community service delivery into an integrated system of care. That package of tools was Cornerstone.

At the beginning of the process, in 1992, the department offered several different MCH programs. These included Women, Infants, and Children (WIC); Healthy Moms/Healthy Kids; EPSDT; pediatric primary care; immunizations; Families with a Future; Drug Free Families with a Future; Parents Too Soon, a teen pregnancy program; and a prenatal smoking cessation program. Statewide, 173 WIC clinics, 104 Healthy Moms/Healthy Kids agencies, 115 immunization sites, and 91 primary pediatric care programs offered services. At that time, several data systems supported the information needs of many of these programs, including the following:

*A statewide WIC system developed in 1989.* This system operated on a personal computer (PC) based network, using a mainframe for support. The system automated the nutritional risk assessment and food coupon issuance functions of the WIC program.

*A case management information system (CMIS) originally developed for the Medicaid-eligible client population.* The CMIS was a PC-based, batch-oriented system for which data were entered locally and submitted for update on disk via mail.

*An HM/HK case management system.* The system had limited functionality and insufficient hardware resources.

*Distributed immunization databases.* As an enhancement to the WIC system, several screens specific to immunization history and current status were created. The immunization data were collected locally and not compiled into a central registry.

The selection of Chicago as a federal Healthy Start Infant Mortality Reduction project site provided an opportunity for Illinois to initiate an integrated information system to support greater coordination, standardization, and sharing of information among community health programs. The requirement of the Healthy Start project to design an information system for collecting evaluation data was also viewed as a way to integrate MCH-related information systems that were not integrated with respect to clients or front-line practitioners and thus led to duplicative intake processes and information collection.

The development of the integrated information system was approached from several key philosophical points of reference. First, to the extent that potential system users were invested in the system from its inception, they would be more likely to use it. Second, to the extent that system developers understood program service delivery, they would better be able to customize it to provider needs. To facilitate this understanding, an individual with a social sciences background served as a liaison between service providers and technical staff during the design process.

An executive steering committee was formed to facilitate planning and ensure diverse representation and contributions to the project. The committee included

*(continues)*

**Case Study 8-B** *continued*

representatives from the then state Departments of Public Health; Alcohol and Substance Abuse; Public Aid; Mental Health and Developmental Disabilities; and Children and Family Services as well as advocates and members of the provider community. The committee met frequently, and several subcommittees and standing committees were responsible for addressing specific areas, such as legal issues, local implementation, program implementation, system support, and funding. As many as 40 individuals participated in the committee work and reviewed the project design.

### Cornerstone

One result of these efforts was Cornerstone. A management information system, Cornerstone supported a case management framework that ensures delivery of prenatal care, well-child visits, nutrition products and education, and immunizations in over 300 separate locations across the state. Its design capitalized on the original WIC service delivery and information system. Cornerstone's features included combined registration, standardized risk assessment, automated care plan development, and consolidated referral and scheduling. Demographic and eligibility information specific to a client was captured once and shared with all other service providers that used the system when caring for the client. The system also provided a client's service history to the various providers responsible for that client. Following is a brief overview of the systems features from the perspective of a system user.

### Registration

When registering a client, a case manager checked the client's enrollment status by searching a locally based statewide index. In this checking process, the case manager could have used the client's identification numbers assigned through Medicaid, WIC, or other community health programs. Potential matches were pulled into the local system and displayed. If no match was found, the case manager enrolled the client and created a Cornerstone participant identification number. During the matching process, the case manager also obtained critical client information through the system (e.g., previously identified medical problems, MCH program status, and contact information).

### Assessment

During an assessment interview, case managers accessed a table of standardized questions designed to assess a client's medical and/or psychological/social risk and prompt either "yes" or "no" or numeric responses. The system compared the responses to a table of normative values for that assessment type, generating a list of goals and recommended services. For example, a "yes" response to the question "Are you pregnant?" automatically generated the goal of adequate prenatal care and a list of recommended services (i.e., prenatal care, prenatal education, WIC, and prepared childbirth education).

### Goals

The risk factors were linked to a set of goals associated with specific services and outlined a recommended care plan. The case manager reviewed the goals and services for appropriateness and had the option, based on professional judgment, to modify these recommendations. The care plan highlighted two dimensions: (1) adult/child services that incorporated MCH elements, prenatal care, well-child care, and injury prevention and (2) a risk assessment that included information on transportation, child care needs, and other requirements.

## Activities and Services

Based on the care plan, a tickler file generated a list of activities and services requiring follow-up or monitoring. To facilitate the referral process, the system offered a localized provider database organized by type of service. The case manager could have selected services based on provider address, volume, or client preference. Provider selection was linked to the client record and documented in the care plan, reminding case managers to follow up to ensure receipt of services.

## Referral and Scheduling

Scheduling within a clinic consisted of matching the client's service needs with the available internal and external providers. The case manager accessed the family's schedule to coordinate all appointments.

Cornerstone technical architecture was based on a PC local area network (LAN) that supported activities in the community health services clinic. The activities, particularly the ones that relied on information sharing between various program providers, were supported by a technical architecture consisting of LANs, wide area networks (WANs), and the state's central computing operation. The LANs supported 2 to 30 workstations (one for each case manager) per service location. Locally collected client information was transmitted to the state nightly for central processing. The WAN enabled local agencies to share appropriate data about clients among themselves. Access to WAN data was accomplished through a "read-only" mode; it can be read but not modified. Access was available on an as-needed basis and was accomplished by a function (or "hot") key built into specific screens. This protocol ensured the autonomy of agency operations in the event of a WAN failure.

As designed, the system consisted of approximately 150 screens and generated as many pre-established reports. It was written in FoxPro, a DOS-based software language, and utilized pulldown menus.

The development and design work was completed in 1995. In May of that year, the long process of installing the system in 300 service locations began. The Healthy Start agencies served as pilot sites where the software and installation processes were tested, reviewed, and documented. The enormousness of deploying Cornerstone across the state—which entailed supplying, installing, and maintaining equipment; providing training on system procedures; and encouraging local program providers unaccustomed to the intricacies of an integrated computer system to accept the new system—prompted a partnership with the Illinois Primary Health Care Association (IPHCA). The association was uniquely qualified for this partnership role because of its widely recognized role as advocate for community health services in Illinois. For the next two years, until December 1997, IPHCA worked side by side with state staff to install over 3,000 computer workstations in 300 locations.

The development of Cornerstone represented an effective response to a situation that was weakening the core functions of public health. Community-based programs provided in a discreet fashion were making uniform assessment, systemwide policy development, and accurate assurance nearly impossible. Underlying Cornerstone's development were a series of guiding principles that in the end ensured the system's successful deployment. These principles included the desirability of listening to diverse viewpoints through a process of inclusion; the benefits of forging partnerships among those involved in service delivery; the interrelatedness of health care problems and social service needs; the necessity of comprehensive solutions rather than

*(continues)*

**Case Study 8-B** *continued*

"bandage" remedies; and the need to promote service integration wherever possible. By adhering to such principles and by incorporating modern technology, the department has operationalized a model that strengthens community health management through efficient and optimal use of available information.

As of 2008, Cornerstone, which is now housed in the Illinois Department of Human Services, is installed in over 3,000 workstations in over 380 sites throughout Illinois. Cornerstone coordinates the delivery of integrated services to over 3,500,000 people. This system is the largest distributed health information system in the United States and has won numerous awards for its innovations.

## Summary

This chapter discussed the key elements of the core function of assessment. It began by describing the assessment process and then went on to consider three assessment methodologies, APEX*PH*, MAPP, PACE-EH, PATCH, and the now-dated model standards approach. These several methodologies, though they overlap, are not mutually exclusive, and elements from all can be combined. Other assessment methodologies were then discussed but not in as much detail. Finally, the chapter considered public health informatics, which involves the collection of data and the use of information system techniques to turn the data into information.

### Discussion Questions

1. What is the relationship among the assessment core function, organizational practices, essential public health services, and performance indicators?
2. What leadership skills are needed for community assessment activities?
3. Why does assessment start the change process?
4. What are the three parts of the APEX*PH* process?
5. Compare and contrast APEX*PH* and MAPP.
6. What is PACE-EH?
7. What are the five phases of the PATCH process?
8. What role can model standards play in evaluation?
9. What are community health report cards?
10. What is public health informatics?

### Exercise 8-1: The Trainerville Gang

*Purpose:* to assess a potential community health problem utilizing community groups

*Key concepts:* assessment, board of health, community advisory board, data protocols

*Procedure:* Trainerville is a small city of 100,000 on the Mentor River in the northwestern United States. There are 10,000 children under the age of 10.

There are also 10,000 young people between the ages of 11 and 18. Citizens have reported that there is a gang presence in the community. Data on gangs are not currently available unless a gang member gets arrested.

Mayor John Snow asked the Trainerville Health Department to develop strategies for getting data on gangs in the community. The director of the health department convenes a community health advisory group to work with him on the mayor's request. The charge to the group is to assess the extent of the gang problem in Trainerville.

Divide into groups of 5 to 10. Each group will develop strategies for determining the extent of the problem in the community. Each group will then present its assessment protocol to the Trainerville Board of Health. The Board of Health includes a representative from each of the groups. The board will then select the protocol that they think will best assess the gang problem. Because the open meetings act is operative, all group members can attend the deliberations and offer citizen comments.

# References

1. J. McKnight, *The Careless Society* (New York: Basic Books, 1995).
2. McKnight, *The Careless Society.*
3. K. G. Keppel and M. A. Freedman, "What Is Assessment?" *Journal of Public Health Management and Practice* 1, no. 2 (1995): 1–7.
4. L. Novick, "Public Health Assessment in a New Context," *Journal of Public Health Management and Practice* 1, no. 2 (1995): v.
5. P. C. Nasca, "Public Health Assessment in the 1990s," *Journal of Public Health Management and Practice* 1, no. 2 (1995): vii–viii.
6. Keppel and Freedman, "What Is Assessment?"
7. Keppel and Freedman, "What Is Assessment?"
8. B. J. Turnock et al., "Implementing and Assessing Organizational Practice in Public Health," *Public Health Reports* 109, no. 4 (1994): 478–484.
9. *Assessment Protocol for Excellence in Public Health* (Atlanta: Centers for Disease Control and Prevention and National Association of County and City Health Officials, 1991).
10. http:/mapp.naccho.org
11. http:/mapp.naccho.org
12. M. W. Kreuter, "PATCH: Its Origin, Basic Concepts, and Links to Contemporary Public Health Policy," *Journal of Health Education* 23, no. 3 (1992): 135–139.
13. Centers for Disease Control and Prevention, "PATCH: Planned Approach to Community Health," draft (Atlanta: Centers for Disease Control and Prevention, 1994).
14. Centers for Disease Control and Prevention, "PATCH: Planned Approach to Community Health."
15. A. Steckler et al., "Summary of a Formative Evaluation of PATCH," *Journal of Health Education* 23, no. 3 (1992): 174–178.
16. American Public Health Association, *Healthy Communities 2000: Model Standards,* 3rd ed. (Washington, DC: American Public Health Association, 1991).
17. American Public Health Association, *Healthy Communities 2000: Model Standards.*

18. American Public Health Association, *Healthy Communities 2000: Model Standards.*

19. American Public Health Association, *The Guide to Implemented Model Standards* (Washington, DC: American Public Health Association, 1993).

20. American Public Health Association, *The Guide to Implemented Model Standards.*

21. S. Randolph and J. Ford, *Community Strategies for Health: Fitting in the Pieces* (Washington, DC: American Public Health Association, 1994).

22. Randolph and Ford, *Community Strategies for Health.*

23. L. M. Anderson et al., "Design and Use of the Behavioral Risk Factor Surveillance System," *Illinois Morbidity and Mortality Quarterly* 1, no. 3 (1994): 16–23.

24. J. M. Bacon et al., "A Consortium Approach to Local Behavioral Risk Factor Assessment," *Illinois Morbidity and Mortality Quarterly* 1, no. 3 (1994): 1–3.

25. J. I. Staff and J. Zimmerman, "Adams County Behavioral Risk Factor Survey Project," *Illinois Morbidity and Mortality Quarterly* 1, no. 3 (1994): 9–11.

26. E. Prez-Stable et al., "Behavioral Risk Factors: A Comparison of Latinos and Non-Latino Whites in San Francisco," *American Journal of Public Health* 84, no. 6 (1994): 971–976.

27. J. Studinicki et al., "A Community Health Report Card: Comprehensive Assessment for Tracking Community Health (CATCH)," *Best Practices and Benchmarking in Healthcare* 2, no. 5 (1997): 196–207.

28. L. Potts et al., *The Growth of Managed Care* (Washington, DC: Association of Schools of Public Health, 1998).

29. K. Jennings et al., *Changing Health Care* (Santa Monica, CA: Knowledge Exchange, 1997).

30. Potts et al., *The Growth of Managed Care.*

31. T. Norris and L. Howell, *Healthy People in Healthy Communities: A Dialogue Guide* (Chicago: Coalition for Healthy Cities and Communities, 1998).

32. A. Friede et al., "Public Health Informatics: How Information Age Technology Can Strengthen Public Health," *Annual Review of Public Health* 16 (1995): 239–252.

33. W. L. Roper and G. P. Mays, "GIS and Public Health Policy: A New Frontier for Improving Community Health," *Journal of Public Health Management and Practice* 5, no. 2 (1999): vi–vii.

34. J. K. H. Tan, *Health Management Information Systems* (Gaithersburg, MD: Aspen Publishers, 1995).

35. Friede et al., "Public Health Informatics."

36. J. R. Lumpkin, "Six Principles of Public Health Information," *Journal of Public Health Management and Practice* 1, no. 1 (1995): 40–41.

37. http:/phf.org/research.htm

38. E. L. Baker et al., "CDC's Information Network for Public Health Officials (INPHO): A Framework for Integrated Public Health Information and Practice," *Journal of Public Health Management and Practice* 1, no. 1 (1995): 43–47.

39. E. L. Baker and J. Porter, "Practicing Management and Leadership: Creating the Information Network for Public Health Officials," *Journal of Public Health Management and Practice,* 11, no. 5 (2005): 469–473.

40. http:/www.cdc.gov/phin

# CHAPTER 9

# LEADERSHIP AND
# POLICY DEVELOPMENT

> Leaders are willing to take the blame.
> William Foege, speech to Public Health Leadership Society

Through assessment activities, public health leaders evaluate the community's health status and identify health problems and risks that need to be addressed. The task they next face is to determine how to deal with the identified problems and risks. The activity of devising effective courses of action (or plans) for problem resolution and risk reduction is known as "policy development," and it constitutes the second core function of public health. The final task is to implement the policies that have been designed. This task is known as "assurance," because by implementing effective policies and enforcing laws and regulations, public health leaders help to ensure the health of community residents.

All state health departments are involved with policy formulation at some level. State health department activities related to policy development include health planning; policy analysis; and the setting of regulations, standards, health objectives, and disaster and emergency public health procedures. Peripheral activities include building coalitions, empowering community organizations, and determining health priorities.

In his 1991 presidential address to the American Public Health Association (APHA) , William Keck argued that the public health community must change its thinking about policy if it is ever to meet the health needs of the American public.[1] The public health community has tended to let market forces and political expediency shape American public health policy rather than look for techniques for maximizing health status. Keck also claimed that American political leaders have a responsibility to develop sound public health policies for the nation. When they fail in their responsibility, they must be held accountable. Methods must be found for getting our leaders to move in different directions. Finally, Keck emphasized the importance of creating linkages between academics, practitioners, and the public in order to empower communities to assess their health status and set health priorities and in order to foster community-based demands for humane decision making.

In her 1992 APHA presidential address, Joyce Lashof stated that public health has made its greatest advances through its commitment to the common good and its strong support for the principles of social justice.[2] Despite these commitments, progress has been erratic, and there continue to be disparities in the health status of socioeconomically, racially, and ethnically diverse communities. The American economic policies of the 1980s and early 1990s have made these disparities worse. Lashof also said that health reform is needed in our society to improve its record in the areas of health promotion, health protection, and disease prevention.

In order to put the issue of policy formulation in perspective, we can build on the discussion in Chapter 6 and Figure 6-1 on agenda setting. Figure 9-1 graphically shows that the policy-making process begins with the fact that a policy agenda grows out of the agenda-setting activities of public health agencies and their external partners.[3] Out of this collaboration comes an awareness that policy is needed to back up the public health agenda. The policy agenda leads to the necessity of formulating policy. Data are needed to support the proposed policy. It is useful to develop alternative scenarios in order to test public and political reactions to proposed policies. A determination must be made about the need to have politicians create the policy or whether the policy can be made by the public health leader and the public health agency without political intervention. Once the policy is created, it is necessary to develop goals and objectives for the policy. If you think of the new policy as a variation of a vision statement, then the steps involved in the Leadership Wheel will be followed (Figure 7-3). Except for the government

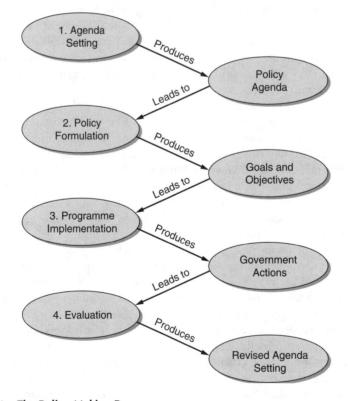

**FIGURE 9-1   The Policy-Making Process**
*Source:* From G. Anderson and P. S. Hussey, "Influencing Government Policy: A Framework," in D. Pencheon, C. Guest, D. Melzer, and J. A. Muir Gray (Eds.), *Oxford Handbook of Public Health Practice* (London: Oxford University Press, 2001). With permission of Oxford University Press.

intervention step, if necessary, in policy development, the Leadership Wheel and the policy-making process are quite similar in that both involve strategic planning and action planning activities.

Exercise 9-1 is an experiment in policy development. It concerns an issue that a local health department and the county board may both have an interest in trying to resolve through the creation of a new policy. Public health departments often recognize potential problems before they become fully mature, giving public health and community leaders the opportunity to deal with the problems before they become unmanageable.

It would be possible for most public health leaders to create a list of the critical policy issues that will face public health over the next 10 years. Table 9-1 lists some of these policy concerns. Social justice and health equity concerns seem always to be critical issues in public health. We fight vigorously to protect the health of the public. Many local health departments struggle with the general issue of access to care and the role of public health in making sure that all residents get the medical care they need. All discussions related to universal health care address access-to-care issues. In order to improve the quality of work of our public health agencies, many discussions are under way about the accreditation of public health agencies. The importance of health issues tied to public health preparedness and response have major policy considerations. How the United States will implement the new International Health Regulations will also affect policy development because the agreement for following these regulations will require state legislation. Certification of public health workers is also a policy concern for the future. The final three issues in the list are also being addressed.

## Institute of Medicine Policy Development Recommendations

In 1988, the Institute of Medicine issued its report *The Future of Public Health*.[4] The report, which listed recommendations regarding policy development, emphasized that public health agencies, in constructing policies, need to balance political realities and professional practice concerns and should always try to serve the interests of community constituents. Agencies also need to provide leadership in policy development, promote the use of scientific knowledge in decision making, and use a strategic planning approach based

**Table 9-1    Selected Public Health Policy Issues**

| |
|---|
| Social justice |
| Access to care |
| Health disparities |
| Accreditation of health department |
| Public health preparedness and response |
| International health regulations |
| Certification |
| Global warming/Environmental health |
| Mental health/Substance abuse |
| Public health systems research |

on the democratic principles. Specific recommendations contained in the report include the following:

1. Public health leaders need to develop relationships and positive partnerships with legislators. They also need to inform politicians and other public officials of the community assessment results. The education of public officials should include an explanation of the strategies being employed by the health department to address health priorities.
2. Agency personnel need to learn the skills of constituency building as well as citizen participation techniques. Citizen involvement in program development needs to be encouraged.
3. It is important to create partnerships between the public health agency leaders, the medical community, and other private sector health entities.
4. Agencies need to cultivate relationships with other professional and citizen groups involved with public health. Such groups might include voluntary health organizations, groups concerned with improving social services, environmental organizations, and economic development organizations.
5. Public health agencies must educate the public on public health issues.
6. Public health agencies need to ensure that the quality of their contacts with grass-roots organizations and community residents is cooperative in nature as well as productive.

The follow-up report on the future of public health pointed to the importance of states taking the lead in policy development.[5] States will need to support the collection of data to better plan for public health programs. States will also need to assure that there are appropriate laws and regulations on the books to support public health programs and activities. State health objectives and workforce development strategies also need to be developed. States need to support the 10 essential public health services throughout their jurisdictions. Local governments also need to carry out the core functions and essential public health services.

## Essential Public Health Services

Three essential public health services are associated with the policy development core function. The first involves informing, educating, and empowering people about health issues. Some potential performance indicators for this service might include the following (adapted from Turnock and his colleagues):[6]

1. The local health department develops social marketing and health communication strategies.
2. The local health department disseminates information to the local media on a regular basis.
3. The local health department provides health information to the residents of its jurisdiction on a regular basis.
4. The local health department informs the public of state and local laws, rules, and regulations.
5. The local health department works with its partners on the development of health education programs.

The second essential service relates to the mobilization of community partnerships. The performance indicators for this essential service include (adapted from Turnock and colleagues):[7]

6. The local health department builds coalitions with community groups.
7. The local health department meets regularly with health-related organizations.
8. The local health department mission is given a public review every five years or less.

The third essential service is the development of policy and plans that support individual and community health efforts. Ten possible performance indicators include the following (adapted and extended from Turnock and colleagues):[8]

9. States need to support leadership development at all levels of the public health system.
10. The local health department prioritizes community health needs based on the size and severity of the needs.
11. The local health department prioritizes needs based on the possible interventions.
12. The local health department takes into account community input when prioritizing needs.
13. States and localities need to track health trends.
14. Consistent policies need to be followed in the development of laws, regulations, and protocols.
15. The local health department develops action plans to address priority health needs.
16. The local health department fosters public participation in the development of the action plans.
17. The local health department incorporates policy analysis into the development of the action plans.
18. The local health department develops a long-range strategic plan that is linked to community action plans.

Policy development guidelines for public health leaders include the following:

- Stress the importance of governance and its implications for the effectiveness of the public health system
- Develop policies that build the core functions and essential services of public health into a community-based public health system
- Learn to share power
- Put policies into action

## The Politics of Public Health Policy

Policy development is a complex process in which the participants consider alternatives for action and decide which alternatives to implement. It is a team process, and many individuals and organizations can be involved, including state and local boards of health, elected officials, community groups, public health professionals, health care providers, and private citizens. Factors that the participants typically need to take into account in their decision making include budgetary considerations; federal, state, and local regulations; and program and organizational operating procedures.

The infrastructure of public health is currently at risk because of the general attack on social and public health programs in Congress and in state legislatures throughout the United States. The discontent with social programs in the United States can be traced back to the 1960s, when many of them were created. Since then, the American public seems to have grown increasingly disenchanted with such programs, largely because of the supposed negative effects of the welfare state as well as doubts about the effectiveness of current programs.[9] There is evidence that the public will no longer tolerate increases in taxation to support health and social programs, including public health programs, and indeed in the mid-1990s public health programs appeared to have come under special assault.

Part of the discontent with federally operated social programs is based on skepticism regarding the competency of the federal government. "Decentralization" was a watchword of the 1990s, and state and local governments took over many programs that had been run by the federal government. On the other hand, part of the discontent is probably based on the idea that social programs act as replacements for traditional groups devoted to problem solving and helping people live better lives.[10] Furthermore, so goes the thinking, social programs, by weakening the authority of traditional groups and encouraging people to become dependent on the government for help, create a demand for more social programs, which foster a higher level of dependency, and on and on in a vicious cycle.

> **Leadership Tips**
>
> *Because most of your work will occur outside the agency with community residents and external stakeholders, make sure you have good managers running the agency.*

It is easy to see the appeal of the view that communities should redefine themselves, re-establish traditional values, and become less dependent on government. Yet it is also easy to see that public health programs are importantly different from other programs. Whereas individuals arguably should assume more responsibility for protecting their own health, surely some type of public health system is necessary to assess terrorism and disasters on health, control health hazards, educate the public about these hazards, and provide population-based services designed to help individuals shed harmful behaviors. Public health leaders need to become advocates for their own agencies and for a population-based approach to health promotion and disease prevention. They also need to distinguish public health programs from other types of social programs and make a strong case that public health programs should be supported no matter what other programs the public chooses to dispense with.

According to one definition, politics is the process of putting the moral consensus of the community into practice.[11] In democratic politics at its best, interested parties discuss the issues face to face, reach a consensus, and develop and implement policies. Yet in this country conflict always enters the picture, because the ideology of self-interest (the American ethic of individualism and search for personal success) is at odds with the strong concern Americans have for promoting and protecting the community. The ideology of self-interest leads to the development of special interest coalitions, and one of the challenges faced by public health leaders is to find ways to promote the community and satisfy special interest groups at the same time.

Among the strategies that can be used to meet this challenge are the following:[12]

- Community leaders and organizations and special interest groups should be involved in policy development.
- The policies developed and implemented should include some that tie together medical care and public health activities. Health promotion is a shared responsibility and calls for interagency collaboration in the pursuit of population-based goals.
- The policies should also include some that will help build a community-oriented continuum of care. Primary prevention programs clearly need to be community based. Examples include programs to reduce the prevalence of lead paint, provide acquired immune deficiency syndrome (AIDS) education, and get people to stop smoking.

Some guidelines related to the politics of public health policy development include:

- Consideration of national health and social policy trends when developing local policies.
- Make a case for the importance of having a governmental public health presence in the community. Moore has called this the process of creating public value.[13]
- Use special public health interest groups in public health policy development.
- Develop integrated and interdependent health and social policies for the community.
- Partner with elected officials to promote public health programs.

## Policy Trends

Policy development, far from being a modern invention, is a universal requirement of community living, and it is affected by the historical circumstances in which it occurs. Many social science theorists have looked at historical trends and studied the social and cultural principles tied to these trends. Indeed, with the coming of the new millennium, there has been increasing interest in understanding where we are and where we are headed.

As discussed in Chapter 6, Alvin Toffler claimed that civilization had undergone three major periods of change, which he referred to as three waves. Assuming that this is a defensible way of looking at human history, the third wave (the information age) will probably be followed by a fourth wave, which, according to Maynard and Mehrtens, will be a period in which humans will attempt to integrate all aspects of life and show an increased concern and sense of responsibility for the whole.[14] People will also attempt to tap into their full range of perceptual and cognitive abilities. The concepts of global stewardship and cultural diversity will grow in importance. Organizations will become strongly oriented toward service, they will become collaborative systems in which power is shared by everyone, and partnership development will be the key to organizational success.[15]

Toffler's theories became extremely influential in the mid-1990s. In early 1995, Newt Gingrich, speaker of the House of Representatives, assigned the recently published *Creating a New Civilization*[16] by Alvin Toffler and Heidi Toffler to newly elected congressional representatives. This book appeared to influence congressional agendas over the next few years, although the prestige of the Toffler model and futures planning seem to have waned recently.

In the preface to *Creating a New Civilization,* Gingrich stated that the present structure of the federal government is tied too closely to the industrialism of the past. The government needs to redefine itself in light of third-wave changes. In his own book, *To Renew America,* Gingrich said that the United States needs to move forward into the information age and to recognize how technology has changed our lives.[17] If the United States does not change the way it does its work, the standard of living of the American people will deteriorate. Whether or not everyone agrees with Toffler's theory of historical waves, no one can escape from the fact that change is a constant.

Furthermore, the way problems are handled changes as the rules of the game change. This means that the field of public health will need to change as well. In all likelihood, the relationship between personal health care issues and population-based services will be expanded and redefined. Some local health departments will become managed care entities. Most public health activities will be team based. The horizontal organization will become a reality, and the old vertical bureaucracies will continue to break down. Community health coalitions will encompass all stakeholders. Public-private partnerships will increase in number, and privatization will become more prevalent. Public health responsibilities will become increasingly decentralized. Public health will be viewed as the community's business, and different groups will take responsibility for different activities. Governance will finally become community-wide, not just limited to the few stakeholders or politicians at the top.

Public health leaders, besides acting as protectors of community values, will need to help the community redefine its values and generate new values that reflect current realities. Political structures will change as more people become involved in political activities. Public health leaders will work in the community more and be less agency-bound than in the past. The community will become stronger and its residents more empowered. Universal access to a multitude of services will be the rule rather than the exception. The quality of life for most people will improve.

In order to increase their understanding of social and economic trends, public health leaders will need to learn the techniques of forecasting. Public health leaders are seen as experts on the health issues of their communities, and public health agency governing boards look to them for guidance on what the future is likely to hold and how to prepare for future developments.

Quantitative forecasting involves applying a set of statistical techniques to present data sets. Statisticians usually do the actual manipulation of numbers. Quantitative forecasting techniques include regression and time series analysis, which can be used to predict public health trends over a period of time and into the future.[18] A regression model mathematically predicts the effect of change in one factor on other factors. For example, immunization compliance for children under two years of age increased during the 1990s. A regression model could help determine the impact of immunization compliance on other health status indicators. Finally, econometric techniques can be used to forecast future program costs.

Qualitative forecasting uses experts to make predictions.[19] One qualitative forecasting method is to survey a number of experts (a so-called opinion jury) and analyze their responses statistically. Another method is to survey clients and evaluate their responses. Reviewing similar case studies to identify trends is a third method. As an example of qualitative forecasting, imagine that a local health department in a rural area is concerned about the potential impact of a new community health center. The health department administrator might hire a consulting organization with expertise in working with primary care organizations and the effects that the entry of a federally qualified health center is likely to have on existing health care, the local public health agency, and social service providers in the community.

Futurists are experts in predicting the future, or at least experts in painting pictures of different possible futures, and considering the scenarios they devise can be helpful for "testing" alternative policies. Public health leaders can see what will be the overall outcome if one policy is chosen and one scenario occurs, if the same policy is chosen and a second scenario occurs, and so on. Together with estimations of the likelihood of the various scenarios, this type of review of different outcomes can help public health leaders make rational decisions as to which policies to implement.

In order to make good policy decisions, public health leaders need to:

- study their community's past from a systems perspective
- understand how local and state public health agencies have affected health outcomes over time
- learn forecasting techniques
- explore national trends and compare them with local and state trends
- apply forecasting techniques in a rational way to best reflect social and economic realities
- develop policies that take cost as well as community values into account
- modify forecasts or develop new ones if new information becomes available

## Advocacy and Empowerment

During the 1970s and 1980s, public health advocacy was viewed as an important tool for social change. The assumption was that people with all types of problems benefited from having professionals speak for them and protect their rights. Public health leaders took on the responsibility of protecting the health of community residents and pushing for the appropriate interventions to be made available to residents facing health problems or health risks. In recent years, the advocacy movement has been criticized for being too paternalistic. Community leaders have argued that they understand their communities better than the health professionals who work there (partly because the latter often live elsewhere). Advocacy without personal community involvement leads to credibility loss within the population supposedly being protected.

Public health leaders have reduced their advocacy efforts not only because they have become frustrated by their inability to gain acceptance within the communities they serve but also because advocacy has been confused with lobbying.[20] Lobbying is an activity pursued by special interests—usually an organization or group of related organizations—in order to influence the enactment or administration of laws. Advocacy is much broader in scope. Advocacy in support of public policy change involves research, policy statement development, action planning, implementation, and evaluation.

Advocacy activities are also to be distinguished from the enforcement of rules and regulations. Advocacy focuses on policy changes necessary to improve the health of the public, not the administration of existing policies. Public health leaders thus need to balance their advocacy efforts, in which there is room for passion, and their enforcement efforts, which should be dispassionate. If they have been successful in building trust and credibility in the local community, they will be able to involve the community in both health regulation and advocacy. One requisite for engaging the community in advocacy for policy changes is to communicate the reasons the changes are necessary.

One disadvantage of advocacy by professionals is that they tend to be oriented toward the weaknesses of the community rather than its strengths.[21] Emphasizing the negatives often leads to fragmented problem solving and partial solutions. In addition, the community's culture, which is typically intertwined with its problems and will have an effect on attempted solutions, is often neglected. Thus, there is a strong argument that people need to become self-advocates and not rely on third parties to protect their interests. Additional support for this conclusion is that policies developed and implemented without community involvement have historically failed. Therefore, at the very least, professional advocacy and community self-advocacy need to be combined. Each group—the professionals and the community residents—brings different strengths to the partnership and contributes to the total impact of the advocacy.

Becoming an effective advocate for health not only protects the health of the advocate, but it can also affect the health of others.

There are five steps to being a successful health advocate:[22]

1. It is necessary to clearly identify whom you want to persuade.
2. It is critical that you know the facts of the issue.
3. It is important to lay the groundwork for advocacy through letters, faxes, or e-mail.
4. It is important to meet the individual you want to persuade—make an appointment.
5. Plan to follow up on your face-to-face meeting.

In a leadership exercise called the elevator speech, you have to deliver your message in a concise manner and do it before the elevator reaches the floor where the person you are trying to influence leaves the elevator.

In their efforts to empower community residents to become self-advocates, public health leaders need to understand that empowerment will not work if it is treated as a fad.[23] Empowerment means that someone will have to give up power and dominance. Public health leaders, by virtue of their skills and their leadership positions in public health organizations, tend to have more prestige as public health advocates and more control than community residents. They need to give up some of their power if empowerment is to occur. Furthermore, empowerment should be system-wide and not restricted to the community leadership. The object is to give all residents in the community a sense that they have some say over public health policy.

There are four aspects to personal empowerment. First, each individual must have a vision for him- or herself and for the local community. Second, the individual needs to identify and manage the other constituencies with which the individual has a relationship. Third, the individual needs to give up a personal wish for dependency on others (this is exceedingly important). Finally, the individual has to have the courage to make the community vision come to life. In empowerment, there is a belief that change is possible and that, through strength, problems will be solved. Empowered people believe that they can make a difference and affect policy decisions.

Table 6-3 presented a list of 10 principles of empowerment that public health leaders can use in their attempts to empower community residents. Public health leaders should also consider taking on a mentoring role in the community. The people they are trying to empower have not, for the most part, exercised power before, at least in the public health area, and they will need guidance as they learn new behaviors.

People to be empowered need to be given authority equal to the responsibilities that they have accepted or that have been assigned to them.[24] Next, they need to learn the appropriate standards of excellence and the skills they must have to meet these standards. Mediocrity is not the goal. Public health professionals and community residents can clearly work together to improve the quality of life, but the residents need information on healthy lifestyles and the skills to bring these healthy lifestyles into reality.

Public health leaders must provide community residents with feedback on the progress they have made toward meeting their goals. They could, for instance, develop a community report card or some other mechanism to report to residents any public health successes and failures. They should also recognize the community's successes in some special way. If the teenage pregnancy rate were to drop significantly in a community, this should be publicized or otherwise specially noted.

The issue of trust plays an important role in community empowerment. Not only must community residents be given the power to make decisions on their own behalf, but they must be trusted to make good decisions. Community leaders often have difficulty recognizing that all residents are entitled to trust. Residents are also entitled to make mistakes. Life includes good decisions as well as bad. Finally, residents have the right to be respected and to be able to maintain their dignity in the community. Public health agencies sometimes struggle to respect these citizen rights fully, especially in situations where cultural diversity is present.

Social and behavioral scientists often wince at the softness of the issues being raised here. A better reaction would be for them to study the advocacy and empowerment process and determine whether empowerment increases the chance of attaining health objectives in a community. They could also investigate whether people with severe mental and physical disabilities, immigrants who do not speak English, homebound individuals, high-risk mothers, chronically ill individuals, persons with AIDS, alcohol or substance abusers, suicide- or homicide-prone individuals, abusive families, or the homeless can become successful self-advocates. These issues need to be studied in order to understand the complexities of empowerment.

Following are advocacy guidelines for public health leaders:

- Build trust and credibility with community constituents.
- Empower others to be advocates.
- Do background research on health issues and draft policy statements in the form of legislative bills.
- Work with elected or appointed officials on the enactment of appropriate legislation.

## Collaboration

Citizen and community empowerment lays the groundwork for the collaboration among organizations, constituencies, and individuals to influence the policy development process. Collaboration can take many forms, and collaborative groups come in many types. Cohen and colleagues identified five.[25] Advisory committees offer suggestions and provide technical assistance to leaders, programs, or organizations. Commissions are usually composed of citizens appointed by official bodies. (The problem with commissions is that the appointments are often political.) Consortia (or alliances) are semi-official in nature. They tend to have broad policy-oriented goals and may cover large geographic areas. A single consortium may include several coalitions. Networks, which are fairly loose in organization, are created for the purpose of resource or information sharing. Finally, task forces are short-lived groups created to address a specific issue.

For our purposes, we will divide collaborative groups into coalitions, which are loosely structured; alliances, which are structured around a specific organizational agenda; and partnerships, which are highly structured (and often contractual). Each type of collaborative group is discussed in turn.

### Coalitions

A coalition is the coming together of people and organizations to influence outcomes related to a specific problem or set of problems.[26] The synergism of joint action allows a coalition to accomplish a broader array of goals than could the participants acting on their own. (See Chapter 6 for a discussion of the importance of coalitions for the assessment core function. Table 6-4 presents an eight-step approach to coalition building.)

The collaborative relationship that sometimes forms among a public health agency, other health and human service-related organizations, and various community constituencies is typically coalition-like.[27] Such coalitions are created to get the organizations and constituencies involved in addressing community health needs and issues. They tend to be less structured than other types of collaborative groupings, and participants move in and out of the coalition as situations and priorities change.

To establish a coalition, a public health agency must make use of a number of strategies, including the following three.[28] First, it needs to establish a dialogue on health service delivery and policy with possible partners. Second, it needs to create a pool of groups willing to collaborate on the resolution of public health issues. This pool might include:

- at-risk groups affected by the health issues
- allies with whom the agency shares common interests
- experts knowledgeable about the issues
- associates that the agency works with on a day-to-day basis
- opposition groups that may challenge agency positions on the issues
- third-party groups indirectly affected by the issues
- state and local government officials who have influence on public policy
- media organizations

Third, the agency needs to establish a communication network for the purpose of exchanging information. Communication is essential for promoting the coalition and mobilizing the members to take action to meet the community's health needs, which is, after all, the whole purpose of creating the coalition.

Coalitions have several significant advantages:[29]

- A coalition can conserve resources, because the participants cooperate in promoting the coalition's agenda and avoid duplication of efforts.
- A coalition is an excellent communication tool, because its member organizations can send out its message to many more people than any single organization can.
- A coalition, through synergy, can achieve more objectives than could the participant organizations acting alone. For example, it possesses greater power to influence political decision makers.
- A coalition has a credibility advantage over its individual members. There is clearly strength in numbers.
- A coalition provides a mechanism for sharing information. For instance, one coalition member can provide information to others not able to attend a meeting, and the entire coalition or individual members can develop releases to provide to the media.
- A coalition typically has a lead agency that most of the coalition members provide with advice, guidance, and direction. In the case of public health coalitions, the lead agency is usually the local health department or public health agency.
- A coalition helps the representatives from member organizations by improving their self-esteem, giving them personal satisfaction, and developing their understanding of their organizations' roles in improving the health of the public.
- Finally, a coalition can foster cooperation among the members and can strengthen the community by concentrating on the community's strengths.

On the downside, a public health coalition takes some effort to sustain. Over time, the community and the community's health needs will change, and the coalition must change in concert. In addition, conflicts over turf occasionally occur, and schisms within the coalition can make it more difficult to deal with public health issues than if the coalition did not exist.

## Alliances

A community health alliance is a group of health care and public health organizations that have combined forces to address key public health risks and problems for the population of a specific geographic area.[30] Although the participating organizations may benefit from the alliance, the purpose of the alliance is to meet the needs of the community residents. A community health alliance might include the local public health agency, health care providers, payers, purchasers of services, advocacy groups, community social service agencies, and neighborhood groups.

Alliances can be divided into three types.[31] An opportunistic alliance is created to increase the knowledge and expertise of organizations in a new field of operation. This new information may be used to develop a new type of program in a community. For example, a local public health agency may collaborate with a number of health maintenance organizations to learn how their managed care programs work and then use this information to develop a Medicaid managed care program of its own.

A resource dependency alliance is created to provide a needed service or resource for multiple health care organizations. For example, a local health department may agree to immunize all children less than two years of age in the community, preventing other health care organizations from having to develop immunization programs.

A stakeholder alliance is developed by organizations willing to work together to achieve a common objective. For example, the alliance members may jointly develop a trauma registry to better document trauma-related problems in the community.

## Partnerships

In the early 1990s, partnership became a favored type of collaborative relationship. The partnering process requires each partner to show respect for the other partners and put personal or organizational agendas aside. The partners, whether from the public or private sector, treat each other as equals. That means that all partners engage as equals in the decision-making process. In an effective partnership, the partners share a vision, are committed to the integrity of the partnership, agree on specific goals, and develop a plan of action to accomplish the goals. A partnership may have a partnering agreement, which is like a contract, to guide its activities.

## An Example

Case Study 9-A looks at a coalition created to develop a policy on leaf burning. Parents of asthmatic children, county public officials, and concerned citizens wanted an ordinance passed that would restrict leaf burning in the county, and by working together they were able to achieve their goal, although not all members of the coalition were perfectly happy with the regulations resulting from their efforts.

To promote the public health agenda, public health leaders should:

- identify potential collaborators among community organizations
- engage in discussion with potential collaborators to determine whether enough commonality of interest exists to justify creating a coalition, alliance, or partnership
- for each collaborative relationship, establish goals that all parties in the relationship are committed to achieving
- use the type of collaborative relationship that is most appropriate for addressing the issues of concern
- show respect for the other members of a collaborative relationship

---

## Case Study 9-A
## Leaf-Burning Policy

*Helene Gottesmann and Michael Tryon*

### Background
Previous leaf-burning legislation in Acorn state had neither been enforced properly nor validated by the courts. In 1974, the Tree County board approved the Nuisance Section of the County Public Health Ordinance, which limited open burning only when adverse health effects could be demonstrated. This was hard to enforce. The state of Acorn also had an open-burning law for counties over 400,000, which was challenged in the courts in 1986, after which any municipality could burn. The state environmental protection agency's stance was that open burning was a local decision. Until January 1995, one could burn any kind of landscape anywhere in the unincorporated areas of Tree County as close as 25 feet from neighboring houses.

### Health Effects of Leaf Burning
The ban on the disposal of yard waste in landfills in 1990, the subsequent increasing costs of solid waste disposal, and an increase in the county population have all contributed to the increased air pollution in Tree County. Air pollution accounts for as many as 60,000 deaths a year. Open leaf burning has been established as a significant source of air pollution and causes a significant increase in carbon monoxide levels, hydrocarbons, and total suspended particulates, which are injurious to the population.

Open leaf burning represents a significant health hazard for asthmatics and other high-risk groups—newborn infants, children, the elderly, and people with chronic respiratory, cardiovascular, and allergy problems. In 1986 and 1987, in Tree County, respiratory diseases, such as emphysema, bronchitis, and asthma, became the third leading cause of death, while they were the fourth leading cause of death in the United States. Bronchitis and asthma were the second leading causes of hospitalization in the 0–14 age group in Tree County during the same time period.

In the fall of 1991, a 14-year-old girl died as a result of an allergic reaction to leaf burning. The following February, another young girl died from asthma when moldy

*(continues)*

**Case Study 9-A** *continued*

yard waste from the previous fall was being burned. During this same season, another child almost died of an asthmatic attack after being exposed to the smoke from burning leaves and had to live with relatives in another town until the air cleared. With support and facts from other parents of asthmatic children in neighboring towns with leaf-burning bans, parents attended several Smokey village board meetings to express their worries about the health hazards of open burning. As a result, in the fall of 1992 a total burn ban was passed by one vote after it was vetoed by the village president. Simultaneously, another parent with an asthmatic child in the neighboring town of Ashes went to her village board with a packet of information concerning the health hazards of leaf burning. The board decided to form a committee to investigate the issue. Not taking no for an answer, mothers continued attending village meetings, networking, and educating the community about the health hazards of leaf burning. Parents also received TV and news coverage.

### Coalition Building
Frustrated by the lack of action by the village board, in the spring of 1992 the concerned parents from Ashes and neighboring towns formed a coalition. In October, the Ashes village board said they wanted to wait 5 to 10 years to investigate and decide the matter.

In the response to this, the coalition circulated a petition and wanted a burning ban by the state pollution control board. "Please don't burn your leaves" fliers were distributed. In November 1992, the burning ban failed. The coalition grew larger, began publishing a newsletter, and called a meeting to devise a plan of action. Individuals from the local and state lung associations and councils, public health workers, emergency department nurses, state and local environmental groups, and lawyers joined forces. The parents received some support from the board of health, which was willing to write letters on their behalf, but it was not known whether the county board members supported the ban and how they stood on the leaf-burning matter.

### Lobbying on the State Level
The coalition felt a policy or law banning leaf burning was needed at the state level because villages and towns with leaf-burning bans were being affected by smoke from unincorporated areas and municipalities without bans. A former state pollution control board member who had received yearly complaints about leaf burning instructed the coalition on how to introduce a state bill. In the spring of 1993, the senate and house introduced a bill against leaf burning that included the 17 counties in Acorn. Dedicated coalition members actively lobbied their senators and representatives. Opponents of the bill tried to kill the legislation, but it finally passed. However, the governor vetoed it in December 1993, claiming it was an "unfunded mandate."

### County Level Involvement
Simultaneously, in 1993 leaf-burning ban activists expressed their concerns not only to local and state officials but also to Tree County board representatives, members of the county board public health services committee, and members of the county board of health. County board members decided not to impose an open-burning restriction on municipalities and the rural areas. Both the board of health and the public health services committee planned to address the leaf-burning issue in the future. The president of the board of health thought the county should launch a massive education effort about the health hazards of leaf burning and alternative disposal methods and start encouraging residents to voluntarily stop burning leaves. The Tree

County public health services committee was scheduled to consider a "voluntary ban," but the politicians said the proposal would be ineffective because it had no enforcement measures. In November 1993, the Tree County public health services committee tabled the issue because the general assembly was considering this legislation. (In the fall of 1993, while parents were in the midst of lobbying the state for a leaf-burning ban, the village of Ashes finally voted to ban leaf burning.)

In January 1994, in response to the governor's veto of the leaf-burning bill in December 1993, lobbyists pressured the county board of health to consider a countywide ban on open burning. In the spring of 1994, the county board of health sought a voluntary burning ban; however, lobbyists against leaf burning continued to pressure board members to oppose it.

**Policy Controversies**

In developing a policy (or ordinance) for leaf burning, the chair of the public health services committee of the county board acted as a bridge between the county board of health and the county board, the legislative body. His main objectives were to build a consensus around the various opinions of the county representatives and develop a balanced policy. In order to develop a balanced policy, the committee needed to consider the following issues: (1) Should grass and other yard waste be included with leaves? (2) What months or days can individuals burn leaves? (3) What educational efforts are needed? (4) What are enforcement alternatives? In addition, the chair wanted to communicate and share his vision of the challenges of a rapidly growing community: "Tree County is the fastest growing county in the state and the issue of open burning will not go away. As the county continues to grow, the issue of open burning will become more serious" (minutes of May 11, 1994, committee meeting).

Policy development and consensus building were done gradually and methodically. The chair of the public health services committee was very specific about steps he had to pursue to accomplish his goal. His first objective was to listen to all conflicting points of view concerning leaf burning before a policy was drafted. For this purpose, the public health services committee held open meetings in the spring and summer of 1994 to obtain the public's input as well as that of the various county officials. In addition, the chair tried to determine what type of ordinance could be passed by the county board by personally talking to every county board member and other significant individuals.

The public health administrator of Tree County health department provided assistance to the public health services committee chair in developing a leaf-burning policy. One goal of the board of health was to reduce respiratory diseases in the county by addressing the issue of open burning. The public health administrator participated in the public meetings held by the public health services committee and presented morbidity and mortality statistics regarding respiratory diseases in the county. He pointed out that the board of health is "an organization that exists in most counties throughout the state for the primary purpose of preventing diseases in the county by addressing the issue of open burning. The board of health had as one of its goals to reduce respiratory disease and disability and improve the health status of the community. In this role, the board of health needs to know what the disease problems are" (minutes of May 11, 1994, committee meeting). In view of this, the provision of epidemiological data becomes critical in policy development.

*(continues)*

### Public Meetings on Leaf Burning

The following section briefly summarizes opposing viewpoints shared at the Tree County board public health services committee public meetings on leaf burning. Developing a policy based on these opposing views was a challenge for the chair of the health services committee and required effective leadership skills.

### Opponents to the Ban

The following are issues raised by those opposed to the leaf-burning ban.

### Big Government versus Individual Freedom

Being one of the most politically conservative counties in the nation, Tree County citizens did not want the government interfering in their lives. They felt that the leaf-burning ban was an "unfunded mandate." The main issue was their right to burn leaves.

### Local versus State Government

If there had to be a ban, individuals felt that it should be imposed locally and not by the county or the state.

### High- versus Low-Density Areas

Individuals felt that the committee needed to differentiate between high- and low-density areas. People were opposed to banning leaf burning in the rural areas or the country because the smoke dissipated before it reached any of the neighbors. Also, unincorporated areas do not have the same waste disposal options as city residents.

### Incorporated versus Unincorporated Areas

The ordinance should not include incorporated areas, only unincorporated areas. Municipalities wanted to decide for themselves.

### Expense of Waste Disposal

Opponents were against the additional cost for waste disposal if leaf burning was banned. Some cities include leaf pickup at no additional cost.

### No Adverse Health Effects

Some opponents did not believe that the smoke from leaf burning had any ill effect. One individual noted that other allergens (such as ragweed) had not been eradicated.

### Proponents of the Ban

The following are issues raised by proponents of the leaf-burning ban.

### Individual Property Rights versus Right to Breathe

Opponents of leaf burning expressed the need to act on behalf of one's fellow humans—and the right to breathe. It was pointed out that the constitution of Illinois requires the government to protect the health, safety, and welfare of the citizens and provide a healthful environment. Therefore, leaf burning, a health hazard, should not be allowed.

### Adverse Health Effects versus No Effect

Citizens with asthma and parents of asthmatic children testified as to the adverse health effects leaf burning has had on their lives and their children's lives. Some opponents of the ban did not believe leaf burning caused asthma and wanted "proof." Medical personnel reported the increasing number of children and adults they treated with respiratory diseases and concluded that a ban on leaf burning would save medical costs as well as lives. It must be noted that some opponents of the ban and their children also had asthma, but apparently they did not feel a ban was necessary.

### County or State Legislation versus a Local Piecemeal Solution

Proponents felt a countywide solution was needed. Though some towns have burning ordinances, people live along borders where leaf burning is allowed. Children may live in one village with a ban but go to a school in a town with leaf burning and are exposed to the air pollution.

### Education or Referendum versus Legislation

Proponents of the leaf-burning ban felt education was extremely important but not a substitute for legislation. They were also against holding a referendum, for they felt people would vote according to their emotions and not the facts.

### Other Burning Issues

The following are some additional concerns expressed at the public meetings on leaf burning.

What kind of waste disposal would there be? How much would it cost and how much responsibility would the county take for doing it? How much would bagging leaves cost? Citizens wanted to be provided with alternatives such as composting, vacuuming of leaves, or collecting leaves for farmers. High schoolers reported that they picked up leaves for free and delivered them to farmers. People wanted to know how the county would respond to complaint calls (the fire department would respond to the calls) and who would enforce the ban. They also wanted to know whether overnight campfires and bonfires would be prohibited.

In May 1994, another open-burning meeting was held by the public health and human services committee of the Tree County board to discover how individual communities and fire districts felt about open-burning regulations. Invited were representatives of the 27 municipalities, 17 townships, and 16 fire districts. The issues brought up were similar to those that had been discussed at the April meeting: assurance of leaf disposal before a ban was enacted and methods of enforcement. Individuals felt that the leaf-burning problem should be resolved by local units of government.

### Consensus Building: Drafting a Balanced Policy

In June 1994, county board members met to discuss and then vote on whether to draft a leaf-burning ordinance. The chair of the public health services committee felt he needed the board to reach a consensus in order to devote staff time and energy to drafting an ordinance. County board members said they wanted options, facts, and documentation of the health effects of leaf burning and of large composting sites. One of the members wanted it stated that the right to clean air had precedence over the right to burn leaves. Another member felt people should be more sensitive to the needs of their neighbors. Some individuals supported extensive educational efforts. A county ban may give locals more control if and when the state passes legislation. County board members voted 19 to 5 for the public health committee staff to draft a balanced policy regulating leaf burning.

At this point, the board was far from a consensus on how to regulate leaf burning. Some board members wanted a total ban, others a partial ban only in the unincorporated areas, and others regulation rather than a ban. They did not want to adopt legislation for municipalities that already had an ordinance. They felt the county could not enforce a ban anyway.

The chair felt he had to resolve the clash of conflicting opinions by means of a compromise. He knew he did not have the votes for a total ban. The committee used

*(continues)*

**Case Study 9-A** *continued*

a conservative approach in formulating the proposal (a "balanced" policy). In order to develop a balanced, integrated policy, the staff addressed the following issues: (1) density (distance between homes), (2) type of waste, (3) disposal alternatives, (4) enforcement, and (5) time of day and year.

In January 1995, the committee presented the following ordinance to the county board for a vote (it passed 13 to 10). It would restrict burning to assigned weekends. The burning ordinance is an amendment of the National Fire Prevention Code, Building Officials and Code Administrators (BOCA) Ordinance. The amendment limits burning of yard waste to weekends between dawn and dusk during the months of October, November, April, and May. Open fires would not be allowed within 30 feet of a structure or within 500 feet of a neighbor's home. The ordinance excluded municipalities.

The leaf-burning policy is an example of governance sharing and collaborative policy development, for three different departments were involved: the health department, the fire department, and the building department. Assurance or enforcement of the BOCA amendment would be provided by all three departments, with the fire department taking the lead. The health department would educate citizens on alternatives to leaf burning and already has a burning ordinance that can ban leaf and yard waste burning if it affects the health of the citizens. The building department would also be responsible for enforcing a fire and safety code that would include the leaf-burning regulation.

The BOCA amendment had a good chance to pass the county board because it is a regulation, not a ban. It provides a mechanism to let people know when the burning is occurring so they can take precautions and adjust their schedules accordingly. The BOCA amendment also exempts municipalities, whereas a public health ordinance would not. A leaf ban would not have passed because the county had no mechanism for leaf pickup. If the chair would have submitted a pickup cost of $75,000, the ordinance would never have passed.

**Conclusion**

In 1993, after the leaf-burning ban was vetoed by the governor, concerned parents and citizens went to the Tree County board and board of health for a countywide ban. The public health services committee of the Tree County board held two open meetings to allow the public to air their opinions on this matter. After receiving the "go ahead" from the county board, the public health services committee researched the matter and developed what it considered was a "balanced" policy on leaf burning.

The parent activists have mixed feelings about this ordinance because it still allows leaf burning on weekends in the fall and spring in densely populated areas. They feel that the regulation should be a health ordinance rather than an amendment to the BOCA (fire) ordinance. The proposed ban treats burning as a fire hazard, not a health hazard. Burning supporters say it was a compromise. The chair says that the BOCA compromise "is the best way of protecting the public by reducing fire hazards without also denying individual property rights." He feels that this is an effective ordinance, because it limits the amount of days leaf burning is permitted.

The coalition has introduced a bill to the state legislature that would give the state pollution control board authority over open burning in the state. Parents say they will continue to try to get stricter measures passed. Concerned citizens have noted the approach used by parents in the Quad Cities, where they plan to argue that local governments that allow leaf burning discriminate against residents with breathing ailments and thus infringe on the Americans with Disabilities Act.

## Priority Setting

The community assessment process ends with the setting of priorities. In fact, priority setting is a link between assessment and policy development, because which policy issues are chosen to be worked on is determined by the priority-setting process.[32]

Setting local public health priorities should be a community-wide activity.[33] The process should include major health agencies, community organizations, key community constituencies, and individuals. Elected and appointed officials will need to put their stamp of approval on the chosen list of priorities, and they might demand changes in the list. For example, public health leaders concerned about an increase in teenage pregnancy in the community may recommend the distribution of condoms in high school clinics. If the community is politically conservative, the condom distribution recommendation may be overridden by elected or school officials.

According to Dever, those engaged in priority setting should follow these eight guidelines:[34]

1. Set realistic goals to maintain credibility.
2. Formulate the goals in understandable terms for the public at large.
3. Set goals that combine process and outcome.
4. Set quantitative and qualitative goals that are able to be evaluated.
5. Evaluate progress toward the achievement of health goals at regular intervals.
6. Set goals that can be pursued in compatible ways across geographic boundaries.
7. Develop techniques to handle data constraints.
8. Set goals that reflect the concerns of all interested parties.

Three other guidelines are worth considering. First, those who are establishing the priorities must determine the magnitude of each problem and the ability of the public health agency to address the problem given the existing staff and budgetary constraints. Second, they must estimate the seriousness of the consequences if the problem was not addressed or only partially addressed. Third, they must decide whether it is feasible to resolve the problem at all.

In the priority-setting process, public health leaders have the responsibility to:

- work with coalitions, alliances, or partnerships
- set health priorities that will be acceptable to elected and appointed officials
- set realistic goals and objectives
- make goals and objectives measurable
- tie action plans to the budget

## Leadership Challenges

Researchers who have investigated the advances in clinical medicine over the past 60 years estimate that only 5 of the 30 years of increase in life expectancy can be tied to clinical breakthroughs.[35] Most of the increase in life expectancy instead is due to changes in public health policy. The last half of the 20th century saw the virtual elimination of polio, the elimination of smallpox, declines in dental decay due to fluoridation in water supplies, and reductions in childhood blood lead levels. If society continues to invest in the public health system, substantial financial savings will accrue, assuming past history is any guide. It is the public health system that prevents epidemics; protects the environment, workplaces, housing, food, and water; promotes healthy behaviors; monitors the health status of the population; mobilizes communities to take remedial action; responds to disasters; ensures the quality, accessibility, and accountability of medical care; reaches out to link high-risk and hard-to-reach people to needed services; performs research to develop new insights and innovative solutions; and leads the development of sound health policy and planning.[36]

Despite the impressive record of achievement by the public health system, financial support for public health programs has recently declined. The result is likely to be an increase in disease and injury—and an increase in health care costs. Major public health problems, including human immuno-deficiency virus (HIV), AIDS, cancer, cardiovascular diseases and stroke, diabetes, teenage pregnancy, substance abuse, and community violence, remain to be dealt with. Following are several examples of the impact that public health agencies, in collaboration with other organizations, can have on public health issues.

**Leadership Tips**

*Keep a leadership journal where you record your personal notes on work-related events. Take notes on articles and books as well.*

Public health professionals have consistently argued that tobacco use is the greatest single preventable cause of premature mortality in the United States.[37] With the harmful effects of tobacco use in mind, the *Healthy People 2000* objectives, reinforced in *Healthy People 2010,* called for the development, enactment, and enforcement of laws prohibiting the sale of tobacco products to adolescents.[38,39] Further, the report stated that in order to reduce access to tobacco by adolescents, vending machine sales should not be allowed.

The tobacco industry fought the *Healthy People 2000* proposals and came up with a proposal for requiring electronic locking devices. In 1990, Forster and colleagues drew a random sample of vending machine locations in St. Paul, Minnesota, where a law mandating the use of locking devices on cigarette vending machines had been passed.[40] The researchers found that the rate of noncompliance by merchants was 34% after three months and 30% after one year. For sites in which a locking device was installed, the purchase rate of cigarette packages from the machines dropped from 86% before the law went into effect to 30% after three months. However, the rate rose again to 48% after one year. The effectiveness of the law deteriorated in all types of businesses over the course of the year. The researchers demonstrated that banning cigarette vending machines, together with other methods to improve compliance, will be necessary in the future. If businesspeople are not committed to a change in policy, its level of effectiveness will be low.

In a second example, a local health advisory board in a small Illinois city decided in 1997 that it was no longer willing to tolerate cigarette vending machines near the local high school. The board recommended a bill to the local city council, which not only agreed with the board but passed a more comprehensive antismoking law. This story indicates how leadership can be required in different places if a policy is to be developed and put into action. It was first needed in the health department (which addressed the question of how to reduce access to tobacco by adolescents), then on the board (which took action on a potentially volatile issue), and then on the city council (which passed a bill that had the potential to be unpopular). In 2006, this town passed a bill to outlaw smoking in restaurants and bars. In January 2008, the entire state of Illinois went smoke-free.

The challenge for public health leaders is to bring different groups in a community together when a critical public health issue needs to be addressed. There are clearly risks involved in trying to influence the political process. The public health community and local, state, and federal governments may have conflicting agendas. Special interest groups often try to undermine the public health agenda through contributions to the political parties as well as by lobbying to prevent a bill from getting passed.

In cases where public health leaders have been instrumental in passing a bill, they need to monitor the effects of the legislation. In 1989, a cigarette tax increase of 25 cents per package went into effect in California, partly because of a public health campaign.[41] Flewelling and colleagues evaluated the impact of this increase one year after its implementation.[42]  Comparing adult per capita consumption data from 1980 to 1989 in California and the United States, they showed that a sharp decline in cigarette consumption in California had occurred at the same time as the tax increase. They concluded that a 5% to 7% decline in consumption was attributable to the tax increase.

The long-term effect of the legislation is, of course, hard to determine. Undoubtedly, educational strategies and other policy mechanisms will be required if further reductions in tobacco use are to occur. Public health leaders must continue to take an active role in the antismoking movement. The battle against tobacco use will not get any easier because the tobacco industry has more money to spend on promoting smoking than public health agencies have to spend on antismoking activities. However, the public is getting the message, and antismoking legislation is becoming more acceptable.

Another example of public health–driven policy development consists of the efforts to deal with the HIV/AIDS epidemic of the 1980s and 1990s. Reducing HIV transmission is still entirely a matter of changing behavior because no vaccine or cure is yet available. Because changing behavior is such a difficult process, the challenges for public health are significant. Although the public health community has been criticized for what it has done and when it has done it, public health practitioners have been on the front lines in the public's education about HIV and AIDS. The only other critical advocacy group has been made up of people with AIDS.

The Ryan White Act stands as a premier example of what legislation can do. However, mustering the resources to deal with the mounting crisis has not been easy. During the 1980s, many policy makers, for political reasons, tried to play down the AIDS epidemic. For example, the evidence is strong that budget considerations were put before the health needs of the American public and that research scientists were sometimes more concerned with their personal reputations than with saving lives.[43]

Public health leaders at the local, state, and federal levels have taken leadership roles in promoting better methods of AIDS surveillance, creating policies to help the afflicted, raising concerns about the cost and accessibility of new treatments, and promoting an increasing number of programs to prevent the disease from spreading. Public health leaders took a strong position in favor of confronting the crisis head on, even when it was not popular to do so. The result is that the quality of life of many people with AIDS has improved substantially.

Success sometimes creates political enemies. Public health leaders need to take risks for the important health issues they think need to be addressed. The consequences for them could include political retaliation, budget cuts, and loss of leadership positions. Public health leaders may also find themselves in conflict with community leaders. To reduce the risk of conflict, they need to work with community leaders, lobbyists, and special interest groups on common agendas. At the same time, they need to realize that deal making has its own risks, because collaboration with lobbyists and special interest groups in particular may compromise their community oversight activities.

Community leaders have a strong voice in community affairs. They usually have a vision of what the community should be like and want others to share it. They may, therefore, be unwilling to accept the public health leaders' view of the community, especially its health priorities. Yet without the support of community leaders, public health leaders may find it impossible to implement the health policies they think are needed. As much as possible, health policies should emanate directly from community groups. When community leaders with credibility join forces, they are usually able to convince most community residents that there is a problem that must be addressed immediately.[44] Unless the community leadership, the public health leadership, and the political leadership come together and work collaboratively, change will not be possible.

Public health leaders are often in a situation in which they have to increase their own knowledge as a prerequisite to policy development. Case Study 9-B describes a possible biological disaster and the community politics and coalition building that were necessary to avert it. All individuals involved needed to learn new things to better understand the nature of disaster planning. The interesting issue in this case is that it predates the events of September 11, 2001.

Judicial decisions have increasingly played a major role in the area of health policy. Public health leaders have found themselves as witnesses in trials or proponents of health policies being evaluated by the courts. Because courts must interpret the law, the outcomes are not always predictable. During the 1990s, class action suits were brought against tobacco companies, and the courts have ruled that these companies must pay enormous damages to the states. How to use the tobacco settlement money has become a new issue. The public health leaders want the money used to prevent smoking and promote smoking-cessation programs, but many states see this tobacco money as a windfall and want to spend large amounts of it on other state priorities. Dealing with the courts and even the happy results of court decisions thus constitutes another challenge faced by public health leadership.

In the area of policy development, public health leaders must:

- collaborate with managed care organizations and community health centers
- collaborate with state legislatures and the U.S. Congress
- create policy agendas in conjunction with community leaders
- work to implement policies even if they are opposed by special interest groups
- understand the relationship between politics and policy
- encourage cooperation between local, state, and federal health organizations
- prepare for retaliation when pushing unpopular issues
- incorporate judicial decisions into policy development

---

### Case Study 9-B
### A Department of Health Learns about Its Role in Emergency Public Health

*Linda Young Landesman*

In the spring of 1995, the commissioner of health of a large metropolis was informed by federal officials that massive amounts of biological chemicals might be released somewhere in his community. This agent was highly toxic and had the potential to cause high levels of morbidity and mortality among those exposed. While the Smithtown Department of Health had a disaster plan, the plan was inadequate to meet the needs that would follow such a release. Further, there was a range of interest among the leadership in the department regarding the need to prepare for and respond to disasters.

**Background**

Tom Asher, MD, MPH, commissioner of health in Smithtown for 5 years, hung up the phone and closed his eyes to think. He wasn't sure if he had heard correctly. There were stockpiles of biological chemicals here in Smithtown. Millions could be killed if there was an accidental release. As health officer, he was responsible for protecting the public's health. Protecting public health against a hidden enemy was not an easy task, especially in this time of shrinking resources.

Smithtown was a large metropolis in the northern section of the country. It was a hub of activity, and millions of people came in and out of the city every day. They came in to work, to shop, to play. Controlling egress within the city was difficult on a good day. There were hundreds of transportation routes involving bridges, trains, buses, ferries, and airplanes. It was an international port of entry by land, sea, and air. A terrorist could slip through easily.

John Thompkins had been elected mayor of Smithtown by a slim margin the year before. His vocal constituency was demanding cutbacks in government service. The mayor was particularly sensitive to this message, because his political adversaries were eager to see his tenure limited to one term. Betsy Reardon, his predecessor, had been a popular mayor. She had served three terms as head of Smithtown, and the local "spin doctors" felt that she lost the election because the city was paralyzed by a major winter storm the previous December. It didn't matter that the citizens of

*(continues)*

**Case Study 9-B** *continued*

Smithtown had voted down the last two transportation bond issues or that it was a 100-year storm. Betsy was blamed because it took almost a week for transportation to move smoothly again. The situation was made worse because the storm occurred the week before the Christmas holiday. Retailers suffered throughout the city. But Betsy was still a political heavyweight in the region. And she and Thompkins had never been friends.

The impetus to "do more with less" came at a time when the state and federal governments were also retrenching and reducing support for government programs. The department of health had already been hit hard. When Tom and his deputies met six months earlier to review the implications of the cuts, they realized that they had to eliminate 10% of their staff and programs. Most of these reductions had already taken place. So resources in the department were scarce.

The health commissioner believed that he was fortunate in other ways. During their mayor-commissioner get-togethers, Tom felt that the mayor was responsive to his message. In these meetings, Tom highlighted how public health professionals were really part of the public safety network. In this city, where public officials were used to dealing with the "crisis of the week," there had even been a recent opportunity for the commissioner of health to educate the mayor about the importance of vigilance against biological agents.

A strain of the bubonic plague had erupted in India. Villagers, fearful of getting sick and trying to avoid the illness, moved from one village to another. It was days before the public health officials there issued a quarantine. As a result, it was very difficult to contain the epidemic. Thousands of people had died. Indian officials suspected that exposed villagers had boarded planes and traveled abroad. Health officers around the world went on alert. When Tom learned about the possibility of plague being brought to the United States by an international traveler, he met with the mayor to discuss what should be done to protect Smithtown.

"This is the end of the 20th century. What do you mean we could have an outbreak of bubonic plague in Smithtown?" asked the major.

"We both realize that Smithtown is an international port," Tom said. "We have visitors coming here from countries where the public health laws are not as vigorous as ours. We need to take a defensive stand by increasing surveillance at all ports of entry and by alerting hospitals and clinics around the region. If we learn of any patients with plague, we'll jump on it immediately."

Mayor Thompkins was insistent: "Do whatever it takes. We cannot have an outbreak happen here."

Tom Asher left that meeting feeling relieved that he had administrative support for an all-out effort to contain an outbreak of the plague if it appeared necessary. At the time, he didn't realize that he'd be calling on that support so soon.

**Solutions**

The next day he returned to his office and was hoping to spend the morning responding to correspondence and returning phone calls when he received the call about the biological agents stockpiled in Smithtown.

"Get Jayne, Jack, and Sid on the phone stat," Tom ordered. "Tell them that I need them in my office in 30 minutes." His secretary, Glen Oaks, ran into the room.

"Only Sid is in the building. What's up?" Glen asked.

"We may have a potential terrorist situation on our hands. We've got to come up with a plan as soon as possible."

"Jayne's at a meeting at the chancellor's office downtown," Glen reported. "Jack took a few hours' leave to take his daughter to the dentist. It may be a while before they can get back."

"Beep them. Tell them to get back here now!"

Glen hurried back to his desk and hoped that Jayne and Jack could get back soon. Jack was at least two hours away if he traveled by public transportation. It would be prohibitively costly for him to take a taxi back to the office. Besides, there was a city rule that travel by taxi was strictly forbidden except in a municipal emergency. Glen wasn't sure that this qualified as an emergency. He was used to the commissioner calling these types of meetings with his deputies. Last month there was that tuberculosis scare. The month before the media reported that the water wasn't safe to drink because of a death due to *Cryptosporidium*. It turned out that the patient was immunosuppressed and had been living in Milwaukee during the outbreak in that city. He had just come home to die. But the resources of the department sure rallied around until the facts were clear.

So how important was this threat? Glen couldn't tell from the commissioner's demeanor, but he felt that he had to do his best to bring the deputies back to the office. And he was in luck: both were on their way and able to meet with the commissioner within the hour.

Tom started the meeting by asking if there was anybody in the department who knew about disaster planning for biologicals. The deputies looked at each other and shook their heads. They knew about monitoring for infectious disease in shelters and guaranteeing the safety of the water supply, but they knew nothing about preparing for biologicals.

The department had a disaster plan, as required by law, but they all knew that it hadn't been tested in the types of event happening around the country. Perhaps more importantly, Jayne, the deputy commissioner for environmental affairs, had come to realize that the health department should be more involved in planning with other agencies in the city than it currently was. Emergency medical services (EMS) had a lock on responding to disasters. Yet EMS didn't have the expertise that was needed to assess and respond to public health issues. They couldn't identify hazardous materials. They couldn't identify infectious agents. They didn't have the skills to conduct surveillance or monitor the safety of those who responded to an event. With EMS as the lead health agency, there were lots of limitations in the current city plan. It was clear to Jayne that EMS was not the agency that should have lead responsibility. She had told Tom that this was a potential problem for the department. But federal dollars for disaster preparedness and response seemed to be flowing to EMS. And so the commissioner and his deputies planned the best that they could and tried to increase their influence in the system.

"What are we dealing with?" Sid asked.

"I received a call from the chief medical officer of the Office of Foreign Disaster Assistance. Remember him? We met him at the public health annual meeting last November. He called to say that he'd just returned from investigating the sarin release in the subway in Japan. While investigating the extent of the cache of chemicals over there, the U.S. team learned that there is a stockpile of hundreds of gallons of sarin somewhere in the Smithtown metropolitan area. There could be a release at any time."

"That would be disastrous," exclaimed Sid, the deputy for infectious disease. "How can we get ready for a Bhopal-type accident? All of our available staff are

*(continues)*

**Case Study 9-B** *continued*

working around the clock as it is, just trying to keep up. Besides, what do we know about planning for these things?"

"I think that we should call Dan Nickels, chief of EMS. They have the manpower and the resources to respond to this thing," Jack insisted. Jack, deputy director for maternal and child health, could be depended on to support only those efforts that affected mothers and infants. He felt that with shrinking resources, he had to fight to ensure that services weren't diverted form this group.

"That's not a bad idea," Sid agreed.

"Wait a minute. Why should we shove this thing over to EMS?" Jayne asked. "We all know that they can't do the job that is needed to guarantee public health. Besides, if we don't know how to prepare for this thing, there must be people across the country that we can use as resources. This can't be the first time any health department in the country has had to deal with this. Besides, I don't think we should work in isolation. We should be sitting at the table where the interagency response is discussed."

Jack used this as an opportunity to complain about his current staffing. "I don't have enough staff to monitor the child health stations. We can't get newborns in for their first checkup until they are 10 weeks old, and you are talking about using staff to scrounge around the country for someone who knows something about preparing for a Bhopal here in Smithtown. I say call Dan Nickels. If you don't want to call him, then call the CDC. But let's not get over our heads."

"Jack's got a point. If we let another agency do it, it's their problem if something goes wrong," echoed Sid.

"I'm not sure I agree," said the commissioner. "I think that our responsibility is very clear. EMS doesn't have the capability to handle the public health issues. And if this thing blows, it will be our necks out there. It happens that I met with the mayor about the plague threat just yesterday. He was very clear. He wants the city prepared, and that means us. If we need to be prepared for plague, we need to be prepared for biologicals."

Jack asked, "Who's going to do it? I don't have anyone to spare."

Sid and Jayne agreed that there was no one on their staff who could be released from current responsibilities to develop a disaster plan for biologicals.

**Conclusion**

Tom looked around the room and pondered what to do. He knew that Jayne would find the time to supervise someone so that the department could better prepare for this thing. But how could he make this happen? More importantly, should he use valuable resources—resources that could be used to meet other public health responsibilities—to become an active player in citywide disaster preparedness?

---

## Summary

Policy development is the core function that, in a sense, follows assessment, for only after public health problems have been identified can policies be created to deal with them. Yet in the normal course of agency operations assessment and policy development are occurring continually and often simultaneously.

The chapter first presented policy development recommendations publicized by the Institute of Medicine in its 1988 and 2003 reports. It then discussed essential public health services associated with policy development and listed performance indicators for each practice. Additional topics covered included policy trends, advocacy and empowerment, and collaboration. Finally, the chapter discussed leadership challenges related to policy development, including the challenge of bringing diverse groups together to address significant public health risks and the challenge of preparing for retaliation when pushing unpopular positions.

## Discussion Questions

1. What are the two essential public health services associated with policy development?
2. What leadership skills are required for developing policies?
3. What is the difference between politics and policy development?
4. In what ways can politics influence policy development?
5. What is a futurist and why should public health leaders pay attention to what futurists say?
6. How do advocacy and collaboration contribute to empowerment?
7. What are similarities and differences among the three main types of collaborative relationship?
8. What are the main advantages of a collaborative relationship?
9. What is the role of priority setting in policy development?

## Exercise 9-1:  Tattooing in Mid-America

*Purpose:* to explore how policy development occurs and how a policy can affect the relationship between a local public health agency and the county health board

*Key concepts:* board of health, policy development, strategic planning

*Procedure:* The number of tattoo parlors in Tolbert County has grown. Tolbert High School Superintendent Violet Davis calls Tolbert Health Department Director Doris Martinez about the significant increase in tattoos among high school students—an increase that has understandably upset the students' parents. Martinez researches the subject and comes up with similar findings. There is no law in the county related to tattooing.

The class should divide into teams of 8 to 10 members. Half the members of each team will act the role of Tolbert County Health Department professionals and stakeholders. The other half will act the role of members of the Tolbert County Board of Health. The health department members, as a way of addressing the issue of tattooing, develop a proposed anti-tattooing law and devise a strategy for convincing the board of health to support the proposed law. The board members invite the health department representatives to a board meeting to present their arguments favoring the proposed law, and the two groups debate the merits and limitations of the proposal, ultimately focusing on whether it should be enacted.

## References

1. W. Keck, "Creating a Healthy Public," *American Journal of Public Health* 82, no. 9 (1992): 1206–1209.
2. J. C. Lashof, "Commitment to the Common Good," *American Journal of Public Health* 83, no. 9 (1993): 1222–1225.

3. G. Anderson and P. S. Hussey, "Influencing Government Policy: A Framework," in *Oxford Handbook of Public Health Practice*, D. Pencheon, C. Guest, D. Melzer, and J. A. Muir Gray, eds. (London: Oxford University Press, 2001).

4. Institute of Medicine, *The Future of Public Health* (Washington, DC: National Academy Press, 1988).

5. Institute of Medicine, *The Future of the Public's Health* (Washington, DC: National Academies Press, 2003).

6. B. J. Turnock et al., "Implementing and Assessing Organizational Practices," *Public Health Reports* 109, no. 4 (1994): 478–484.

7. Turnock et al., "Implementing and Assessing Organizational Practices."

8. N. Glaser, *The Limits of Social Policy* (Cambridge, MA: Harvard University Press, 1988).

9. Glaser, *The Limits of Social Policy*.

10. R. N. Bellah, "The Quest for the Self," in *Interpretive Social Science*, eds. P. Rubinow and W. M. Sullivan (Berkeley: University of California Press, 1987).

11. L. A. Aday, *At Risk in America* (San Francisco: Jossey-Bass, 1993).

12. M. H. Moore, *Creating Public Value* (Cambridge, MA: Harvard University Press, 1995).

13. H. B. Maynard Jr. and S. E. Mehrtens, *The Fourth Wave: Business in the 21st Century* (San Francisco: Berrett-Koehler, 1993).

14. J. L. Marrioti, *The Power of Partnerships* (Cambridge, MA: Blackwell Publishers, 1996).

15. A. Toffler and H. Toffler, *Creating a New Civilization* (Atlanta: Turner Publishing, 1994).

16. N. Gingrich, *To Renew America* (New York: HarperCollins, 1995).

17. S. P. Robbins and M. Coulter, *Management,* 8th ed. (Upper Saddle River, NJ: Prentice Hall, 2005).

18. Robbins and Coulter, *Management*.

19. M. Siegel and L. Doner, *Marketing Public Health: Strategies to Promote Social Change* (Gaithersburg, MD: Aspen Publishers, 1998).

20. J. P. Kretzmann and J. L. McKnight, *Building Communities from the Inside Out* (Evanston, IL: Northwestern University Center for Urban Affairs and Policy Research, 1993).

21. Trust for America's Health, *You, Too, Can Be an Effective Health Advocate* (Washington, DC: TFAH, 2004).

22. P. Block, *The Empowered Manager* (San Francisco: Jossey-Bass, 1987).

23. D. Tracy, *Ten Steps to Empowerment* (New York: Morrow, 1990).

24. L. Cohen et al., *Developing Effective Coalitions: An Eight Step Guide* (Pleasant Hill, CA: Contra Costa County Health Services Department Prevention Program, 1994).

25. Cohen et al., *Developing Effective Coalitions*.

26. M. T. Hatcher and J. K. McDonald, "The Constituency Development Practice in Public Health Agencies" (Atlanta: Centers for Disease Control and Prevention, 1994).

27. Hatcher and McDonald, "The Constituency Development Practice in Public Health Agencies."

28. Cohen et al., *Developing Effective Coalitions*.

29. G. P. Mays et al., "Collaboration to Improve Community Health: Trends and Alternative Models," *Joint Commission Journal of Qualitative Improvement* 25, no. 10 (1998): 518–565.

30. Mays et al., "Collaboration to Improve Community Health."

31. Public Health Service, *Healthy People 2000* (Washington, DC: U.S. Department of Health and Human Services, 1991).

32. Public Health Service, *Healthy People 2000.*
33. G. E. A. Dever, *Community Health Analysis* (Gaithersburg, MD: Aspen Publishers, 1991).
34. Public Health Service, *For a Healthy Nation: Returns on Investment in Public Health* (Washington, DC: U.S. Department of Health and Human Services, 1994).
35. Public Health Service, *For a Healthy Nation.*
36. Centers for Disease Control, *Reducing the Health Consequences of Smoking: 25 Years of Progress,* Report of the Surgeon General (Washington, DC: U.S. Department of Health and Human Services, 1989).
37. Public Health Service, *Healthy People 2000.*
38. Public Health Service, *Healthy People 2010* (Washington, DC: U.S. Department of Health and Human Services, 2000).
39. J. L. Forster et al., "Locking Devices on Cigarette Vending Machines: Evaluation of a City Ordinance," *American Journal of Public Health* 82, no. 9 (1992): 1217–1219.
40. M. Siegel and L. Doner, *Marketing Public Health: Strategies to Promote Social Change* (Gaithersburg, MD: Aspen Publishers, 1998).
41. R. L. Flewelling et al., "First Year Impact of the 1989 California Cigarette Tax Increase on Cigarette Consumption," *American Journal of Public Health* 82, no. 6 (1992): 867–869.
42. R. Shilts, *And the Band Played On* (New York: St. Martin's Press, 1987).
43. D. D. Chrislip and C. Larsen, *Collaborative Leadership* (San Francisco: Jossey-Bass, 1994).

# CHAPTER 10

# LEADERSHIP AND ASSURANCE

Be sure it's done well by you or others.
K. Gebbie, Speech to the Illinois Public Health
Leadership Institute

The core functions of public health, for the sake of explanation, can be viewed as a series of interactive steps. First comes assessment—the evaluation of the health status of a community, including the health risks it is facing. Next comes policy development—the creation of plans to deal with the community's health problems, or at least those that are given a high priority because they have serious consequences and can be dealt with effectively. Finally comes assurance, which largely consists of the implementation of the plans developed during the second stage. Assurance, in a phrase, involves ensuring that the public's health is protected and, hopefully, even improved.

Of course, these three core functions are all ongoing, interactive, and overlapping. Changes occur in a community and new problems arise, so evaluations of the community's health status must occur regularly. Newly uncovered problems call for new solutions, so policies must be developed continually as well. And assurance is obviously a continuous function, for it involves the development, implementation, and maintenance of public health programs. Because assurance is a community-wide set of activities, public health leadership is needed to coordinate it.

## Overview

### Prevention

Assurance activities focus on disease prevention and health promotion. Primary prevention involves creating an environment in which disease will not come into being—the ultimate public health goal. Secondary prevention involves intervening when problems occur and implementing major initiatives to prevent the consequences from becoming worse. Tertiary prevention involves stopping the progression of a disease or disability in order to prevent dependency. As one writer put it, prevention of health problems is essentially equivalent to public health.[1]

The three levels of prevention are usually presented linearly, but a circular representation would seem to be more appropriate (Figure 10-1), because an intervention initiated at one level will affect activities at the other two

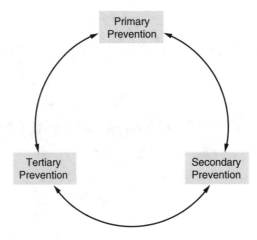

**FIGURE 10-1    The Cycle of Prevention**

levels. For example, the discovery of a new vaccine to prevent a childhood disease will lead to an immunization strategy at the primary prevention level. If the strategy is successful, the disease will become less prevalent, making secondary and tertiary strategies for dealing with the disease less critical, perhaps to the point where they can be abandoned. A new treatment for a disease (secondary prevention) may lead to the discovery of a vaccine to prevent the disease (primary prevention) as well as reduce the long-term harmful effects of the disease, lessening the need for rehabilitation (tertiary prevention). The virtual eradication of polio shows how scientific research, leadership, and prevention can work together creatively.

## Infrastructure

Public health agencies provide services to their communities on a regular basis, but they also are responsible for maintaining the capacity to respond to critical situations and emergencies. The term "capacity" is used extensively in public health. In 1994, the Washington State Department of Health's *Public Health Improvement Plan* defined "capacity" as the ability to perform the core functions of assessment, policy development, and assurance on a continuous, consistent basis, made possible by maintenance of the basic infrastructure of the public health system, including human, capital, and technology resources.[2]

A public health charter was presented in a 1990 report that laid out an agenda for strengthening the infrastructure of public health in Illinois. Two articles of the charter[3] are relevant to the assurance function:

Article III: Categories of Public Health Services to Be Assured
Public health workers in Illinois have established five categories of public health services that further the mission of public health and are appropriate to the governmental role in public health. These are: Health Promotion; Primary Care; Environmental Health; Infectious Disease Control; and Health Care Regulation.

Article IV: Guiding Principles for Restructuring the Public Health System in Illinois

The following principles . . . should guide the restructuring of governmental public health responsibilities in Illinois. The principles enumerated below are predicated on the belief that most services to public health clients are most efficiently and effectively provided at the local level by local health units:

1. The delivery of public health services in the State of Illinois should be improved.
2. The societal benefits derived from public health services should be more effectively communicated.
3. The quality of public health services provided in Illinois should be improved and standardized.
4. The funding of public health services should be increased.

The implementation of these principles has required leadership to drive the implementation of these principles. There was a clear shift in these principles from a program-oriented model to the core functions approach. Leadership is also required to keep the principles in force and to enhance the state requirements for local health department certification with the new national voluntary accreditation program.[4]

# Barriers

The Institute of Medicine report on public health described a number of barriers to carrying out the assurance function.[5] To begin with, the roles of the state and local health departments vary from state to state, and the patterns of assurance activities performed by these departments differ as well. Four states did not even have official local health departments (Delaware, Hawaii, Rhode Island, and Vermont).[6] In seven states, the state health department operates all the local health departments (Arkansas, Florida, Louisiana, Mississippi, New Mexico, South Carolina, and Virginia), whereas the remaining states either possess completely decentralized systems or use a mixed approach.

Differences in funding sources also contribute to the variation in the types of assurance activities performed.[7] One result of the variation in assurance activities is that universal access to services is not a reality for many segments of the population. Even in the case of population-based initiatives, such as communicable disease control, the benefits are inequitably distributed.

Public health agencies and their leaders need to be proactive rather than reactive in the area of assurance. Public health leaders often seem to sit on their hands and allow other entities to decide what the role of public health agencies is to be. One difficulty they face is that, in the United States at least, public health and politics are so intertwined that it is often impossible to know which is which. Nonetheless, they need to make certain that the communities they serve receive the services that are needed to attain agreed health objectives,[8] either by having the public health agencies provide the services or ensuring, through regulation, that they are provided by other public or private health organizations. Assurance of adequate services is guaranteed by social contract. Living up to the guarantee can be difficult, for it often requires subsidization or direct provision of personal health services for those who cannot afford them.

At the federal level, assurance involves making services available that are needed to deal with nationwide problems, such as human immunodeficiency virus (HIV) transmission, and, at the state level, it involves providing public health services that are needed statewide. Local public health agencies have the responsibility of ensuring "that high quality services, including personal health services, needed for the protection of public health in the community are available and accessible to all persons; that the community receives proper consideration in the allocation of federal and state as well as local resources for public health, and that the community is informed about how to obtain public health, including personal health, services, or how to comply with public health requirements."[9(p.143)] These same points are reiterated in the 2003 Institute of Medicine report on public health.[10]

Public health leaders must:

- ensure the development of priority public health programs
- explore multiple public and private funding sources for programs
- stress population-based and evidence-based program development
- start programs with a primary prevention focus
- use governance to support prevention activities
- encourage capacity-building activities in local health departments
- build community partnerships to support programs

## The Role of Leadership in Assurance

There are four essential public health services associated with the assurance core function. A fifth essential service, the research dimension, is a systems integrating service but also can be considered part of the assurance function. It will be included under assurance in order to complete our discussion of the three core functions.

The first essential service is related to the enforcement of laws and regulations that protect health and ensure safety; it has important leadership implications. This essential service is also an interface between the core functions of policy development and assurance. This essential service includes the following three performance indicators.[11]

1. The local public health system reviews existing laws and regulations related to public health in the community.
2. The local public health system is involved in the improvement of laws, regulations, and ordinances.
3. The local public health system recognizes the necessity of enforcement of laws, regulations, and ordinances.

The second essential service involves connecting people in the community to needed personal health services and the necessity of ensuring that necessary services are provided. The leaders in the system need to coordinate their efforts in searching for new resources and restructuring the public health agency and the public health system to better meet community health needs. Utilizing the two performance indicators in the National Public Health Performance Standards Program[12] with the two performance standards discussed by Turnock and colleagues on organizational practices,[13] the multidimensional aspect of this essential service can be seen:

1. The local public health system is able to identify the personal health needs of the local population.
2. The local public health system is able to ensure the linkage to needed community services.
3. The local public health system addresses its programs.
4. The local public health system provides services to meet priority health needs.

The third essential service relates to the important issue of ensuring that there is a competent public health and health services workforce to serve the needs of people in the community. There are four performance standards enumerated in the National Public Health Performance Standards instrument for local public health systems.[14] To this list of four must be added the additional standard discussed by Turnock and his colleagues on professional and regulatory standards.[15] The five performance indicators are:

1. There is a need to do workforce assessments at the national, state, and local levels and then plan for recruiting new professionals into public health.
2. The local public health system needs to demonstrate compliance with professional and regulatory standards.
3. The local public health system will develop and maintain public health workforce standards required at the local level.
4. The local public health system will require public health professionals to get any special training necessary to carry out their jobs. They will support a lifelong learning model.
5. Public health professionals will get management and leadership training.

The fourth essential public health service related to assurance involves evaluation to measure effectiveness of programs, accessibility to these programs, and the quality of population-based services. Feedback data are gathered and looked at to determine if programs need to be revised or resources redirected in order to deal with problems that have arisen during implementation. The behavioral and social sciences have developed many methodological techniques for evaluating public agencies. Public health leaders need to support program evaluation, be involved in evaluating data, and adopt a system of performance monitoring. All these activities will strengthen the functioning of the local agency. There are four program indicators for this essential service:[16]

1. The local public health system evaluates population-based services and programs.
2. The local public health system evaluates personal health services and programs.
3. The local public health system evaluates the system.
4. If changes in programs are necessary, the agency revises programs based on evaluation and quality assurance activities.

The final essential service involves research related to new insights and innovations for addressing public health challenges. This final essential service can be seen as an assurance function as well as a system integrating function. There are three performance indicators for this essential service:[17]

1. The local public health system fosters innovation.
2. Linkage with institutions of higher education and with researchers.
3. Determination of the capacity to initiate or participate in research activities.

Whether a public health agency engages in the assurance essential services described here indicates whether it is meeting its public mandate. Of course, it can be questioned whether the essential services are comprehensive and properly defined and whether the performance indicators are a good gauge of the extent to which the practices are being adhered to. For one thing, the essential services seem to overlap, in the sense that some of the activities associated with a given essential service are associated with others as well.[18]

Furthermore, because program implementation demands more than two-thirds of the resources of local public health agencies, it might be beneficial to subdivide the essential service and local health agency organizational practices in order to take account of the diversity of programs provided. Another issue is the allocation of staff time to the activities associated with each essential service and organizational practice.[19] For example, not much staff time and not many financial resources are devoted to the practices associated with assessment or policy development, and the role of technical assistance is not clearly defined in the core function practices model. These issues need to be addressed if the model is to be workable over the long run. Many of these criticisms are also applicable to the organizational practices approach.

In a national sample of local health departments, Turnock and colleagues investigated the rate of use for the 10 organizational practices.[20] The overall rate was 50% (this figure was calculated using weighted responses from 208 local health departments). The rate of use was highest for the practices associated with assurance and lowest for practices related to policy development. The researchers also found that about 40% of the U.S. population was being served by health departments utilizing the core functions approach to public health during 1993. The rate of use for the essential services model is currently unknown except in the states and localities using the Mobilizing for Action through Planning and Partnerships process or National Public Health Performance Standards.

Illinois has been so committed to the core function practices model that the Illinois administrative code was changed in 1993 to reflect the new commitment.[21–23] Table 10-1 shows the activities required for the certification of local health departments before and after adoption of the 10 essential public health services as part of the administrative code. This move to a core function–based system meant that all local health departments, and by extension the local public health system, would be held to the same standards and a more consistent approach to community-based public health.[24]

Case Study 10-A shows the benefits of creating community partnerships—including a partnership between the local state university and the community—as a way to enhance the implementation of community health activities. (Note that the neighborhood health advisors program described in the case study is oriented toward leadership development, an added plus.)

**Table 10-1   Activities Required for Certification of Local Health Departments in Illinois, Before and After July 1993**

Before July 1993
 1. Food sanitation
 2. Potable water
 3. Maternal health and family planning
 4. Child health
 5. Communicable disease control
 6. Private sewage
 7. Solid waste
 8. Nuisance control
 9. Chronic disease
10. Administration

July 1993 and later
 1. Assess the health needs of the community
 2. Investigate health effects and hazards
 3. Advocate and build constituencies
 4. Develop plans and policies to address needs (includes analyzing for determinants and setting priorities)
 5. Manage resources
 6. Implement programs
 7. Evaluate and provide quality assurance
 8. Inform and educate the public

*Source:* Reprinted from Illinois Administrative Code, Title 55, Sec. 600, 1993, State of Illinois.

---

## Case Study 10-A
## Big City Neighborhood Health Advisors

*Adam B. Becker, Barbara A. Israel, and Rose Hollis*

In today's context of decreasing budgets and increasing disparities in health status among U.S. population groups, health departments are faced with a serious challenge in trying to ensure the delivery of adequate and appropriate services to communities. Given the complex needs of communities and the differences between professional and lay experiences and perceptions, health department services often fail to be as relevant to community issues as they could be. To create more relevant services, some health departments are finding creative ways to involve community members in meeting the diverse needs in the community.

The Big City Health Department (BCHD) developed the Big City Neighborhood Health Advisor (BCNHA) project with the assistance of a local community-based organization (CBO) and a nearby school of public health. The project was funded for four years under the umbrella of a larger, multisite project aimed at increasing the capacity of communities, bringing stronger community influence into the practice of public health, and changing the public health curriculum in universities to strengthen the community focus. Developing the BCNHA project was one strategy adopted by the BCHD to meet community needs and ensure that appropriate quality services were available locally.

*(continues)*

## About Big City: The Project Setting

Big City is one of the largest cities in the United States and has a population well over 1,000,000. Among the 77 U.S. cities with populations above 200,000, Big City has at times been ranked first in the percentage of people below the poverty level (as high as 32%). Big City has also been ranked first in unemployment rate (as high as 13% overall). In certain sections of the city, the unemployment rate is as high as 36%. Within Big City, 19% of all households are female headed, and 55% of these live below the poverty level. In addition, more than 40% of all children under the age of 18 live below the poverty level.

There is an increasing amount of racial and ethnic segregation in Big City, with extreme differences in health and income status between European Americans and people of color. Racial and economic segregation in Big City is linked to decreasing access to social and structural supports within the local communities, as jobs, stores, and other community institutions relocate to suburban areas and as the city's major industries downsize or disappear altogether.

## "Big City Health Department: Your Partner in Good Health"

As federal, state, and local budgets for health and human services decline, the BCHD finds it more and more difficult to ensure that quality services are available to the residents. Many residents are not aware of the services that are available, or how to access them. Those services that are available, because they are fewer in number and spread out, are often hard to reach for those who need the services the most.

In attempting to fulfill the three core functions of public health as defined by the Institute of Medicine (assessment, assurance, and policy development), the BCHD made an intensive effort to form partnerships with the communities it serves. The BCNHA project was one means by which the BCHD formed such partnerships. This kind of relationship with the communities was not new for the BCHD, nor was the BCNHA project the only example of a project it had implemented. The health department's openness to such partnerships was one of the factors that contributed to the success of the BCNHA program. This openness is evident in the BCHD's motto— "Big City Health Department, Your Partner in Good Health"—and its mission statement: "The overall role of the department is to prevent disease, promote health, and protect the environment. This is accomplished through partnerships and other types of collaboration with schools, hospitals, churches, physicians, health insurers, businesses, and other community-based agencies . . ."

When university faculty, members of a major community-based organization, and staff of the BCHD sat down to determine the role of the health department in the umbrella project in which they were all engaged and the project activities it would take on, the BCNHA project seemed a natural fit for the BCHD. The BCNHA project would help the BCHD achieve its mission by strengthening and expanding the role of Big City community members in the delivery of services aimed at meeting community needs.

## Developing the Big City Neighborhood Health Advisors Project

The first step in developing the BCNHA project was to establish a steering committee to oversee the project. This committee consisted of university faculty and students, community members, and staff from the CBO partner and the health department. The committee developed criteria for identifying and recruiting neighborhood health advisors (NHAs), established goals and approaches for training NHAs, and determined the relationship of the NHAs to the health department.

The steering committee based the BCNHA project on the lay health advisor concept. Within communities, there have always been people who are trusted and respected and whom others rely upon for care, advice, and support. The support given is often informal, spontaneous, and so much a part of everyday life that it may go unrecognized. In most cases, the informal support is given by one person to another within a preexisting relationship: friend to friend, coworker to coworker, neighbor to neighbor, or family member to family member. These special community members are knowledgeable about their community and well respected by friends, family, and neighbors. Others frequently turn to them for advice and assistance, and they are responsive to the strengths and needs of others. The NHA Steering Committee established these characteristics as the criteria for identifying potential NHAs.

In determining the relationship between the NHAs and the BCHD, the steering committee wanted to differentiate the roles of the NHAs from the roles that community members played in other BCHD projects. Health departments and other types of health and human service agencies often rely on members of their target populations to assist in the provision of services. Community members may provide information and education to others with similar backgrounds and life experiences (e.g., peer educators), extend the agency's access into the community and increase community awareness of agencies and services available to them (e.g., community outreach workers), or provide agencies with input into the types and quality of health services available (e.g., community advisory boards). These roles are extremely helpful in improving services and breaking down barriers to care.

The steering committee felt that the NHA role should be broad enough that the NHAs could provide services to their community in some or all of the capacities mentioned above. The distinction made between NHAs and other community members in BCHD projects was that NHAs would be identified, not created; would work with the BCHD and according to their own perceptions of priorities within their communities and not for the BCHD and according to its objectives; would not be paid employees of the health department; and would live or work in the settings in which they would provide help and assistance, perhaps facing issues similar to those faced by the people who would receive their support.

**The Role of the Big City Health Department**

Although the NHAs would not be employees of the BCHD, the steering committee decided that the BCNHA project headquarters should be housed at the health department. The health department's role, therefore, would be to hire a program coordinator and provide support and resources wherever possible. The BCHD hired Sue Siloh as the program coordinator. At first, Ms. Siloh felt out of place at the BCHD. The characteristics that made her a perfect fit for the job of coordinator meant that she was a unique health department employee. Ms. Siloh lived in the community served by the BCNHA project, had spent some time living in public housing, and did not have public health training. Initially, Ms. Siloh often felt that others did not take her or her program seriously.

The BCHD's deputy director, who was a strong supporter of both the BCNHA project and Ms. Siloh, saw that something needed to be done to create a support system for the project within the health department. Ms. Siloh was made a member of the administrative team of the BCHD, which had traditionally consisted only of the director, deputy director, and division heads. As a result of her inclusion on the team,

*(continues)*

**Case Study 10-A** *continued*

Ms. Siloh was able to develop personal relationships with all the division heads, and they in turn learned more about the BCNHA project, how they could help support the project, and how the project could help the community and thus strengthen the department's relationship with the community, benefiting all of BCHD's programs. As needs arose for training or delivery of services (e.g., satellite immunization clinics, health screenings in community centers or churches), Ms. Siloh could now personally contact those in the BCHD who could help her to meet those needs.

### The Role of the Coordinator: Recruiting, Training, and Supporting NHAs
Sue Siloh's official title was community health coordinator. As coordinator of the BCNHA project, she was given many responsibilities. Ms. Siloh was responsible for recruiting and selecting NHAs, training new NHAs (she coordinated the eight-week training programs and additional in-service trainings and also served as a trainer for some sessions), supporting the trained NHAs (she coordinated monthly meetings, assisted NHAs with special projects, and maintained contact with each individual NHA), and starting up new NHA projects in other target areas of the city as requested (she assisted several CBOs in developing similar projects). In addition, Ms. Siloh presented the BCNHA project at professional meetings and conferences, advised other agencies in the development of NHA projects, and worked with members of the university on publications about the BCNHA project. Ms. Siloh also participated in grant-writing activities to bring in new money to sustain the project.

### Recruiting NHAs
The recruiting process for NHAs was somewhat informal and combined several strategies. The coordinator contacted local block clubs, churches, and other community groups in order to spread the word about the project. Flyers were posted throughout the community. Ms. Siloh also contacted community members she knew from her work as a community organizer and advocate. For subsequent cohorts, previously trained NHAs played a recruiting role by bringing in interesting friends and neighbors. As for qualifications, NHAs were expected to have the trust and respect of people in the community, an interest in learning about the community, and an eagerness to work to improve the health and quality of life of community members.

### Training the NHAs
Once the NHAs were identified, they participated in eight sessions of "core" training. This initial training covered three broad areas: health education, community resources and referrals, and community problem solving and organizing. Health department staff provided most of the training in health education (topics included diabetes, high blood pressure, and HIV/acquired immune deficiency syndrome (AIDS). Representatives from local agencies provided information about the resources available to the NHAs and their neighbors, and faculty from the university provided the community problem-solving and organizing training.

Once trained, NHAs also participated in training subsequent cohorts. They worked in teams with trainers to give the NHA perspective on the training topic and to provide "real-life" examples of how NHAs could put their skills to work.

Although the initial training content was, for the most part, determined by the steering committee, the trainees determined the training schedule as a group to fit their needs. They also had opportunities to select priority areas on which to focus during the core training. After the core training, NHAs had opportunities to go on to specialized training in areas they selected, such as cardiopulmonary resuscitation organizing block clubs, substance abuse, and parenting. Over 40 NHAs participated in three core trainings.

### Neighborhood Health Advisors at Work

Once they graduated from the training program, NHAs had increased skills to continue the help they were providing in their communities. NHAs became involved on a daily basis with individuals and groups in their own neighborhoods—helping friends and family to access needed services, assisting block clubs to organize and address community issues, providing day care to families, transporting neighbors to appointments, and providing education on health issues to church and community organizations and businesses.

Health was not the only human service sector with which BCNHAs were involved. Several NHAs began to work with a local police precinct through the Safe and Healthy Neighborhoods Program to educate neighborhood residents about crime and safety and to assist police in learning to work with community members in a way that would foster trust and cooperation.

In addition to these helping roles, NHAs developed some dynamic programs in their neighborhoods. Examples include the Community Cupboard, a neighborhood food and clothing pantry; Together We Can, a grief support group for those experiencing loss; and Facing the Challenge, a parenting program that builds skills and provides support for pregnant women. In addition to these programs, NHAs participated in other ongoing programs, such as the Peterson Clinic Advisory Council, a community board that assisted a local health clinic in developing programs for the community, and the Violence Task Force, a group that worked to provide alternative activities for youths at risk. NHAs participated in these projects according to their interests and the needs in their neighborhoods. In addition to these projects, the NHAs distributed a monthly newsletter to over 5,000 individuals and families in Big City. The newsletter included information about health issues and services, local business news, and community events.

### Special Program Issues

*Recognition and Reimbursement*

Given the number of activities in which NHAs were involved and the limited resources available to the program, the question of reimbursement was one that continued to arise for the BCNHA project. Many of the NHAs had full- or part-time jobs. Some did not want to be paid because they considered helping friends and family as part of their responsibility to the community or to God or as part of being a member of a family and community. There were other NHAs who wanted to have a full- or part-time job, and their hope was that the training and activities they did in conjunction with this program would lead them to a job. Regardless of whether NHAs wished to be paid, their work needed to be recognized. Whenever possible, portions of new grant monies brought in to sustain the NHA project were designated for reimbursement for travel (e.g., gas and mileage), reimbursement for meals (e.g., dinner during training sessions), to provide incentives (each NHA received a printed cloth carrying bag with the NHA logo), or as stipends for hourly work on special neighborhood projects. For most of the NHAs, these forms of compensation were enough to support and encourage them as they engaged in their work.

*(continues)*

**Case Study 10-A** *continued*

In a few cases, NHAs were hired by the BCHD or affiliated organizations for full- or part-time positions. Although employment was welcomed by these NHAs, formalizing their work as NHAs was not without challenges. Along with a salary came an obligation to the paying agency. Some of the NHAs who received jobs found that they had less time to work with groups in their own neighborhoods. Others found that they were limited in the scope of health issues with which they could work, because their training was specialized to fit their new jobs.

To some extent, those who became employed through their work as NHAs lost a modicum of the community's trust when they became agency employees. They were seen by some as "part of the system" rather than part of the community, and their loyalties became suspect. Because an open, trusting relationship between an NHA and the local community was essential to the work of the NHA, employment actually decreased the ability of some to provide individualized support and assistance.

Though the steering committee and the program coordinator had varying opinions on the subject of compensating NHAs, decisions about paying stipends to BCNHAs or hiring them into agencies followed two basic principles: (1) the work of NHAs had to be recognized and compensated in some way, and (2) NHAs themselves had to be involved in the decision regarding their compensation.

### Evaluating the Work of the NHAs

Assurance of service delivery and the quality of those services requires public health departments to evaluate programs to determine whether they are meeting community needs appropriately and sufficiently. Several challenges faced the BCNHA program when it came to evaluation. First, designing an evaluation plan for such a diverse set of activities was extremely difficult. Some NHAs worked more with individuals and others more with groups, some worked with certain agencies and others worked independently, some participated in all monthly meetings, and others attended only when they needed materials or to meet with the coordinator. In addition, all NHAs possessed unique styles of helping. Given the diversity, could an evaluation plan be developed that would be appropriate to all NHAs?

Second, collecting data on BCNHA activities was a challenge. The often spontaneous and informal nature of the work of NHAs made observation by evaluators difficult if not impossible. Likewise, NHAs found it difficult to keep records of their activities because they took place during a phone call from a friend or a chance meeting in the grocery store. Much of the "helping work" done by NHAs was seen by project staff and evaluators as program-related work. NHAs, however, saw their work as part of daily life and therefore not appropriate for documenting. Confidentiality and trust issues, as well as the sheer number of people in contact with NHAs, made "client" interviewing a challenge as well.

Given the above challenges, the steering committee, the coordinator, the evaluator, and the NHAs themselves knew that whatever evaluation methods were used would not be able to capture an entire picture of the BCNHA project. Talking with NHA "clients" who were willing to be interviewed helped the program evaluators form an idea of how the NHAs were interacting with other community members and what that interaction meant for the community. Community members were less likely, however, to talk about weaknesses of the program because of the relationships they had with the NHAs.

Looking at community outcomes was also extremely difficult. Could NHAs be credited with a drop in infant mortality rates or a decrease in visits to the emergency department? Could they be held accountable for a rise in criminal activity or incomplete immunization rates? With so many other activities going on in Big City, how would evaluators determine what changes were effects of the project? The steering committee felt that using communities without NHAs as comparisons was also a problematic strategy. The ethical responsibility of the BCHD to all the communities in which it works, the difficulty of matching diverse communities, and a shortage of resources were among the reasons why the project chose not to implement a quasi-experimental evaluation design.

The effects of participation on the NHAs themselves were, however, assessed through the evaluation. NHAs completed a profile form when they joined the program. They were asked to indicate employment status, education level, skills and talents, interest in and commitment to empowering their neighborhoods, organizational affiliations, and availability. Changes in these items for each NHA were assessed either through having the NHA complete a profile form after a certain amount of time or through an interview.

In addition, documentation gave those involved with the project a good idea of how program activities were being carried out. The program coordinator used several strategies to encourage NHAs to document their work. NHAs were given documentation forms to keep track of activities, needs, challenges, and ideas for priority projects in the community. Once a month the NHAs jointly met with the coordinator to discuss project ideas and challenges, to learn about new resources in the community, to give each other support, and sometimes to receive additional training. The first portion of these meetings was devoted to discussing and providing assistance in completing the documentation forms.

### The NHAs and Assurance

The BCHD takes very seriously its responsibility to the community. In order to fulfill part of the assurance function, the BCHD implemented and supported the BCNHA project. The project helped the BCHD to carry out assurance activities in several ways:

- by disseminating information throughout the target area regarding health issues, resources, and services available
- by strengthening the connection between the health department and the community and expanding the role that community members play in the delivery of health services
- by providing training to community members that strengthened their ability to solve problems, gain access to resources, voice their needs and concerns, and transfer these skills to other community members

This program is an excellent example of how one health department approached the function of ensuring the delivery of quality services to the community in a time of decreasing budgets and increasing needs for services.

---

Public health leadership activities tied to assurance include:

- building a strong agency managerial team
- delegating authority for programmatic decisions
- restructuring agency activities to address health priority needs
- encouraging feedback to all constituents
- supporting program evaluation on an ongoing basis
- mentoring and training staff
- developing a technical assistance team

- working with external partners on community-wide population-based public health programs
- promoting a systems orientation to public health

## Population-Based Services and Personal Health Services

Public health leaders and their professional colleagues are often confronted with the question of how public health differs from health care. The usual answer is that public health practitioners provide services oriented toward the population at large and do not routinely provide personal or direct services to individuals. Population-based services are programs intended to promote health and prevent disease in a community or a larger geographic entity. Public health practitioners are concerned about the factors that affect health. Some of these factors are in the control of each person in a community and some are not.

The major determinants of health are biology, environment, lifestyle, degree of wealth, and health organizational matters.[25] All of these key determinants have psychosocial components, such as social status; ties between people (e.g., family ties), social networks, and ties to voluntary organizations; and relationships to the neighborhood or community.[26]

The relationship between the provision of population-based services and the provision of direct health services is complicated. The medical care system in the United States reserves the right to provide personal health- and illness-based direct services, and the medical care infrastructure has been built up to support this medical care approach. Yet, although the public health system often takes a backseat to the medical care system in the United States, many people who need help cannot get services, even when government financial support is available, and as a consequence public health agencies sometimes act as service providers of last resort.[27]

Table 10-2 shows some of the population-based services that local public health agencies provide, such as surveillance, environmental health and control, communicable disease control, aging programs, and maternal and child health programs. Personal health services include community health clinical services, primary health care, case management services, dental health services, and clinical counseling programs. Some services mix elements of both, such as immunization, health screening, and dental sealant programs.

Regardless of the changes that occur in the health care field in the future, population-based programs will probably still mainly be a public health responsibility. The configuration of personal health services constantly changes in response to changes in health policy. The mixed services may remain unchanged or become reconfigured in some way. Assurance is interconnected with the whole public health system, so it causes changes and also responds to changes in other parts of the system. Currently, the three major areas of assurance arguably are personal health service provision, environmental control, and behavior modification,[28] but undoubtedly a new list will be needed for the 21st century because local public health agencies will probably be less involved in the direct delivery of personal health services.

**Table 10-2    Examples of Assurance Activities in State and Local Health Departments and Leadership**

| Population Based | Mixed | Personal Health Based | Leadership Activities |
|---|---|---|---|
| Public health surveillance | Community health nursing | Community health clinical services | Delegation of programmatic responsibilities to others<br>Evaluation of collected data for decision making |
| Environmental health and control (air and water quality, waste disposal, toxic substances control, etc.) | Health screening programs | Clinical services for children with lead toxicity | Program oversight<br>Translation of environmental health goals into action |
| Occupational health and safety | Immunization<br>Substance abuse screening<br>Accidents | Clinical services for workers | Development of treatment partnerships with other health providers |
| Injury control | Infant car seat laws<br>Violence prevention<br>Teen peer support | Deliver donated car seats to people who cannot afford them | Education of the public<br>Enforcement of laws and regulations |
| HIV/AIDs surveillance | Screening programs<br>Reporting laws | AIDS counseling | Enforcement of laws and regulations<br>Use of data for decision making |
| Communicable disease control | Immunization programs | Primary health care | Monitoring of health issues in the community<br>Study of global health trends<br>Education of the public |
| Family planning | Statistical monitoring of lack of prenatal care by pregnant teens | School clinics | Education of the public<br>Development of partnerships with the community |
| Maternal and child health programs | Metabolic/genetic screening programs Women, Infants, and Children (WIC) eligibility | Case management services | Enforcement of laws and regulations |
| Aging programs | Medicaid eligibility | Long-term care | Collaboration with other agencies that serve older populations |
| Nutrition programs | WIC eligibility | Nutrition counseling | Placement of emphasis on innovation<br>Program oversight |

*(continues)*

**Table 10-2** *(continued)*

| Population Based | Mixed | Personal Health Based | Leadership Activities |
|---|---|---|---|
| Disaster preparedness | Community disaster plans | Disaster clinics (emergency public health) | Advocacy of a role for public health in disasters<br>Creation of disaster teams |
| Health promotion and disease prevention | Educational programs | Clinical counseling | Creation of a vision and mission based on primary prevention<br>Development of goals<br>Translation of goals into action<br>Development of academic linkages |
| Dental health | Dental sealant programs | Dental health clinics | Delegation of responsibility to dentists<br>Program oversight |
| Vector/animal control | Observation of community health standards | Maintenance of animal shelters | Enforcement of laws and regulations<br>Delegation of responsibility to other professional staff |
| Restaurant inspection | Monitoring of food-borne health problems | Community health clinic services | Enforcement of laws and regulations<br>Creation of partnership with local restaurant association |
| Health hazard appraisal | Evaluation of community health hazards | Community health clinic services | Placement of emphasis on innovative program development<br>Support and evaluation of data collected |
| Train and educate the workforce | Leadership development programs | Application of learning to clinical programs | Mentoring and training<br>Health communication<br>Social marketing |
| Population-based managed care | Development of managed care model(s) for all community residents | Running of public health maintenance organization by a local health department | Development of partnerships with local health providers |
| Laboratory activities | Privatization of some laboratory activities | Personal testing for problems | Support for laboratory directors' involvement in public health decision making |

Public health surveillance is a marriage between the core functions of assessment and assurance, and epidemiology serves as the minister who joins these two functions together.[29] In turn, surveillance connects research to service needs and monitors the linkage routinely.[30] Public health surveillance involves the collection, interpretation, and use of data (for purposes of policy development and decision making). Thacker listed 11 reasons for surveillance:[31]

1. health planning
2. monitoring changes in public health practice
3. quantitatively estimating the extensiveness of a health problem in a community
4. determining the natural history of a disease
5. detecting epidemics and disasters
6. determining the spread of disease in a population
7. facilitating epidemiological and laboratory investigations
8. hypothesis testing
9. evaluating assurance activities
10. monitoring changes in infectious agents
11. monitoring isolation activities

It is imperative to link the population-based health objectives to the assurance activities of the local public health agency at the community level.[32] Assurance of vital services is a governmental function. However, the community needs to define its own process for tying goals to services.

The state of Washington tied the population-based assurance activities of local health agencies to capacity standards that identified what the agencies and their governmental and community partners needed to do on a regular basis to protect and promote health and prevent disease.[33] Appendix 10-A presents the list of health promotion, health protection, and quality assurance activities contained in the Washington State Public Health Improvement Plan during the early 1990s.[34] Quality assurance is defined in the plan as monitoring and maintaining the quality of public health programs and services. Quality assurance includes licensing and training health professionals, licensing health facilities, and enforcing standards and regulations. Quality assurance is discussed in detail in the next section. Although this classification is no longer used in Washington in its original forms, it still provides us with a useful classification of assurance capacity indicators.

Public health leaders must:

- utilize creative techniques to maintain population-based programs during a downsizing period
- provide clinical services that are not accessible to segments of the population for lack of insurance or other reasons
- tie public health issues to personal health issues
- learn to interrelate surveillance to program development
- support quality assurance
- integrate public health preparedness activities into the assurance activities of the local public health system

## Quality Assurance

The U.S. General Accounting Office (GAO) was asked in 1989 to review the issue of quality assurance in health care.[35] In a briefing report to the chair of the U.S. Bipartisan Commission on Comprehensive Health Care, the GAO pointed out the multidimensional factors associated with quality measures. Part of the difficulty in quality assurance is that quality means different things to different people and organizations. For the individual, health improvement is the measure of quality. If the improvement can be tied to a particular treatment intervention, then quality is implied in the techniques used. For health care leaders and providers, such factors as accurate diagnosis and treatment, the clinical content of care, and technical skill are viewed as related to quality. Purchasers tie quality to factors such as cost-effectiveness, the appropriateness of the care setting, and the frequency and duration of services. For the public health leadership, quality can be tied to meeting health objectives, declines in rates of disease and infant mortality, and increases in healthy behaviors.

The GAO report also argued that quality assessment and quality assurance are sometimes confused with each other:

> Quality assessment involves the use of measures of quality, based on either explicit or implicit criteria, to assess the structure, process, and outcomes of care and to monitor levels of quality over time. Quality assurance goes beyond the simple assessment of quality to include its improvement. This requires identifying and confirming problems in the quality of medical care, planning interventions to lessen or eliminate the problems, monitoring the effectiveness of the interventions, and instituting additional changes and monitoring where warranted. . . . Quality assessment is a prerequisite to quality assurance.[36(p.7)]

Because quality assurance is an important part of the core function of assurance, developing a national strategy to address concerns about quality assurance may be required. The GAO report raised the issue of equity and people's need to gain access to services that are able to improve their well-being. Equitable access to services depends to a degree on how services get reimbursed. It is also related to the different health needs of different subpopulations. Older people, for example, have different concerns than young mothers with sick children. A national strategy may also be required to deal with the issue of comprehensiveness of health care services.[37] The services available in a community are partially determined by the service models in use in the community.

A comprehensive national strategy for quality assurance would likely include:

- national practice guidelines and standards of care
- enhanced data to support quality assurance activities
- improved approaches to quality assessment and assurance at the local level
- a national focus for developing, implementing, and monitoring a national system[38]

Quality of care is affected by a number of factors, including demographic factors, such as the age, gender, race or ethnicity, socioeconomic status, education, and occupation of those who use the services. Poor people, for instance, tend to be sicker and have more trouble getting the services they need. Economic factors, of course, play a role in determining the quality of care as well. It is common to hear that there is not enough money to provide universal access to services, keep the quality of care at a high level, or hire enough health professionals to provide the needed services. Finally, politics, including the political orientation of the party in office, can have an impact on the quality of the health care system. Indeed, the direction of health care policy may be largely determined by the lobbying of powerful groups such as the American Medical Association or the various managed care organizations (MCOs).

One of the keys to quality assurance is the accreditation process, in which special review organizations, most notably the Joint Commission on Accreditation of Healthcare Organizations, evaluate the care provided by health care organizations. One problem with present accreditation procedures is that the focus is on structural and staff performance requirements rather than treatment outcomes. Moreover, health care organizations, in order to improve their services, must be motivated by more than a desire to receive accreditation; they must be motivated to engage in improvement efforts out of an inner need to offer the public the best care they are capable of providing.

Public health agencies may undergo an accreditation review for some of their clinical programs, such as home care or ambulatory care services. A voluntary public health accreditation program for local public health agencies will be implemented in 2011. Also, state and federal money is given to local agencies to provide certain mandated programs, and sanctions, including loss of funds, are applied if the mandated programs are not implemented, although the use of sanctions is inconsistent.

> **Leadership Tips**
>
> *Recognize your direct reports for work well done, but fit the type of recognition to the desires of the people recognized.*

There is a built-in quality assurance process related to health objectives. If one of a local public health agency's objectives is to increase the immunization rate to the point where 90% of children under a certain age are receiving immunizations, the agency, by developing indicators of success, can determine the extent to which the objective is being achieved and also which segments of the population are being reached effectively. Partnerships with academia are useful in evaluating progress toward the attainment of objectives, and business techniques associated with continuous quality improvement or total quality management can be applied to uncover the reasons for the failure to meet objectives. Also, publicizing the success of community programs can strengthen the local public health infrastructure by demonstrating to residents that the public health agency is an effective social service organization.

Public health agencies need to monitor community assurance activities. The fear among public health professionals is that MCOs will take over the assurance function from local agencies. Public health leaders need to make sure that all public health agency and private health organization programs are of high quality.

Public health and mental health agencies have become program partners in many communities. Quality assurance is an important issue for mental health agencies as well, and it is likely to become even more important with the likely continued growth in third-party payers, governmental regulations, and national organization involvement.[39] Quality assurance methods need to be used not only in program operations but also in the training of public health and mental health professionals. Agency leaders need to support the training of the public health and mental health workforce in innovative approaches to solving problems and making decisions.

In the area of quality assurance, public health leaders must:

- develop local guidelines for practice
- promote high-quality programs
- meet or surpass proposed health objectives
- increase access to care for underinsured and underserved populations
- engage in quality assurance activities, such as those necessary to gain accreditation
- support continuous quality improvement procedures
- promote a consumer- and community-driven public health system
- train the public health workforce in quality techniques
- work to integrate public health and mental health quality assurance activities

## The Greatest Leadership Challenge

The greatest challenge for public health leaders in the coming years will be to work out a viable relationship between governmental public health agencies and MCOs. Public health leaders have become defensive on the issue of partnering with MCOs and in fact have tended to ignore the MCOs in their communities under the mistaken assumption that they will eventually disappear.[40] As pointed out above, public health leaders are concerned that MCOs will take over many of the assurance responsibilities that currently belong to health departments. They are also concerned that MCOs will increase their community penetration by serving more and more community residents, with the result that public health agencies will suffer a reduction in operating funds for mandated services and core function activities.

It is important to point out that the assurance activities of government public health agencies will not diminish but will rather expand, especially in light of the increased emergency preparedness and response activities now required of health departments.[41] These agencies also will continue to have the responsibility of ensuring that necessary programs and services are available to all residents of the community. Each local public health agency will need to come up with unique solutions for meeting this responsibility. For example, an agency in some cases may be the managed care provider for certain segments of its community. Case Study 10-B presents an interview conducted in 1995 with Dr. Jean Malecki who as a director of a Florida public health unit helped to develop a unique managed care program for her county. This interview shows the importance of creativity in leadership and how a local health unit can benefit from collaborating with local service providers. The interview now includes a postscript public health quiz where Dr. Malecki brings her perceptions up to date.

---

### Case Study 10-B
### A Leadership Interview with Jean M. Malecki

*Louis Rowitz*

Jean M. Malecki, MD, MPH, is the director of the HRS/Palm Beach County Health Unit. She holds a doctor of medicine degree from New York Medical College and a master of public health degree from the University of Miami. Dr. Malecki is also a graduate of the Public Health Leadership Institute in California. She has been one of the leaders in the development of unique models for public health service at the county level and talks about these programs during the interview, which occurred on February 17, 1995.

**How have you helped your health unit reinvent public health for the county?**
We have begun a countywide total quality improvement project where we initially used APEX as our tool and then brought in outside consultants on visioning and team building for all staff. In so doing, we decided as a health department that we would continue to do traditional public health but that would be the foundation for a major effort in prevention and primary care in the managed care arena. Currently, we are putting in an application for a commercial health maintenance organization (HMO), which would use only public dollars—both Medicaid and tax dollars. The HMO will be called Healthy Palm Beach. It will be housed in the health department. We currently have a Medicaid HMO. We are thus applying for a commercial HMO so that we can use some of the same tax dollars that are currently received to a taxing entity to provide the same level of care to the working poor that we provide to the Medicaid clients. It will be a single payer. Any willing provider can be part of the system. This proposed program provides a healthy competition environment.

**Are the three core functions still relevant in a reinvention environment?**
The core functions are even more relevant in a reinvention environment. You have to have the core functions in place whether the health department directly provides the care or not. The health department has to oversee healthy outcomes. It is necessary to ensure that any health care reform that takes place achieves what it is supposed to. In Florida, what we are seeing, unfortunately, is that the cost factor is number one to policy makers. Costs—and not quality—are driving the system. Having the core functions are extremely important if we are going to work out what we need to on the local level. Both the new model of essential public health services and the model of core functions are needed. They need to be integrated. The critical issue relates to a continuum of services and functions that need to be applied in a rational manner.

**Where is public health going during the next five years?**
The answer to your question depends on how rapidly and influentially we can educate our policy makers. We got a reprieve last year (1994) when national and state

*(continues)*

**Case Study 10-B** *continued*

health care reform legislation was not passed. We need to intensively educate our public because education was neglected at the national and state level. First, we need to educate our policy makers one on one in terms of what public health is. The idea of core functions is not part of the message to policy makers because the terms are misleading. It is necessary to be very concrete rather than abstract with policy makers. The arguments need to not only be concrete, but also the messages given must be very simple and strong. For example, we might say that the mission of public health is to prevent epidemics and the spread of disease, protect against environmental hazards, prevent injury, promote and encourage healthy behaviors, respond to disasters and assist communities in recovery, and ensure the quality and accessibility of health services. Specific local examples will strengthen the arguments. The important message to give is that the health reform plans will not work unless we have a strong public health foundation.

**How do we do more with less money?**
This depends on the decisions of the organization. In Florida, health departments are doing three things. First, they are downsizing completely and doing nothing except traditional public health activities totally out of the prevention/primary care arena. Other health departments are downsizing but are doing things in the contractual arena with local HMOs to provide some prevention and some primary care. There are other departments like us that are competitive, entrepreneurial, and will compete for the primary care dollar in just as businesslike a manner as the private entrepreneur. The money that we get and save goes into public health. There may be less money through categorical funding, block grant funding, or whatever, but there is a way to make money to fund public health. We chose the latter road.

**How do we become more entrepreneurial?**
Public health professionals need to learn how to be more creative. They need to learn how to create a vision that defines what public health should be. This needs to be done by working with the community as well as other colleagues in the health department. Then, it is necessary for the public health department leader to market itself. You first create the vision. To achieve it, you must become more businesslike and accountable. You don't market yourself only to get more business, but market in terms of health promotion activities and successes. Thus, you need to market yourself to the community and all the way up to the policy makers. I can tell you what we did to attract the attention of our entire legislative delegation. They are impressed with our mobile clinics that go to migrant camps, as well as the fact that we serve clients at night and on weekends. We are not always as good at tooting our horns as we should be. That is a mindset that hasn't been in public health.

**What is public health's role in managed care?**
I look at it three ways. Number one is you are doing it yourself. Number two is that you are participating with other managed care groups. Third, if you are not in the business yourself or participating with other managed care entities, you do have to oversee the assurance piece. If you are in the business, you are going to have to monitor assurance anyhow. Assurance of the managed care activities in your jurisdiction is a critical public health activity for the health department whether the department is doing the managed care or not.

**What aspects of health care reform will pass Congress in the near future?**
I don't think anything is going to pass soon. If anything does pass, it will probably be something related to insurance reform. It will be tough because the insurance

lobby is strong. With a great amount of discussion now on welfare reform, we are more likely to see action here that might relate to the tightening up of Medicaid benefits. I don't see that much change is going to occur in Florida either.

### What is the relationship between strong leadership and restructuring the field of public health?

It's everything. We can't stress this more. How come we don't have a public health political action committee? Everybody else does. Public health professionals don't seem to fight for public health like other special interest groups do. Leadership development should not be separated out from professional education. It should be part of the educational experience of our public health students. Leadership training should also be available for residency training directors. Leadership training is clearly important for preventive medicine residents. Fellowship training is good, but leadership development needs to occur earlier in the educational process.

### Postscript: Comments from Dr. Jean Malecki (February 2008)

Since 1995, the most critical question public health faces today is how do we champion an assurance role in the area of health care access when the existing health care delivery system is in disarray and imploding right in front of us? A system does not exist for the delivery of appropriate, acceptable, and integrated care that incorporates prevention, early intervention, and primary and specialty care as a continuum for the individual patient. The disease-based model that is procedure driven and promotes the hospital/emergency department as the "hub" of clinical care remains the status quo. This model is antiquated and wasteful and will continue to provide no potential future health improvements for all Americans. Other critical issues that face public health today include the ability to rapidly respond to emerging health threats and recognizing the aging and neglected critical public health infrastructures that have been the primary success of public health for the past 100 years, such as water treatment facilities and wastewater plants. The globe is warming, disparities continue, and our behaviors are out of control. A third of school children in Palm Beach County are either obese or overweight. The plate of local public health is full!

The first Medicaid HMO in the state of Florida was created by the Palm Beach County Health Department. It continues to exist and is called Healthy Palm Beaches. It is now run by the Health Care District of Palm Beach County, which is the public health funder for trauma, indigent care, and public health programs. As the director of the local health department, I am a member of the Health Care District Board. This model, an HMO housed in a governmental entity, is both productive and efficient. Its focus is on prevention and early intervention. I propose that national health care reform consider Public Health Managed Care as its central doctrine.

Emergency preparedness and response initiatives are now part of everyday behavior of local public health agencies. Our mission statement now includes four "P's": Prevention, Promotion, Protection, and Preparedness. Fortunately, the money we receive funds core public health such as epidemiology, risk communication, and active disease surveillance. These had "unfunded mandates" in the past. We have used those dollars at the local level to test response capabilities utilizing real-life scenarios, such as distribution and provision of Flumist to up to 30 schools, over 1,000 children within a one-week period of time. The coalition of "preparedness and response partners" has proven to be very effective. Again, public health is all about sustained relationships and a shared commitment to the public's health and well-being. Public health is everyone's business in a society that cares about its community.

Managed care can be defined as "a system of administrative controls intended to reduce costs through managing the utilization of services. Managed care can also mean an integrated system of health insurance, financing, and service delivery that focuses on the appropriate and cost-effective use of health services delivered through defined networks of providers and with allocation of financial risk."[42(p.371)] This definition does not mean that public health agencies will be without a direct service role in the future. Strong partnerships between public- and private-sector organizations will provide a synergy that could well lead to more effective public health initiatives at the community level—with more citizens being served as a result of the collaboration.

Strong leadership on both sides is necessary if improvement in the community's health is to occur, and everyone involved with improvement efforts needs to be aware that public health leaders, managed care leaders, and legislators have different priorities.[43] The highest priority for managed care leaders and legislators is to keep costs down. The highest priority for public health leaders is to increase access to services, the next highest is to ensure that the services are of high quality, and third in rank is keeping costs low. Managed care leaders put quality second and access third. Legislators put access before quality. Thus, partnership is sometimes difficult because of the differences in priorities.

One thing that public health leaders and managed care leaders can agree on is the importance of prevention, for preventive activities are essential for keeping the demand for managed care services low (which of course keeps MCO costs low). Novick[44] reported on an interesting partnership between the public health agency in Onondaga County, New York, and the four Medicaid MCOs that were providing services to county residents. The partners:

- set up a system for monitoring the delivery of preventive services in the MCOs and in the community at large
- created linkages between managed care clinical services and population-based prevention services (e.g., programs to reduce the prevalence of sexually transmitted diseases, tuberculosis, and HIV infection)
- worked together to facilitate disease surveillance, health-promotion and disease-prevention programs, and behavioral and environmental interventions

The relationship between public health agencies and MCOs can take many forms. It can range from complete independence through various levels of interaction to complete integration. In my study of public health leaders (see Case Study 2-A), most of the leaders believed that governmental public health agencies need to remain independent if they are to serve their communities well, perhaps because it is not possible to delegate responsibility for program oversight to nongovernment organizations.

Whatever the relationship between a public health agency and local MCOs (except for complete independence), public health leaders need to create a process for creating and maintaining it. One such process, developed by Leviss and Hurtig, encompasses the following 10 steps:[45]

1. Conduct assessments of both the inside and outside of the organization.
2. Evaluate and redefine the mission and vision of the agency in order to create viable assurance activities.
3. Review partnership models and start implementation.

4. Create collaborative relationships with MCOs.
5. Develop formal structures to undergird the collaboration.
6. Create new policies and regulations to support the collaboration.
7. Market materials to demonstrate the partnership.
8. Build an infrastructure to support the partnership.
9. Not only choose models of collaboration, but implement the models.
10. Evaluate the process.

The Institute of Medicine Report on Healthy Communities discusses the evolving relationship between government public health agencies and the MCOs.[46] Three recommendations from the report are relevant to the present discussion:

1. Local public health agencies should ensure that there are high-quality services and programs available in their jurisdiction, including personal health services, and that these are accessible to all residents.
2. The leadership of local public health agencies, MCOs, and other stakeholder organizations must agree on their proper roles and responsibilities.
3. Public health agencies need to increase the level of their oversight of the health services system in their jurisdiction. For purposes of oversight, they need to collaborate with insurance regulators and state Medicaid agencies. If they perform their oversight activities effectively, they will have the opportunity to define the integrated health care system of the future.

The evolving relationships between public health agencies and MCOs will continue to present formidable challenges. Whether public health leaders like it or not, managed care will not go away. Furthermore, putting your head in the sand is never a good strategy. It is clear that managed care will be part of any comprehensive system of health services.

Public health leaders must:

- make public health promotion the number-one community action priority
- work proactively with MCOs and not ignore them
- redefine the health care delivery system to include primary prevention programs
- reorganize local public health agencies (e.g., by creating new programs and revising current ones)
- develop a public health leadership toolkit

Public health leaders need to take an active role in developing assurance programs and services. Exercise 10-1 is based on a leadership credo exercise discussed by Kouzes and Posner.[47] Discuss your credo in relation to the percentage of time that you allocate to each of the three core public health functions.

## Summary

Finding out what problems exist (assessment) and figuring out what to do about them (policy development planning) would be pointless without the final step: doing what needs to be done (assurance). In public health, the overall goal of assurance is to prevent disease and promote health in the community. This chapter began with a discussion of disease prevention and the barriers to carrying the assurance function. It then went on to discuss the essential public health services associated with this core function.

Oddly, even though managed care may become more prevalent and take over the provision of direct services in most communities, the assurance activities of government public health agencies will expand rather than diminish. These agencies will continue to have oversight duties and will need to come up with new ways of meeting their responsibility to ensure that necessary programs and services are available to every community resident. Indeed, working out a viable relationship between public health agencies and MCOs will be one of the main challenges for public health leaders in the early part of the new century. One important lesson of the past decade is that all health system programs and services are subject to change. If public health constantly changes, then we can expect that MCO models will also change as political and social changes occur. A universal health care model will also change public health and the health delivery system.

## Discussion Questions

1. What are the differences between primary, secondary, and tertiary prevention?
2. What are the program responsibilities of public health agencies in primary, secondary, and tertiary prevention?
3. What are some of the main barriers that public health leaders face in meeting their assurance responsibilities?
4. What are the five essential public health services of assurance?
5. Are the assurance activities of government public health agencies likely to diminish or increase? Explain why.
6. How do public health agencies benefit from creating community partnerships?
7. What are the differences between population-based services and personal health services?
8. What are some of the factors that affect quality of care?
9. The greatest challenge that public health leaders will face in the immediate future is dealing with the growing prevalence of managed care. How can public health leaders meet this challenge?
10. Why is prevention likely to play a large role in the relationship between public health agencies and MCOs?

## Exercise 10-1:  Leadership Credo

*Purpose:* to develop a set of guidelines for agency staff that reflect the agency leader's beliefs, values, and concerns

*Key concepts:* core public health functions, delegation of responsibility, leadership credo, leadership values

*Procedure:* Each student is to pretend that he or she is the head of a public health agency and has been given a six-month leave of absence to luxuriate on a tropical island that lacks all modern means of communication, including mail service. Before departing, the leader of the agency must give general guidance to the staff. The staff need to know the leader's values and beliefs—in short, the leader's credo. The leader must write a one-page memorandum that expresses that credo. After the credos are written, they are read to and discussed by the entire class.

*Source:* J. M. Kouzes and B. Z. Posner, *Credibility,* pp. 62–63. 1993, Jossey-Bass.

# References

1. B. J. Turnock, *Public Health: What It Is and How It Works,* 4th ed. (Sudbury, MA: Jones and Bartlett, 2008).
2. Washington State Department of Health, *Public Health Improvement Plan: A Progress Report* (Olympia, WA: State of Washington Department of Health, 1994).
3. Roadmap Implementation Task Force, *The Road to Better Health for All of Illinois* (Springfield, IL: State of Illinois, 1990).
4. E. J. Bassler, B. J. Turnock, and L. Landrum, "Sustaining Leadership in Public Health Improvement in Illinois over Five Decades," *Leadership in Public Health,* 7 (2007): 2–5.
5. Institute of Medicine, *The Future of Public Health* (Washington, DC: National Academy Press, 1988).
6. G. Pickett and J. J. Hanlon, *Public Health: Administration and Practice,* 9th ed. (St. Louis: Times Mirror and Mosby College Publishing, 1990).
7. Institute of Medicine, *The Future of Public Health.*
8. Institute of Medicine, *The Future of Public Health.*
9. Institute of Medicine, *The Future of Public Health.*
10. Institute of Medicine, *The Future of the Public's Health* (Washington, DC: The National Academies Press, 2003).
11. Centers for Disease Control and Prevention, National Public Health Performance Standards Program: Local Public Health System Performance Assessment Instrument, Version 2.0 (Washington, DC: U.S. Department of Health and Human Services, 2007).
12. Centers for Disease Control and Prevention, Local Public Health System Performance Assessment Instrument, Version 2.0.
13. B. J. Turnock et al., "Implementing and Assessing Organizational Practices in Local Health Departments," *Public Health Reports* 109, no. 4 (1994): 478–484.
14. Centers for Disease Control and Prevention, Local Public Health System Performance Assessment Instrument, Version 2.0.
15. Turnock et al., "Implementing and Assessing Organizational Practices in Local Health Departments."
16. Centers for Disease Control and Prevention, Local Public Health System Performance Assessment Instrument, Version 2.0.
17. Centers for Disease Control and Prevention, Local Public Health System Performance Assessment Instrument, Version 2.0.
18. J. Studinicki et al., "Analyzing Organizational Practices in Local Health Departments," *Public Health Reports* 109, no. 4 (1994): 485–490.
19. Studinicki et al., "Analyzing Organizational Practices in Local Health Departments."
20. B. J. Turnock et al., "Local Health Department Effectiveness in Addressing the Core Functions of Public Health," *Public Health Reports* 109, no. 5 (1994): 653–658.

21. Illinois Administrative Code, title 77, sec. 600.
22. Turnock et al., "Implementing and Assessing Organizational Practices in Local Health Departments."
23. Turnock et al., "Local Health Department Effectiveness in Addressing the Core Functions of Public Health."
24. Bassler, Turnock, and Landrum, "Sustaining Leadership in Public Health Improvement in Illinois over Five Decades."
25. Pickett and Hanlon, *Public Health,* 9th ed.
26. L. A. Aday, *At Risk in America* (San Francisco: Jossey-Bass, 1993).
27. L. Breslow et al., Preface, in *Annual Review of Public Health* 1, eds. L. Breslow et al. (Palo Alto, CA: Annual Reviews, Inc., 1980).
28. Breslow et al., Preface.
29. K. Gebbie, Redefining the Assurance Function (speech) (Chicago: Illinois Public Health Leadership Institute, 1995).
30. S. B. Thacker, "Historical Development," in *Principles and Practice of Public Health Surveillance,* eds. S. M. Teutsch and R. E. Churchill (New York: Oxford University Press, 1994).
31. Thacker, "Historical Development."
32. American Public Health Association, *Healthy Communities 2000: Model Standards* (Washington, DC: American Public Health Association, 1991).
33. Washington State Core Government Public Health Functions Task Force, *Core Public Health Functions* (Olympia, WA: State of Washington Department of Health, 1993).
34. Washington State Department of Health, *Public Health Improvement Plan: A Progress Report* (Olympia, WA: State of Washington Department of Health, 1994).
35. U.S. General Accounting Office, *Quality Assurance: A Comprehensive National Strategy for Health Care Is Needed* (Gaithersburg, MD: U.S. General Accounting Office, 1990).
36. U.S. General Accounting Office, *Quality Assurance.*
37. U.S. General Accounting Office, *Quality Assurance.*
38. U.S. General Accounting Office, *Quality Assurance.*
39. J. Zusman, "Quality Assurance in Mental Health Care," *Hospital and Community Psychiatry* 39, no. 12 (1988): 1286–1290.
40. G. P. Mays et al., "Managed Care, Public Health, and Privatization: A Typology of Interorganizational Arrangements," in *Managed Care and Public Health,* eds. P. K. Halverson et al. (Gaithersburg, MD: Aspen Publishers, 1998).
41. I. Rowitz, *Public Health in the 21st Century: The Prepared Leader* (Sudbury, MA: Jones and Bartlett, 2006).
42. Turnock, *Public Health.*
43. C. P. McLaughlin, "Managed Care and Its Relationship to Public Health: Barriers and Opportunities," in *Managed Care and Public Health,* eds. P. K. Halverson et al. (Gaithersburg, MD: Aspen Publishers, 1998).
44. L. P. Novick, "Managed Care and Public Health," *Journal of Public Health Management and Practice* 4, no. 1 (1998): vi.
45. P. S. Leviss and L. Hurtig, "The Role of Local Health Units in a Managed Care Environment: A Case Study of New York City," *Journal of Public Health Management and Practice* 4, no. 1 (1998): 12–20.
46. M. A. Stoto et al., eds., *Healthy Communities: New Partnerships for the Future of Public Health* (Washington, DC: National Academy Press, 1996).
47. J. M. Kouzes and B. Z. Posner, *Credibility* (San Francisco: Jossey-Bass, 1993).

# APPENDIX 10-A—STATE OF WASHINGTON ASSURANCE CAPACITY STANDARDS

## Health Promotion Capacity Standards

All public health jurisdictions, both state and local, must:

- Bring about needed changes in laws, regulations, ordinances, and policies.
- Develop health promotion programs that are culturally and linguistically appropriate for the community.
- Provide education about and intervention to prevent specific infectious and noninfectious diseases such as dental caries, vaccine-preventable diseases, hypertension, cancer, and heart disease.
- Provide education about and intervention to address specific personal and environmental risk factors such as substance abuse and hazardous materials in the home.
- Provide assessment data to the community about the incidence and causes of intentional and unintentional injury.
- Provide education in the community to help create healthy living environments.
- Provide public and professional education and other interventions to reduce intentional and unintentional injury.
- Provide services and education that enhance the formation of healthy family relationships, promote normal child growth and development, and foster appropriate child health care practices.
- Provide education about reproductive health and family planning methods and strategies.
- Provide education about noninfectious disease to affected individuals and their families, especially regarding disease progression, treatment, and support services.
- Provide publications, presentations, programs, and media releases on a routine basis that inform and educate the public on the health status of the community, relevant health issues, and positive health behavior.

Each local public health jurisdiction must:

- Address prioritized public health risk factors in the community through a planning process, developed in collaboration with the community that identifies appropriate intervention strategies for specific issues and populations.
- Maintain an information and referral system concerning available health facilities, resources, and services.

- Give community members access to information and training regarding appropriate actions that enhance their living, working, school, and recreational environments.

The state must:

- Help agencies develop education strategies, including media releases and hotlines, aimed at reducing behavioral and environmental public health risk factors.
- Provide staff and technical expertise and support where local level resources are temporarily or permanently unavailable to ensure that health promotion plans and programs addressing health risk factors are fully implemented statewide.
- Serve as the lead agency for coordinating public health activities during emergencies.
- Develop intervention strategies, education materials, and classes for specific needs of caregivers, health professionals, and other public and private partners on a statewide basis.
- Design model health education and related organizational, environmental, and economic interventions to address public health risk factors.
- Help develop public health curricula in K–12 school health education.
- Develop or provide information and referral mechanisms, including hot lines, for statewide services (for example, oral health, mental health, and environmental health issues).
- Coordinate with local health agencies and other state organizations to draft and promote statewide legislation aimed at reducing public health risk factors and promoting healthy behaviors.
- Work with the higher education system to ensure that health education/promotion personnel and training is available to address health promotion needs in local and state agencies.

## Health Protection Capacity Standards

All public health jurisdictions, both state and local, must:

- Maintain appropriate monitoring, inspection, intervention, and enforcement activities that eliminate or reduce the exposure of citizens to communicable disease, environmental health, and emergency hazards.
- Coordinate protection efforts with many other local, state, and federal agencies and groups.
- Develop protection programs, in accordance with federal guidelines and scientifically identified risk factors that address prioritized health risk factors.
- Ensure that communicable disease contact investigation and follow-up are done in a timely and appropriate manner, in adherence to guidelines of the federal Centers for Disease Control and Prevention.
- Ensure that persons with communicable diseases are identified, treated in a timely, appropriate manner, and given information regarding treatment protocols and appropriate behavior to reduce the spread of disease.

- Take appropriate legal or other action if treatment protocols or behavior changes are not followed through.
- Ensure that individuals, especially children, are immunized according to recommended public health schedules.
- Provide surveillance, diagnosis, and treatment of infectious diseases of public health significance.
- Analyze and interpret data regarding environmental and personal risk factors.
- Provide maternity services such as outreach, case management, and support services.
- Provide nutrition intervention services for children and childbearing women that include education and provision of specific foods.
- Regularly screen and assess children who are at risk or who live in high-risk families.

Each local public health jurisdiction must:

- Conduct ongoing inspections and provide oversight consistent with state and local board of health rules and regulations.
- Respond to concerns expressed by the public regarding health problems.
- Conduct surveillance and manage the data generated so that program efforts can address community needs and problems.
- Enforce compliance with public health regulations whenever a voluntary compliance strategy is not effective or appropriate.
- Train operators of facilities (for example, water treatment plants and food service establishments) in order to ensure that facilities are properly operated and maintained on a day-to-day basis.
- Identify and control small animal, insect, and rodent populations that present potential and actual hazards to public health.
- Determine the nature and impact of public health emergencies and mobilize resources to control or prevent additional illness, injury, or death.
- Provide public health information services on a 24-hour basis to inform and help coordinate responses of local, state, and federal organizations to public health emergencies.
- Maintain an inventory of local medical and health personnel, medical equipment, facilities, and other resources that might be needed during emergencies, noting availability and response criteria.
- Provide or have access to laboratory services that can, during emergencies, support the local detection, identification, and analysis of hazardous substances that may present threats to public health.
- Maintain required potability and quality of domestic water supplies affected by emergencies.
- Provide for the public health concerns of the rescue workers and care providers in emergency situations, including needs for shelter, food, and sanitation equipment.
- Provide ongoing public health staff training in emergency response plans, including participation in practice exercises on a routine basis.

The state must:

- Facilitate and provide periodic training to local health agency staff and operators of facilities (for example, hotels, hospitals, restaurants, water treatment plants, public swimming pools, sewage disposal plants) on new and emerging issues.

- Routinely coordinate with federal rule-making agencies and the Congress to ensure that they take into account the effects of federal rules and statutes on the health risks, protection needs, and resources of Washington State.
- Develop, in cooperation with local health agencies, consistent uniform statewide regulations and policies that guide the public health activities of direct service providers, the local public health jurisdictions, and state agencies.
- Support the day-to-day efforts and provide assistance in the crisis response efforts of local agencies.
- Carry out the direct regulatory responsibilities over the largest public water supplies and certain community on-site sewage disposal systems.
- Assume appropriate service, consultative, and coordination responsibilities for emergency response efforts.
- Serve as the lead agency for coordinating all public health activities during emergencies in the State Emergency Operations Center.
- Provide public information support to the Office of the Governor and to other state or federal emergency management agencies during emergency and disaster recovery operations.
- Support local health agencies in the provision of laboratory services, food and water inspection, radiological assessment, and disease identification and testing during emergencies.
- Help coordinate and incorporate local emergency response plans into a statewide plan.
- Help coordinate the transfer of needed personnel, resources, and equipment to emergency sites.

## Quality Assurance Capacity Standards

Each local public health jurisdiction must:

- Ensure that communicable diseases are being appropriately treated in the community.
- Ensure that prevention and intervention efforts for communicable diseases are being appropriately implemented, including tracking the immunization status of children in the community.
- Evaluate the health status of populations who receive public health services and the impact of those services on their health status.
- Recognize and respond to unmet community needs, especially those related to high-risk conditions or behaviors.
- Gain access to data systems to provide long-term trend analyses, including being a participant in the Health Services Information System.
- Monitor and ensure the competence of people such as food handlers whose activities can affect the health of the public and who are not otherwise licensed or monitored by the state.
- Develop strategies to ensure that individuals and families can be linked with needed providers.

- Help inform providers regarding public health interventions, areas of concern, and recommended standards of care.
- Evaluate access to personal health services, especially for low-income and special populations. Where applicable, the evaluation should include a measure of the cultural appropriateness of services.
- Educate providers about specific public health interventions or areas of concern and recommended standards of care.
- Support strategies to ensure linkages between providers, families, and individuals.
- Evaluate the efficacy, costs, and benefits of prevention services as compared to medical treatment.
- Recognize the need for and establish criteria for competency assessment and assurance of health professionals.
- Design, implement, and evaluate licensing and certification programs and methods for health professionals and facilities and providers of other public services.
- Ensure compliance with appropriate regulations and standards in health care sites and facilities.
- Periodically review local health agency and community programs to ensure compliance with state standards.
- Assess and monitor state-funded public health programs for outcome results.
- Conduct quality assurance activities and operate state-mandated regulatory programs necessary to ensure that all laboratories produce high-quality outcomes. Work with agencies to correct deficiencies and provide appropriate training programs.
- Ensure that laboratories that provide data for public health purposes are linked through a common information management system that ensures consistent laboratory performance and ready access to analytical and diagnostic data.

# Leadership Skills and Competencies

# CHAPTER 11

# LEADERSHIP AND COMMUNICATION

> There was an inimitable cadence, an emphasis on certain
> words, an exaggeration of certain phrases, a kind of intoning
> here and there which made his telling unforgettable.
>
> A. Thirkell on Rudyard Kipling, *Three Houses*

Part III of this book looks at the tools and skills that leaders need to apply in carrying out their responsibilities. This chapter is concerned with communication skills. Leading, after all, is an interactive process involving leaders and followers, and obviously good communication among all participants in the process is absolutely essential.

Communication is the transfer of information and meaning,[1] and it has become even more important over the last decades—the start of the so-called information age—than it was previously. Information makes situations orderly, promotes change and growth, and defines reality. The importance of meaning and how the messages are perceived and processed by the recipient of the message is extremely important. It plays an important part in the leadership process, as does the communication of information in all the various forms that such communication takes, from face-to-face conversation to electronic transfer of data. In learning organizations, it is communication that drives the process. Leaders are teachers as well as learners. Their personal experiences lead the way into their vision of the future. Tichy and Cohen stated that it is ideas, values, and energy that drive the learning and teaching process.[2] These three skills give leaders an edge in solving problems and making decisions. This energy and passion gets communicated through many mechanisms that are discussed in this chapter.

## The Communication Process

It may be difficult to communicate effectively, but it is impossible not to communicate at all.[3] Each person's life is based on developing and using language to interact with other people.

A communicative act involves the transmission of two messages. The first message is about the topic of the communication. The second message concerns the hidden or real agenda of the parties to the communicative act. Communication is an ongoing process throughout our personal and professional lives. It does not solve all our problems itself but must be accompanied by action.[4]

## Barriers to Communication

There are many barriers to effective communication.[5] Communication can be blocked by forces within the participants as well as external forces. Nonverbal behavior—in the form of facial and hand gestures—can influence how a message is received, as can conscious and unconscious thoughts and distractions such as noise and motion. In addition, men and women have different conversational styles that can either enhance communication or create barriers to communication.

The intended recipient's state of mind can be a major barrier to receiving a message. How many of us have found ourselves daydreaming in a public health agency staff meeting when the agency director or our supervisor asks our opinion on an issue. Other reasons for not listening to a conversation include anxiety about talking, lack of interest in the topic, thinking about what to say, confusion from trying to make sense of overly complicated discourse, lack of understanding of the professional lexicon, dislike of the speaker and his or her principles, and a desire to be somewhere else.[6] Lencioni has warned of the problems of boring and uninteresting meetings.[7] We need to be wary of death by meeting.

Sometimes a person says things in order to upset the listener, and the message does not completely reflect the ideas of the sender.[8] This type of behavior can create tensions in a marriage—or an agency. Suppose the director of a program says to a staff member, "John, I need further infant mortality data from the state. Please call the state epidemiologist and get me the infant mortality data for the last five years for our county. Would you also ask her to evaluate the data for us?" The true message might be this: "I don't trust John's interpretation of the data. John probably did it wrong." John may understand the underlying message, and his response—"I'll do it immediately"—might have as its underlying message, "Why doesn't he do it himself? I did the analysis correctly."

Other barriers include injecting into the communicative process a judgment that discredits the other party to the process and avoiding the concerns of the other party.[9]

## An Interactionist Model of Communication

Hulett[10,11] built a communication model based on the symbolic interactionist approach used by some social scientists, including Robert Sears, who had developed a model of communication as a dyadic action system.[12] According to Sears, each individual brings a personal history to each communicative interaction. Hulett, who thought that most communication models were simplistic, claimed that communication needs to be seen as a natural social process that encompasses what takes place within each participant as well as what takes place between the participants and that every act of communication occurs within a multilevel social system that it influences and by which it is influenced.

Hulett analyzed an act of communication into a number of steps, which he called the "instigation action sequence." Each step involves one of five types of act or event: a motivating stimulus, a covert rehearsal, an instrumental act, an environmental event, or a goal response (Figure 11-1). Each participant in a communicative act brings to it a cognitive map that affects the motivating stimulus. The initiator of the act evaluates the stimulus and mentally rehearses the proposed communication (covert rehearsal; see

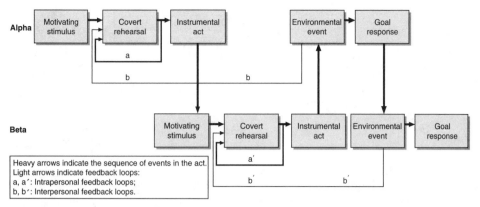

**FIGURE 11-1    Block Diagram of a Social Act Between Two Interacting Individuals, According to Symbolic Interactionist Principles**
*Source:* Reprinted with permission from J. E. Hulett Jr., A Symbolic Interactionist Model of Human Communication Part I, *AV Communication Review,* Vol. 14, No. 1, p. 14, © 1966, AECT.

Figure 11-2). The initiator then performs some action or says something (instrumental act) that triggers the motivating stimulus for the recipient of the interaction, who then mentally goes through the covert rehearsal phase. The recipient performs an instrumental act (answers the sender), which becomes the environmental act for the initiator. If the initiator is satisfied, then the goal response will be positive. If the recipient sees the response as positive, the interaction is complete. Feedback loops in the process allow the initiator and the sender to clarify issues and then finish the process.

According to Hulett, the covert rehearsal is the stage at which the individual role-plays his or her actions and tries to determine how the other person will respond. The self-concept of each participant, the values that guide each person, and the person's perceptions of the other's role influence the communicative process. For example, a public health leader will approach communication differently depending on whether the intended recipient is an agency staff member, the leader of another agency, or the president of the board of health. Further, a public health leader from a middle-class, suburban background will likely have different expectations when dealing with the residents of a working-class community than would a public health leader from a working-class background.

The model devised by Hulett concerns personal communication between two people. However, leadership also occurs at the team, agency, community, and professional levels, and the communicative process at each of these levels is complicated by the fact that a multitude of individuals are involved, each of whom comes to the process with a unique agenda and a unique interpretation of the same set of facts. A public health leader addressing a coalition, for instance, must discuss the issues with each coalition member individually at another time to ensure that the communication of ideas or information is successful.

### Communication Skills

Table 11-1 lists the communication skills needed by leaders at the five levels of leadership. It indicates that a public health leader requires at least 19

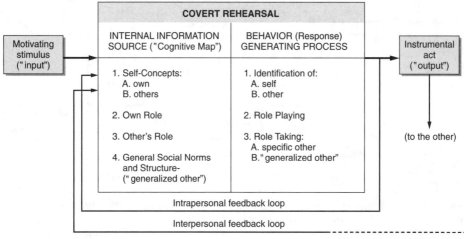

**FIGURE 11-2   The Covert Rehearsal of Either Participant in a Social Act, According to Symbolic Interactionist Principles**
*Source:* Reprinted with permission from J. E. Hulett Jr., A Symbolic Interactionist Model of Human Communication Part I, *AV Communication Review,* Vol. 14, No. 1, p. 18, © 1966, AECT.

communication skills. Most are discussed in this chapter, but conflict resolution and negotiation are discussed in Chapter 14; cultural sensitivity is discussed in a wider context in Chapter 15; and coaching, mentoring, and facilitation are discussed in Chapter 16.

To be effective communicators, public health leaders must:

• fully develop their communication skills as part of their lifelong learning agenda
• respect the different agendas that coalition members or partners bring to the table
• use the core functions of public health to guide communication with others
• use their communication skills to guide the transfer of knowledge
• be on the lookout for barriers to communication

## Interpersonal Communication

According to Hulett, interaction between two individuals is the basic unit of communication. In the workplace, critical communicative interactions include giving instructions, asking and answering questions, listening to the concerns of others, and, especially in the case of leaders, publicizing the organization's mission and vision.[13]

There are advantages to oral communication.[14] First, talking is the quickest form of communication. Ideas and thoughts can be relayed in a simple form that others can understand. Quick feedback is also possible. An important disadvantage is that the potential for distortion is great. Even with the best of intentions, community leaders may misinterpret the statements of

**Table 11-1   Communication Skills and Levels of Leadership**

| Skill Categories | Personal Leadership | Team Leadership | Agency Leadership | Community Leadership | Professional Leadership |
|---|---|---|---|---|---|
| Interpersonal communication | X | X | X | X | X |
| Active listening | X | X | X | X | X |
| Public speaking | X | — | X | X | X |
| Interviewing | X | X | X | X | X |
| Written communication | X | X | X | X | X |
| Computer skills | X | X | X | X | X |
| Media advocacy | X | X | X | X | X |
| Cultural sensitivity | X | X | X | X | X |
| Feedback | X | X | X | X | X |
| Delegation | X | X | X | X | X |
| Framing | X | X | X | X | X |
| Dialogue, discussion, and debate | X | X | X | X | X |
| Meeting skills | X | X | X | X | X |
| Health communications | X | X | X | X | X |
| Social marketing | X | X | X | X | X |
| Coaching, mentoring, and facilitation | X | X | X | X | X |
| Conflict resolution | X | X | X | X | X |
| Negotiation | X | X | X | X | X |
| Storytelling | X | X | X | X | X |

public health agency leaders. Communication will have to be continuous if agreement on goals and programmatic interventions is to occur.

## Communication Styles

Different conversational styles exist, and the differences in style can have social ramifications.[15] It is not uncommon for residents in a nursing home to be called by their first names by the staff, but this kind of informality may disturb some older residents, who might see the use of first names as indicative of a lack of respect. Also, major differences in conversational style exist between men and women, shown by the fact that men and women often seem to talk at cross-purposes. In addition, although the public health workforce is mostly female, most of the agency heads are men, and this may have something to do with the fact that women have different public speaking styles than men. Women must speak without the appearance of submission or of lack of a strong position. Women tend to not be overly aggressive,[16] but they will need to face conflict squarely in order to convince others of the truth of their beliefs.

In general, leaders need to avoid being too submissive or too aggressive in their communications.[17] Assertiveness is the most effective strategy. Assertive leaders fight for their beliefs and thus gain the respect of others without antagonizing them by being aggressive. Many public health leaders believe that they possess finely honed interpersonal skills, but in fact observation shows that these leaders frequently have trouble communicating with their staff and with community partners. Learning interpersonal skills is a lifelong process.

## Types of Formal Communication

There are three types of formal communication within an organization.[18] The first type is downward communication, from a superior to a subordinate. Among its benefits, it allows a supervisor to correct problems, and it keeps communication channels open, which tends to increase employee satisfaction. The second is upward communication, in which a subordinate initiates a conversation with someone at a higher level. This type of communication has the potential of preventing problems as well as solving existing problems. The final type of communication is horizontal or lateral, as occurs when colleagues at the same level communicate among themselves. The benefits include cooperation across sections of the organization. Cooperation between public health leaders and community leaders involves the last type of communication.

Informal communication networks are based on personal friendships, similar personal interests, shared career interests, and the closeness of working together in the same organization.[19] Informal communication networks focused on community health issues can be built on love of community and a desire to help the community by strengthening the infrastructure of public health.

## Interpersonal Communication Guidelines

Effective interpersonal communication requires talking to people in a way that will be meaningful and about topics that will be meaningful for them.

For example, public health leaders might talk to agency staff about the importance of the core functions of public health. In talking to a community group, on the other hand, they might discuss putting on a health fair or implementing a Healthy Communities 2020 program.

Leaders need to be careful not to let hostile feelings interfere with their judgment. Expertise should drive their conversation, not their organization titles. And they should always respect those with whom they are talking. Each conversation needs to be based on mutual trust. Judgment is critical to effective leadership. According to Tichy and Bennis, judgments relate to people, strategy, and reactions to crisis events.[20] There are three stages to judgment from a preparation stage to the judgment call itself and then to execution. Communication is critical during all three stages.

Leaders should use language that is understandable to their audience, which in many cases means forsaking the specialized language of public health. They should speak from the heart and take a positive perspective. Credibility is important to communication, which may fail without it. Sometimes the maintenance of credibility requires a leader to abandon his or her own agenda and replace it with an agenda favored by others.[21]

To ensure that their interpersonal communication is effective, public health leaders should:

- converse with other people in a meaningful way and on meaningful topics
- be assertive, not aggressive
- control hostile feelings
- allow their expertise, not their titles, to be the basis for paying attention to what they say
- make judgments carefully
- be open to considering new ideas
- respect the agendas of others and know when to abandon their own agenda
- use understandable language, speak from the heart, and take a positive perspective

Personal communication is the most important means of sharing a mission and vision with others. In the 21st century, it will be impossible for leaders without personal communication skills to sustain their credibility with colleagues, teams, agency staff, and community stakeholders.

## Active Listening

Public health leaders must be not only proficient speakers but also active listeners. Active listening takes concentration. The goal is to understand what the other person is saying and what it entails. Four critical skills are needed for active listening:

1. intensity of involvement in the interaction
2. empathy for the other's message and meaning
3. acceptance of the other person's message without judgment until the other person finishes talking
4. willingness to get all the information needed to make a decision[22]

Passive listening is listening without much involvement.[23] Passive listening is sometimes the appropriate listening style at a public presentation, for example. How many of us have taken courses or attended conferences where we were talked at rather than with. Passive listening may be interrupted by questions from the audience.[24]

The classification of listening styles into active and passive is somewhat simplistic. Alessandra and Hunsaker divide listeners into four types.[25] First comes the nonlistener, who does not pay attention to the message being sent. The second type is the listener who only marginally listens to the message. This listener is always rehearsing what to say or is preoccupied with other thoughts. The evaluative listener, the third type, listens to the entire message but misses the intent. The final type is the active listener. Scharmer has discussed four types of listening.[26] First, downloading is where confirmation is made of previous information, judgments, and decisions. Second, factual listening is where we listen for new facts or information that goes against previous decisions or judgments. Third, empathic listening is where we are trying to understand the feelings of others; this is closely allied to the concepts of emotional intelligence.[27] Finally, generative listening is when we relate to systems issues and a view of the world that is more expansive than our usual view.

To be an active listener, a person must ask good questions that will clarify both the content and the intent of the message.[28] Open-ended questions allow the respondent to go into detail about the meaning and intent of the message, whereas close-ended questions are meant to elicit short answers that will illuminate specific comments. One strategy, the so-called funnel technique, involves starting with global, open-ended questions and then gradually moving toward focused, close-ended questions.[29]

Consider this example: A new health department administrator is asked by the local board of health to explain the core functions and essential services of public health and why they are important. The administrator gives a 15-minute informal presentation on the topic. Board members start with broad questions, indicating that they still do not understand the core functions model, or why the administrator favors this model. The administrator answers these broad questions as best he or she can. As he or she clarifies his or her position, the board members narrow in on specific details by asking close-ended questions.

A listener can use questions to offer advice or attack the speaker for holding a position contrary to the listener's. In addition, the listener, in asking questions, may have a hidden agenda of which the speaker is unaware. The questions asked should be sincere and intended to elicit information the questioner truly needs in order to understand the speaker's meaning.

Walton listed five rules governing conversational etiquette:

1. Don't hog the floor.
2. Don't change the subject.
3. Don't step on the sentences of others.
4. Do hold your tongue.
5. Don't forget—there's always tomorrow.[30]

In active listening, the listener should make eye contact with the speaker and pay close attention to the speaker's words as well as any nonverbal message the speaker is conveying. Active listening is intense and requires an expenditure of energy. The speaker expects the listener to pay attention and not do distracting things, like answering the telephone or shuffling papers. When the speaker is finished, the listener should ask questions that show that attention was paid to the speaker's comments. The questions, however, should be as brief and to the point as possible. The author has been to talks in which an audience member got up and gave a 10-minute exegesis on his or her personal views—hardly a sign of active listening.

Active listeners:

- make eye contact and listen with all their senses
- avoid distracting actions, like answering the telephone or shuffling papers
- ask questions
- do not interrupt
- do not talk too much
- use positive gestures as part of their listening behavior

## Public Speaking

Public health leaders may have a clear vision of the future, but the effort they spent developing the vision will be all for naught unless they can publicize their vision and inspire others to share it. One of the best ways of publicizing it is to speak in different public venues, from local PTA meetings to national conferences, such as the annual meeting of the American Public Health Association. And to speak effectively, no matter what the venue, additional skills are needed beyond those required for effective personal communication.

At some state universities, public speaking is a university curriculum requirement. But even in these states, students tend not to understand the benefits to be gained by acquiring public-speaking skills. Public speaking helps teach the individual not only how to conceptualize an issue concisely but also how to integrate words with gestures to make a more effective argument in support of a particular point of view. Further, the more a person speaks in public forums, the easier public speaking tends to become.

Leaders know how to use language that strengthens the message given. Leaders tell stories as is discussed later in this chapter. President Reagan always added inspirational stories to his talks, and President Clinton did the same. Leaders also use analogies and metaphors in their talks. A public health leader might say, for example, "We must be careful not to let the ship of public health founder in the stormy debate over proposed cuts in federal programs." Body language is important. Holding on to the podium, for instance, does not communicate confidence. A speaker's nonverbal language should correspond with the speaker's words. In addition, the speaker should be aware of the pitch of his or her voice, especially when using a microphone.

Speakers should tailor each speech to the needs of the audience.[31] If the members of the audience cannot identify with the issues raised, they will tune out or forget the message fairly quickly. Speakers need to have a message that is realistic and focused. Unfocused presentations confuse the audience. Speakers also need to include supporting information.

Speakers need to appear credible to the audience.[32] They can maximize their acceptance by proving they are competent to discuss the chosen topic. They also need to earn the trust of the audience, which they can do partly by impressing the audience with the fact that they and the audience are basically alike and partly by appearing sincere. Also, using names of people in the audience sometimes increases the degree of acceptance of both the speaker and the speech.

Speakers are often viewed as mentors or teachers[33] and as entertainers. It has been suggested that public speaking is 25% knowledge and 75% charisma. Consequently, a speaker may find it worthwhile to rehearse the presentation ahead of time.[34] Dressing appropriately is important as well. A speaker in blue jeans does not go over well when the audience is in suits and dresses. If possible, speakers should leave time for questions, which is a good strategy for appearing human before the audience and gaining its acceptance. Of course, in some cases acceptance is hard to obtain, and so speakers should develop the skills necessary for dealing with a hostile audience. Humor usually helps when confronting hostility—and in most other cases as well.

Speakers need to know their audience but also be flexible enough to modify the prepared text if it is not appropriate for a particular audience. They also need to take note of the layout of the room because it can have an effect on the acceptance of the message.

Public health leaders who are required to do a lot of public speaking should familiarize themselves with the speaker aids that are currently available. Overhead projectors or liquid crystal display devices, for instance, allow speakers to present information concisely. One danger with overheads and slides is that they often contain so much information in such small type that they cannot be read beyond the second row or in a reasonable amount of time. (The so-called six-second rule is that every overhead or slide should be able to be read by the audience in six seconds.) Another danger is that, when many overheads or slides are displayed, the audience may become frustrated trying to keep up with the overheads and slides by taking notes on what they contain. A good solution is to provide copies of the overheads and slides to the audience in order to lessen the information overload. Slides and computer-based slide presentations tend to be better in large groups, at least if the remote control switch works. Handouts can be used in conjunction with slides to good effect, for they help the audience to remember the information after the talk is over. Running a short video may enhance a presentation. New computer presentation software and new projection devices can be useful, though buying or renting the necessary equipment at meeting sites can be costly. Further, since this equipment may break down, it is important to have a backup set of slides or overheads.

Which are the best speaker aids to use in a given situation depends to a degree on the speaker's speaking technique. If the speaker reads from a prepared draft, slides can be easily coordinated with the words. When using an overhead projector, the speaker may have to leave the podium and come down to the projector. This kind of interruption can lend the presentation an informality that some audiences seem to prefer, but it can also act as an irritant.

Case Study 11-A is a public health practice quiz with Toni Rowitz. Ms. Rowitz has been teaching public speaking at Oakton Community College in Illinois for over 35 years with over 12,000 students. She looks at public speaking as a critical set of skills for an effective leader.

---

## Case Study 11-A
## Public Health Practice Quiz for Toni G. Rowitz

### Why do leaders need to be good public speakers?

In their roles as advocates for good public health, leaders need to be effective speakers for a variety of reasons. First, though it's called "public" health, the concerns are with the well-being of individuals: vaccinations for children, mammograms for women, awareness of the propensity for high-blood pressure in African American men, crisis management in catastrophic situations, etc. Second, most public speeches are "one-shot deals." They need to be clear, thorough, and open to minimal misinterpretation. Even assuming that information is valid and current, the discussion needs to be interesting so that people will listen. Unfortunately, listening skills are poor; we tend to listen in 15- to 20-minute attention spans. Most persons listen at only 25% efficiency, and most of what is remembered is distorted or inaccurate.[1] Third, a speaker needs to be committed and focused on the specific needs of the audience(s). Speeches need to be "tailored" to make a good fit with the listeners. Finally, and perhaps most relevant, the credibility and commitment of a speaker carries more weight with audiences than the actual content. How the audience perceives a speaker will make all the difference. If you are a good speaker, you're a good leader because the information gets out where it needs to be.

### What are the major types of public speeches?

The basic types of public speeches most likely to be used by a public health leader are information, demonstration, and persuasion. Of course, all speeches are informational; the difference is the kind of information, the way it's used, and the speaker's intention. There may be overlapping of types, but it's easier to organize a presentation, and more important, it's easier for an audience to listen intelligently if there is basic grounding.

The first question a good leader asks is, "What is the purpose of this speech?" There are two sides to this question; the speaker's purpose in delivering the presentation has to coincide with the listeners' reasons for being there. A good leader puts a great deal of consideration into achieving the goals of the audience; they are always the primary component in any speaking situation.

Information speeches "tell," making the words primary in communicating the content; visual aids are helpful in delivering the message. The demonstration speech "shows" what it looks like/how it functions, how the parts connect, etc. Visual materials are primary in developing the content; however, there needs to be a fairly steady running dialogue as well for clarification and connection. These two speeches require the audience to listen, understand, and possibly offer feedback or participate in question/answer afterward. What they do with the information may not be directly communicated to the speaker.

The most challenging of the speeches is the persuasion. Its purpose is to encourage the making of different choices in behavior and practice. Sometimes, a member of the audience is in a "show me" frame of mind and asks questions beginning with "I may not be the expert here but . . ." In other instances, though they listen to the speaker ostensibly to examine and evaluate present programs and practices, as well as to seek expert advice, listeners may be limited by legitimate questions of money or facilities or personnel. A speaker can't do anything about those circumstances. Unfortunately, sometimes it's personalities that interfere: a speaker

*(continues)*

## Case Study 11-A *continued*

will have some say in this area. Energy and good will, as well as preparedness and expertise, are necessary for successful presentations, as well as for effective leadership.

### What techniques can engage an audience?

We've all listened to speakers who were learned and well meaning and so boring we wanted to jump-start their motors. Remember the teachers who practically put you to sleep, or the ones who were so disorganized that you never knew quite where you were? There are no guarantees for audience engagement, but there are some basics that can help to shape a successful presentation, for both speaker and audience.

First, being prepared is absolutely essential. The preparation does not only include materials, notes, etc. It's necessary to view a speech in terms of before, during, and the after. Speakers are speakers before they ever get up to the lectern. Personal interactions in the hallway or at receptions create impressions that will positively affect how listeners perceive and react to a speaker.

Intelligent listeners are better listeners. It's hard to listen intelligently if a speaker is disorganized, uneven, or unclear about the direction of the presentation. Initial engagement starts with the comments that capture the audience's attention and put them in the "ballpark"; an organized development of the topic makes listening easy and prevents confusion and subsequent inattention or dissatisfaction. During the speech, a smooth-flowing, natural delivery style does much to engage an audience. Eye contact, appropriate tonal variations, and response to feedback are all behaviors that encourage an audience to listen and to participate. To account for differences in learning styles and attention spans, use various support materials to increase interest and comprehension and to help listeners stay on track. Encourage active listening by assigning group or individual tasks or exercises (not busywork) that coincide with the topic. It is important to include a summary of the discussion, either on slides or hard copy, and take questions from the audience.

In short, the adept speaker/leader is confident in his expertise, respects the audience, is well prepared for all parts of the presentation, and makes a deliberate effort to communicate with, not talk at, the audience. At no time does a good speaker/leader get caught up in arguing or posturing. A confident, well-intentioned approach is maintained, and in cases of disrespect or deliberate misunderstanding, keeping one's cool is imperative. After the presentation, speakers need to be available for a reasonable length of time to answer questions, provide referrals, clarify concepts, etc. Presentations don't necessarily end according to the clock; leadership never does.

### How can speakers use slide presentations to enhance their speeches?

We are living in an age of visual stimulation; it's fast, in color, and so much a part of every aspect of life—entertainment, education, communication, and advertisement—that it's expected during presentations. In fact, a presentation devoid of PowerPoint or slides or videos is often regarded as less than excellent. One picture may represent more than a thousand words, but the words have to be there as well as the person speaking them. The term used to be "visual aid," with the operative word being "aid" as in assistance or support. Now, in many instances, the speaker has become the mechanic who works the equipment.

Several mistakes are consistently made in the use of slides or other visual aids. Most predominant is the mostly "absent" speaker, or the mechanic, who just turns on the projector, steps aside, and reads the slides to the audience. It's not interesting or engaging and worse does not fulfill one essential requirement of effective speaking—the speaker as focal point.

That's not to say that visual materials cannot contribute to an excellent delivery style. The first secret of successful slide presentations is having hard copies for listeners, so that they can make notes as the speaker discusses—NOT READS—the slides. Pictures, diagrams, and enhanced imagery need to be interesting and pertinent, and presented on the screen in an outlined or bulleted or numbered format. The details and information that flesh out the outline are presented as the speaker weaves in and out, using the visual materials to explain or reinforce the spoken commentary, sometimes when the slide is on, sometimes in between slides. The speaker always remains the focal point, in direct contact with the listeners. Any time that a slide isn't being used or referred to, the screen should be blank. If images remain on the screen, a listener is torn among watching the screen, looking at the speaker, and writing notes; it becomes a visual triangulation that breaks concentration and disconnects speaker from audience. Keep the informative slides simple and succinct. In between, for fun or interest or as attention-getters, use the "fancy" slides. Don't combine them—it diminishes effectiveness of both the slides and the discussion objectives. Keep in mind the original term, "visual aid"; it was never "visual crutch."

### What kind of clothes makes a difference in different types of speaking venues?

Dress is a matter of taste and common sense . . . good taste and uncommon sense, in considering fashion, etiquette, special circumstances. All the information about the effect of first impressions and about your appearance shaping a person's perception of you is true. The crucial point is that speakers don't want to diminish their ethos and effect because an audience is distracted by the way they look; no speaker wants listeners to pay more attention to appearance than to presentation. Because most speeches are delivered at conferences or other professional meetings, it would be in order to ask a couple of questions: Where are you going to be speaking? Who will be there? What are you talking about?

On one hand, the safest assumption to make is that any speaker is a professional person and is expected to dress as such. For men, that means suit or jacket and slacks, and tie . . . no jazzy jacket or hat or reeking aftershave. Common sense—maybe a great tie is an asset. Women need to wear a dress or skirt (not a "mini") with jacket or tailored blouse. A tailored pant suit may also be acceptable . . . no wild-print scarf or glitzy jewelry or heavy cologne. Common sense—a small scarf or understated piece of jewelry can work.

On the other hand, there is what's appropriate for a particular venue. Usually, no hats are worn at the lectern. Of course, if you are talking to a group of Little League baseball coaches about regional funding, and they give you a baseball hat with a logo on it, probably you should wear it, at least for a little while. Perhaps, instead of a dress with black pumps, a gaily colored lab coat and sneakers may be worn if the objective of the discussion is to effect a change in the way nurses dress in pediatric wards. Cultural and traditional apparel is always appropriate.

There are always alternatives to the "basic" dress. Sandals might be appropriate—thongs never. Jacket off may be okay, but T-shirt is out. Sleeveless blouse could be okay—tank top, not okay. Perhaps your best guide is to imagine yourself as speaker. As hard as it is, try to see yourself as others will see you . . . and go from there.

*(continues)*

**Case Study 11-A** *continued*

**Because leaders often need to be able to communicate with audiences from other cultures, are there special techniques needed for multicultural presentations?**

Multicultural presentations present an array of variables with which to deal, including language, acceptable/not acceptable body behavior, goal and style of presentation, appearance, time, behavior when not speaking, etc. There are so many cultural variations that the best advice is to get a good book, one that deals with "how to do it—don't do it" in other countries, such as Joseph DeVito's *Messages: Building Interpersonal Communications* (6th edition, Longman). Additionally, for a real-life personal perspective, if you know someone from the particular country, ask questions especially about speaking situations. When I am up there, what is an appropriate address to my audience? Is humor a good idea? If so, what kind? Do I get straight to the point or do I have to dance around it for a while? Do I open the floor for questions or do I lead the questioning by targeting specific areas?

Do not make any assumption about another culture, based on what you've been told or have been led to expect. A classic example is the situation explained to me by a Japanese colleague, whose husband is Caucasian. Whenever they dined out, the wait person would discuss after-dinner beverage preferences, asking her if she would like tea and if her husband would like coffee. As a matter of fact, he is the tea drinker and she drinks coffee. That's minor, but a speaker cannot afford to err in any direction. Something as small as a hand gesture, or looking into the eyes of someone whose culture determines that to be disrespectful, or a casual remark that is offensive, or a mannerism that is improper, will affect an audience's perceptions to the point of making the entire presentation an exercise in disrespect. Above all, the words and phrases used will carry the most weight—be careful to be able to correctly pronounce names, places, and terms. (I shudder when somebody pronounces it "Illinoiz.")

The special technique in the area of multicultural presentations is simple and precise: recognize that you have to be diligent in the tedious, but absolutely imperative, exploration of how a leader/speaker would perform and behave in a country not his own.

[1]J. Daly and I. Engleberg, *Presentations in Everyday Life—Strategies for Effective Speaking.* (Boston, MA: Houghton Mifflin, 2005).

---

In preparing a speech and giving it in front of an audience (Exercise 11-1), a public health leader should:

- become extremely knowledgeable about the topic of the speech
- find out the nature of the audience
- make the speech informative, persuasive, and entertaining
- integrate feelings and facts
- be candid and tell stories
- harmonize the verbal message and the message conveyed by body language
- blend theory and practice

## Interviewing

Interviewing skills are used by public health leaders when interviewing job seekers, agency staff for membership on self-directed work teams, and representatives of community organizations for partnership development.

As regards job recruitment, public health leaders must develop not only protocols for recruitment but also strategies for helping selected candidates keep their jobs.[35] Those responsible for job interviewing need to specify the qualifications for each job and follow a schedule in interviewing candidates so that all candidates are evaluated objectively.

A distinction can be made between direct and indirect recruiting. Direct recruitment is tied to defined positions that are currently vacant. Indirect recruitment is aimed at expanding the pool of potential job candidates through internships, school presentations, community health promotion programs, community lectures, and so on.

When interviewing a job candidate, the interviewer should cover a range of topics, from the job description to the way the candidate might fit into the agency. Table 11-2 lists 12 topics that should be explored in an interview.[36]

The interview format can be structured or open-ended. In a structured interview, the interviewer works from a set of standardized questions. The problem with this strategy is that the set of questions lacks application beyond the selection of a candidate for the particular job. An open-ended interview uses a general outline and allows the interviewee to structure his or her responses. The two format types can be combined to create an instrument that includes some of the best features of each.

Where the interview is conducted is also important. Interview questions asked from behind a desk will elicit different responses than if asked in a conference room or a more casual setting. In conducting the interview, the interviewer needs to establish rapport with the interviewee and control the direction of the conversation so that the necessary topics are covered.[37] The interviewer should urge the interviewee to give concise and thoughtful answers and make clear what his or her goals are. In addition, the interviewer should indicate to the interviewee the basis on which he or she will be evaluated.

The interviewer should either take notes during the interview or, if the interviewee agrees, audiotape the interview.[38]

---

**Table 11-2    Issues in Interviewing Job Applicants**

1. Job requirements and expectations
2. Department and institution characteristics (including patient and staff demographics)
3. Department and institution strengths
4. Management's unique vision of health care delivery
5. Mission of the institution
6. Applicant's technical level of skill
7. Opportunities for advancement within the department and institution
8. Applicant's career goals
9. Salary expectations
10. Applicant's personal and professional assets and liabilities as they relate to the worker role
11. "Fit" between the institution and the individual
12. Benefits

---

*Source:* Reprinted from J. G. Liebler and C. R. McConnell, *Management Principles for Health Professionals,* 4th edition, pp. 235–236. © 2004, Jones and Bartlett Publishers.

Checking the candidate's references is essential, because not all résumés are accurate and not all letters of recommendation are truthful.[39] Telephone reference checks are especially useful if done after the interview because they then allow the interviewer to delve into issues raised during the interview. In fact, the author has found telephone conversations with references to be more useful than letters of recommendation. Candidates sometimes develop fears about reference checks, whether or not those fears are legitimate. They also can be concerned to keep their present employers from finding out that they are applying for other jobs.

Public health leaders, though usually acting as the interviewer, do occasionally take the role of interviewee, such as when applying for a job as administrator at another agency and being questioned by the agency's governing board.[40] In interviews for leadership positions, the board must define the relationship between the administrator and the board as well as the boundaries of the administrator's authority. A candidate should not accept a position if convinced that he or she will not be able to function within the parameters set by the board.

One cautionary note: board members rotate off the board and some of today's members may not be on the board in a year. A candidate for a position as administrator should try to identify the challenges that exist and determine whether it is worth accepting the appointment on the chance that things will improve in the future.

Interviewers need to follow these guidelines:

- Prepare a series of questions ahead of time.
- Select the appropriate interview structure.
- Arrange the setting for the interview.
- Learn different interviewing techniques and when each is appropriate.
- Maintain high ethical standards.
- Keep each job candidate informed about the process of selection.

## Written Communication

Leaders need to be masters of all types of communication. The written word can have a major impact on readers. Leaders sometimes use the words of others to guide their vision and actions. The Declaration of Independence and the United States Constitution, both written more than 200 years ago, still provide the framework for political and social life in the United States.

Written communication in a modern organization encompasses, among other things, memoranda, letters, periodicals and books, e-mail, electronic bulletin boards, blogs, personal notes, grants, contracts, statistical and technical reports, overheads and informational slides, and performance appraisals. One of the major advantages of written communication is that it contributes to the creation of a permanent tangible record[41] and thus allows verification of past activities and events. Another advantage is that the written word is often clearer than the spoken word, largely because it can be reviewed and revised until the author is satisfied.

On the negative side, good written communication takes time. A telephone call takes but a moment and the feedback is immediate, whereas a letter takes time to write and reception of the response can be delayed for days or weeks. Of course, a telephone call leaves no permanent record unless it is followed up with a memo or letter. One-day mail delivery service and facsimile transmission do speed up the process of getting written feedback more quickly, but the process still lasts many times longer than a phone conversation.

Successful written communication demands preparation. The writer needs to plan the communication by organizing the underlying facts and developing the message prior to putting down words. If the organizing step is left out, the communication will almost certainly fail to be clear, specific, accurate, and concise.

Some writers find outlining a useful technique. Some can do this mentally. Wycoff suggested using a technique called "mindmapping."[42] This technique, in which possible approaches to an issue are diagrammed, can clarify the purpose of a written communication and provide a focus (a focus is important for the reader).

In the actual writing, choosing the right words is of the utmost importance. The use of jargon may undermine the effectiveness of the written communication and obscure the information to be disseminated. The promotion of health among community residents through written materials requires language that the residents understand. The writer should always keep in mind the recipients and how the message may be received. It is also important to follow up on the impact of the written materials over time.

Writers usually possess more facts than they are able to use. Part of the task of writing is to winnow out those facts that are unnecessary and focus on those that are critical to the intended message. The written product should of course be grammatically correct and contain no typographical errors—an easily attainable goal now that virtually all word-processing programs have a spelling checker. The importance of writing coherently cannot be overemphasized, and it is a good idea to have a peer check the writing for clarity. The reviewer should point out places where the writing is obscure or confusing and should offer any other advice he or she thinks might be helpful.

Public health leaders engaged in producing written health promotion materials or any other kind of writing should pay attention to the following guidelines:

- Use proper English and restrict yourself to a vocabulary that the intended audience understands.
- Master different writing techniques and use the appropriate technique for each piece of writing.
- Create an outline for a piece of writing prior to writing it.
- Check spelling and correct typographical errors.
- Avoid the incorporation of extraneous material into written materials.
- Write in the same way you talk, although choose your words more carefully.

## Computer Communication Skills

The personal computer has added some new wrinkles to communication and the transfer of information. Now we trade e-mail messages rather than letters. One advantage is that send-and-respond times are appreciably reduced. Further, although most e-mail messages are short, informal, and limited in scope, e-mail programs allow the sender of a message to attach large document files, such as for a report or research paper.[43] Personal computers can now also be used to do research on the Internet, by using search engines or by tapping into various databases.

One of the latest trends in high technology is the integration of personal computers, fax machines, cellular phones, and pagers.[44] The integration of computer technology and communications technology is allowing organizations to become even more interconnected. For example, any person connected to the Internet can create a network of colleagues around the world devoted to discussing topics of common interest. One way that this communication occurs is through blogging. Blogs are Web sites where people with common interests can communicate with each other in a narrative fashion.[45] Blogging has become a major tool of businesses, and it appears to be spreading to people working in public health.

The new technologies have some negative consequences, however.[46] One problem is the difficulty of ensuring the security of the messages that are sent. Another is e-mail overload and the decrease in responsiveness that sometimes results. Many of us go on a one-day business-related trip to come back to 100 e-mail messages or more. All of them have to be at least perused to see which are worthwhile reading and which need a response—a time-consuming process. Reviewing and answering messages on a daily basis can eat into valuable work time, as can listening to and answering phone messages. The transfer of e-mail or phone messages over the phone lines occurs virtually instantaneously, yet it is still the same old sluggish human brain that has to interpret each message and figure what to do in response. Shipley and Schwalbe pointed to the need to be careful about e-mails being unclear in their content, inadvertently insulting, possibly criminal, cowardly, inappropriate, too casual, or sarcastic.[47]

Public health agencies are struggling to acquire the technology necessary to enter the information age. Small rural health departments with limited budgets may not be able to purchase more than one or two personal computers, which will need to be shared. Even when computers are available, public health professionals complain that the necessary training is not. Public health leaders need to convince their governing boards of the importance of computer technology, including new advances.

One recommended strategy is to chart communication activities in order to determine how much time is spent talking, listening, reading, and sending e-mail messages.[48] Public health leaders may find it necessary to reorganize their communication activities so as not to impair their ability to carry out their main responsibilities. Leaders need to remember that computers are tools for dealing with problems, not complete solutions to them. And something else they should remember is that computer communication systems are not substitutes for personal communication.

Any important new tool brings with it a need to redefine work. The advent of computer and communications technology has made it necessary, for instance, to change interorganizational and intraorganizational structures,[49] and changes in technology will continue to affect the field of public health and the way public health leaders go about doing their job. To keep pace with the computer and communications revolution, public health leaders must:

- learn how to use e-mail and the Internet to increase effectiveness
- understand the advantages and disadvantages of e-mail as compared with other forms of communication
- learn e-mail etiquette
- master the art of blogging
- monitor advances in computer hardware and software
- train staff in the use of personal computers and the Internet

## Media Advocacy

During the 1980s and early 1990s, public health leaders had to learn how to talk to the media. They had to learn, for instance, how to condense a message into a 20-second sound bite, how to use letter-writing campaigns, and how to dress for television—all with the goal of promoting the goals and objectives of public health by using the media to bring pressure on policy makers in order to influence policy.[50] Public health leaders are the leaders most likely to view public health issues from a systems perspective, taking into account social, cultural, psychological, economic, and political dimensions, and they have a duty to use media advocacy to get the message out.[51] Media advocacy can be viewed as a form of empowerment in which public health leaders galvanize the community residents to fight for policies that will directly benefit them.

Major planning efforts need to be undertaken to create a coordinated approach to using the media to help solve community health problems. Public health leaders, in publicizing a public health concern, should urge the importance of developing a policy to deal with it and should involve community partners in any publicizing and policy development activities. In promoting a given policy, public health leaders must make sure the facts are researched and verified and must get key stakeholders to support the policy.[52] One of the tasks required for media advocacy is to foster good relationships with media representatives so that channels are open for important public health messages to get out to the community.[53] In developing support for public health initiatives, the use of each of the various media should at least be considered.

There are important differences between traditional public education and media advocacy (Table 11-3).[54] In traditional health promotion programs, the individual is the target, and the goal is to alter the individual's behavior. In media advocacy, the individual becomes empowered by becoming involved in the push for health policy changes. Advocacy is aimed at policy makers, and the goal of advocacy is to get beneficial policies legislated and put into action. The advocates, besides public health practitioners, are people who are affected by the health problem at issue and are willing to fight to ensure that the necessary changes are made.[55]

Media advocacy is most effective when it is community based. At its best it includes collaborative efforts at framing issues, setting agendas, developing talking (or writing) points, and monitoring the progress of policy proposals. Those collaborating in the media advocacy process must also keep the general public up to date on the various happenings.

A caution regarding media advocacy needs to be raised here. According to Fallows, the media often undermine the American political system by

**Table 11-3 Comparison of Media Advocacy and Public Education**

| Media Advocacy | Public Education |
| --- | --- |
| Individual as advocate | Individual as audience |
| Advances healthy public policies | Develops health messages |
| Decentralized and opportunistic | Problem and approach fixed |
| Changes the environment | Changes the individual |
| News and paid advertising | Relies on public service |
| Target is person with power to make change | Target is person with problem or at risk |
| Addresses the power gap | Addresses the information gap |

*Source:* L. Wallack and L. Dorfman, Media Advocacy: A Strategy for Advancing Policy and Promoting Health, *Health Education Quarterly*, Vol. 23, No. 3, pp. 293–317, copyright © 1996 by Sage Publications, Inc. Reprinted by permission of Sage Publications, Inc.

generating a sense of hopelessness about the future.[56] He stated that the media need to become more public spirited, support the American political system, and empower the public to influence policy. Those who use the media must recognize their limitations and the difficulty of controlling media reactions to local health problems. Case Study 11-B describes a situation in which the press overreacted to a potential private well contamination problem. It shows how the media need to be handled in the context of public health surveillance activities and how public health leaders should communicate these activities to policy makers and the public.

---

### Case Study 11-B
### Leadership Opportunities in Private Well Contamination with Volatile Organic Compounds

*Lillian Mood*

### Introduction
One of the emerging public health problems of our time is the actual or perceived risk of disease, particularly cancer, as a result of exposure to toxins in the environment. Two factors make protecting the health of the public from the dangers of environmental toxins particularly difficult. One is that the science of acceptable risk is still young; standards are developed as chemical compounds are identified as being harmful or potentially harmful to human health. The second factor is that the period of time between exposure and illness is measured in years and sometimes decades rather than the few hours to several days that has been the norm for communicable diseases.

The whole concept of "acceptable risk" is a dilemma in itself. Persons who willingly take risks, such as not wearing a seat belt, exceeding the speed limit, living a sedentary life, and even smoking, want and expect their environment to be free of any contamination from sources outside their own home. To them, any chemical that can be detected at any level is harmful and must be eliminated; many insist on limits for chemical compounds in air, water, and soil that are below detectable levels. The assessments are made in parts per billion, a quantity hard for the average citizen to conceptualize. Making the acceptance of reasonable risk even more complicated is the feeling people have about risks over which they have no control. The thoughts are something like this: "I can choose to eat a diet filled with foods that increase my risk of heart disease, but I have a horrible fear of and outrage about what that industry down the road is putting into the air or into the nearby river. Someone may be doing something to harm me that I can't see or feel, and I'm not at all sure that I can trust the government to protect me."

This is the general climate in which the state health department works toward its goals of minimizing health risks, preserving the quality and safety of the environment, and being responsive to citizens' concerns.

**Case Chronology**

In early September 1990, a resident of the Regal Oaks community contacted Al Brown, director of the Midlands Environmental Quality Control (EQC) District of the state health department, to register a complaint about his water. The resident, Mr. Bell, was experiencing itching and a skin rash that he was sure was due to contamination of his well from a nearby industry. Because Regal Oaks is not on Capital City's public water system, groundwater is the source of water from the private wells in the neighborhood.

*Surveillance (Assessment)*

Because contaminated groundwater could affect the quality of water in the Regal Oaks' wells, on September 12, 1990, scientists from the Midlands EQC District took groundwater samples in response to the resident's complaint. Samples were taken from the complainant's home on the 700 block of Fore Avenue and at another home on the 200 block of Fore Avenue. They were analyzed for volatile organic compounds (VOCs), pesticides, and herbicides, drinking water metals, and general water chemistry.

Analytical data received September 14 indicated the presence of three VOCs, including tetrachloroethene (PERC), trichloroethene (TCE), and cis-1,2-dichloroethene from one well in the 200 block of Fore Avenue. The level of PERC was 5.04 parts per billion (ppb), exceeding the maximum contaminant level (MCL) of 5.0 ppb that has been proposed for this compound and is in the process of negotiation by the federal Environmental Protection Agency (EPA).

The sample from the 700 block of Fore Avenue, Mr. Bell's home, was clean. More samples were taken from the 200 block of Fore Avenue and four other homes upgradient of that location. Analytical results from these samples confirmed VOCs above MCLs on the 200 block of Fore Avenue and identified detectable levels on the 100 block of Fore Avenue. A detectable level does not necessarily mean that levels are unsafe but shows the need for more testing. For this reason, the staff began an ongoing sampling program at Regal Oaks to determine the extent and source of the groundwater contamination and the resulting risk to the resident population.

On September 17, 1990, confirmatory sampling for VOCs was conducted at the previously sampled private well in the 200 block of Fore Avenue and four wells that appeared to be upgradient of the contaminated well. Analytical data received September 26, 1990, confirmed previous sampling results of PERC at 5.09 ppb and identified these same VOCs below established or proposed MCLs at a second well. The other wells sampled were free of contamination.

*Political Inquiry*

Meanwhile Lee Steele, the deputy commissioner for environmental quality control at the state health department, received a letter from the Reed County Council chair,

*(continues)*

**Case Study 11-B** *continued*

Jim Moore, dated September 18, 1990. Mr. Moore asked for an assessment of the air and water in Regal Oaks because residents were complaining to him that "the drinking water was often green in color and that an unpleasant smell can be frequently found in the air." The residents suspected that the air and water were being contaminated by the Woodbranch Subdivision's wastewater treatment plant, which was adjacent to Regal Oaks. Mr. Steele's response of September 25 indicated that inspectors had found problems at the treatment plant that accounted for the odors, and corrective action was being taken with the operator. Bacterial analyses of the groundwater, however, did not show contamination indicative of the presence of sewage. He also updated Mr. Moore on the status of the sampling for the VOCs.

*Surveillance Follow-up*

On October 3, 1990, department personnel obtained groundwater samples for VOC analysis from 17 additional wells. Analytical data received October 19, 1990, found three additional wells with the identified VOCs above the MCLs. Two other wells had detectable levels of VOCs but below the MCLs.

When the results were received for each sampling, each resident received a letter giving the analytical data for his or her well. If an MCL was exceeded, the resident was advised not to use the water for drinking or cooking.

Between September 1990 and February 1991, concurrent with the private well samplings, EQC personnel pursued identification of a potential source, or sources, for the identified contamination. Activities included review of project files and monitoring data, site inspections and interviews with staff personnel, and review of tax maps and property records. Review of the file for Diamond Board, Inc. (formerly Wheeler Trace, Inc.) indicated that Mitchell Jones, state health officer, had responded on September 19 to an August inquiry from Mr. Moore on behalf of his constituents in Regal Oaks.

The residents were concerned that an industry (Wheeler Trace, Inc.), formerly located adjacent to the subdivision, was believed to have used or disposed of hazardous chemicals at its site, and if this were true, those chemicals may have contaminated the environment. The state health officer's reply indicated that a consent order in January 1990 required the present industry on the site (Diamond Board, Inc.) to install two groundwater monitoring wells. Two rounds of samples from these wells allowed department staff to determine that groundwater was not adversely affected by the historical discharge of wastewater.

*Media Response*

A local newspaper reported the investigations on November 1, 1990. The options for well owners with water problems included digging new wells, treating their existing wells, using bottled water for drinking, or tapping into the city lines. Some residents had begun using bottled water, and Mr. Moore had approached city officials about extending the city's water system to the area. The city's estimate of the cost at that time was approximately $1 million; the cost to each resident would be slightly over $3,000 for the tap-in fee.

On November 2, 1990, two existing monitoring wells located on the former Roberts and Mixon facility property were sampled for VOCs, general water chemistry, and drinking water metals. Analytical data received December 7, 1990, revealed no detectable levels of VOCs from these wells.

On February 28, 1991, EQC personnel installed a temporary well on the property at 10260 Two Notch Road located apparently upgradient of private wells previously identified as being contaminated. Sampling results received April 18, 1991, revealed no detectable levels of VOCs.

On April 25, 1991, a news article reported the status of the investigation to the public.

*Department Action*

A May 10, 1991, internal department memo to the managers of the Facilities Compliance Section and the Assessment and Development Section of the Bureau of Drinking Water Protection from Pat Bissell, Midlands District hydrologist, summarized the activities and findings of the investigation and requested additional sampling between residences #144 and #224 along Fore Avenue. It was Mr. Bissell's opinion that, given the configuration of the affected wells, if a single source of contamination existed, it should manifest itself in that area.

On July 3, 1991, two additional private wells were sampled for VOCs (161 Fore Avenue and 232 Wynnette Way). Analytical data received August 8, 1991, indicated both wells had detectable levels of the identified compounds, with one well exceeding the MCL for PERC (11 ppb).

On August 22, 1991, an EQC district memorandum to the Bureau of Drinking Water Protection summarized the analytical data obtained to date: "Groundwater contamination appears to approximate an elongate plume which has (or is) emanating from an unidentified point south-southwest of the subdivision. Currently, the apparent contaminate plume is undefined both in vertical and lateral extent, which indicates additional receptors may be utilizing impacted groundwater at this subdivision."

Mr. Bissell urged a meeting as soon as possible to discuss actions necessary to resolve the matter expeditiously. On August 27, 1991, Mr. Bissell met with the director of the Division of Drinking Water Quality and Enforcement, three staff members from the Groundwater Protection Division, and a representative of the Enforcement Section of the Bureau of Drinking Water Protection. The staff agreed to continue efforts to identify the source of contamination and to extend the sampling to additional wells to determine if they were affected. The division director agreed to contact the state health department's legislative liaison to discuss funding alternatives for city water in this subdivision.

On August 29, 1991, a site discovery form listing the Regal Oaks subdivision was sent from the Bureau of Drinking Water Protection to the manager of site screening at the Bureau of Solid and Hazardous Waste. The Site Screening Section is funded by the EPA to conduct investigations at sites that may potentially qualify for the National Priorities List (NPL) for federal "Superfund" action. If Regal Oaks site qualified for the NPL, federal monies might be available to assist in remediation of the plume.

In September and October of 1991, additional water samples were collected from individual wells in an effort to identify all potential receptors of affected groundwater; 19 samples were obtained on September 4, 1991; 7 samples on September 12, 1991; 19 samples on September 30, 1991; and 8 confirmation samples on October 8, 1991. Analytical results indicated that 7 samples exceeded the MCL for PERC or the MCL for TCE.

On October 22, 1991, seeking more information about potential sources of the groundwater contamination, EQC personnel sampled the sanitary septic tank (sludge bottom) at Diamond Board for VOCs. Analytical data identified three VOCs

*(continues)*

normally associated with petroleum products. None of the VOCs found in ground-water within Regal Oaks were detected by this sampling. In another attempt to locate a possible source, on October 23 Midlands EQC District hydrogeologists met with university agricultural experiment station employees to explore the history of use of the station property. Experimental station employees of many years (15 and 32 years) were not aware of any spills, landfills, or landfilling activities on the station property during their tenure.

On October 25, 1991, health department staff met with state, county, and city officials to discuss the necessity for an alternative water source for the subdivision. In addition to providing an update on the status of the investigation, department personnel informed attending officials that the department has no funding, nor does it know of any funding source, to assist in the development of an alternative water supply.

On November 15, 1991, EQC staff installed and sampled three temporary wells, two on property directly across Two Notch Road from the subdivision and one on the corner of Two Notch Road and Fore Avenue. Detectable levels of two VOCs were identified in the two wells across Two Notch Road, but the compounds and levels needed to be substantiated through additional sampling. No VOCs were found in the sample collected from the corner of Two Notch Road and Fore Avenue.

*Legal Interest*
On December 3, 1991, Pat Bissell wrote a letter to Jim Moore updating him on the status of the well sampling and enclosed maps of the area. Mr. Bissell also wrote a letter to the Perdy law firm in response to a Freedom of Information Act request for information on the investigation. The Perdy law firm was also referenced in a letter sent by a resident of Regal Oaks to other residents on January 17, 1992. The law firm had been retained for a class action suit. Other citizen initiatives to get action on their concerns were described.

Informally, citizens reported that persons indicating they represented a law firm were knocking on doors in the neighborhood and asking if residents were experiencing health problems and needed legal assistance.

*Funding for a Public Water Supply*
On January 30, 1992, EPA officials informed the health department that no source of funding was available to assist in providing a public water system for the Regal Oaks subdivision.

On January 31, 1992, department personnel met again with state, county, and city officials to provide additional information in an effort to assist in obtaining grants to fund a public water source for the affected area of Regal Oaks.

On February 5, 1992, 15 additional water samples were collected from individual wells in an effort to track the location of the suspected contaminant plume. As of February 12, 1992, the department had collected 94 samples from 73 water supply wells in the Regal Oaks subdivision. Also the department had installed and sampled four temporary monitoring wells and sampled four existing monitoring wells at two facilities in the immediate area. Of the 73 wells sampled, data indicated that 30 wells exhibited detectable levels of VOCs, principally PERC and TCE. Twelve of the wells exceeded the established and/or proposed maximum contaminant levels for PERC and/or TCE, which are 5.0 ppb.

*Communication with Residents*
Each time sampling was done, a copy of the results and a letter of explanation were provided to each resident whose well was sampled. Residents were invited by the

Midlands EQC District director and the Reed County Council chair to a public meeting on February 12, 1992. A large number of Regal Oaks residents attended. Al Brown, EQC District director, welcomed the group, introduced the others who would be speaking, and explained a number of the terms (e.g., ppb, VOC, and TCE) in a fact sheet furnished to each attendee. Overhead projections of maps were used to show exactly the area affected and the points beyond which no contamination had been found.

Pat Bissell, hydrologist, described the patterns of groundwater migration in the area, which provided the basis for ruling out certain industries as potential sources of the contamination.

Mac Monroe, division director of the Drinking Water Protection Bureau, explained how standards for MCLs are reached and the boundaries of authority of the drinking water program. Bill Marks, MD, director of Health Hazard Evaluation, talked about what is known and not known about exposures to VOCs and what people can do to minimize their risk of exposure.

There were a number of questions from residents about health symptoms ranging from itching to rashes and about some residents' impression that the neighborhood had too many cases of cancer. Information was given on the usual effects of toxic doses of the VOCs identified. Liver damage and tumors of the liver occurred but only after long exposure to high concentrations. Well samples had been taken from the residences of persons with health complaints and no VOCs were found.

Jim Moore, county council chair, spoke of the efforts of elected officials to find funding to provide city water to Regal Oaks. He explained the availability of funds from the governor's office if the subdivision qualified. Because qualifying was dependent on the income levels of residents, attendees were given forms to fill out documenting their income. They were assured that the confidentiality of the information provided would be maintained.

*The Media Turn Up the Volume*
The meeting and some of the residents' reactions were reported in the local newspaper. A letter to the editor dated February 20, 1992, cited the Regal Oaks investigation as an example of "Power Failure," a term coined by the newspaper to support the governor's initiative to restructure state government into a cabinet organization of state agencies. One part of the proposal was to separate the health and governmental protection functions into two separate departments.

A March 25 letter to the editor from the district EQC director attempted to clear up some misunderstandings of the department's actions.

*Interim Measures*
On March 30, 1992, residents with contaminated wells were notified that money had been made available through the Superfund program to install granular activated charcoal filters in their homes as a temporary measure. The filters would allow residents to use their well water safely until the city water system was extended to the subdivision. The filters would then be removed by the health department staff.

Obtaining a filter was voluntary; residents were told how to request a filter. After some follow-up, 7 of the 11 residents contacted requested filters, 1 said he would give permission for additional monitoring, and 1 declined the filter. No reply was received from 2 residents.

*(continues)*

**Case Study 11-B** *continued*

About the same time Reed County provided a single tap into the city water system with a faucet so residents would have access to safe water, making it no longer necessary for them either to buy bottled water or go outside the area to fill bottles of water.

On May 14, 1992, a letter was sent to all Regal Oaks residents giving them current information, and on August 6, 1992, a news article reported the status as of that date.

**Present Status**

The last sampling by Midlands EQC District staff occurred in March 1992. Sampling by the state Superfund staff is scheduled to begin on September 22, 1992.

Funding for the public water supply is progressing. A public hearing on funding through the community block grant is scheduled for September 23, 1992. A meeting with county officials is scheduled in order to pursue the local matching funds required by the block grant.

There has been no further word on the class action suit. The resident who made reference to the suit in her letter to other residents has sold her property in Regal Oaks and moved out of the neighborhood.

The news media has been relatively silent on the issue recently. There was one recent TV news spot that presented a very negative view of the situation. The emphasis of the story was on funding a public water supply, and the implication was that people were suffering severe health problems. The health department was not contacted by the TV news prior to or for comment on the story. The spot generated only one follow-up call to the department from a citizen.

Jim Moore was defeated in his primary bid for re-election to the Reed County Council in August 1992. He had served on the council since 1984 and as its chair for one year.

---

One media advocacy issue is how to publicize health risks. Public health leaders should involve key stakeholders in discussions of the technical aspects of health risks. For one thing, a given risk must be evaluated from social, psychological, economic, and political perspectives.[57]

In publicizing a health risk, public health leaders should explore the various media options and choose a presentation format appropriate to the level of concern. All the media should be used to inform the community about a health risk. See Table 11-4 for a list of risk communication rules.

Public health leaders should:

- use their media advocacy skills to influence policy makers
- include key stakeholders in the media advocacy process
- follow the seven cardinal rules of risk communication
- write a letter on a public health issue to the local newspaper twice a month
- dress conservatively for television events
- learn to present messages concisely
- select appropriate communication channels for advocacy and risk communication
- rehearse before any oral presentation of advocacy positions
- make sure they are the appropriate spokesperson for a media interview

**Table 11-4   Seven Cardinal Rules of Risk Communication**

1. Accept and involve the public as a partner. Your goal is to produce an informed public, not to defuse public concerns or replace actions.
2. Plan carefully and evaluate your efforts. Different goals, audiences, and media require different actions.
3. Listen to the public's specific concerns. People often care more about trust, credibility, competence, fairness, and empathy than about statistics and details.
4. Be honest, frank, and open. Trust and credibility are difficult to obtain; once lost, they are almost impossible to regain.
5. Work with other credible sources. Conflicts and disagreements among organizations make communication with the public much more difficult.
6. Meet the needs of the media. The media are usually more interested in politics than risk, simplicity than complexity, danger than safety.
7. Speak clearly and with compassion. Never let your efforts prevent your acknowledging the tragedy of an illness, injury, or death. People can understand risk information, but they may still not agree with you; some people will not be satisfied.

*Source:* Reprinted from V. Covello and F. Allen, *Seven Cardinal Rules of Rush Communication,* 1988, Office of Policy Analysis, U.S. Environmental Protection Agency.

## Communication and Cultural Sensitivity

American society has always been diverse, ethnically and racially as well as in other ways, but it is becoming even more so. For example, women and minorities are increasingly assuming leadership roles in the workplace. Because protection against health risks is a right of all citizens, the makeup of public health programs should reflect the makeup of the larger society. This entails that public health leaders need to learn to be students of culture and develop the interpersonal skills needed for relating to staff and community residents of different social and cultural backgrounds.[58]

A culture is a type of social system that encompasses a shared language, shared values, and a shared set of behaviors. A person's culture to a large extent determines how the person acts and reacts, and thus public health leaders need to understand the cultures of the community they serve and eliminate their prejudices if they want to work for the good of the community.

Diversity can be an obstacle to communication and cooperation among agency staff or with community partners.[59] Fortunately, public health leaders can use a number of techniques to evaluate how an agency is responding to the issue of diversity. First, they need to study how the agency treats job applicants from different backgrounds as well as clients or community partners from different backgrounds. They also need to explore the power relationships that exist between staff from diverse backgrounds and to read all printed materials related to the organization in order to determine if the messages given are discriminatory. They should walk around the agency to see how people from diverse backgrounds are treated by staff and interview staff about instances of mistreatment that may have occurred or patterns of discrimination that may have developed. Finally, they should build a "web of inclusion."[60] As a prerequisite, they need to ensure that a system of open communication is in place and that information flows freely throughout the organization, allowing, among other things, power relationships to become realigned.

With regard to gender differences, the increase of women in the workplace has led to an increase in sexual harassment laws and new approaches to affirmative action.[61] In the late 1990s, there was a backlash against affirmative action laws and regulations that will affect organizations well into the 21st century. The legality of these affirmative action programs is being debated in the courts. One thing to keep in mind is that many Americans believe that the only way to create change is through opposition. As one author put it, ours is an "argument culture."[62] Yet it is best to move away from debate to more of a dialogue between equal partners. Equality and dialogue are critical if we are to understand each person, no matter what gender, race, or ethnicity, and be able to listen to him or her with an open mind.

Public health leaders will need to become multicultural in the 21st century,[63] which is to say that they will need the skills to communicate effectively with diverse social groups. In general, they will need to increase their cultural sensitivity by investigating the reasons diverse groups act in certain ways. Cultural sensitivity leads to mutual respect and to the empowerment of previously marginalized groups. It also allows public health leaders to find innovative ways to increase the health literacy of people from different backgrounds.[64]

Culturally sensitive public health leaders:

- remain objective
- learn to control gender, racial, and ethnic prejudices by clarifying values
- understand the different expectations that men and women bring to leadership
- learn the spoken and gestural languages and behavior patterns of different racial and ethnic groups
- adjust the way in which they convey messages in light of the culture of the audience and the situation
- build a web of inclusion
- become familiar with sexual harassment laws, affirmative action laws, and other laws and regulations relevant to the issue of diversity

## Feedback

Completion of an act of communication requires feedback from the respondent, whether in the form of a spoken statement, printed data, graphics, or a videotape. Communication strategies, including strategies for giving feedback, change to reflect the expansion of technology,[65] but certain principles remain unaltered. For example, feedback may be positive or negative, but most people seem to respond better to positive messages than to negative ones.[66] Negative feedback, however, can lead to positive results when there is potential resistance. The response is affected by the credibility of the person giving the feedback and the ability of the person receiving the feedback to evaluate what has been said objectively.

In the case of a group, such as a team or even a whole organization, the receivers of a message can engage in a conspiracy of silence in which they subvert the message without informing the sender. Leaders need to become expert at determining whether lack of feedback is a reflection of acquiescence or silent resistance.

The solicitation of feedback should be planned and not left to chance.[67] In fact, leaders need to develop continuous feedback loops between themselves and staff and organizational and community stakeholders.[68]

Feedback can be divided into various types.[69] Verbal feedback is extremely interactive, and it often affects the total process of communication. Nonverbal feedback involves the use of body language and facial gestures. Fact-based feedback presents relevant information for dealing with a specific situation. In a fourth variety of feedback, the receiver of the message expresses his or her feelings, sometimes nonverbally, about the message. Public health leaders need to be empathetic and pay attention to the feelings of those they are communicating with.

The symbolic interactionist model developed by Hulett (see Figure 11-1) includes feedback control.[70] The person initiating a communicative process performs an instrumental act that motivates the other person to become involved in the communicative process and eventually perform his or her own instrumental act, which can be viewed as a response to the message (or as feedback). The person receiving the return message may then go through the covert rehearsal phase for a second time in order to clarify the message received and perform another instrumental act, leading to further feedback. Hulett identified two feedback loops: an intrapersonal loop (part of the covert rehearsal stage) and an interpersonal loop. The interpersonal feedback loop is used to relay information from the receiver of a message back to the sender.

In performance evaluations, feedback on specific behaviors is preferable to feedback on general behaviors.[71] Specificity makes the feedback seem more personal, as if the individual giving the feedback took an active interest in the individual receiving the feedback. At the same time, the feedback should be objective. It should not consist of criticisms of the person, but of an evaluation of job-related behaviors. If the evaluator must give criticism (negative feedback), the critique needs to focus on behaviors that the individual can change. Feedback on performance should be oriented toward the goal of improving the person's performance and achieving desired outcomes, which of course means that the message must be understandable to the receiver. The timing of feedback is important as well. It should be given to an individual as soon as possible after the occurrence of the behaviors being evaluated.

In giving feedback, including feedback on a person's work performance, public health leaders should:

- accentuate the positive but point out ways in which performance could be improved
- concentrate on specific rather than general behaviors
- be objective and goal oriented (aim at improving work performance)
- provide the feedback in a timely fashion
- offer negative feedback only in regard to behavior that is controllable
- create ongoing feedback loops

## Delegation of Authority

To delegate is to give others, including individuals and teams, both the responsibility for certain actions and the power to ensure that the actions are performed. There is a strong communication component in delegation, and the delegators need to be cognizant of the communication factors that can enhance the delegation of responsibility and the factors that can obstruct its delegation. One way to look at delegation is that it is a shift in the power to make decisions and to act from one level to a lower level of the organizational hierarchy.[72] Delegation is not shared decision making. Rather, if decision-making authority is truly delegated, the decision made by the delegatee will be put into force. This entails that the boundaries of the delegated authority must be made clear to the delegatee, which of course requires good communication between the delegator and the delegatee.

When responsibility is delegated, the delegator must nonetheless act as an overseer to ensure that the delegatees are moving in the right direction. If the delegator loses confidence in the ability of the delegatees to carry out their assigned responsibilities, the delegator may accept their recommendations while taking back final decision-making authority.

Because a public health agency usually has many specialized public health programs, the agency leaders tend to delegate responsibility for these programs. Sharing power can increase agency effectiveness and can generate trust and credibility.[73] Among the best activities to delegate are those that a leader has done over and over but that are still needed for the smooth functioning of the organization.[74] Because the leader has extensive experience with these tasks, he or she can give detailed instructions to staff members on how to perform them. Also, because a leader cannot attain expertise in all areas under his or her purview, he or she would do well to delegate certain specialty areas to the appropriate experts. In the information age, the need for delegating responsibilities will increase in line with the expansion of technology, including information-processing technology.

Leaders should not delegate the responsibility for attending meetings that require their presence, nor responsibility for activities related to personnel or other confidential matters. They need to control the policy-making function, and although delegatees may influence policy development, the leaders need to make the final policy recommendations. All organizations occasionally face crises, and the leaders need to monitor any mounting crisis and maintain tight control over the efforts to resolve it.

All leaders struggle with the issue of too much responsibility and too little time. Each new task that a leader accepts brings with it new duties and often a new set of constituents. As the number of tasks grows, the leader experiences role overload.[75] On the other hand, sometimes staff members feel that they do not have enough to do—an example of role underload. Thus, delegation can lead to interesting results. If assignments are delegated to public health practitioners lower down in the organization, those staff members will experience a reduction in role underload. Conversely, the leader should feel relief because pressure is being removed. The leader, however, might also feel insecure as a result of the transfer of responsibility. Hopefully, the leader will gradually become more secure as he or she sees the positive results of the delegation of activities. Delegation involves a balance between trust and control.

Hersey and colleagues treat delegation as one of four leadership styles.[76] The ability of a leader to delegate authority is determined by the abilities and backgrounds of others in the organization. New employees may need specific instructions on how to perform tasks as well as supervision during the learning process. Gradually the leader moves from discussing decisions with the staff to delegating decision-making authority. During this process, the leader should provide continual feedback.[77] Empowered staff members need information on how they are doing, and good performance should always be recognized.

As mentioned earlier, the delegator of an activity needs to make the assignment clear to the delegatees. The best strategy is to be as specific as possible and yet leave room for the delegatees to use their creativity to address the problems presented by the assignment. If a whole task is not within the realm of authority of delegatees, they need to know the limits of their authority. Further, the delegator should inform others in the organization or community about the delegation of responsibility. This is another place where communication plays an essential role in delegation.

In delegating authority and responsibility for activities and outcomes, public health leaders must:

- define the dimensions of the assignment
- specify how much freedom the delegatees possess to do the task
- delegate the whole task to an individual or a team
- include potential delegatees in the whole decision process
- let other staff or partners know about the delegation
- set up feedback channels

## Framing

A paradigm is a set of rules that define boundaries and act as guidelines for action.[78] Followers of a professional paradigm are generally accepted by other professionals in their field. Given that science and practice continue to change, paradigms do not last forever. If a paradigm reaches its operational limits, then a new paradigm will evolve to take its place.

There is a strong communication component in paradigm building. Once the new paradigm has been constructed, the leader has to communicate it to the various public health stakeholders. Their response to it is a form of test. Following is a set of guidelines for creating a new paradigm for public health:

- Create a mission and vision or adopt existing ones.
- In developing the paradigm, take into account the perspective of key stakeholders.
- Promote individual leadership development.
- Promote organizational change on the basis of core functions and essential public health services.
- Develop public health coalitions built on a team-based model and a community-defined agenda.
- Improve transorganizational relationships (meta-leadership).
- Move toward an integrated community-wide model with strong prevention components.
- Increase interaction among local governmental boards, local agencies, state health and health-related agencies, and the local health department.

According to Goffman, framing consists of a series of acts that integrate primary frameworks (or paradigms) and actions.[79] Primary frameworks, which create a culture of understanding in teams, organizations, and communities, include such things as values and beliefs. Communication is the mechanism for monitoring the framing process. In addition, communication, as well as new perceptions, can add new information to past experience and thus clarify a current framework or require a reframing.[80]

A framework is a tool, and like any tool it can be used well or poorly.[81] If the right framework is used in a given situation, the framework will be supported or extended. If the wrong framework is used, it may become undermined.

If a crisis occurs, mechanisms must be found for renewing the organization.[82] The leaders of an organization might even precipitate a crisis in order to break down the frameworks that do not work. Because the leadership role includes acting as a change agent, leaders need to master transformational change methodologies, people management skills, and framing skills.

It is through framing that reality gets defined.[83] Framing creates an action language that serves as an aid to understanding situations. This language helps in classifying information within the context of the framework used. Leaders tend to be more effective when they recognize framing opportunities and take advantage of them to create frameworks for self-guidance and the guidance of others. Table 11-5 identifies several types of framework, describes their functions, indicates when to use them and when not to use them, and gives examples of each.[84]

Public health leaders need to:

- develop or adopt frameworks (paradigms) to guide action
- become familiar with the frameworks of those with whom they interact
- learn reframing techniques
- coordinate their vision and their primary frameworks (governing paradigms)
- learn how to use metaphors, jargon, contrast, spin, and stories for purposes of framing

## Dialogue, Discussion, and Debate

Imagine that several public health leaders come into a room and take chairs organized in a circle. All preconceived notions and professional credentials are left at the door. The rules governing the ensuing conversation are that each person gets to talk without interruption and that no one should be concerned about the output of the group process. The kind of discussion that will result—if the leaders talk freely—is what has been called dialogue. It can be a means of uncovering hidden values and agendas[85] and exploring the way these values and agendas control the behavior of the participants. Further, it can change the way people work because it diffuses information throughout the dialogue group and eventually throughout the organization and community.[86]

Dialogue, because of the group's synergism, is a communication process in which everyone can win.[87] The participants often find out things they were unaware of, such as the fact that they share patterns of thought. They might

**Table 11-5  Framing Techniques**

| | Metaphors | Jargon/ Catchphrases | Contrast | Spin | Stories |
|---|---|---|---|---|---|
| Function | They show a subject's likeness with something else. | They frame a subject in familiar terms. | It describes a subject in terms of its opposite. | It puts a subject in a positive or negative light. | They frame a subject by example. |
| Use it because | You want a subject to take on new meaning. | Familiar references can enhance meaning. Jargon and catchphrases help communicate a vision's "god" and "devil" terms. | It is sometimes easier to define what your subject is not than state what it is. | It can reveal your subject's strengths or weaknesses. | Stories attract attention and can build rapport. |
| Avoid it when | They mask important alternative meanings. | A word or phrase is in danger of overuse. | Meaning can be skewed by a poor contrast. | The ratio of spin to reality is excessive. | They mask important alternative meanings. |
| Example | "I feel our relationship is formal, like punching a ticket." | "We've got to break the squares today." | "It's a choice between raising my hand for the teacher to ask if it's okay or just telling it like it is." | "Which Ray will show up? The one who's cooperative and generous, or the egotist who constantly reminds others of his successes and what is due him." | "In my first three or four years here, I was a lot like you. I thought . . ." |

*Source:* Reprinted with permission from G. T. Fairhurst and R. A. Starr, *The Art of Framing*, p. 101. © 1996, Jossey-Bass Inc., Publishers.

also identify shared areas of concern, common causes of conflict, ways to heal fragmented perspectives, and new approaches to personal and organizational development.[88] However, a dialogue group might find itself struggling because of the lack of objectives, even to the point where emotions flare up. Therefore, a facilitator is often used to guide the dialogue process. The goal is to prevent participants from getting angry at each other and instead get them to feel enthusiasm for the process.

The first step in holding a dialogue session is to contact potential invitees to gauge their willingness to attend a session. The invitees should be apprised of the guidelines for the session. For example, in order for the dialogue process to be effective, the participants must actively listen to what others are saying and must observe themselves as well as the other participants. In addition, the participants should suspend assumptions and judgments for the period set aside for the dialogue (usually two hours). One recommendation to give participants is that they should try to provide concrete examples of what they are talking about. Concrete examples clarify abstract language and aid in coming to a shared understanding.[89]

Following a dialogue session, the participants can begin discussing ways to implement ideas coming out of the session. Discussion is perhaps the primary mechanism for problem solving and decision making. One of the dangers of discussion is that personal agendas can undermine the activity.[90] Another is that the participants might not listen respectfully (or at all) to the opinions of others and might tend to interrupt each other. If a dialogue session is held first, the participants would have a better chance of using discussion to develop and implement action plans because their different perspectives would have already been addressed. Further, discussion is the form of discourse in which attempts are made to come to agreement on the issues, whereas dialogue is intended to be only exploratory.

We live in a society full of turmoil and change.[91] There are arguments and stresses related to all our communication. A debate allows extreme views to be presented and evaluated in a controlled forum, reducing the chance of emotional flare-ups. A good example of a debating forum was the television show *Crossfire* on the CNN network, where parties on both sides of a controversy could present their views. A debate can help to clarify positions and change opinions, but, despite its value, debating as a technique for acquiring information is often ignored in organizations.

As an example of the appropriate use of debate, imagine that a group of community residents come to a county board meeting to convince the board to do something about the contaminated water supply. Their testimony might be followed by the testimony of a local chemical company claiming that it cannot clean up the local river because of the high expense. The board thus hears both sides of the story and is in a better position to make a rational decision as to what to do.

Table 11-6 contrasts dialogue with discussion and debate. All three types of discourse are valuable if used appropriately.[92]

Public health leaders should:

- engage in dialogue rather than discussion or debate at the first level of interaction whenever possible
- be open to changing their views as a result of dialogue, discussion, or debate

- invite, not force, potential participants to come to a dialogue session
- use dialogue to strengthen relationships
- use discussion to problem solve
- use debate to explore both sides of an issue

## Meeting Skills

Public health leaders spend a large amount of their time in meetings. When I held a university administrative position, more than 30 committees required my time. It is amazing how little time 30 committee assignments leave to get noncommittee work done.

Most public health leaders attend internal staff committee meetings, team meetings, board meetings (which are often open meetings), community meetings, partnership and coalition meetings, and professional meetings, among others. One way they can increase their effectiveness as leaders is to cut down the number of meetings they attend, and they can do this by delegating committee assignments to staff members who exhibit leadership ability.

For a meeting that a leader does have to attend, the goal is to run the meeting as efficiently as possible. A good strategy for preparing for a meeting is to review the results of the previous meeting as soon after it occurs as possible.[93] The idea is to review successes as well as the failures in order to judge whether improvements need to be made.

Problems that arise need to be addressed from a systems perspective.[94] For example, one problem may be that there are too many meetings. If so, consolidation or elimination of some committees needs to occur. Another problem may be that attendees are seldom prepared, forcing those who are prepared to educate those who are not, thereby wasting valuable meeting time. Still another common problem is the tendency of a small number of attendees to try to take over meetings. And another is the tendency of meetings to drag on past the scheduled time. It is important to set an end time and stick to it.

Each meeting should have, besides a chairperson, a facilitator (to help the group to maintain its focus) and a recorder (who should remain objective so as to be able to record what happens accurately). This means that the recorder often does not participate in discussion and may not have a vote or an official membership role on the committee. The other participants should be actively engaged in what is going on. The regular chair may decide to delegate

**Table 11-6    The Conversation Continuum**

| Dialogue | Discussion/Debate |
|---|---|
| Seeing the *whole* among the parts | Breaking issues/problems into *parts* |
| Seeing the *connections* between the parts | Seeing *distinctions* between the parts |
| *Inquiring* into assumptions | *Justifying/defending* assumptions |
| *Learning* through inquiry and disclosure | *Persuading, selling, telling* |
| Treating *shared* meaning among many | Gaining agreement on *one* meaning |

*Source:* L. Ellinor and G. Gerard, eds., Dialogue. Copyright © 1998, John Wiley & Sons. Reprinted by permission of authors. All rights reserved.

the role if it will lead to a more successful outcome or if he or she prefers to take an active part in the discussion of issues. It is the chair's responsibility to create a sociable climate in which sharing of thoughts can occur and objective decisions can be made. Good minutes will remind members of where the group is in dealing with the issues before it. Members may find that a review of several months of minutes will provide insights into the meeting process as well as the specific issues. Participation by all members is important. Passive members may silently disagree with decisions that are made and subvert these decisions in the normal course of their work.

The purpose of an official meeting is to solve problems, make decisions, and meet organizational challenges. Thus, the facilitator must keep the meeting on track while encouraging members to present all sides of an issue and argue in favor of the positions they sincerely hold. The facilitator's other main task, of course, is to get the members to reach a decision on each issue (even if the decision is merely to continue consideration of the issue at the next meeting).

Not all meetings are the same, and public health leaders need to adjust their role according to the type. Organizational meetings deal with issues related to the running of the agency and its programs, and they should cover the diversity of activities in which the agency is engaged. In a team meeting, the agency director may transfer the role of chair to a staff member who is expert in the issues under examination. In a meeting of the governing board, the agency director may collaborate with the board chair in running the meeting. At a community meeting (or any open meeting), the director will have the task of listening carefully to issues raised by community residents.

In carrying out their meeting-related responsibilities, public health leaders should follow these guidelines:

- Keep committee meetings to a minimum.
- Make community and other extraorganizational meetings as information based as possible.
- Use communication skills appropriate to the meeting format.
- Hold extraorganizational meetings in a neutral place if possible.
- Use round tables to increase interaction, and do not assign seats.
- Keep the number of attendees to fewer than 15 if possible.
- Plan the agenda carefully.
- Encourage both dialogue (exploratory discourse) and discussion (problem-solving discourse) in meetings.
- Start and end meetings on time.
- Allow a few minutes for socializing.
- (Then) Keep meetings focused on the issues.
- Serve refreshments.

## Health Communication

Specific skills must be learned to translate health information into understandable messages. Not only must these messages be developed, but they must be marketed. There is controversy over the relationship between health communications and social marketing. In this book, these two communication activities are presented separately. In an interview with the media expert

Robert Howard, Shirley Randolph explored some of these issues (Case Study 11-C).[95] Howard said that the concepts of health communication and social marketing are closely related. In health communication, the target audience is typically the community or population at risk, and the long-term goal is to help people in this population increase control over and improve their health. Social marketing, which is discussed in the next section, is aimed at increasing the acceptability of an idea, social practice, or social cause among the target audience. The desired goal of public health-oriented social marketing is to induce the public and policy makers to support disease prevention and health promotion concepts and programs.

---

### Case Study 11-C
### A Leadership Interview with Robert Howard

*Shirley F. Randolph*

*Robert Howard was the director of public information at the Centers for Disease Control and Prevention (CDC), Atlanta, at the time of the interview. He is now a private consultant on disaster communication models who has presented health communications workshops at the Mid-America Regional Public Health Leadership Institute over the last 15 years. Dr. Howard brings a wealth of experience to his presentations about effective health communications. Prior to joining the CDC, he was a career Navy officer assigned to public and media relations in a variety of settings. This interview took place immediately following a workshop conducted by Dr. Howard in September 1995.*

**"Communications" and "marketing" are words that frequently are used interchangeably. What is the difference between health communications and health marketing?**

I think that health communications and marketing are almost interchangeable. Marketing is a management tool whereby you determine exactly what your market is, who the message is directed toward, who the audience is, who the communication is to go to. First, identify what your communication point is . . . your single overriding communication objective . . . your SOCO. Then go back and carefully examine who you are delivering this message to; who you are marketing this information to . . . what works with this audience . . . what works with this market. Then, decide how to deliver the health message to the audience to which it is directed. I think, to a great extent, "communications" and "marketing" are interchangeable. They cannot be separated. You cannot have good marketing without having good communication . . . and vice versa. If you come up with a health message, you really do have to think about who you are communicating this message to. So, I think to a great extent the two terms are interchangeable.

**Many public health practitioners have never had training or developed skills relative to working with the media. Can you speak to how the "average Jane and the average Joe," working day to day in a local health department, can improve their media relations skills?**

The very first thing you have to do is you have to know *who* your local media representatives are. I think that as the local health officer or health administrator, it is important for you to get out and know these people. If you haven't already done it,

*(continues)*

**Case Study 11-C** *continued*

you need to visit with your local media folks and introduce yourself. You need to find out who they are; they need to know who you are. It's important to know the individuals on the editorial boards of the local newspapers. You should also know the local assignment editor at the newspaper and the local television station and the news directors of the local radio stations. Let them know what use you can be to them and when they can call you. Let them know who they should call at the health department if there is an issue dealing with public health. Let them know what resources are available to them within public health. You do that by going around and getting to meet these people. There is nothing wrong with calling a reporter who covers a health beat consistently and does it very well and saying, "You did a really great job covering that story. We really appreciate your effort." Everybody likes an occasional stroke, and it's important to say, "You did a super job on that story." At the same time, if a reporter gets something wrong, gently help that reporter get it right! Understand, the newspapers and radio stations are a medium through which you can market your communication message. It's important that you develop a relationship with them. The most important thing that a local public health official can do is to establish that base relationship with his or her media. Get to know them and discern and understand what works. Understand how you can best deliver your information locally. Public health workers at the local level are truly the core of public health practice. You are where the rubber meets the road. You are out there on a day-to-day basis dealing with issues locally. You are the ones that Dr. David Satcher, director of the Centers for Disease Control and Prevention, has been pointing to and saying, "We need your help to get a better understanding of the issues and problems that face local public health."

**Many of the local health departments in Illinois, as well as in the nation, have small staffs and do not have a media expert or a public relations expert. Do you think that it is important to have one person in the agency designated as the media contact?**

I think that it is very important for the media to have a single number that they can call or a single person they can contact if they have questions. There ought to be a single or central clearinghouse or clearing point that the media can go to. It is very important that you, in your agency or office, have a policy that tells the staff this is the procedure that you need to follow in responding to media inquiries. If you don't have a plan or a policy in place, develop one quickly to establish what should happen if you're not available. Designate the person who should respond to media inquiries in your absence. Your staff won't know what to do if there is not a policy. You need to develop a policy that works, that is unique to your specific area and your specific situation . . . develop that policy; identify that person. And, most important, make sure that everybody in the agency understands what the policy is. Go over it occasionally; share it and make sure that people don't violate it.

**How can public health practitioners who use public health "lingo" on a daily basis translate our "language" in order to better "sell" our products to the media and the community?**

I found that what works best at CDC is that the decisions about developing appropriate health messages are best not made in a vacuum. You need to put together a team of people in your office. Even if you have only four or five people on your staff, you will usually have one or two people who are pretty good at communication. It might be a nurse practitioner or somebody who is out there on a daily basis dealing with the public and who understands the best way to communicate with them. The public is not going to understand "risk" or "needs assessment," they're not going to understand "acute" and "chronic," or they're not going to understand "immunization schedules." Look to get your people who are working with the public to be a part of your communications team. Develop a team concept. Use the team to develop messages that the public will understand. These decisions cannot be made and communications messages cannot be developed in a vacuum by one person. It has to be a team approach.

**What are the most important factors to keep in mind when preparing for an interview with someone from the media?**
First, any time you give an interview, you ought to know *why* you are doing the interview, and you ought to know *exactly* who your target *audience* is. You ought to remember to tell yourself, "These are the people who brought me to this dance. These are the folks I'm representing, and I need to direct my message to them. I need to remember that they are the reason why I'm here, and I'm representing this agency or this office." You need to develop that communication point . . . your SOCO . . . your single, overriding communication message. What is the "take-home" message for people when your public turns off the television that night? What is the "take-home" message . . . the thing that you want them to remember from having seen your message? You can only develop that message if you sit down ahead of time and plan. You can't get from Chicago to Indianapolis without knowing the route; you have to plan your trip and plan your route; and you do that by sitting down with a map and thinking about how you're going to get there. You do the same thing when you're trying to market or communicate a message.

**Sometimes media interviews become somewhat hostile. Is there any way to prepare for that? How do you deal with a hostile reporter?**
If a reporter becomes hostile, I take that opportunity to absolutely "stay within my zone" as much as I can. You really do need to remember that if a media person becomes hostile, it does not mean that you have to become hostile. As soon as you become angry, remember that you're the person being quoted . . . you're the person being seen on camera. If you lose your cool, if you fall off the beam, that is all that will be seen . . . not the fact that the reporter became hostile. It is really important that you keep your focus and that you remember that your body language, your image, what you project, is going to be seen by people. If you are seen as hostile, that is what is going to be portrayed; so just stay within your zone. If a reporter asks you a hostile question or creates a hostile situation, don't buy into it. *Keep your cool!* If the question is inappropriate or improper, just say, "I'm not the person to address that issue" or "I don't share your feelings on that one" or "That's not what this agency represents." *Keep your cool!* Don't terminate an interview. Don't rip off a microphone and throw it down or storm out of the room. There is no quicker way to guarantee that you will see yourself on television than to do one of those things. The moment that you lose your cool, the moment that you lose control, is the moment I can guarantee that you will be quoted.

**Is there any way to anticipate all or a majority of the questions that you might be asked to address during an interview?**
No. You cannot anticipate all of the questions, but you *can* anticipate many of them by knowing local issues, by knowing local sensitivities, and by sitting down ahead

*(continues)*

**Case Study 11-C** *continued*

of time with that communications team and developing some questions and answers and thinking about where the interview might go. For instance, what does the community really think about this issue? What are some of the sideline issues that might impact on this? You can't think of *every* question but you can sure think of *most* of them. There will be an occasional surprise question. Occasionally a reporter will surprise you, but you need to handle surprises as best you can. I find that generally you can predict around 80% of the questions you are going to get. Generally, the ones that you don't predict are relatively simple questions. If a reporter is coming to your shop to do an interview, there is probably some local tie-in or local issue to be explored. Try to keep your focus local. Try not to look at everything from a global or national perspective. Remember, once again, who brought you to the dance . . . who am I directing this interview to? Am I talking to doctors? Am I talking to nurses? Am I talking to teachers or to public health practitioners? Am I talking to the Hispanic community? Who is my audience? Factor your audience into all of your answers.

**What should you do when the reporter keeps asking you the same question(s) over and over or tries to lead you down a path that you really don't want to go?**
That is a frequent technique used by reporters. The most important thing to remember is the right answer is the right answer the first time and it's the right answer the tenth time. Don't change your answer just because you are asked the question again or asked the same question a little differently. If the reporter keeps doing it and becomes incessant, there is nothing wrong with saying, "I've already answered that question, but I'll be happy to answer it for you again." Then, if it gets to be too much, say, "I would really ask that we move on to something else. I've answered that question and I think I've answered it fairly, and I would like to move on to something else." But, *don't lose your cool!*

**What should you do if the reporter won't accept that answer. Do you just repeat, "I've answered that question . . . we've talked about this issue . . . we need to move on"?**
That's exactly what you do. It doesn't matter if you're asked that question 20 times. And, finally, when you've reached the allotted time you have established in advance for the interview, you say something like, "If you don't have any other questions, I have another appointment. I have something else I really have to get on to and it is time for me to go now, and I *have* answered your questions." When you agree to an interview, you should establish the parameters, including the amount of time you have available, where the interview is to be held, what the background is going to be, what subject(s) will be discussed, and the area(s) of questions. You establish those parameters at the beginning of the interview. You get the reporter to buy in to that. You say, "I have about 30 to 45 minutes to spend with you; is that all right?" When you reach the time period you have established, it's okay to say, "I really do have something else I need to attend to."

**What can or should a public health practitioner do if a media representative just shows up on the doorstep to do an interview? Something is happening in the community, and a reporter is sent to the public health department to "get a story" or a statement and says, "This is the situation . . . do you have a comment?" Is it better to go ahead and "get it over with," even if you're not prepared, or are there other strategies that are effective in such situations?**
If a reporter just shows up, the very first thing you need to do is to make sure you are the right person to talk to the reporter on the subject she or he wishes to discuss.

First, have a policy in place as to who will comment on issues as they arise. Get in touch with that person, make sure the person is briefed on the situation, get a handle on what's going on locally that would cause that reporter to show up on your doorstep. Why is this reporter here unannounced? What has brought the reporter here? Sit down with that reporter and make a determination about what it is the reporter wants to talk about. Buy yourself as much time as you possibly can to think about your comments before you go on camera or begin a taped interview. If the cameras are already rolling, if they catch you and "ambush" you, then it's very important for you to say, "The public health concerns of this issue are of great importance to us . . . it's important to us that we get the right message and the right information to people. You have just 'shown up on our doorstep' and I have not had an opportunity to take a look at this issue yet. We're going to do that, and as soon as I find out what the situation is, we will get back to you immediately."

**What should you do if the media tries to "pit" you against other levels of government, such as a local health official against a state health official, or a state health official against a federal health official, or vice versa?**

Remember that you should only address issues that are appropriate for you to address and that you ought to be addressing. It is appropriate to say, "I don't have those specifics in front of me and I cannot address a subject for which I do not have the specifics. I didn't know we would be doing this interview." Don't hesitate, particularly in a live situation, to let the public know you have been blindsided and to let the people on the other end of the camera or microphone know that this is the first time you have seen or heard this information. Let the public know that this is not a prepared interview. Don't hesitate to say, "You caught me without my information available. I didn't know we would be chatting today. I would like very much to address this issue or get you to the right person to get this issue addressed."

**If you had to write the three top rules to follow when preparing for an interview, what would they be?**

The very first thing to do is to establish a team within your public health department. You need to have a communications team—people who will sit together and discuss and review the issues prior to the interview. It's the difference between fire prevention and firefighting. Everything should not be a firefighting situation. You shouldn't have to break out the hoses every time something goes wrong. It's a lot better to have that smoke detector in place. It's what your communication team is . . . it's your smoke detector. It's your team that smells the smoke and gets together to determine what you're going to do. Have a communications team in place. Make sure everyone knows what to do when something goes bad.

Number two: on any given issue, develop your communication point . . . your SOCO . . . your single overriding communication objective. Sit down, communicate, identify who your market or media segment is, who you are delivering this message to within the population. Share this information within your agency. Make sure that everybody within your office understands what the SOCO, the single overriding communication objective, is. Finally, write that down and take it with you when you do the interview. I mean *take it with you physically and mentally.* Be thinking about the SOCO during the interview. Think about delivering that message over and over. And always, particularly when you're dealing with broadcast media, think visually. What can we do to best communicate this through the visual media? What can we best do to communicate this in the way of background video or how

*(continues)*

**Case Study 11-C** *continued*

can we portray this best, either in a picture or on camera? Try to think, what do the broadcasters want? Try to think that this is what they're going to want . . . they'll want a laboratory shot or they'll want an immunization shot. Then make sure that your people in those clinics or in those areas look appropriate and appear appropriate and they know about the SOCO and the press visit. It's all part of that process of your communications team sharing that information internally and externally.

Finally, deliver your message. That always sounds so simple, but on more occasions than I can count I have seen people prepare for interviews, write the SOCO down, take the SOCO with them, and go to the interview. But because they get so caught up in the excitement or the nervousness of the interview, they fail to deliver the message. They never take the opportunity to grab hold of that interview and say, "I'm here today to say . . ." It is really good to frame your answers with those kinds of attention-grabbing devices. And, most importantly, use what works for you. Everyone is an individual; not everything works for everybody.

Finally, *practice, practice, practice*! You only get good at these things by practicing. *Good communication does not come naturally to anybody.* You get good at communicating because you work at it and you do it a lot. You need to practice.

---

The CDC perspective on health communication is that it "is the crafting and delivery of messages and strategies, based on consumer research, to promote the health of individuals and communities. . . . Effective health communication activities will be an integral component of all programs designed to promote health, improve quality of life, and foster healthful environments."[96(p.2)] The CDC developed 10 guidelines for increasing the effectiveness of health communication. They are as follows:

1. Review background information. (What is out there?)
2. Set communication objectives. (What do we want to accomplish?)
3. Analyze and segment target audiences. (Whom do we want to reach?)
4. Develop and pretest message concepts. (What do we want to say?)
5. Select communication channels. (Where do we want to say it?)
6. Create and pretest messages and products. (How do we want to say it?)
7. Develop promotion plan/production. (How do we get it used?)
8. Implement communication strategies and conduct process evaluation. (Let's do it!)
9. Conduct outcome and impact evaluation. (How well did we do?)
10. Provide feedback to improve communication. (Where do we go from here?)[97(pp.2–4)]

These 10 guidelines can be applied in Exercise 11-2, which concerns the development of a team-based health communication strategy.

Despite the fact that more than 500,000 individuals are employed in public health programs nationally, the public health system is not routinely promoted as an essential provider of health-related services of importance to all constituencies. As a result, public health practitioners are at a disadvantage in getting funds for programs in the highly competitive health services arena.

It is almost as if they do not want to talk to the various media and broadcast their accomplishments.

Because of the restructuring in health service delivery and financing, the future role and functions of public health are now uncertain. The uncertainty is not necessarily to be decried. New opportunities for public health agencies to address community health issues are becoming apparent. Primary among these are opportunities to promote healthy behavior through health communication initiatives. The first step in creating an initiative is to build a coalition of equal partners for the purpose of defining, planning, operationalizing, and evaluating health communication (and social marketing) strategies. The second step is to acknowledge existing barriers to full operationalization of the coalition, including the difficulty of creating a coalition in which no one partner controls the components of the process or its outcomes.

Figure 11-3 shows the essential components and partners in any action partnership for health.[98] Each partner has a vested interest in ensuring that the health communication initiatives will succeed. In addition, each partner brings unique resources and expertise to the coalition. Once the action partnership is established and the responsibilities of the partners are negotiated, the first order of business should be to achieve a consensus on the initiatives to be pursued and to develop action plans for implementing the initiatives at the community level.

Creating action partnerships for health is one of the best ways available to public health agencies of addressing community health issues. Further, by establishing such coalitions, public health agencies can maintain

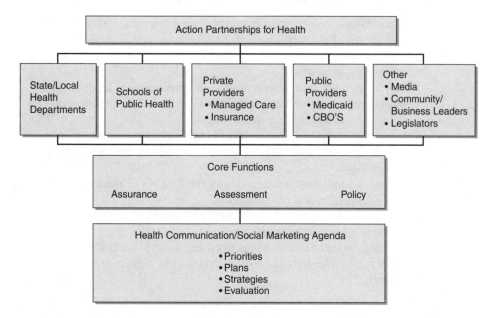

**FIGURE 11-3    Coalition Components and Partners**
*Source:* Reprinted from L. Potts and L. Rowitz, Social Marketing/Health Communications: Leadership Opportunities for the 1990s, *Journal of Public Health Management & Practice*, Vol. 2, No. 4, p. 75, © 1996, Lippincott, Williams, & Wilkins.

an important leadership role. On the other hand, if they fail to work with community partners, they may face a future of lost opportunities.

Public health leaders must:

- build coalitions of equal partners capable of defining, planning, operationalizing, and developing health communication strategies
- set communication objectives, select communication channels, and determine how to use programs
- identify single overriding communication objects
- identify and respond to barriers to full operationalization of coalitions

## Social Marketing

Social marketing has been defined as "the application of commercial marketing technologies to the analysis, planning, execution, and evaluation of programs designed to influence the voluntary behavior of target audiences in order to improve their personal welfare and that of their society."[99(p.7)] The purpose of public health–oriented social marketing is to increase the general acceptance of certain health practices so as to induce the public and policy makers to support health promotion and disease prevention concepts and programs. This kind of social marketing depends on mass communication, because mass communication is the easiest and surest means of informing the public of the behavior changes that are necessary to improve the health status of the community.[100]

A social marketing campaign, according to Winett and Wallack, has seven essential characteristics:[101]

1. It possesses a consumer orientation geared toward meeting the needs and values of the target audience.
2. It places an emphasis on the audience's voluntary exchange of resources for products.
3. It rests on a strong research base, including audience analyses and market segmentation studies that indicate the needs, preferences, and values of various target populations.
4. It uses formative research to test the audience's acceptance of messages, concepts, campaign design, and products prior to full implementation.
5. It seeks an optimum balance among the four P's of marketing (product, price, place, and promotion).
6. It uses channel analyses to test the appropriateness and effectiveness of the campaign delivery systems.
7. It evaluates campaign components using built-in feedback systems in order to discover how to modify them during implementation (if necessary).

To understand how the four P's of marketing apply to social marketing, consider a situation in which public health practitioners are trying to promote dietary changes to reduce fat intake.[102] *Product* encompasses the foods that the public will have to give up or consume in a different form. If people are addicted to pizza, they might have to give up pizza altogether or convince the local pizzerias to offer low-fat varieties. *Price* relates to the cost to the public of making the necessary changes. Will people be willing to pay three dollars extra for a low-fat pizza and put up with the loss in flavor? *Place* is where the activities occur. Perhaps the only place to get low-fat pizza is at the supermarket, so that reducing fat intake means eating at home. *Promotion* involves activities intended to convince the public to accept the message and alter their behavior. (Note that social marketing has a fifth P, *politics*. Part of a social marketing campaign may be devoted to convincing politicians to pass or revise a law.)

Case Study 11-D is intended to clarify the relationship between health communication and social marketing. Note that it is possible to have a health communication success and a marketing failure. It will be hard, for instance, to convince pizza lovers to give up the high-fat food. Public health issues tend to be controversial, and people's views are closely related to the values that they hold dear. Think of the pipe smoker who believes that smoking a pipe is safer than smoking cigarettes. Also, people do not see the results of lifestyle change for years and do not project forward their increased risk for disease as a result of present activities. Another social marketing challenge is that priorities differ in different segments of our communities, such as among the affluent and the poor. And still another is that local public health agency leaders have limited budgets for social marketing and must choose their battles carefully.

---

### Case Study 11-D
### HIV Prevention: Communications Success, Marketing Failure

*Fred Kroger*

"America Responds to AIDS" is the campaign banner for the federal government's campaign to inform the American public about human immunodeficiency virus (HIV) and acquired immune deficiency syndrome (AIDS). Campaign planners have employed marketing techniques that have resulted in its messages being seen or heard by more Americans and with greater frequency (e.g., more than 7 billion audience impressions estimated for 1993) than for any government-sponsored public service health campaign to date. Yet, its CDC sponsors consider it more a health communications program than a social marketing effort.

In 1993, a panel of health communications experts external to the CDC was asked to assess its national efforts to promote HIV prevention and to recommend strategies for improvement. The principal elements of the effort have been a national media campaign, national toll-free hotline services, a national clearinghouse for distributing materials and managing databases on HIV services and programs, grant programs for national partnership development, grant programs to support state and local information activities, and communications research and evaluation.

The panel gave favorable marks for the program's marketing efforts to media gatekeepers and for its success in nurturing effective collaborations among its many and diverse national partnerships. Aggressive, sustained interaction with national and local public service directors helped place HIV prevention high on their list of concerns. The national partners advised CDC on its "product" development processes but also became its sales force in delivering materials and programs to constituencies

*(continues)*

**Case Study 11-D** *continued*

at organizational and community levels. The communications program was recognized as an integrated system that allows information to flow bidirectionally, and that had mass, institutional, community, and individual elements to it.

Its shortcomings, however, fell within two dimensions that most social marketing practitioners consider essential—audience segmentation and product definition. Undergirding these two deficiencies, the fifth "p" of government-based marketing programs, "politics," was described as the major impediment to effective marketing in HIV prevention.

### Audience Segmentation

Congress had been clear in designating the general public as the primary audience for the CDC's mass communication efforts on AIDS. An informed and supportive population is recognized by behavioral scientists to be an important ingredient for causing healthy behaviors to be initiated and sustained. The "America Responds to AIDS Campaign" was criticized by the AIDS Action Council, the Gay Men's Health Crisis in New York City, by other AIDS advocacy groups, and by the review panel for not meeting the needs of high-risk audiences, such as gay men, by not providing sexually explicit behavioral messages.

### Product

"America Responds to AIDS," though viewed by some as a public service advertising and pamphlet distribution campaign, was designed to be a sophisticated communications system that includes online computer databases; toll-free, live telephone hotline services; and a network of national organizations to mediate and deliver education programs and materials. The product was seen by campaign planners as value-free, technically accurate information. AIDS activists called for condoms promotion as the principal product. Congress and media critics expected proof of prevention effects. In assessing this confusion over product specificity, the review panel called for a more behaviorally focused product—for example, "health information with an attitude." Disease-preventing behaviors, including condom use, should be aggressively promoted.

Evaluation efforts have been undertaken to position the HIV prevention "product" in more consumer relevant terms. Just as athletic footwear is sold as aids to "soar through the air, slam dunk, in your face" feats of athleticism rather than as canvas covers for the feet, such prevention products as condoms, monogamy, or abstinence still lack similar consumer-oriented positioning.

---

The awareness task has been judged by experts to be complete. It has been accomplished primarily through communication tools. Can the adoption of risk-reducing behaviors now be sold to persons at highest risk and will the body politic be supportive? This more challenging goal will require better application of core marketing principles. Will the second decade of HIV prevention marketing improve upon the first? Stay tuned. Kotler and Roberto developed a hierarchy-of-effects model (Figure 11-4) that takes into account that not all of the target audience will accept the message of a social marketing campaign.[103] It is important, therefore, to provide reinforcement for people who have made a commitment to change or have assimilated the new knowledge gained from the campaign.

Public health leaders need to know how to develop health communication programs and monitor the effectiveness of these programs. Creating

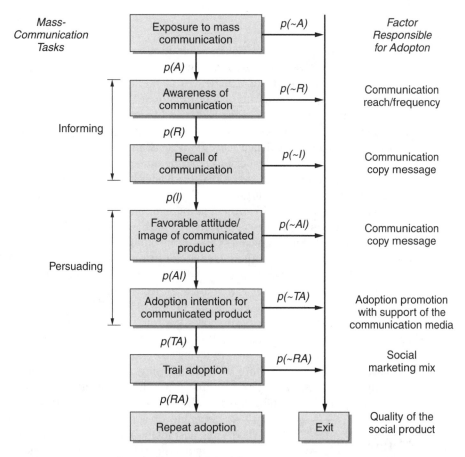

**FIGURE 11-4   Hierarchy-of-Effects Model of the Mass-Communication Process**
*Source:* Reprinted with permission of The Free Press, a Division of Simon & Schuster, from *Social Marketing* by Philip Kotler and Eduardo L. Roberto. Copyright © 1989 by The Free Press. Reprinted with permission of authors.

effective programs is complicated by the fact that many communities want to maintain the status quo or at least contain community groups hostile to the message of such programs.[104] In order to market public health information more effectively, public health leaders need to conduct surveys on consumer health knowledge, investigate different behavior change strategies, target programs at appropriate population segments, and modify programs as necessary.

Public health leaders should:

- use social marketing as a process to increase the acceptance of an idea, social practice, or social cause among a specific audience
- develop strategies for promoting health promotion and disease prevention initiatives in the community
- learn techniques for fostering behavioral change
- identify the various population segments within the overall population
- conduct research on the use of different strategies and their outcomes
- create innovative funding mechanisms for health communication and social marketing campaigns

## Storytelling

Leaders tell stories. Tichy and Cohen have discussed the role of leaders as teachers and leaders need to present a teachable perspective.[105] This perspective utilizes personal stories or experiences of the leader. At the basic story level, there are the stories that tell about the life of the presenter. Then, there are stories that define the role of the leader and the relationships between the leader and his or her audience. The final type is a story about the future. Stories also engage an audience more than facts and numbers do. In storytelling, it is critical for the leader to know the audience. It is also important for colleagues and other staff to see that the leader lives the life portrayed in the story. Gardner has argued that it is through stories that leaders are able to reach out to others and affect them at an emotional and practical level.[106]

Stories take many different approaches to the basic typology listed above. However, people working in business and in the public sector often react negatively to someone who says they have a story to tell. Public health leaders often struggle to show that a story can have as great an impact as facts and numbers. I suppose the answer is that a leader needs to know when and how to tell a story and when to present factual information. It is useful to tell stories, but it is critical that the right stories get told. Denning has stated that leadership is often about persuasion. It is about getting your audience to buy into the lessons or plans that you are trying to create.

Narrative patterns are quite diverse. Denning presents a rationale for eight different narrative patterns.[107] First, there is the springboard pattern that is used to mobilize and motivate others to action. These stories use an example of a change that occurred in the past in an organization or a community and how that experience is relevant to a challenge of today. The past serves as a springboard to the future. The second narrative pattern is about building trust. The leader tells a story about his or her personal life in terms of strengths or vulnerabilities. The third story narrative is used to build trust in your organization. You are creating a brand narrative to show how effective your organization is or has been in promoting the health of the public. The fourth narrative involves stories that demonstrate the values of public health for your organization. The fifth narrative is about collaboration. In public health, this would be a story that you or one of your partner organizations tells about how your collaboration is helping the public health of your community. Next, there is the knowledge-sharing narrative that focuses on a problem and how it was handled. Alternative scenarios can also be presented to demonstrate how different solutions may have led to different outcomes. The seventh narrative involves humor or other methods to deal with rumor and gossip. The final narrative involves vision and how the leader wants to move his or her organization forward.

Denning has also stated that stories are critical in transformational leadership situations.[108] He does warn that these stories have dangers. The goal behind the story may not be clear. The commitment to change may not be readily accepted. Body language is not consistent with the verbal narrative. The leader does not correctly understand the audience. There is a lack of what Denning calls narrative intelligence. The story may be too abstract or theo-

> **Leadership Tip**
>
> *Be prepared for any crisis that your agency may encounter.*

retical for the audience. It may be clear that the storyteller is not being truthful. The audience is clearly not listening to the story or its message. The leader is not able to get the audience to accept that change is important or is even the real issue. The leader's story may get a reaction opposite of what the leader wanted. Finally, the audience feels the storyteller is not willing to discuss the story. Monologues create boredom for the audience. Telling stories is useful and provides the leader with a useful set of skills for mobilizing others.

Public health leaders need to:

- Learn the art of storytelling
- Utilize different types of stories for different reasons or for different audiences

## Summary

Communication is central to leadership. For example, the leader of an organization may be able to develop a compelling organizational vision, but if that leader is unable to communicate the vision to others in the organization in a way that inspires them, the work of visioning will have been all for nought.

This chapter began by discussing the nature of the communication process and the barriers to communication, which include the fact that people in a communicative situation can have different communication styles. As was pointed out, one means of getting around the barriers that exist, at least in the case of oral communication, is to engage in active listening. Of course, not all communication is oral, and the chapter presented the advantages and disadvantages of oral communication and those of written communication as well.

Advancements in communication technology bring with them new communication skills that need to be learned. The most obvious example is the widespread use of computers for the transfer of data and for sending messages in a timely fashion and the corresponding need to master computer skills. Technological advancements also typically bring with them new problems, such as the e-mail overload that public health leaders frequently experience.

Public health leaders must communicate not only with their colleagues but also with the public, for part of their responsibility is to educate the public about public health issues and act as advocates for public health. In short, they need to publicize pertinent information and promote the public health agenda. The only way to do the latter is to communicate the agenda to policy makers who have a direct say in whether the agenda gets implemented or not. Therefore, among the communication skills that public health leaders need are media advocacy skills. They also need to learn the various skills associated with health communication and social marketing. Finally, the importance of storytelling as providing a useful approach to communicating with others was presented.

### Discussion Questions

1. As a public health leader, how would you develop a health education program to increase the health literacy of the people in your service area?

2. What are the barriers to successful communication and how have you personally overcome them?

3. What would be a workable communication strategy to get more funds for an expanded childhood immunization program?

4. What strategies might you use to increase your interpersonal communication skills?

5. What are the advantages and disadvantages of oral communication as opposed to written communication?

6. What are the characteristics of active listening?

7. What are Walton's five rules of conversational etiquette?

8. What speaker aids can be used to enhance a public talk and what are their advantages and disadvantages?

9. What are some guidelines for interviewing job candidates?

10. What are the differences between media advocacy and public education?

11. What are the advantages of engaging in dialogue before engaging in discussion or debate?

12. What are the differences between health communication and social marketing?

13. Why is storytelling important? Describe the different types of stories.

### Exercise 11-1:  Using Persuasion

*Purpose:* to learn how to use public speaking for purposes of persuasion

*Key concepts:* persuasion, public speaking, strategic planning, team consensus

*Procedure:* The class should divide into teams of 8 to 10 members. Each team has the task of preparing a speech intended to persuade community residents of the benefits of a particular project. It seems likely that federal funds will become available to the community for the development of a teen clinic at Margaret Sanger High School. The team, during 30 minutes of discussion, should first identify a strategy for convincing an audience made up of community residents that the teen clinic will benefit the community and should then develop a speech based on that strategy. After the speech is completed, the team selects a spokesperson to give a five-minute presentation at a community meeting in support of the teen clinic.

### Exercise 11-2:  Creating a Health Communication Strategy

*Purpose:* to understand the process of developing a health communication strategy to address a local health problem

*Key concepts:* epidemiology, health communication

*Procedure:* A group of children who had eaten hamburgers and drunk milkshakes at a local fast-food restaurant, Old Mother Hubbard Eatery, become seriously ill. The health department calls in the state epidemiologist, who investigates the problem and determines that a salmonella outbreak has occurred. The epidemiologist also finds evidence of E. coli contamination. The local health department is called in to develop a health communication strategy to get the word out to the public. The class should divide into teams of

8 to 10 to develop the communication strategy. Following the CDC guidelines, each team should draft a brief document that outlines this strategy, including the communication skills to be used by each team member during the process.

## References

1. S. P. Robbins and M. Coulter, *Management,* 8th ed. (Upper Saddle River, NJ: Prentice Hall, 2005).
2. N. M. Tichy and E. Cohen, *The Leadership Engine* (New York, Harper Business, 1997).
3. R. B. Adler and J. M. Elmhorst, *Communicating at Work,* 5th ed. (New York: McGraw-Hill, 1996).
4. Adler and Elmhorst, *Communicating at Work.*
5. J. G. Liebler and C. R. McConnell, *Management Principles for Health Professionals,* 4th ed. (Sudbury, MA: Jones and Bartlett, 2004).
6. D. Walton, *Are You Communicating?* (New York: McGraw-Hill, 1989).
7. P. Lencioni, *Death by Meeting* (San Francisco: Jossey-Bass, 2004).
8. D. Tannen, *That's Not What I Meant* (New York: Ballantine, 1986).
9. R. Bolton, *People Skills* (New York: Simon & Schuster, 1979).
10. J. E. Hulett Jr., "A Symbolic Interactionist Model of Human Communication. Part 1: The General Model of Social Behavior; the Message Generating Process," *AV Communication Review* 14, no. 1 (1966): 5–33.
11. J. E. Hulett Jr., "A Symbolic Interactionist Model of Human Communication. Part 2: The Receiver's Function; Pathology of Communication; Non-Communication," *AV Communication Review* 14, no. 2 (1966): 203–220.
12. R. R. Sears, "A Theoretical Framework for Personality and Social Behavior," *American Psychologist* 6 (1951): 476–482.
13. N. L. Frigon Sr. and H. K. Jackson Jr., *The Leader* (New York: AMACON [American Management Association], 1996).
14. Robbins and Coulter, *Management,* 8th ed.
15. Tannen, *That's Not What I Meant.*
16. D. Tannen, *The Argument Culture* (New York: Random House, 1998).
17. Bolton, *People Skills.*
18. Adler and Elmhorst, *Communicating at Work.*
19. Adler and Elmhorst, *Communicating at Work.*
20. N. M. Tichy and W. G. Bennis, *Judgment* (New York: Penguin Portfolio, 2007).
21. R. Pitino, *Success Is a Choice* (New York: Broadway Books, 1997).
22. S. P. Robbins and M. Coulter, *Management,* 5th ed. (Englewood Cliffs, NJ: Prentice Hall, 2006).
23. Robbins and Coulter, *Management,* 5th ed.
24. Adler and Elmhorst, *Communicating at Work.*
25. T. Alessandra and P. Hunsaker, *Communicating at Work* (New York: Simon & Schuster, 1993).
26. C. O. Scharmer, "Uncovering the Blind Spot of Leadership," *Leader to Leader,* 47 (2008): 52–59.
27. D. Goleman, *Emotional Intelligence* (New York: Bantam Books, 1995).
28. P. R. Scholtes, *The Leader's Handbook* (New York: McGraw Hill, 1998).
29. Alessandra and Hunsaker, *Communicating at Work.*
30. Walton, *Are You Communicating?*
31. Adler and Elmhorst, *Communicating at Work.*
32. Adler and Elmhorst, *Communicating at Work.*
33. Walton, *Are You Communicating?*

34. Alessandra and Hunsaker, *Communicating at Work.*
35. J. G. Liebler and C. R. McConnell, *Management Principles for Health Professionals,* 3rd ed. (Gaithersburg, MD: Aspen Publishers, 1999).
36. Liebler and McConnell, *Management Principles for Health Professionals,* 3rd ed.
37. Liebler and Mcconnell, *Management Principles for Health Professionals,* 3rd ed.
38. B. D. Smart, *The Smart Interviewer* (New York: Wiley, 1989).
39. Smart, *The Smart Interviewer.*
40. J. Carver, *Boards That Make a Difference,* 2nd ed. (San Francisco: Jossey-Bass, 1997).
41. Robbins and Coulter, *Management,* 5th ed.
42. J. Wycoff, *Mindmapping: Your Personal Guide to Exploring Creativity and Problem-Solving* (New York: Berkeley Books, 1995).
43. Adler and Elmhorst, *Communicating at Work.*
44. B. Nelson and P. Economy, *Managing for Dummies* (Foster City, CA: IDG Books Worldwide, Inc., 1996).
45. R. S. Scobel and S. Israel, *Naked Conversations* (Hoboken, NJ: John Wiley and Sons, 2006).
46. Robbins and Coulter, *Management,* 8th ed.
47. D. Shipley and W. Schwalbe, *Send* (New York: Alfred A. Knopf, 2007).
48. Walton, *Are You Communicating?*
49. S. M. Shortell et al., *Remaking Health Care in America* (San Francisco: Jossey-Bass, 1996).
50. L. Wallack and L. Dorfman, "Media Advocacy: A Strategy for Advancing Policy and Promoting Health," *Health Education Quarterly* 23, no. 3 (1996): 293–317.
51. L. B. Winett and L. Wallack, "Advancing Public Health Goals Through the Mass Media," *Journal of Health Communications* 1 (1996): 173–196.
52. S. Iyengar, *Is Anyone Responsible? How Television Frames Political Issues* (Chicago: University of Chicago Press, 1989).
53. M. Siegel and L. Doner, *Marketing Public Health* (Gaithersburg, MD: Aspen Publishers, 1998).
54. Wallack and Dorfman, "Media Advocacy."
55. Wallack and Dorfman, "Media Advocacy."
56. J. Fallows, *Breaking the News* (New York: Pantheon Books, 1996).
57. M. R. Lum and T. L. Tinker, eds., *A Primer on Health Risk Communication: Principles and Practices* (Washington, DC: U.S. Department of Health and Human Services, Public Health Service, 1994).
58. Robbins and Coulter, *Management,* 8th ed.
59. Adler and Elmhorst, *Communicating at Work.*
60. S. Helgesen, *The Web of Inclusion* (New York: Doubleday, 1995).
61. D. J. Breckon, *Managing Health Promotion Programs* (Gaithersburg, MD: Aspen Publishers, 1997).
62. Tannen, *The Argument Culture.*
63. A. J. DuBrin, *The Complete Idiot's Guide to Leadership* (New York: Alpha Books [MacMillan Reference USA], 1998).
64. DuBrin, *The Complete Idiot's Guide to Leadership.*
65. L. M. Harris, "Differences That Make a Difference," in *Health and the New Media,* ed. L. M. Harris (Mahwah, NJ: Lawrence Erlbaum Associates, 1995).
66. Robbins and Coulter, *Management,* 5th ed.
67. Liebler and McConnell, *Management Principles for Health Professionals.*
68. P. R. Scholtes, The *Leader's Handbook* (New York: McGraw-Hill, 1998).

69. Alessandra and Hunsaker, *Communicating at Work.*

70. Hulett, "A Symbolic Interactionist Model of Human Communication. Part 1: The General Model of Social Behavior; the Message Generating Process."

71. Robbins and Coulter, *Management,* 5th ed.

72. Robbins and Coulter, *Management,* 8th ed.

73. M. DePree, *Leading Without Power* (San Francisco: Jossey-Bass, 1997).

74. C. L. Brown, *Techniques of Successful Delegation* (Shawnee Mission, KS: National Press Publications, 1988).

75. C. Handy, *Understanding Organizations* (New York: Oxford University Press, 1993).

76. P. Hersey et al., *Management of Organizational Behavior,* 9th ed. (Upper Saddle River, NJ: Prentice Hall, 2007).

77. DuBrin, *The Complete Idiot's Guide to Leadership.*

78. J. A. Barker, *Future Edge* (New York: Morrow, 1992).

79. E. Goffman, *Frame Analysis* (Cambridge, MA: Harvard University Press, 1974).

80. D. Tannen, *Talking from 9 to 5* (New York: Morrow, 1994).

81. L. G. Bolman and T. E. Deal, *Reframing Organizations,* 3rd ed. (San Francisco: Jossey-Bass, 2003).

82. D. K. Hurst, *Crisis and Renewal* (Boston: Harvard Business School Press, 1995).

83. G. T. Fairhurst and R. A. Starr, *The Art of Framing* (San Francisco: Jossey-Bass, 1996).

84. Fairhurst and Starr, T*he Art of Framing.*

85. D. Bohm et al., *Dialogue—A Proposal* (Gloucester, England: Dialogue, 1991).

86. L. Ellinor and G. Gerard, eds., *Dialogue* (New York: Wiley, 1998).

87. D. Bohm, *On Dialogue* (Ojai, CA: David Bohm Seminars, 1989).

88. J. C. Lammers, "Building Learning Communities to Expand Public Health Resources and Effectiveness" (paper presented at Association of State and Territorial Directors of Health, Promotion and Public Health Annual Meeting, Washington, DC, April 27, 1996).

89. M. R. Weisbord and S. Janoff, *Future Search* (San Francisco: Jossey-Bass, 1995).

90. Bohm, *On Dialogue.*

91. Tannen, *The Argument Culture.*

92. Ellinor and Gerard, *Dialogue.*

93. M. Doyle and D. Straus, *How to Make Meetings Work* (New York: Jove Publications, 1982).

94. Nelson and Economy, *Managing for Dummies.*

95. S. Randolph, "A Leadership Interview with Robert Howard," *Leadership in Public Health* 3, no. 4 (1995): 7–11.

96. K. S. Lord, "Issues in Health Communications," *Leadership in Public Health* 3, no. 4 (1995): 1–4.

97. Lord, "Issues in Health Communications."

98. L. Potts and L. Rowitz, "Social Marketing/Health Communications: Leadership Opportunities for the 1990s," *Journal of Public Health Management and Practice,* 2, no. 4: 75.

99. A. R Andreasen, *Marketing Social Change* (San Francisco: Jossey-Bass, 1995).

100. Winett and Wallack, "Advancing Public Health Goals Through the Mass Media."

101. Winett and Wallack, "Advancing Public Health Goals Through the Mass Media."

102. Winett and Wallack, "Advancing Public Health Goals Through the Mass Media."
103. P. Kotler and E. L. Roberto, *Social Marketing* (New York: The Free Press, 1989).
104. Siegel and Doner, *Marketing Public Health.*
105. Tichy and Cohen, *The Leadership Engine.*
106. H. Gardner, *Leading Minds* (New York: Basic Books, 1995).
107. S. Denning, *The Leader's Guide to Storytelling* (San Francisco: Jossey-Bass, 2005).
108. S. Denning, *The Secret Language of Leadership* (San Francisco: Jossey-Bass, 2007).

# CHAPTER 12

# LEADERSHIP AND PEOPLE DEVELOPMENT

Really great people make you feel that you too can become great.

Mark Twain

At its essence leadership is about the building of relationships. Leadership is more than about the personality of the person seen as a leader; it is about the behavior of that person.[1] In discussing the five practices of a leader, Kouzes and Posner stated that leaders guide others by being role models, inspire others to follow and share their vision, challenge the way things get done, empower and enable others to behave in positive ways, and encourage and reward others for their work. As pointed out earlier in this book, we can find leaders everywhere. Leaders garner trust and respect in the people they encounter. However, leadership has to be more than follow the leader. Williams has pointed out that real leadership requires that leaders need to face reality in their activities.[2] Leaders help their colleagues and followers to understand situations by developing strategies to address challenges and problems and learning how to take advantage of opportunities.

Many of the activities to be discussed in this chapter involve the necessity of understanding who we are as people and as leaders. As we discussed in Chapter 6, leaders have to develop their personal leadership talents and abilities. This level of leadership requires an understanding of what self leadership means. A leader needs to accept responsibility for his or her actions rather than blaming others. Blanchard and his colleagues have stated that empowerment gives a person the responsibility to make things work.[3] Mind reading is not realistic and it is very often incorrect. It is often our own perceptions that limit our activities. Blanchard and his colleagues call this "assumed constraints." These constraints are really the ways in which we let our mental models limit our choices. These constraints are also about the barriers we put up that limit our choices. DeBono discussed the importance of the way we let our attention limit our perceptions.[4] A paradigm limits our attention by setting up boundaries to what we observe. Freedom is exploring all the possible ways that a challenge can be addressed, and a lack of freedom is letting our personal views of the world limit our choices.

An important aspect of the perception factor is the related aspects of legacy and sustainability. Leaders want to believe that their work makes a difference and will affect public health beyond their tenure in a particular public health organization. Some of these issues can be explored in exercise 12-1 which has been adapted from an article by Laur and Schlag.[5] This exercise looks backward, then forward, and finally to the present and how our perceptions affect our mental models and our concerns related to sustainability.

In discussing power, Blanchard and colleagues argued that it is necessary for a leader to define the different "points of power" that affect our personal leadership.[6] They discussed five major categories of power. First, there is personal power in which a leader can influence the work of others in a positive manner by encouraging them and keeping them involved in the work activities. This is different from position power where a leader uses position to guide others. In other words, I am doing this because my supervisor says I have to. Knowledge power comes from expertise on a subject. Task power is power that comes from the ability to do specific types of work. The fifth type of power that is critical to the subject matter of this chapter is relationship power, which involves the ability to work with others. An important aspect of building relationships is the ability to collaborate.

When we talk about relationships, it is important to look for guideposts. First, it is important to develop relationships with intelligent people. Robbins stated that this is controversial, although most evidence points to intelligence as being critical for leaders and the people with whom they relate.[7] Second, it is easier to relate to people with a positive perspective than those that tend to be negative. Third, past experience with others is often a good indicator of relationships in the future even though it is important to compare differences related to the past situation and contrast it to potential differences in the new job or collaborative relationship. Fourth, leaders know when to use different forms of communication that will expedite action. Fifth, the ability to develop solid relationships with others can help the leader to influence many areas of his or her life.[8] It is important to develop credibility with others. Regardless of the structure of the interactions from individual relationships to group situations, it is always critical to interact with people on an individual level. Relationships are thus built on mutual respect, common experiences that are shared, mutual trust, reciprocity (transactional leadership relationships), the ability to enjoy the relationship, and humor.

Many of us would argue that our agencies do good work. This important issue is how to move our agencies forward from just being good to being a great agency. Collins has stated that it is Level 5 leadership that makes the difference.[9] Level Five Leaders blend knowledge, talents and skills as well as good work habits (Level 1), contribute and work well in teams (Level 2), manage people well (Level 3), and are effective leaders (Level 4). Level 5 leaders are humble and put their organizations and communities ahead of their personal egos. They are experts in relationship building and are concerned about the needs of the people with whom they work. All prepared leaders need to be committed to promoting healthy communities.[10] This chapter will explore the importance of building relationships with our agency staff, our community residents, and our external stakeholders. Figure 12-1 shows these relationships as interactive. The dimensions of this figure will be explored through the rest of this chapter.

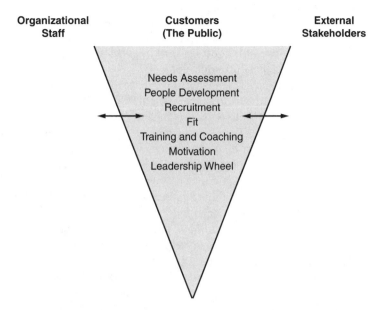

| Organizational | Customers | External |
| Staff | (The Public) | Stakeholders |

FIGURE 12-1    Relationships—Developing Interaction Model

## Organizational Staff Relationships

The field of human resource management has developed over the years to address the issue of management of the people who work in our organizations and agencies. As staff and as managers and leaders, our responsibility is to put our strengths to work.[11] The role of managers is to help people find the right fit for their talents. Nurturing and supporting our work colleagues is critical. In public health, our agency colleagues need to be seen as partners in the public health enterprise. Robbins and Coulter saw human resource management as tied to improving the knowledge, skills, and abilities of staff through education and training; working to motivate people so that work is a positive experience; dealing with difficult or nonproductive colleagues; and increasing retention rates for excellent staff.[12]

Large businesses and agencies tend to have human resources departments. These departments are in charge of recruitment, interviewing, hiring, firing, performance evaluations, probationary decisions, maintaining civil service requirements in the public sector, and supporting a agency environment oriented toward retention. In addition, they protect confidentiality, provide advice when relationships with supervisors are contentious, react to problems, and deal with job-related harassment situations.[13] Human resource professionals need behavioral science training as well as training in sound business practices. An important set of concerns arises when it appears that the human resources techniques and protocols interfere with the work of the agency. These departments need to be cognizant of the culture and practices of the agency and not superimpose different human resource concepts on the staff of the agency. It sometimes appears that the human resources specialist takes authority away from the direct management staff of the agency or organization. This is a danger in that the management and leadership individuals work with both internal staff and community customers. They know when interactive situations are working well and when they are not. Human resources specialists often do not.

In small agencies, managers take on the responsibility for human resource issues related to their direct reports. This clearly has the advantage of having managers and their direct reports in sync with the goals and objectives of the agency as a whole. The Gallup Organization has pointed out that it takes an engaged manager to help develop engaged employees.[14] Who better than an excellent manager to best fit the talents of an employee to the jobs that need to be done and the people that they will serve in the community?

However, talent without application is not advantageous to an agency. According to Maxwell, talented people have to believe in their talent.[15] Engaged employees need to have passion for their work and the work of their agency. Passion helps to energize people to use their talents in a positive way. Talented people need to take the initiative to make their talents work for them. Focus is also important. Maxwell also discusses the importance of preparation. Without preparation and practice, it is hard to put your talents to work. It is easy to get discouraged. It is important to persevere. Taking risks requires courage. Teaching others also provides a way to verbalize how we use our talents. Our relationships also reinforce our strengths.

Although talent alone does not make an employee engaged, personality alone does not either. In reviewing many studies on personality factors in success at work, Robbins pointed to the conscientious employee as one who would be most likely to succeed in the workplace.[16] He also stated that extraversion is a good personality trait for managers, and I would add leaders. These are the people with high emotional intelligence. Low emotional stability may prevent a person from getting a job in the first place. Thus, engaged employees are excited by the opportunities to learn and develop friendships in the agency, are encouraged to develop their talents and skills by their supervisors, and feel that they have the resources necessary to carry out their jobs in an effective manner.[17]

Figure 12-1 lists several dimensions of better understanding and improving our relationships with our organizational colleagues. The V figure also points to the fact that our relationships inside and outside our agencies are based on a set of similar issues. It is also important to recognize that our agency staff is interacting with both our community customers and our external stakeholders in many different initiatives. If a staff member lives in the service area of the public health agency, he or she may be both employee and customer. Public health is mostly about people. When a local agency looks at the issues related to the public health workforce, its managers and leaders need to determine not only what types of workers it will need, but also the scarcity of certain categories of workers in today's environment. For example, we read about nursing shortages. The collection of data related to need is important. The question of what incentives need to be given to encourage people to enter public health or to work in public health is critical. We clearly have to distinguish need from want here. We need certain types of workers but may want to expand our staff into new areas if financial resources become available.

People development, which for the agency involves public health education and training, needs to keep the agency staff up to date on cutting-edge issues related to the health of the public. The agency needs to have a commitment to lifelong learning for its staff. Because public health is always changing, this is a requirement. Educating and training are requirements for staff from the top leadership, managers, public health professionals, and the nonprofessional staff. There are many places to get this knowledge, from online to face-to-face training opportunities. Graduate education in public health should also be encouraged.

Whether the agency is guided by civil service or not, recruitment is an important issue. Present recruitment processes are not the most effective. People tend to be hired on the basis of their credentials and not on the basis of whether they have the talent, knowledge, and skills to carry out the responsibilities of the job. The credibility of the manager who is hiring a staff member is affected by poor selections.[18] It is the job of the recruiter to select talented people, successfully recruit people who will be high-level performers, address potential performance issues in a timely manner, develop appropriate training opportunities that will improve performance, and retain the excellent employees. If a staff member does not wake up in the morning excited about going to work, it is going to be difficult to retain this worker. Work has to be more than just work.

> **Leadership Tools**
>
> *Be a role model to your staff and show good ways to balance work and home.*

Many people have difficulty in defining their own strengths. Buckingham used the acronym of SIGN to help individuals define their personal strengths.[19] The "S" refers to an awareness of those times when we are aware of our successful experiences as one clue to our personal strengths. Instinct is another factor in that we seem drawn toward certain types of activities. The "G" or growth indicator is evidence that we seem to get better at doing certain types of things than others. The "N" stands for need. We find that sometimes we just need to engage in certain types of activities. People need to put their strengths to work. When we do, we seem to get great satisfaction. Managers and leaders just love what they do.

All of these activities of managers and their direct reports relate to creating a good fit between an individual and the organization's culture and subcultures, values, activities, and overall direction. Thus, it is not technical skills alone that create the fit; it is personality, talent, knowledge, skills, emotional reactions, vision of the leader, administrative skills of the manager, organizational culture, community relationships, social justice, and commitment to improving health and preventing disease that combine within a systems framework to make the fit work.[20] Coaching and mentoring help in this process and create teachable moments for managers and their direct reports. With this in mind, it is important to recognize that people will fit some organizations and agencies and not others.[21] In looking at the perspective of a staff member and how they evaluate their activities in an agency, there are three signs of a miserable job.[22] First, there is the concern with being seen as a contributing person in the agency by managers and supervisors (anonymity factor). Second, performance measures have to be clear. Staff who think they are not being measured appropriately will evaluate their jobs negatively. Finally, people need to see their jobs as relevant to the mission and vision of the agency.

It should be clear by now that motivation of colleagues is critical to making the job worthwhile and reinforcing the fit of the employee to the organization. It is also clear that many of us are in public health because of our strong beliefs in social justice and not primarily for the salaries that we receive. It is not that salary is an unimportant factor, but it is not the most important. Motivation is about the activities and the processes that affect our commitment to public health and its mission to promote health and prevent disease in our communities and the factors that guide us to work hard to reach the goals of our agencies and our community relative to our mission. The critical relationship in the workplace is the one between a supervisor and the direct report. Motivation is personal and is derived from this critical relationship. If this relationship is not built on trust and collegiality, then motivational techniques will often not work. Leaders and managers all need to strive for these solid relationships if we want to engage staff members in our agencies.

Performance level is not the same as motivation, although motivation can increase performance. Ramundo and Shelly pointed out that motivated people want to do their work, and leadership is inspiring others to want to work to help the agency reach its organizational goals.[23] Managers and leaders need to be careful not to be pessimistic, stifle creativity, gossip, be uncommunicative, discourage friendships and teamwork, and criticize staff in front of others. These behaviors and other negative behaviors will stifle and decrease motivation in others. Motivation is an emotional thing that affects the individual at a personal level. Ramundo and Shelly have created a list of 25 ways to motivate an employee.[24] As can be seen in Table 12-1, these motivational tips are also relevant to our community residents and our external stakeholders.

It is also important for our agency colleagues to support the core functions and essential public health services. This does not mean that every employee is involved in all the functions or all the essential services. We need to collaborate with our community to make the public health functions work. The leadership wheel gives some structure to our work and leaders, and managers incorporate motivation into the work that needs to be done.

## Community Relationships

If organizational staff is not engaged in its agency work and does not feel motivated by managers and leaders, work with community clients and residents will be adversely affected. The external environment is also critical in defining the service community for human services agencies. If public health is all about the system, the public health agency is embedded in its community and needs to be seen relative to its customers (residents of the community), its agency competitors (other community stakeholders), public pressure groups (also community stakeholders as well as elected officials), and suppli-

**Table 12-1    Twenty-five Ways to Motivate People**

1. Listen!
2. Be sincere.
3. Use incentives.
4. Be a coach.
5. Promote camaraderie.
6. Encourage ideas and discussion.
7. Set clear goals.
8. Get rid of routines.
9. Develop a purpose.
10. Discipline fairly.
11. Be a mentor.
12. Be a confidant.
13. Keep secrets.
14. Recognize achievements.
15. Award achievements.
16. Create security.
17. Inspire!
18. Offer a challenge.
19. Make work fun.
20. Encourage!
21. Recognize what's important to your team.
22. Be friendly.
23. Invest people in the cause.
24. Be optimistic.
25. Create satisfaction.

*Source:* M. Ramundo and S. Shelly, *The Complete Idiot's Guide to Motivating People* (Indianapolis, IN: Alpha Books, 2000). Used by permission of Alpha Books, an imprint of Penguin Group (USA) Inc.

ers (public health technology and public health experts external to the community).[25] The specific community is also strongly influenced by its neighbors, the state, the federal government, and the global public health community. Broad economic, political, social, legal, and technological concerns affect the local community.

For public health agencies, the relationship with community customers is a primary relationship. The concept of Human Sigma has been formulated to show the importance of this relationship.[26] There are five key components or rules that define the Human Sigma model. The first rule requires good management of public health agency staff by local administrators and good relationships with community clients and all community residents. Staff and customers need to be seen in terms of the relationships that are generated between them. In fact, these relationships need to be seen as primary to the work of public health. If the agency staff is not engaged in its work, then the community clients will also be affected. This rule and the other three rules work synergistically in that staff and customer interactions are affected by the positive and negative consequences that come from the interaction as well as customer feedback. It is often impossible to predict these synergistic outcomes, but it is possible to learn from them to help in future encounters.

If I take my child to the public health agency to be immunized and my child and I are kept waiting for several hours for the nurse, then I will be upset. If the nurse is patronizing, my negative experience gets compounded. I will complain and I may also tell others in the community about my negative experience. The second rule of Human Sigma is the necessity of paying attention to the emotions aroused in an encounter between an agency staff member and a community resident. Emotions become facts in relationships.[27] The third rule addresses the issue of thinking globally and acting locally. Public health is a local phenomenon but is clearly affected by health issues in other parts of the world. If staff and customer interactions are mostly positive, then the chances increase that these positive occurrences can affect future budgeting considerations. The fourth rule points out that successful staff and customer relationships will affect the financial bottom line of the organization. These solid relationships will lead to the better utilization of the finances of the agency. The final rule states that intentions are not enough. Action will be the criterion for success. Despite these rules, all people have good and bad days. Exercise 12-2 explores this dimension.

There are many factors that can help to build customer loyalty. In addition to building good relationships between agency staff and community residents, leaders look for such things as consistency in services that are provided, caring and helpfulness, authenticity, positive attitude, professionalism, orientation to detail, responsiveness to complaints, good communication and follow-up, knowledge of other service providers to address special needs of clients, humor when appropriate, and community health days to celebrate improvements in the health of the community.[28] Good customer relationships are affected by always knowing why and for whom you are doing your work, treating your clients the way you want to be treated, supporting staff as discussed above, and providing leadership in support of the public health enterprise.[29]

As shown in Figure 12-1, part of the responsibility of the local public health agency is to monitor the health needs of the public and provide the technology and programs necessary to address those needs. Sometimes, things do not work out as expected. Case Study 12-A explores this situation of unanticipated events or anticipated events that are ignored when there is not enough influenza vaccine to go around. In addition to the needs assessment process, public health agencies have to determine how to help community residents understand public health and how their behavior affects their health. Education and training of the public is one way to increase knowledge of the public about public health. Recruitment of community residents to serve as volunteers in public health is also a useful process. Another interesting approach used by business is to use satisfied customers as spokespeople for successful public health programs. The development of the Medical Reserve Corps to address a community crisis is another example.

---

### Case Study 12-A
### Facing the Long Shot: Out of Vaccine, Out of Time

*Steven Curatti, Devon "Tony" Dede, Troy C. Hedrick, Veronica Halloway, Gwendolyn Mitchell, Tom Szpyrka, and Jerrod Welch*

#### Introduction
Emerald County lies along the shores of the Ohio River, and its borders encompass plentiful farm fields and orchards, as well as multiple communities, including the rapidly growing city of Thumbsville, with a population of just over 125,000. The county's ideal location along the river has created a busy riverfront with high-volume

barge traffic to ship goods from a growing manufacturing base and grains from large agricultural farms. This strong economic base has drawn many young urbanite professional families, as well as many Hispanic families. Combined with the pre-boom farming community population, this has led to a diverse county demographic. The majority of the county's Spanish-speaking population lives in the town of Greensboro, which is typically considered a part of Thumbsville, but has its own borders and government.

The Emerald County Health Department (ECHD) was established as a certified local public health department in the 1950s. Its structure is similar to that of many county health departments in that it has a governing board, a public health administrator, and multiple divisions with division directors reporting to the administrator. With the population boom Emerald County has experienced in recent years, election to the Board of Health has become very competitive because it is a prestigious post and a springboard for future political ambitions. Despite this, the board displays remarkable knowledge and flexibility and maintains a strong relationship with the administrator and most of the health department's staff.

ECHD is by all accounts highly effective in protecting the public's health through its various programs. The board, the administrator, and the department staff all take pride in ECHD's reputation for quality and effective service to all residents of Emerald County. Residents of the county rely heavily on many of these services and, in recent years, have come to know ECHD as "the" provider of flu vaccine each influenza season. ECHD's clinics have always run early in October, and the philosophy of Ima Lamduk, the longtime director of nursing (DON), has been that protection of the public from seasonal influenza is much more important than making money on seasonal clinics. This view is shared by the Board of Health, and in recent years the cost of adult and pediatric flu shots has remained stable even as surrounding providers have increased their prices regularly.

This fall it was expected that vaccine would arrive during the first week of October, as it always had. Ima had placed her vaccine order in March, and the Centers for Disease Control and Prevention (CDC) reported throughout the spring, summer, and early fall that more doses would be available this year than ever before. There was no reason for concern that ECHD would be short on doses; it never had before, and after all, it was a public agency and a participant in a statewide ordering group that would lobby on its behalf should vaccine distribution bog down. Advertisements for the first clinic had been placed in both of Thumbsville's major newspapers, as well as in the Greensboro Spanish-language newspaper. Radio and television ads and public service announcements were running daily, and Ima was confident that the community was receiving the message and that it would be no problem giving most of the 18,000 doses of Flu-Goo that had been ordered. Staff were actively promoting clinics, as were community advocates such as Diego Verde, the director of the Hispanic Cultural Center of Greensboro and a prominent and influential member of the Spanish-speaking community. Clinics would be held periodically throughout October and November, beginning October 10 at the Emerald County Courthouse.

**The Call—October 1 and Beyond**
In the mid-morning of Thursday, October 1, Ima had just met with her administrator, Guy Newman, in a regularly scheduled biweekly update meeting. Among the topics they had discussed were the bioterrorism grant budget, the implementation of

*(continues)*

**Case Study 12-A** *continued*

a new continuing education policy, and final details of the seasonal flu kickoff clinic at the courthouse. Mr. Newman had been through only one previous flu season as ECHD's administrator, and it had gone very smoothly. Ima reported that everything was in order and they were waiting on the arrival of Flu-Goo, which they expected any day. There was no reason for concern, just business as usual.

The meeting ended and Ima headed back to her office. She noticed her phone message light was blinking but had a few e-mails to read before checking the message. Nitus Flourengale, Ima's immunizations coordinator, dropped in to chat, and before Ima knew it, lunchtime had arrived. She grabbed her jacket and was just about to head out the door before she remembered the phone message. Though she could feel her stomach growling, she decided to listen to the call just to make sure it was nothing urgent.

"Ms. Lamduk. This is Mordy Lemmas from the SVOC (Statewide Vaccine Ordering Consortium). I wanted to touch base with all of our members about some vaccine distribution problems we are experiencing. It seems that there have been some problems with the vaccine distribution chain and we aren't going to be receiving all doses of Flu-Goo until at least late October. We are going to make every effort to get at least some doses out to all consortium members before next Friday, but right now we just aren't sure if that is feasible. I'm sorry for the inconvenience, and please don't hesitate to call me if you have any concerns. Thanks, and talk to you later."

It took a moment for Ima to register what she had just heard, and all of the possible fallout from the news. Her first reaction was to call the SVOC and tell them that ECHD already had clinics scheduled and needed priority. After thinking about it for a second, she reconsidered, knowing that many other health departments were also scheduling or had scheduled clinics for the second and third weeks of October. It would do no good to make that call, though Ima decided to write a letter later on to voice her frustration and concern. Now, she thought, was the time to think through the implications of having a limited and undefined vaccine supply.

The first thing that came to mind was her conversation just hours ago with Mr. Newman. "Everything is going as planned," she had told her boss. Now what would she tell him? That was really the least of her concerns considering all of the problems this would cause with the Board of Health during an election year, with the media and public trust in ECHD, and especially with the impact on general public health during what was predicted to be one of the worst flu seasons in recent years. She knew action was needed quickly to get this information out, but she wanted to get her thoughts in order before discussing this with Mr. Newman and her staff. She began to write down these thoughts.

### Public Health: Who will be affected most?

1. *CDC says young will be especially vulnerable this year, as will the elderly.*
2. *We also need to keep medical and first-responder personnel protected so they can report to work to assist others.*

### Who else provides in the county?

| | |
|---|---|
| *County General (NFP)* | *Who has vaccine?* |
| *Eastside Medical Center (NFP)* | *Priority groups?* |
| *Greensboro Medical Group (private)* | *Can we purchase?* |
| *Green-Wal Pharmacy (private)* | *Can we coordinate?* |

**Who have we told about our clinics?** *We'll have to get the word out that they are either postponed or that we may not have enough vaccine.*

*Staff and Board of Health*
*Volunteer nurses planning to show*
*Courthouse staff*
*Media: get the public notified quickly*
*Senior population and schools*
_____ *who else???*

**PR and Damage Control:** *Message must be consistent, up to date, and honest. We need to give viable alternatives to the clinics we planned (e.g., refer to other providers). Set up phone line and Web site for updated info.*

Ima thought that she had covered most immediate concerns in her written thoughts, though she felt like she was missing something. She just couldn't remember what. Well, she thought, it would come to her once she started talking things out with Mr. Newman and her staff.

Early that afternoon, Mr. Newman returned from lunch to find a hastily written e-mail from Ima telling him they needed to meet ASAP about flu vaccine delivery. He was curious, but not overly concerned, and wanted to get settled in and check his other messages before calling Ima. In the meantime, Ima had decided lunch was not all that important, and that she would get in touch with other providers in the community to assess their current supply and distribution plans. She found that County General had received 500 doses, which they were planning to give to CDC-defined high-risk individuals and key staff. Eastside Medical Center, the area's federally qualified health clinic, had received 2,000 doses of the 5,000 they had ordered. The clinic's 2,000 doses were Flu-Squirt, the inhaled version of the seasonal flu vaccine, and they were earmarked for distribution to pediatric populations to avoid giving kids injections. Eastside was happy to work with ECHD, though, and would take any recommendations to better serve the community. Vaccine price varied based on ability to pay, but most individuals were asked to pay $20 per dose. Greensboro Medical Group, the large private-practice clinic in the area, had received its full order, 1,500 doses of Flu-Goo and 500 doses of Flu-Squirt. Though the director of patient services said to Ima that they would help in any way they could, she could detect that their plan was to preserve the vaccine for their own staff and patients. They planned to charge $35 per dose for either vaccine and did not take the state medical card. Ima spoke with the pharmacy manager at Green-Wall, the chain pharmacy in Thumbsville, but couldn't get any useful information about the plans Green-Wall had for its vaccine (nor how much had been ordered, because that was proprietary information). Through the grapevine, Ima heard from one of her nurses who knew a Green-Wall pharmacist that the business had received 7,000 doses of Flu-Goo and 2,500 of Flu-Squirt and would be charging $18.50 per dose and would accept some Medicare. It seemed to Ima that Green-Wall was trying to undercut other providers, either to pick up a larger chunk of customers or as a political maneuver. Ima knew that the owner of the Green-Wall store in Thumbsville was currently running against a Board of Health incumbent for a seat at the board table, and it would look good politically to be able to tout this public service in his campaign.

By the time Mr. Newman called Ima, it was 2:00 PM, and Ima was starving. She had a little bit of hypoglycemia and was shaking slightly. As she broke the news that ECHD's order would be delayed, Mr. Newman noted her shaking and perceived it to mean she was very worried and nervous about the developments. As Ima went over her thoughts on the delay, he mentally registered what she was saying, but also

*(continues)*

**Case Study 12-A** *continued*

began thinking about the major political ramifications for the Board of Health and how that might affect him. Board members, already touting the reputation of ECHD in delivering reliable and broad flu vaccine coverage to the county, had begun e-mailing him to inquire about the arrival of the vaccine. He had assured them it was scheduled to arrive on time. He also thought about the February board meeting, where he had proposed that ECHD continue to order through the consortium to save money, even though Ima had recommended that for an additional 20 cents per dose, they could order directly from the manufacturer and receive a guaranteed delivery. This was never really a consideration, though, because never before had there been a problem with arrival of vaccine in plenty of time for the first public clinic. As Ima finished her summary, Mr. Newman voiced these concerns. It was decided to notify the chairman of the Board of Health of this situation, and to begin an active effort to notify the media that vaccine would not arrive on time and that clinics were postponed until further notice. Mr. Newman was to talk to the chairman, and Ima was to talk with her staff and begin drafting a press release that would notify county residents. She would also have to pull all advertising immediately.

By the end of the day on October 1, Ima had contacted all local media and made sure that all advertising for ECHD's public clinics was pulled. She asked the Supportive Services Division to be prepared to change the phone message to reflect information that she would provide them in a press release. She also asked that they designate one phone line, (123) 444-5678, to play the pre-recorded message in English and Spanish, with the option of being transferred to the switchboard once the message was completed. She contacted Mordy Lemmas at SVOC to see if anything else was known at present, but Mordy could only tell her that from what he understood, the manufacturer of Flu-Goo had all the vaccine produced, but there was a problem with the packaging. Mordy also felt that there would be a partial shipment by Tuesday, October 6, and that ECHD could consider keeping the first clinic scheduled. Ima asked how sure Mordy was about this, and he said, "Off the record, 100%. I can get you 1,800 doses, shipped Monday by FedEx." Ima discussed this with Mr. Newman and the chairman of the board on a conference call, and together they decided that ECHD would keep the October 10 clinic scheduled, but "postpone" all other clinics. With that information at hand, Ima had Nitus Flourengale draft a press release to fax (Appendix 1).

October 2 turned out to be a much busier Friday than ECHD staff and management had hoped for. Ima's entire staff was busy contacting churches, schools, nursing homes, and other groups that had made arrangements to receive flu shots through ECHD. Ima and Mr. Newman were busy fielding calls from the media, from concerned citizens, and from various board members who wanted to be kept directly informed of the situation. One staff member was assigned the duty of monitoring television and radio media for misinformation. At one point, conflicting statements were discovered between information on Channel 10 and Channel 12. Ima suspected that Mr. Newman might have misspoken to the Channel 12 newscaster that the clinic would run extended hours to accommodate school children (after all, it was on a Saturday). Ima quickly ensured that the information was corrected and suggested to Mr. Newton that she be the public information officer to ensure a consistent message. He quickly agreed, relieved to be able to focus on the Board of Health concerns.

By late afternoon on Friday, Ima had been asked a number of times by various individuals and media why there appeared to be no vaccine supply problems at

Green-Wall or Greensboro Medical Group, the two private providers in the area, but that all of the public providers were without their full vaccine orders. She had no strong answer and alluded to the type of vaccine ordered and the fact that vaccine supplies, especially flu vaccine supplies, were always vulnerable to manufacturing and distribution problems. Green-Wall had stepped up its media advertising campaign, stating that it had plenty of vaccine, plenty of staff ("average wait times are shorter than a fast-food drive through," the ad stated), and an affordable price. Ima and Mr. Newman discussed partnering with Green-Wall by offering staff and a location but elected not to because it may have stepped on the toes of the current board members facing re-election. Instead, Ima contacted the chief medical officer at County General and the director of nursing at Eastside Medical Center to form a "County Emergency Flu Response Strategy." The goal of the group was to assess the current countywide situation and determine level of coverage for vulnerable populations, medical personnel, and community first responders and how best to utilize the available combined vaccine (currently approximately 4,300 doses, including the promised shipment from SVOC). The group was to meet Tuesday, October 6. Ima didn't call Greensboro Medical Group for this planning committee, because she had already decided that its administration would not cooperate.

Monday, October 5, was much like the previous Friday, with Ima's staff busy fielding calls and making last-minute plans for the October 10 clinic. All supplies were ready, and if Flu-Goo arrived as promised by SVOC, there would be just enough doses to cover the clinic unless the media coverage had caused a panic. Ima made a mental note to ask Eastside's director of nursing if it would provide vaccine should ECHD run out at the clinic. In the afternoon, the sheriff's office called Mr. Newman to inquire about security at the clinic. Sheriff Andy Fife had concerns that long lines and possible shortages may have led to some level of civil unrest. He was up for re-election and didn't need a black mark on his record fresh in voter's minds. Mr. Newman agreed that security was not a bad idea, but asked that officers carry their weapons concealed so as not to create an atmosphere of fear, especially in any Hispanic individuals who already distrusted county and city police. Sheriff Fife thought this request was ridiculous and the issue was left unresolved, though two officers were committed to attend the clinic. Late in the day, Ima and Mr. Newman met to make sure everything was proceeding well. They discussed how the media had been handled, the prospect of receiving their 1,800 doses of Flu-Goo the next day, and various other issues. Ima reported that staff had handled all of the public inquiries admirably, and that there didn't appear to be an air of panic within the community. Mr. Newman thought that the Board of Health would be as satisfied as it could be with the situation as it had been handled.

The next morning, the three-member flu response strategy committee met. The Eastside DON agreed to provide up to 500 doses for the October 10 ECHD clinic, as well as three nurses and one support staff. Her only caveat was that Ima make every effort to give Eastside's doses to individuals aged 4 to 18 years, to which Ima agreed. County's chief medical officer stated that he was concerned that there was unrest in the Spanish-speaking community about receipt of timely information related to the current flu vaccine issue. Suddenly Ima had a sinking feeling in her stomach: "Oh no, I didn't call Diego."

"Hello Mr. Verde, this is Ima at the health department. I know you have already heard on the news that we are having some problems with the delivery of vaccine.

*(continues)*

**Case Study 12-A** *continued*

I wanted to touch base though, and give you an update on where things stand at this point. We are still running our October 10 clinic and appreciate your help in promoting it. Right now, our other clinics are postponed, including the one planned on October 14 at St. Mary's Cathedral. We do hope to be rescheduling later in October and early November, and hope that the church will be available at some point during that time."

"Ima, I must be honest. I have already been telling others that the clinics are cancelled, but I am very concerned that we as a community are not being fully informed of the situation. You know, many of us in Greensboro won't be able to have transportation to the courthouse in Thumbsville. We have been banking on the clinic at St. Mary's. In fact, I have been assuring others that there will certainly be a clinic here because I hadn't heard from you yet. I truly appreciate all your department does for our community, but I see a real issue here, and I plan to point it out. Also, I have been told that you have a Spanish-language message on your question line, but that if additional information is needed, no person at the health department speaks Spanish fluently enough to help. I think we have multiple problems that the Board of Health should be addressing in the future if this is indeed a *county* health department."

After the uncomfortable conversation with Mr. Verde, Ima checked in with Nitus, who was happy to report that 1,800 doses of Flu-Goo had arrived. She also reported that in pre-filling syringes, it seemed that nurses could get about 10.75 doses per vial instead of 10, which would yield as much as 1,935 doses. Ima agreed that this was good news indeed and reported the same to Mr. Newman. In the meantime, he had received a call from County Judge Roy Bean (the main man in Emerald County by all accounts), who felt that his family was at high risk for flu and would be coming down on Thursday to receive their shots. Ima was proud that Mr. Newman had told Judge Bean that no exceptions could be made and he should arrive early on Saturday to avoid any delays in receiving vaccine.

On Wednesday, Green-Wall began running daily clinics on a walk-in basis. They appeared to be running smoothly despite reports that some retired nurses volunteering at the clinics might have been working under expired licenses (or as they stated, working under the license of the pharmacy director). Green-Wall even went as far as to rent a bus to travel back and forth from Greensboro to ensure access for the Hispanic population, a move praised mightily by local media (though one political analyst questioned whether the move was mainly political in nature).

The rest of the week went relatively smoothly for ECHD, and by Friday afternoon everyone was ready to get Saturday going. People began lining up at 8:30 AM, and Ima made the decision to begin service at 10:00 instead of 11:00 so that an 11:00 rush would not further add to the line lengths. She assumed that she would hear some negative feedback on this move but felt it was the right thing to do. With the additional Eastside nurses helping, things still ran relatively smoothly. The courthouse had been the site of a "kickoff" clinic for many years, and the layout and flow was well known to staff and patrons. However, at 2:00 PM, Nitus found Ima and reported her concern that the vaccine supply was running low and might not last until 3:00. Ima reminded Nitus that Eastside would give an additional 500 doses, but cringed when Nitus reported that she had included that in her calculations. The clinic had already distributed 2,200 doses and only 250 remained. The nurses were beginning to panic. "Nitus," Ima said, "we've done all we can do. I will go count out the line and at 250 will cut it off. I'm just going to direct the rest of these folks to Green-Wall."

The clinic ended and only about 25 individuals had to be redirected. Everyone breathed a sigh of relief. They had come through without too many problems. Of course they faced the rest of the flu season with the prospect of no additional vaccine unless SVOC came through.

## The Aftermath: Post 10/10

After the Saturday clinic, Ima felt that ECHD had handled the flu vaccine crisis as well as could be expected. Public health had remained her highest priority despite the various pressures from the media, the board, other political factions, and the public in general. She contacted SVOC the next Monday, October 12. Mordy Lemmas had bad news; vaccine would not be available until late November. ECHD would give no more vaccine that flu season, because demand would be nonexistent after Thanksgiving. Green-Wall had already successfully purchased an additional 7,500 doses from another regional provider who had ordered excess and would by default be the primary provider of flu vaccine that season, effectively privatizing this vital public health service.

Flu season did not strike as hard this year as the CDC said it would. Ima and all of the ECHD breathed a sigh of relief at that. The community as a whole had received fairly adequate coverage, only about 5% down from the previous 5-year average. Though a small blow to the ECHD's reputation of being a "premiere" public health department in the state, the whole incident quickly died down in the media and the general populace seemed to forget there was ever concern. By February, ECHD had rapidly and effectively handled a small local outbreak of salmonella and had launched a new after-school program for at-risk youth, and the media had raved at these successes. However, Ima's mind still mulled over the problem-riddled flu season. She decided that this could not happen again and wanted to make sure that multiple stakeholders considered what had occurred and how to plan for the expected and unexpected in future flu seasons. In late February and just before flu vaccine orders would be due through the SVOC, Ima called representatives from her staff, the previously organized "Emergency Flu Strategy" group, the Board of Health (including the two newly elected members, neither of which was the Green-Wall owner), schools, the senior center, and the cultural center (Mr. Verde was definitely remembered this time) together for a planning meeting. The meeting was well attended, and everyone was very appreciative to be included in the process. At the meeting, the following questions and issues arose.

## February 23 Flu Planning Group Meeting: Critical Questions and Issues

1.  What thoughts and facts discussed during the assessment of the situation would lead the coalition to decide who would receive the first doses of vaccines?
2.  What information should be included in the assessment process as the group develops a plan for next year?
3.  Should there be more than one source to purchase vaccine? Should the vaccine be purchased through a competitive bid process involving several manufacturers/providers? Why?
4.  What would be the advantages and disadvantages to public health relinquishing the administration of the vaccines to the private sector? Does it really matter who gives the vaccine?
5.  How can the Hispanic community be better included and informed in this scenario?

*(continues)*

**Case Study 12-A** *continued*

6. Where in the assessment process did Ima go wrong in developing her response to the shortage?
7. Are there other groups that could/should be included in the collaborative assessment of this year's project and in the planning for the coming year's effort?
8. In Ima's assessment of stakeholders, who else could she have included?
9. What role does the assessment of political interests have in the delivery of public health services?

### Appendix 1: Nitus Flourengale's October 2 Press Release

Emerald County Health Department - For Information Contact: (123) 456-7890
PRESS RELEASE—FOR IMMEDIATE RELEASE—October 2, 2006
UPDATED INFORMATION ON EMERALD COUNTY HEALTH DEPARTMENT SEASONAL INFLUENZA CLINICS

Emerald County Health Department (ECHD) was notified today that shipments of seasonal flu vaccine have been delayed. ECHD orders seasonal flu vaccine through a consortium representing multiple local health departments in the state. According to the distributor, it is anticipated that distribution of vaccine to all consortium members will be completed by late October. As a result of the delay in receipt of flu vaccine, changes to ECHD's seasonal flu clinics will occur as follows:

- ECHD's previously scheduled flu clinic at the Emerald County Courthouse on Saturday, October 10, will proceed as scheduled from 11:00 AM to 3:00 PM.
- All other flu clinics previously scheduled are postponed and will be rescheduled upon ECHD's receipt of flu vaccine.
- The United States Centers for Disease Control and Prevention have indicated that seasonal flu this year may be most severe in young children and the elderly. At this time, ECHD will not limit the distribution of vaccine to these target groups but does ask that healthy adults consider waiting to receive their flu shot until more supply arrives.
- A question line has been set up, and anyone with concerns or questions may call (123) 444-5678 and an ECHD representative will address their concern. In Emerald County, influenza typically does not circulate in the community until February-March. Therefore, at this time, a short delay in vaccine delivery does not present a public health concern to Emerald County. Individuals who have specific concerns regarding receipt of an adult flu shot prior to public clinics should call their primary care provider to discuss their concerns. As always, individuals should practice good personal hygiene to minimize their risks from flu and other illnesses. These practices include:
  - Cover your mouth and nose with a tissue when you cough or sneeze. Discard the used tissue and thoroughly wash your hands with soap and warm water. If no tissue is available, sneeze into your sleeve instead of your hand.
  - To minimize the spread of germs, stay home when you are sick and avoid close contact with others who are sick.
  - Parents should ensure that their children wash hands frequently.
  - Practice other good health habits, including getting plenty of rest, eating nutritious food, being physically active, and avoiding stress. ECHD will continue to provide updated information to the community regarding rescheduling of seasonal flu clinics as information on vaccine delivery becomes available.

### References

National Association of County and City Health Officials (NACCHO) Web-based Influenza Vaccine Distribution Survey, October 2006 found at: http://www.naccho.org/topics/infectious/documents/InfluenzaSurveyresults10-10-061_000.doc

Peter Sandman, Crisis Communication: A Very Quick Introduction, April 15, 2004. http://www.psandman.com/col/pandemic.htm

NACHO—www.naccho.org

1. "Issue Brief," Issue 4, Number 1, April 2004, "Local Public Health Agency—Federally Qualified Health Center Collaboration to Improve Health Services Delivery"
2. Primary Care: Audio Conferences
   a. "Important Issues for Smooth Financing of a Community Health Center in a Local Health Department
   b. "Local Health Departments That Have Collaborated with a Federally Qualified Health Center"
   c. "Local Health Departments That Have Received Community Health Center Funding and the Community Health Center Governance Structure"
3. Primary Care - Publications and Tools, "Making Strategic Decisions about Service/Delivery Partnerships Project"

National Association of Community Health Centers - www.NACHC.org, Various topics using the internal search engine

MMWR, Prevention and Control of Influenza Recommendations of the Advisory Committee on Immunization Practices (ACIP), Vol 55, No RR10;1

MMWR, Influenza Vaccination of Health-Care Personnel Recommendations of the Healthcare Infection Control Practices Advisory Committee (HICPAC) and the Advisory Committee on Immunization Practices (ACIP), Vol 55, No RR2;1

MMWR, Influenza Vaccine Prebooking and Distribution Strategies for the 2005–06 Influenza Season, Vol 54, No MM12;307

MMWR, Notice to Readers: Updated Recommendations From the Advisory Committee on Immunization Practices in Response to Delays in Supply of Influenza Vaccine for the 2000–01 Season, Vol 49, No MM39;888

MMWR, Experiences with Obtaining Influenza Vaccination Among Persons in Priority Groups During a Vaccine Shortage—United States, October–November, 2004, Vol 53, No MM49;1153

Johnson, Cheryl, Executive Director/Public Health Administrator, Kendall County Health Department. Personal interview. 4, Jan. 2007.

United States Government Accountability Office (GAO) Testimony—Flu Vaccine, Recent Supply Shortages underscore Ongoing Challenges—November 18, 2004

World Health Organization (WHO) Global pandemic influenza action plan to increase vaccine supply—WHO/IVB/06.13

---

The issue of "fit" requires that there be a solid relationship between the engaged staff member and an engaged community resident. Not all residents choose to go to a public health agency for service. It is necessary to point out that the public health agency is only one partner in the public health enterprise. Fit needs to be expanded to all the community agency and hospital resources. The goal is to strive to find appropriate access to service for every resident somewhere in the community and to even extend the service option to other agencies outside the community when necessary. In many ways, public health is about education. People need to learn how to help make themselves more healthy. Public health leaders need to use their skills to create teachable moments. Community residents need motivation and support for their health. The motivation tips listed in Table 12-1 clearly fit here as well. Finally, strategic and action planning as demonstrated by the leadership wheel requires that the public be involved in public health activities. Their needs and concerns must be addressed as part of all planning activities.

## Community Stakeholders

Public health leaders know that they have to work with other community partners if the public health enterprise is to work. These decision makers outside the public health agency will need to be involved in the overall public health planning and agenda if there is to be successful implementation of public health programs and services.[30] These stakeholders will have to make a commitment and also provide financial resources to the enterprise. As pointed out in Part II of this book, public health leaders carry out their public health mission and vision within the context of the core functions and essential public health services paradigm.

Public health leaders also need to view the community within a systems thinking orientation. The public health system includes the local public health agency and the population of the community; it also includes many stakeholders such as other health and social agencies from the private, public, not-for-profit, and volunteer sectors who will work with the local public health agency in carrying out the essential services. Figure 12-2 views the public health system as a network of interacting partners that includes public health agencies, health care providers, public safety agencies, human service and charity organizations, education and youth development organizations, recreation and arts-related organizations, economic and philanthropic organizations, and environmental agencies and organizations.[31] Community residents have many relationships with these organizations and influence policy through these relationships with community stakeholders.

In strategic planning, which is discussed in Chapter 13, stakeholder analysis is one of the techniques involved. Public health leaders need to study stakeholders to see what the local public health system is like as well as to determine if gaps exist in the service system. There are three steps in stakeholder analysis.[32] The first step involves a determination of the services available. This step involves not only an enumeration of resources, but also what each stakeholder resource can contribute to the overall public health enterprise. Secondly, a determination needs to be made about the level of organizational performance by potential public health partners. Finally, public health leaders need to determine how public health stakeholders will perform relative to the goals and objectives for public health in a given community.

One important dimension that is often ignored is the necessity of stakeholder development. Stakeholders do not always understand what public health does. They need training in public health and need to develop a virtual public health stakeholder learning community if a face-to-face community is difficult to sustain. Public health leaders also need to be on the look

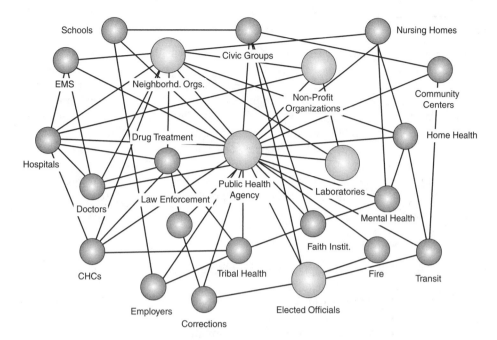

**FIGURE 12-2    The Public Health System**
*Source:* Centers for Disease Control and Prevention, National Public Health Performance Standards Program Users Guide, Version 2.0 (Washington, DC: U.S. Department of Health and Human Services, 2007).

out for new or emerging resources as they develop. Partners from outside the service community are also important. At the transactional leadership level, recruitment of new stakeholders will address reciprocity concerns.

Fit is clearly important as well. A few years ago, a small local health department in a Midwest state applied for a state grant to develop a special maternal and child health program. A local community agency also applied for this same grant. The directors of the two agencies were extremely competitive and did not work well together. The state gave the grant to the community agency, requiring the two agencies to work together on the program. The staff of the two agencies tried to collaborate although the fit was not a good one. Many conflicts ensued.

Because leaders are often dealing with leaders in stakeholder situations, motivation strategies still remain important. Relationships need to be on a person-to-person level. If the relationships are always or mostly position to position, these relationships tend to be conflictual. There has to be both transactional and transformational gains if collaboration is to succeed. Decisions will need to be made about carrying out the 10 essential public health services. Whenever strategic planning activities occur or the public health assessment process is undertaken, community partners need to be involved in the process. As shown in the leadership wheel, public health planning both strategically and in terms of action requires a partnership among the local public health agency, its customers, and its partners.

## Summary

This chapter has presented the subject of relationships in public health. These relationships involve the staff of the local public health agency, its community customers, and its community partners. Public health practice requires a systems view of the community. Public health leaders and managers must strive for good relationships with their staff inside the agency. Public health agency staff need to develop good relationships with their clientele in the community. Good relationships inside the agency often mean that relationships outside the agency have a better chance at success. Public health leaders also need to nurture and develop good relationship with their community stakeholders and bring them together as partners in the public health enterprise.

### Discussion Questions

1. What are the key factors in recruiting new employees into the local public health agency?
2. Why is the relationship between the public health manager or supervisor so important?
3. What are the best methods for motivating agency staff?
4. How does the Human Sigma model apply to public health?
5. What are the factors that increase chances for more solid relationships with the public?
6. Who are public health's partners?
7. What is the relationship between public health customers and the network of public health partners?
8. Why is a systems perspective more viable than an agency-based perspective in public health?

### Exercise 12-1: Journey Through Time

*Purpose:* to see the impact of perception on sustainability

*Key concepts:* perception, sustainability, mental models, visioning

*Procedure:* This exercise will help you to explore how your impact on your agency over the years will be affected by your personal mental models. Divide the class or training group into small groups of four or five people. Answer the journey questions for your group members:

1. Go back 100 years and describe the world of your ancestors. What was their world like and what were their mental models about health and the environment? What would your ancestors want you to learn from their world?
2. Go forward 100 years and describe the world of your descendants. How has the present affected their lives? What is their mental model about health and the environment? What messages do they want to relay to you?
3. Go forward 10 years and describe yourself and your family and co-workers. What did you learn from the you of today about health and the environment? What would you have done differently?

4. Reflect on what you have learned. What do you want to do differently at work and in your community? What must we do to improve the ways we make public health more effective?

*Source:* Adapted from J. Laur and S. Schlag, "A Journey in Time," in P. Senge, J. Laur, S. Schlag, and B. Smith (eds.), *Learning for Sustainability* (Cambridge, MA: Society for Organizational Learning, 2006).

### Exercise 12-2:   Good Days and Bad Days

*Purpose:* to explore our relationships with the public and determine the factors that lead to both positive and negative experiences

*Key concepts:* engaged public health workers, engaged customers, motivation

*Procedure:* Divide the group into dyads. Each person will describe a good day with the community and the factors that made it so. How much of the good day related back to the agency and how much of it was affected by the encounter with the community? Share the experiences with your dyad partner. Repeat the discussion for an example of a bad day in the community. What are the differences in the two types of day? What would you have changed? Return to the large group and report on the things that make a good day and what makes a day not so good. For the large group, have a recorder list the good day and bad day factors.

## References

1. J. M. Kouzes and B. Z. Posner, *The Leadership Challenge,* 4th ed. (San Francisco: Jossey-Bass, 2007).
2. D. Williams, *Real Leadership* (San Francisco: Berrett-Kohler, 2005).
3. K. Blanchard, S. Fowler, and L. Hawkins, *Self Leadership and the One Minute Manager* (New York: William Morrow, 2005).
4. E. De Bono, *Free or Unfree* (Beverly Hills, CA: Phoenix Books, 2007).
5. J. Laur and S. Schlag, "A Journey in Time," in P. Senge, J. Laur, S. Schlag, and B. Smith (eds.), *Learning for Sustainability* (Cambridge, MA: Society for Organizational Learning, 2006).
6. Blanchard, Fowler, and Hawkins, *Self Leadership and the One Minute Manager.*
7. S. P. Robbins, *The Truth About Managing People* (Upper Saddle River, NJ: Prentice-Hall, 2002).
8. J. C. Maxwell, *Relationships 101* (Nashville, TN: Thomas Nelson, 2003).
9. J. Collins, *Good to Great* (New York: Harper Business, 2001).
10. L. Rowitz, *Public Health in the 21st Century: The Prepared Leader* (Sudbury, MA: Jones and Bartlett, 2006).
11. M. Buckingham, *Go Put Your Strengths to Work* (New York: Free Press, 2007).
12. S. P. Robbins and M. Coulter, *Management,* 8th ed. (Upper Saddle River, NJ: Prentice-Hall, 2005).
13. H. E. Chambers, *Finding, Hiring, and Keeping Peak Performers* (Cambridge, MA: Perseus Publishing, 2001).
14. C. Coffman and G. Gonzalex-Molina, *Follow This Path* (New York: Warner Books, 2002).
15. J. C. Maxwell, *Talent Is Never Enough* (Nashville, TN: Thomas Nelson, 2007).

16. Robbins, *The Truth About Managing People.*
17. J. H. Fleming and J. Asplund, *Human Sigma* (New York: Gallup Press, 2007).
18. Chambers, *Finding, Hiring, and Keeping Peak Performers.*
19. Buckingham, *Go Put Your Strengths to Work.*
20. Fleming and Asplund, *Human Sigma.*
21. Robbins, T*he Truth About Managing People.*
22. P. Lencioni, *The Three Signs of a Miserable Job* (San Francisco: Jossey-Bass, 2007).
23. M. Ramundo and S. Shelly, *The Complete Idiot's Guide to Motivating People* (Indianapolis, IN: Alpha Books, 2000).
24. Ramundo and Shelly, *The Complete Idiot's Guide to Motivating People.*
25. Robbins and Coulter, *Management.*
26. Fleming and Asplund, *Human Sigma.*
27. Fleming and Asplund, *Human Sigma.*
28. J. Brandi, *Building Customer Loyalty* (Dallas, TX: Walk the Talk, 2001).
29. K. Blanchard, J. Ballard, and F. Finch, *Customer Mania* (New York: Free Press, 2004).
30. J. M Bryson, *Strategic Planning for Public and Nonprofit Organizations,* 3rd ed. (San Francisco: Jossey-Bass, 2004).
31. Centers for Disease Control and Prevention, *National Public Health Performance Standards Program Users Guide, Version 2.0* (Washington, DC: U.S. Department of Health and Human Services, 2007).
32. Bryson, *Strategic Planning for Public and Nonprofit Organizations.*

# CHAPTER 13

# LEADERSHIP AND
# THE PLANNING PROCESS

> We live in a world where no one is "in charge." No one
> organization, or institution has the legitimacy, power, authority,
> or intelligence to act alone on important public issues and still
> make substantial headway against the problems that threaten
> us all.
>
> J. M. Bryson and B. C. Crosby,
> *Leadership for the Common Good*

No matter what changes occur in the world of public health, planning activities will continue to occupy much of the work time of public health leaders. Because preparing for the future is part of their mandate, public health leaders must devote substantial energy to strategic thinking, which is basically thinking devoted to the resolution of problems and the achievement of desired goals. Strategic thinking is essential for all varieties of planning, such as working out the details of strategic planning, a continuous quality improvement (CQI) program, Six Sigma program, a re-engineering project, or a community partnership scheme. This chapter covers the skills that public health leaders need in order to do the full range of planning they will be responsible for over the next few decades.

## Community Health Planning

As noted, public health leaders work at many different levels, including the community level. Community health planning involves the development of public health goals and objectives and the ordering of the actions necessary to accomplish these. In this type of planning, it is important, first, to use an approach that is able to generate innovative public health strategies and, second, to keep in mind the core functions and essential services of public health for guidance.

Planning is a form of rational decision making.[1] The first step in the process is to decide on goals and objectives. The next step is to determine the constraints on the planning process and the likely changes in the environment that may affect how easy the goals and objectives are to achieve. The third step is to figure out what actions, policies, and programs to implement. A good strategy at this stage is to develop a series of outcome scenarios so that those engaged in the planning have several options to choose from.[2] Note that even if a plan is a good one—that is, its implementation will lead to the achievement of the desired goals and objectives—leaders must remain constantly aware of factors that may undermine the implementation process and sometime will have to modify their activities as a result of unexpected happenings.

Planning is often viewed as a routine task and something that managers do rather than leaders. It has routine aspects to it, but planning, especially strategic planning, must ultimately be driven by the big picture and strategic thinking that leads to the leaders' vision of the future. Therefore, leaders need to remain intimately involved in the planning process because the planning process will be an important set of techniques to help leaders realize their visions.

The planning process can be formal or informal. Formal planning leaves a paper trail, because all critical decisions are documented, whereas informal planning is less organized and more guided by social interaction.

Planning, although time consuming, is almost never a waste of time. It gives structure to the activities that are directed toward achieving desired goals and may also save money by encouraging the monitoring of these activities. Planning does not eliminate change but rather fosters change. It can also foster flexibility in the implementation process, although it has the potential, if done poorly, to act in the opposite way and hinder flexibility.

In public health, planning was not common until the 1920s.[3] The increase in the funds devoted to public health over the years has created a need to plan for and be accountable for the expenditure of the funds. In the mid-1960s, Congress passed a comprehensive health planning act (P.L. 89–749), which required states and local areas to be involved in planning activities. The reasoning was that public health is the responsibility of state and local entities. The act did not work as well as expected. The development of health service agencies (HSAs) led to a duplication of activity. Many local health department leaders, even those involved in HSA activities, believed that the local public health agency should be doing the health planning. With the end of federal funding for HSAs in the 1980s, state and local public health agencies re-absorbed planning into their program portfolios.

Community health planning is key to the promotion of public health services.[4] Planning activities should use epidemiological data and be community based in the sense that they integrate public and private interests for the benefit of the residents. Public health leaders should include community partners in the planning process, and the plans developed should encompass all segments of the community.

Rohrer describes three planning models that are typically used in the field of public health.[5] The rational planning model encompasses "fact finding, problem definition, goal setting, implementation, monitoring, feedback, and evaluation." This model is generally applied to planning directed toward reforming the internal operations of an agency. The community development model is empowerment oriented and promotes local citizen participation in planning activities. Decisions are reached by consensus. The activist model is applicable when community groups threatened by a particular public health danger become mobilized. These models are limited in value. The strategic-planning approach discussed in the next section has the advantage that it applies to both organizational reform and community health planning.

As discussed in Chapter 8, assessment is a prerequisite for planning, although assessment and planning activities are typically ongoing. The gathering of assessment data informs public health leaders about community needs that should be addressed immediately, and they can thus direct their planning activities at developing policies and programs to respond to these needs. Once the programs and policies are in place, their effectiveness should be evaluated, and if they are found to be less effective than expected, the leaders could then engage in further planning in order to improve them (Figure 13-1).[6]

Public health leaders must:

- use the core functions and essential services of public health as a foundation for community health planning
- learn how to use the different planning methodologies and how to choose the appropriate model for a given initiative
- determine the actions necessary to achieve desired community health goals and objectives
- use planning and scenario building to discover innovative public health strategies
- be involved in formal planning activities
- create community partnerships to carry out planning activities

## Strategic Planning

The relationship between strategies and tactics is similar to that between goals and objectives. Both goals and objectives are ends or desired states of affairs. One difference is that goals tend to be broad in scope and objectives relatively less so. Another is that objectives are ends that are sought largely because they lead to the achievement of goals. Improving the level of health in a community is a good example of a goal. Relative to this goal, testing the community's water supply might be one objective. Note that it is relatively narrower in scope and would be one step on the way to achieving the goal.

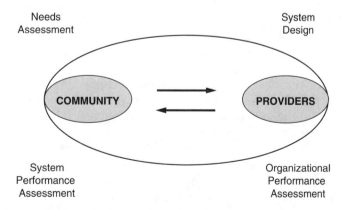

**FIGURE 13-1  Community-Oriented Health Systems Planning**
*Source:* Reprinted with permission from J. E. Rohrer, *Planning for Community-Oriented Health Systems,* © 1996, American Public Health Association.

Strategies are plans or methods that are relatively broad in scope, are often long term in nature, and often involve a significant expenditure of resources. Tactics are methods that are relatively narrow in scope and use relatively few resources. Roughly speaking, strategies are likely to be used in attaining goals, whereas tactics are likely to be used in attaining objectives. (Be warned that there is some looseness in the use of these terms and that many people employ "goal" and "objective" as synonyms and "strategy" and "tactic" as near synonyms.)

Strategic planning is planning directed at the achievement of goals—significant or even ultimate ends. As such, it is an extremely important task and falls largely on the shoulders of the leadership. A list of strategic-planning guidelines and a 10-step strategic-planning model follow. As in the case of any major task, those responsible for completing the task should remain upbeat in order to motivate others involved to do their share. First, the guidelines:

1. Strategic planning is a team process in which the team members need to share the leader's vision. The team members also need to be carefully selected and represent all parts of the organization. The leader needs to be clear about the responsibilities of the team and may want to convene a community advisory board to discuss how the plan meets the health needs of the community.
2. The team needs to set a timeline for the planning process. The process should be short enough to devise a plan and implement it before events have rendered it irrelevant.
3. The team needs to consider how to get the plan accepted after the planning process.
4. The team needs to create a schedule for the planning process.
5. The team must disseminate the results of the process—the plan—following its completion. The team must carefully determine what will be disseminated, but it is generally better to disseminate more rather than less.
6. The team must decide on the techniques that will be used to evaluate the process.[7]

Bryson developed a 10-step procedure for strategic planning (see also Table 13-1).[8] The first step could be called the "planning to plan" stage.[9] According to Bryson, the leader needs to be clear on the reasons that strategic planning was chosen rather than some other technique. A readiness assessment occurs. The leader also needs to communicate with potential stakeholders and to lay the groundwork for a shared vision. The partners will want to know what they are "buying" and how long the planning and implementation process will take. Bryson suggested that partners might do well to start the process by going on a retreat. Strategic planning can be an expensive process, and funds will be needed to carry it out.

Step 2 involves the clarification of organizational mandates. Public health practitioners are constantly bombarded with formal mandates that take substantial time to abide by. Not only that, public health agencies are legally mandated to perform certain functions and are given funds to carry out these functions but might not be funded to implement other public health initiatives closer to the mission of public health as defined by the local health department and the community stakeholders. Stakeholders are persons or

**Table 13-1  Bryson Strategic Planning Model Applied to Public Health**

| Bryson Model | Public Core Functions | Organizational Practices | Essential Services | System Activities |
|---|---|---|---|---|
| Initiation and agreement on a strategic-planning process | Policy development | Constituency building | Mobilization of community partnerships to identify and solve health problems | Coalition building and values clarification |
| Identification and clarification of the nature/meaning of externally imposed formal and informal mandates | Policy development and assurance | Evaluation of programs in accordance with plans and policies | Enforcement of laws and regulations that protect health and ensure safety | Values clarification |
| Clarification of organizational mission and values | Policy development | Not applicable | Not applicable | Values clarification and mission and vision development |
| Assessment of the organization's external and internal environments to identify stengths, weaknesses, opportunities, and threats | Assessment | Assessment of health needs of the community  Investigation of the occurrence of health effects and health hazards | Monitoring of health status to identify community health problems  Diagnosis and investigation of health problems and health hazards in the community | Vision and goals and objectives development (based on assessment data) |
| Identification of the strategic issues facing the organization | Policy development and assessment | Analysis of the determinants of identified health needs  Setting of priorities among health needs | Development of policies and plans that support individual and community health efforts | Development of goals and objectives and action plans |

*(continues)*

**Table 13-1** (continued)

| Bryson Model | Public Core Functions | Organizational Practices | Essential Services | System Activities |
|---|---|---|---|---|
| Formulation of strategies to manage these issues | Policy development | Development of plans and policies to address priority health needs | Development of policies and plans that support individual and community health efforts | Action planning |
| Review and adoption of the strategic plan or plans | Policy development | Management of resources and development of organizational structure | Not applicable | Action planning |
| Establishment of an effective organizational vision | Policy development | Not applicable | Not applicable | Vision development |
| Development of an effective implementation process | Assurance | Management of resources and development of organizational structure  Education of the public | Linkage of people to needed personal health services and assurance of the provision of health care when otherwise unavailable | Action plan development and implementation |
| Reassessment of strategies and the strategic-planning process | Assessment, policy development, and assurance | Evaluation of programs and performance of quality assurance activities | Evaluation of the effectiveness, accessibility, and quality of personal and population-based health services | Evaluation using the systems perspective |

*Source:* Adapted with permission from J. M. Bryson, *Strategic Planning for Public and Nonprofit Organizations* (3rd edition). © 2004, Jossey-Bass Inc., Publishers.

organizations that have an interest in public health programs and how they are implemented. They include concerned citizens, government representatives, other health and social service representatives, governing board members, church representatives, and members of professional associations.

It is critical to include the appropriate stakeholders in strategic planning. For example, major community employers, unions, regulatory or licensing agencies, bankers, and neighbors of the agency are often excluded from community coalitions despite the fact that they can prevent decisions from being implemented.[10] In general, stakeholders expect the agency and its leadership to be responsive to their needs and can even issue what might be called informal mandates. If the agency does not respond to these informal mandates, the stakeholders will look elsewhere for support. The local public health agency must determine whether the formal mandates prevent addressing the informal mandates. Several local public health administrators interviewed by the author said that responding to the formal mandates in their state took almost 90% of their agency's time. Creating innovative programs became virtually impossible because of the lack of time.

In step 3, agency leaders begin to investigate the values that will govern the agency and the agency's community relationships. The agency's mission should refer to its role in the community. By going through the values clarification process and developing a mission, the agency will be in a better position to monitor the strategic-planning process. This step might include the performance of a stakeholder analysis, which will clarify who the stakeholders are, what their values are, what their goals and objectives are, what issues are likely to affect them, and what their degree of commitment is to the status quo.

The fourth step involves the assessment of the internal and external environments in order to identify the opportunities and the challenges arising from the change process.[11] This has been referred to as a SWOT analysis, for it focuses on *s*trengths, *w*eaknesses, *o*pportunities, and *t*hreats. The external assessment looks at forces that may affect agency programs, whether at the local, state, federal, or global level. For example, diseases or disease-causing agents that originate in one portion of the globe may eventually spread to all other parts, as did the human immunodeficiency virus (HIV).[12] The analysis should include key stakeholders who have an agenda that they wish to see implemented and major competitors, such as local managed care organizations (which may want to take over public health roles and responsibilities). Assessing external forces should be an ongoing activity and not be limited to one step in the strategic-planning process.[13]

The internal assessment looks at the agency's resources, the process of carrying out the agency activities, and the performance outputs. Part 1 of the Assessment Protocol for Excellence in Public Health, described in Chapter 8, is an assessment of an organization's internal capacity. This organizational component is not visibly present in the Mobilizing for Action through Planning and Partnerships assessment process, which is a system-based assessment. However, there is nothing that prevents a public health agency from doing an internal capacity assessment.

The collection of information, the clarification of values, the development of a mission, and the assessment of the agency and its environment provide the foundation for the rest of the strategic-planning process. Step 5 is the identification of the issues to be addressed by the plan. In this stage, the stakeholders typically come together to define the issues utilizing a group process approach. The stakeholders need not only to identify the critical issues but also to explain why these issues are critical and to describe what the consequences of not addressing these issues will be.

Another approach to completing this step is to define goals and objectives and then develop issues based on the goals and objectives. Still another approach is for the partners in the strategic-planning process to devise ideal scenarios (descriptions of the way they would like the world to be) and present them to each other and try to come to a consensus. One problem with scenario building is that it is a complex process and requires the participants to be trained in how to create scenarios.[14] Without proper training, the participants may not be able to get results that are valid. In a fourth approach, the strategic-planning team tries to facilitate the formulation of issues by slowly guiding the stakeholders through the process.

Step 6 involves the development of strategies to address the issues delineated in step 5. In short, it is during this step that the strategic plan is actually devised. Possible strategies include the setting of new policies or new rules and regulations, the development of new programs and services, and changes in the allocation of resources. The stakeholders need to determine how the chosen strategies interrelate and thus how the whole system works. Some strategies might involve both the agency and the community, some might involve just the agency or just agency subdivisions, and some might involve agency programs and services.

In step 7, the stakeholders review, modify, and adopt the strategic plan developed in step 6. Here, as in steps 5 and 6, they must consider the actions that will be necessary to carry out the plan. The plan in a sense consists of actions that are intended to achieve the goals and objectives identified by the stakeholders early in the planning process.

Step 8 is the creation or revision of the organizational vision. Strategic planning may lead to changes that affect the vision, and thus visioning is tied to each step of the strategic-planning process. In point of fact, the vision need not be fully determined early on but can be left to evolve during several cycles of this process.[15] The vision should grow out of an integration of past accomplishments and perceptions of the future. The vision also needs to provide inspiration to other stakeholders. However, the agency's mission tends to drive the strategic-planning process more than the vision does.[16]

Step 9 is the implementation of the plan. In prior steps, while developing the plan, the stakeholders need to define their roles in the implementation process. They also should try to ensure that accomplishments, even if small ones, will occur early in the process. Success tends to foster success, because the stakeholders will remain motivated and undiscouraged if they see progress. The stakeholders need to allocate the necessary resources before the implementation process begins. As changes are made, the agency and the other stakeholders need to adjust accordingly and monitor the effects of the changes over time.

Step 10 involves monitoring the implementation and making necessary midcourse corrections.

Each of the 10 steps of the Bryson model is related to one of the three core public health functions (assessment, policy development, and assurance).

The model is in fact compatible with the systems approach to public health leadership (Leadership Wheel) shown in Figure 7-3, and all of the activities in this approach, which is based on the core functions of public health, are included in the Bryson model. The relationships between the model and the organizational practices and essential services of public health are more cloudy. For example, visioning is not included in typical lists of such practices and services. Montgomery has noted that the strategic process should move beyond being a distinctive set of strategies and move to being a dynamic evolving process.[17] The dynamic approach to strategic planning should create an interactive model that ties changes in the community to changes and adaptations within the agency.

As regards strategic planning, public health leaders must:

- learn the benefits of such planning
- determine the readiness of the agency to undertake the strategic planning process
- perform a stakeholder analysis
- expand the strategic-planning process to include stakeholders in the community
- remain optimistic during the strategic-planning process as a means of motivating other participants
- do the necessary homework to prepare for each successive step of the strategic-planning process
- be realistic about what is possible
- perform an assessment of organizational capacity

Exercise 13-1 is intended to give students a chance to use or develop their strategic-planning skills. The task is to use strategic thinking in the planning of a community education program designed to inform the public of the advantages of empowerment and community coalitions. An additional perspective can be seen in Case Study 13-A, which explores the issues raised in border health disputes when strategic processes vary in two different countries.

---

## Case Study 13-A
## Health Issues at the United States–Cannico Republic Border

*Bailus Walker*

### Introduction
One of the tasks of public health is to ensure that services necessary to achieve agreed-upon goals are provided. The assurance function does not always entail the direct supervision of needed services but rather their identification and development, their coordination, and oversight of their accessibility and quality.

As the governmental presence in health, public health has the responsibility for ensuring (1) that every community is adequately served by an emergency health services system, by adequate hospitals with prenatal care, and by appropriate environmental health services and (2) that community residents are properly immunized and are provided with services designed to prevent the transmission of infectious diseases and the occurrence or progression of noninfectious diseases and dysfunction as well.

*(continues)*

**Case Study 13-A** *continued*

The assurance function today requires that state and local health agencies not only merge the pursuit of comprehensive health services with social and economic goals within state or local boundaries but also recognize the transboundary dimensions of public health challenges and opportunities. Massive amounts of goods, services, and capital and large numbers of people flow across international boundaries each day. At the same time, certain human activities continuously increase the risk of disease, dysfunction, and premature death as well as create unprecedented demands on the health services system.

For example, along the 2,000-mile border between the United States and Cannico, U.S. hospitals report that a third of the emergency admissions are Cannico nationals who cannot afford treatment or other personal health services. The health, social, and economic conditions in one border community raise critical issues for policy makers and health service specialists, administrators, and program managers dedicated to making sure their community is adequately served by a comprehensive public health service system.

### Bingo County

Bingo County is in the southwest section of the state of Pennsylcola. It is on the United States–Cannico border. Bingo City has been the county seat since 1871. The chief employment opportunity in the county is manufacturing. Farm production, timbering, tourism, and military installations are major sources of employment.

Bingo County, which is larger than Massachusetts and Rhode Island combined, covers 9,266 square miles, of which 25% are rural. The county includes a population estimated in a special 1990 census to be 1.2 million. Within the county are five incorporated cities: Bingo City (population 669,000), Randolph (101,000), Pickett (94,000), Thompson (78,000), and Edgar (67,000). There are 14 other incorporated towns of less size (with populations ranging from 2,000 to 20,000) and 163,000 people living in unincorporated areas of the county. In the 1990 census, 93.4% of the residents were considered urban.

According to the same census, 80.9% of the county's population was white, 14.6% Hispanic, 3.4% black, and 1.1% Native American.

Estimates furnished by the Pennsylcola Department of Economic Security in 1990 placed the median family income at approximately $12,100, with 15.8% of the population falling below the poverty line. Of the population over age 25, 49.7% had completed high school. In December 1990, 9.3% of the workforce was unemployed.

### Cannico

Within the last five years, the country of Cannico restructured its government, moving from a communist system toward democratization of all aspects of its society, including more liberal migration policies. In the process of this change, Cannico experienced severe social and economic problems. Prices rose and wages fell because the industries no longer received huge allotments of cash from the government for their payroll. Food shortages were pervasive and health services were described by some analysts as "substandard" by U.S. criteria.

There is very little information on demographics and health resources of Cannico because during the upheaval that led to the change in government many valuable records and databases were destroyed. What is clear is that the border with Bingo County has become a favored place of entry for Cannico nationals desiring to get into the United States. This development has been fueled by growth in Cannico's population and shifts in the country's economy.

### Bingo County Health Resources and Services

There are an estimated 900 primary physicians in Bingo County, and several health maintenance organizations (HMOs) serve the county. The state of Pennsylcola has eight programs for Medicaid enrollment, each with its own criteria for eligibility. There are 10 privately owned acute-care hospitals with a combined bed capacity of 3,228. Several of the hospitals in the area provide extensive outpatient services, drawing clientele from the entire region. Five hospitals are tertiary care centers.

The mission of the Bingo County Department of Public Health reads as follows: "To provide for the health care of the people and to protect and promote the health of all persons in the county in a professional and effective manner."

The Bingo County Department of Public Health provides a range of services, including disease control, sanitation, food inspection and licensure, screening, and health education. The department provides direct personal health services, including maternal and child health services; nutrition services, including a Women, Infants, and Children supplemental feeding program; and categorical programs to cope with alcohol and drug abuse. All of the varied activities of the agency are ultimately accountable to the Bingo County health officer, who has statutory responsibility for leadership of the department.

### The County Government

Bingo County operates under an executive-commission nonpartisan form of government. The executive is entrusted with broad powers and appoints most of the administrative officials and department heads, including the head of the local board of health and the county director of public health.

In the state of Pennsylcola, the local health department operates with decentralized authority in relation to the state department of health. The state's guidance and support are regarded as "moderate."

It is the view of the state policy makers that the Bingo County Department of Public Health has three responsibilities: (1) promotion of personal and community health, (2) maintenance of a healthful environment, and (3) prevention of disease and disability.

### Bingo County Department of Public Health Personnel and Services

In 1990, the Bingo County Department of Public Health had a staff of approximately 1,000 people who provided medical care, social services, environmental health services, and nursing, among other services. Of the 20.5 full-time equivalent (FTE) physician employees, 10 were full time. Three of these employees had administrative positions. The other 10.5 FTE physicians were part-time physicians engaged in private practice.

The majority of personal health services are delivered through the department's family primary health care program, which operates three health centers. These clinics provide the following services for all age groups:

- promotion and maintenance of health
- prevention of illness and disability
- basic care during acute and chronic phases of illness
- guidance and counseling of individuals and families
- referral to other health care providers and community resources

*(continues)*

**Case Study 13-A** *continued*

The department also provides dental services. The head of dental services for the Bingo County Department of Public Health, Dr. Bush, DDS, told the Centers for Disease Control and Prevention (CDC), "By definition our department is the provider of last resort in dental care."

Limited laboratory services are provided for water and food analysis and to support efforts in infection control.

Environmental health services include regulatory services in food sanitation, sanitary nuisances, water quality monitoring, housing and recreational sanitation (e.g., swimming pools and air pollution monitoring). The department also participates in land use planning, including the approval of community development (e.g., housing construction).

The department makes modest use of nurse practitioners; they are classified as public health nurse clinicians. Other personnel include family planning specialists, laboratorians, dentists, environmental health specialists, and veterinarians.

The Bingo County Department of Public Health employs approximately 15 community health services assistants. These workers are from disadvantaged backgrounds, lack formal education, and serve as patient advocates, helping consumers interact with other agencies (e.g., social services) and enroll in appropriate programs (e.g., food stamps).

Because the department has a number of categorical programs, staff members are generally employed by specific programs. This practice constrains, to some extent, staff mobility and departmental flexibility.

Encounter data for a number of the department's major activities are shown in Table 13-A-1.

The total budget for fiscal year 1989 was $26,652,351 (Exhibit 13-A-1). The budget is made up of 12 different state contributions or allocations (each representing separate state laws), federal grant programs, numerous fees, and different local actions. From the revenue of $21,283,954, Bingo budgeted a wide variety of services shown under public health control and regulatory programs.

**Other Economic Considerations**

The undocumented immigrant population (from Cannico) of Bingo County costs nearly $172 million a year in local government services.

**Table 13-A-1 Service Encounters (1989–1990)**

| Program | Number of Encounters |
| --- | --- |
| Communicable Disease | 52,172 |
| Immunizations | 10,966 |
| Venereal Disease | 15,229 |
| Chronic Disease | 2,000 |
| Multiphasic Screening | 1,109 |
| Well-Child Conference | 5,063 |
| Prenatal Classes Attended | 6,784 |
| Family Planning | 21,000 |
| Environmental Health Inspection | 19,000 |

**Exhibit 13-A-1 Bingo County Department of Public Health Budget**

| General Revenue Funds (State) | |
|---|---|
| General | $6,330,294 |
| AIDS Patient Care | 379,000 |
| School Health | 205,198 |
| Improved Pregnancy Outcome | 667,513 |

| Federal Funds | |
|---|---|
| Family Planning | $240,136 |
| Child Health | 33,610 |
| AIDS | 129,199 |
| Hypertension | 37,041 |
| Nutrition Program Administration | 250,000 |
| EPA Grants | 128,300 |
| Child Health Improvement Program | 50,000 |
| Sterilization | 11,337 |
| AIDS Testing and Counseling | 31,891 |

| Fees | |
|---|---|
| For Enforcement | $361,784 |
| Personal Fees | 87,280 |
| For Primary Medical Care | 623,475 |

| Other Sources | |
|---|---|
| Interest on Trust Fund | $100,000 |
| Primary Care | 3,000,000 |
| Sexually Transmitted Diseases | 198,675 |
| State Lab Revenue | 561,459 |
| Tuberculosis Control | 95,851 |
| Immunizations | 48,947 |
| Supplemental Food Supplies | 1,763,703 |
| Pharmacy | 452,929 |

| County Support | |
|---|---|
| General Appropriation | $5,611,055 |
| Fees | 1,618,556 |
| Building Rental | 1,595,148 |
| Maintenance of Buildings | 481,134 |
| School Board | 55,000 |
| County Air Pollution | 398,308 |
| County Toxic Substance Control | 83,102 |
| Epilepsy Foundation | 18,000 |
| Primary Care Grant | 716,898 |
| Headstart Dental Program | 1,700 |
| Sabal Palm (Private Grant) | 27,398 |
| Robert Wood Johnson (Grant) | 87,879 |
| Communications | 170,551 |
| Total | $26,652,351 |

| Expenditures | |
|---|---|
| Control and Regulatory Programs | |
| Immunizations | $536,163 |
| Sexually Transmitted Diseases | 353,082 |
| AIDS | 111,156 |
| Tuberculosis Control | 405,393 |
| Private Water Systems | 32,693 |
| Public Water Systems | 379,237 |
| Bottled Water | 26,154 |
| Swimming Pools | 307,313 |

*(continues)*

**Case Study 13-A** *continued*

**Exhibit 13-A-1   (continues)**

| | |
|---|---|
| Individual Sewage Disposal | 496,931 |
| Public Sewage System | 235,388 |
| Solid Waste Disposal | 170,003 |
| Water Pollution Control | 268,081 |
| Food Hygiene | 1,013,478 |
| Group Care Facilities | 379,237 |
| Migrant Labor Camps | 104,617 |
| Housing Safety and Sanitation | 130,771 |
| Mobile Home Parks | 32,693 |
| Occupational Health | 26,154 |
| Consumer Product Safety | 26,154 |
| Sanitary Nuisances | 241,927 |
| Air Pollution Control | 536,163 |
| Radiologic Health | 19,616 |
| Toxic Substances | 111,156 |
| Rabies Control | 13,077 |
| Arbovirus Surveillance | 13,077 |
| Emergency Medical Services | 13,077 |
| Vital Records | 268,081 |
| Personal Health Services | |
| Chronic Disease Services | $286,327 |
| Nutrition Services | 805,293 |
| Family Planning | 702,313 |
| Improved Pregnancy Outcome | 3,684,791 |
| School Health | 2,113,801 |
| Dental Health Services | 1,355,180 |
| Comprehensive Child Health | 2,765,493 |
| Comprehensive Adult Health | 3,032,187 |
| **Total** | **$21,283,954** |

A two-year study conducted by private consultants for the Pennsylcola state auditor general examined the impact of the city's 200,000 illegal immigrants on schools, law enforcement, health care, and social services. Some groups have criticized the report. They suggest that any discussion of the impact of immigrants must include the fact that this population provides a cheap, flexible labor pool that stimulates the creation of new businesses and helps preserve labor-intensive ones in Bingo County and the surrounding region.

The findings also indicate that HIV-related health care provided through the Pennsylcola Medicaid program costs about $2,800 per month per person. The data used to calculate this statistic were from a fixed period and included many persons who were still in the early stages of infection at the end of the data collection period.

Although in theory Cannico has a national health system, in fact there are major gaps in access and quality. Persons with a large income have access to private facilities and practitioners at home and abroad. The middle class, which includes government workers and residents of certain agricultural communities, generally have access only to government clinics and hospitals.

Utilization by Canniconians of health services in the United States takes place on the following levels. First, there are the wealthy, who pay in full or on a fee-for-service basis for their physician and hospital care. Second, there are those who seek care in the United States because of their desire to have a child who is a U.S. citizen, because they hope to find adequate services or because they are responding to an emergency. In urban areas of Cannico, the Health and Welfare Ministry maintains health clinics and hospitals often staffed by recent medical school graduates. Rural areas of Cannico are likely to be served only by a nurse. Hospital access for those who are poor and not covered by the Health and Welfare Ministry programs is often limited to civil hospitals, which are not well staffed or funded.

### Community Health Assessment

In November 1989, Frank Daly was appointed county executive. When the county health officer retired soon afterward, Daly appointed James Verdon Reed, MD, MPH, to fill the position. Concerned about the health problems of Bingo County, Dr. Reed asked the CDC to conduct a community health assessment.

This community health analysis provided indicators of how citizens, activities, and services on one side of the border relate to and influence those of the other side and ultimately both nations. The CDC report suggests that it is unlikely that any other bi-national border has such variety in health status and health care utilization. What follows are relevant findings of the CDC analysis.

### General

While most residents of Bingo are eligible for public assistance, relatively few physicians are willing to accept Medicaid payment and the tangle of paperwork that goes with it. People seeking Medicaid assistance in Bingo County also must go through a complicated set of procedures. The state of Pennsylcola has eight programs for Medicaid enrollment, each with its own eligibility criteria. An indigent, mentally disabled person must negotiate up to 13 different application procedures for federal and state benefits. Many of these programs, the CDC team reports, have periodic review procedures with provisions for termination of benefits for those who do not complete the necessary paperwork. It is not uncommon for persons who are functioning marginally and miss filing deadlines for review of their disability benefits to learn that their benefits have been terminated.

In the county, an estimated 13,000 women are eligible for Medicaid maternity benefits, but only 50 doctors are willing to treat them under the state aid program—a patient doctor ratio that CDC representatives call far too high.

In Bingo County, there are nine nonprofit community health centers, which charge fees based on the patients' ability to pay. The centers served approximately 8,000 patients in 1989, 44% of them children. But many more were turned away because of excessive patient loads. As many as 3,000 people, both from Bingo County and Cannico, are typically on waiting lists for the tight-budgeted health centers. In Bingo County, last winter, amid a heavy viral respiratory outbreak, there were waiting periods up to 36 hours for pediatric care.

The effects of the lack of care are various, according to the CDC report. Pregnant women who have received no prenatal care often suffer severe complications, and many babies are born underweight, contributing to the infant mortality rate of 19 per 1,000 live births (for the past three years) in Bingo County. A separate CDC study of five counties in Pennsylcola, including Bingo County, showed that the chance of a bad pregnancy outcome was 35% greater for women without health insurance, even when income, race, and other factors were controlled for.

*(continues)*

**Case Study 13-A** *continued*

A study prepared by the Bingo Chamber of Commerce reported that, in 1989, 19.9% of the city's residents had no insurance coverage, largely because their employers did not provide it and their wages were so low that they could not buy a policy. The results of the lack of insurance can be seen every day in hospitals along the Bingo-Cannico border where patients whose medical problems might have been prevented or easily treated in the early stages have waited until they have become acute.

The CDC reports that childbirth itself is an issue in Bingo County. Many pregnant Cannico women show up at hospital emergency departments in Bingo County at the last minute, so far along in labor that they cannot be turned away. The children they bear are American citizens eligible for immediate medical and nutritional aid as well as other long-term benefits.

According to the CDC analysis, the Lamplight Medical Center, a private hospital, receives the largest share of what is known as "disproportionate funds" from the state to help compensate for care given to patients from both sides of the United States–Cannico border.

In one lower socioeconomic section of Bingo County, there is only one pediatrician for a population of 170,000 people, and only six physicians in the area accept Medicaid. Of the 900 physicians in the county, only 20 have offices or clinics south of Burlington Highway, the line of demarcation between the poor and middle-class neighborhoods and the entry point for most Canniconians.

These health service problems are developing at a time when rapid population growth shifts have severely taxed the infrastructure of Bingo County. Lured by the possibility of jobs in the United States, hundreds of impoverished Canniconians from the interior of the country have made their way to the border neighborhoods near Bingo.

During the last several years, as the Cannico economy has weakened, the border population has ballooned from 36,000 to more than 500,000, and most of the growth has occurred in the last two years. Shantytowns, without sewers or running water, have become part of the border landscape.

*Cholera*
The CDC report indicates that the Pennsylcola-Cannico border is an ideal setting for an outbreak of cholera that has taken an estimated 5,000 lives in 14 states of Cannico. At least one cholera case has been confirmed recently in Bingo County. A woman contracted the disease from eating contaminated shrimp while on a trip to Borisville, the southernmost city of Cannico.

*Rubella*
From January through June 1989, an outbreak of rubella occurred among Bingo County residents. It was part of a widespread outbreak reported among lower socioeconomic groups in three states in Cannico and the state of Pennsylcola on the U.S. side.

The Bingo County Department of Public Health, in cooperation with the CDC, conducted an investigation to document cases of rubella among pregnant women in Bingo County.

The health department and the CDC identified 89 women from Bingo County and Cannico as having rubella-like illness during pregnancy. Vaccination histories were available for 25 of these women. One (from Bingo County) had a history of prior rubella vaccination. Of the 89 women, 18 (20%) had laboratory-confirmed acute rubella; 31 specimens were insufficient for analysis, and no specimens were obtained from the remaining 40.

Based on the findings for a five-month study period, the rate of congenital rubella infection was 83 per 1,000 live births in the lower socioeconomic groups of Bingo County. The CDC notes that the risk of congenital rubella syndrome is greatest when maternal infection occurs early in pregnancy. When infection occurs during the first trimester, congenital rubella syndrome occurs in up to 85% of births.

### Dengue Fever

Another problem on the Pennsylcola-Cannico border is dengue fever. Indigenous dengue transmission was documented in southern Cannico in the 1980s, where of 63 reported cases at least 27 cases were identified in patients who had traveled outside that country before the onset of the disease. In Bingo County, 10 cases were reported as imported cases. Persistent large-scale outbreaks of dengue fever in Cannico make this area more at risk, but a widespread outbreak could occur in the United States, because the *Aedes aegypti* mosquito is now in the Bingo County region and on the Pennsylcola-Cannico border. There is no eradication program at this time.

### Tuberculosis and AIDS

A review of 2,205 clinical charts for 1985–1989 at the four largest hospitals in Bingo County for patients who had *Mycobacterium* tuberculosis isolated from spinal fluid revealed that 455 patients (21%) also had an HIV infection. Of the 37 HIV-infected patients with tuberculosis meningitis for whom records were available, 24 (65%) had clinical radiological evidence of extrameningeal tuberculosis at the time of admission.

Local officials believe that in recent years men from Cannico have brought acquired immune deficiency syndrome (AIDS) to Bingo County. Doctors and epidemiologists report that official statistics on AIDS in Cannico describe only the tip of the phenomenon, which remains submerged in denial and social taboos.

The nurse in charge of AIDS treatment at a Cannico hospital, having carefully traced the sexual partners of her patients, concludes that a score of local people in Cannico are probably infected. Few of them wanted to be tested for the virus. National health officials in Cannico emphasize that, even when suspicious cases are added to those in which AIDS infection can be clearly traced to the victim's migration to Bingo County, the connection still accounts for only a small fraction of the 9,000 cases of the disease reported in Cannico.

Given the hundreds of Canniconians who cross legally and illegally into Bingo County each year, the number of those who come to Bingo County with AIDS and those who return to Cannico with AIDS appears to be small. But as the epidemic in Cannico has begun to level off among homosexual men and victims of a blood supply that was still poorly screened and badly contaminated less than five years ago, the spread of AIDS among migrants has become a growing concern on both sides of the border.

The concern is fueled by the difficult lives of undocumented workers from Cannico and the different sexual mores of two neighboring societies. While Cannico migration patterns have more women and families joining the flow of male job seekers, it is the archetypal lonely young men who are at highest risk. Almost everywhere these young men land, activities that put them at risk of infection tend to be more

*(continues)*

**Case Study 13-A** *continued*

available than affordable health care, AIDS prevention programs, or information in the Canniconian language. Moreover, sexually transmitted disease on the border has long been a problem, not only because of the cross-border use of red light districts but also because contact tracing is much more difficult.

*Measles*
During the past three years, measles cases and deaths have risen sharply in Bingo County. In 1989, more than 500 cases and 9 deaths were reported, the largest number of deaths in two decades. The epidemic intensified during 1990, with more than 700 cases and more than 11 deaths. The principal cause of the measles epidemic was failure to provide vaccine to children at the recommended age.

According to the CDC, many families in Bingo County have no ongoing relationship with a health care provider. The low immunization rate reflects, in part, inadequate access to health services. The CDC's analysis also showed that many opportunities to provide the needed vaccines were missed. Two types of missed opportunities were particularly noticeable in Bingo County: (1) a child brought to a center for immunization is not vaccinated because of inappropriate contraindications, such as minor illness, or only one of two vaccines is given when, in fact, others are also needed and should be given, and (2) a child in need of vaccination has contact with a health care provider for other reasons but his or her immunization status is not assessed and immunizations are not offered.

*Reproductive and Developmental Problems*
From 1986 to 1989, 102 women in Bingo County gave birth to babies without brains. The rate occurrence in the county of this rare congenital defect, known as anencephaly, is 10 times the national average. No cause has been identified, but some longtime residents of Bingo County suspect toxic emissions from factories above the border in Cannico. Other residents suspect the nuclear power plant accident that occurred inside Cannico several years ago.

On the Cannico side of the border, the infant mortality rate is significantly higher than in Bingo County and in the United States as a whole, although it is beginning to decline. In Cannico, the infant mortality rate has declined from an estimated 59 deaths per 1,000 live births during 1967–1971 to 47 during 1982–1987.

In Bingo County, the infant mortality rate for the period between 1982 and 1987 was 18 per 1,000 live births. Bronchitis and pneumonia, noninfectious gastroenteritis, and intestinal infection disease accounted for 220 deaths in the postneonatal period in Bingo County from 1982 to 1989.

*Chronic Disease*
In 1989, the overall mortality rate for coronary heart disease, stroke, lung cancer, cervical cancer, cirrhosis, and diabetes in Bingo County (age adjusted) was 75.8 per 100,000 population. Of the five risk factors examined—cigarette smoking, hypertension, obesity, alcohol consumption, and "never use Pap screening"—cigarette smoking made the largest contribution to deaths from the six diseases (30%). Examined one at a time, other risk factors also contributed to deaths from these diseases: obesity (25%), high cholesterol level (15 %), hypertension (15%), and diabetes (10%).

*Environmental Health*
Sanitation in Cannico (i.e., water supply, waste water disposal, and solid waste collection and disposal) is far below U.S. standards. There is no evidence of regulatory control of environmental quality—broadly defined—in Cannico. Daily, 12 million gallons of raw sewage flow into the Kopa River, which flows into the Bingo County

area from Cannico. Users of well water in the rural areas in Bingo County have noted increased contamination.

Air pollution in the Bingo–Cannico area has been a continuing problem, and discharges from the smelters on the Bingo side have been cited as a cause of high blood lead levels in both Cannico and Bingo County. More recently, Bingo County has exceeded the Environmental Protection Agency's ozone and carbon monoxide standards, largely because of older vehicular fleets in Cannico, the lack of emission controls, and the poor quality of gasoline used. Depending on wind speed and wind direction, air pollutants discharged in Cannico can add to the pollution load in Bingo County. Emissions in Bingo County may also affect atmospheric conditions in Cannico.

## Continuous Quality Improvement

Whereas strategic planning is a process that can be analyzed into a number of specific steps, CQI involves accepting a whole new philosophy of doing business or providing services. Public health organizations have been slow to adopt CQI methods, and where they have done so, they have not had great success.[18] Part of the explanation for the lack of success is that public health leaders have not kept up with the developments in the field of CQI. In studying public health clinics in California, Scutchfield and his colleagues found that less than 20% of the agencies performed CQI activities.[19] They also found that public health leaders were often unclear when it was appropriate to use specific tools.

Public health agencies have a reputation for providing mediocre service. One problem obstructing the improvement of service is that federal and state funding for new public health programs has been shrinking. Another is that government rules and regulations, as well as union rules, put obstacles in the way of delivering services in a timely fashion. A third problem is that public health leaders often misinterpret quality assurance as a type of CQI. *Improving* quality is more than an assurance issue, and it depends on viewing the public health consumer as entitled to the best that public health professionals have to offer. It requires, in other words, a whole change in philosophy.

The focus of CQI activities in a public health agency is on improving service provision and enhancing relationships with external stakeholders.[20] These activities are based on information about the public health issues to be addressed, the strengths and weaknesses of the public health agency, and stakeholder concerns.

To improve service provision, public health leaders need to utilize a systems perspective, promote a client orientation,[21] and engage in strategic thinking. Some public health leaders have found that they can integrate strategic-planning approaches and CQI, especially if one of the strategic goals of the agency is to improve the quality of service. Quality needs to be a personal issue as well as an agency or systems issue.[22] Each public health staff person has to be personally committed to high quality. A commitment to quality will improve performance. Having talent, knowledge, and skills to do public health's work will go nowhere without a personal commitment to do the best work possible with strong positive relationships with the public and with external stakeholders.

CQI is closely related to another management methodology called "total quality management" (TQM), and in fact the terms "continuous quality improvement" and "total quality management" are often used interchangeably.[23] They will be treated as synonymous here, and the term that appears in each instance below will be the term used by the particular author (or authors) under discussion.

TQM is based on the philosophy of total quality control, first promoted by Feigenbaum.[24] According to Sashkin and Kiser, TQM uses an evolving methodologic toolkit that includes all sorts of ways of measuring quality. The two main principles are that the focus of the organization must be on the customer and that everybody in the organization, not just the leadership, must be committed to quality. In their words, "TQM means that the organization's culture is defined by and supports the constant attainment of customer satisfaction through an integrated system of tools, techniques, and training. This involves the continuous improvement of organizational processes, resulting in high quality products and services."[25(p.39)]

## CQI Models

Five names are tied to the CQI movement: Shewhart, Deming, Crosby, Juran, and Feigenbaum. Shewhart demonstrated that statistical control is critical in CQI activities.[26] Deming, the best known of the CQI theorists, in the 1950s had to go to Japan to test his ideas about quality. To publicize his ideas, he devised a 14-point set of principles (Table 13-2).[27] The focus of these principles is on training the workforce and fostering a total commitment to quality. As Deming was aware, each customer wants high-quality products and services and evaluates the quality of products and services received. Deming also developed the planning, doing, checking, acting cycle.[28]

Crosby argued that the only way to improve quality is to demand zero defects and refuse to accept anything less.[29] After all, customers define quality, and, in the business world, dissatisfied consumers will stop buying defective products. The public health customer, however, has limited service choices and will grudgingly accept less than the best, so it is up to public health leaders to empower their communities and make sure that high-quality standards are maintained. Public health leaders also need to gain support for the CQI approach from both internal and external stakeholders and must be prepared to cope with resistance.

CQI requires total commitment and involvement.[30] Crosby outlined a 14-step process for implementing TQM in organizations.[31,32] The process starts with a commitment by the leadership to the pursuit of quality and all that this entails. Most of the steps involve the core functions of policy development and assurance. There is only one step in which assessment plays the major role.

The Crosby model applies to intraorganizational change, whereas the kind of assessment public health agencies must perform encompasses both internal operations and community needs. The focus on intraorganizational change is a characteristic of the Deming model as well (Table 13-2). Note, however, that, in the case of a public health agency, an assessment of community needs provides critical data for determining what intraorganizational changes are required and for integrating complex systems of health care in order to provide high-quality programming.

**Table 13-2    Deming's 14 Points**

1. Create constancy of purpose toward improvement of product and service with the aim to become competitive and to stay in business and to provide jobs.

2. Adopt the new philosophy. We are in a new economic age. Western management must awaken to the challenge, must learn their responsibilities, and take on leadership for change.

3. Cease dependence on inspection to achieve quality. Eliminate the need for inspection on a mass basis by building quality into the product or service in the first place.

4. End the practice of awarding business on the basis of price tag. Instead, minimize total costs. Move toward a single supplier for any one item on a long-term relationship of loyalty and trust.

5. Improve constantly and forever the system of production and service to improve quality and productivity and thus decrease costs.

6. Institute training on the job.

7. Institute leadership. The aim of leadership should be to help people and machines and gadgets to do a better job. Leadership of management is in need of overhaul as well as leadership of production workers.

8. Drive out fear so that everyone may work effectively for the company.

9. Break down barriers between departments. People in research, design, sales, and production must work as a team to foresee problems of production and use that may be encountered with the product or service.

10. Eliminate slogans, exhortations, and targets for the workforce asking for zero defects and new levels of production.

11. Eliminate work standards (quotas) in the organization. Eliminate management by objectives. Eliminate management by numbers, numeric goals. Substitute leadership.

12. Remove barriers that rob the hourly worker of rights to pride of workmanship. The responsibility of supervisors must be changed from sheer numbers to quality. Remove barriers that rob people in management and engineering of their right to pride of workmanship. Abolish annual or merit rating and management by objective M.B.O.

13. Institute a vigorous program of education and self-improvement.

14. Put everybody to work to accomplish the transformation.

*Source:* Reprinted from *Out of the Crisis* by W. Edwards Deming. Copyright 1986 by the W. Edwards Deming Institute.

The fourth theoretician in the quality revolution is Joseph M. Juran. Juran pointed out that quality does not occur by chance.[33] It requires a planned process that encompasses planning, quality control, and quality improvement (known as the Juran trilogy). Juran also believed that leaders need to organize information for the purpose of monitoring the process. Finally, Feigenbaum held that quality is involved in every activity of an organization, from direct service activities to marketing and finance, and that an organization must determine the cost of quality improvement programs before embarking on them.[34]

Building on the work of the founders of the TQM approach, Creech identified what he called the five pillars of TQM: product (service), process, organization, leadership, and commitment.[35] According to Creech, TQM has been more effective in Japan than in the United States because Japanese businesses seem to accept the concept of quality more readily than American businesses do. Creech has further pointed out that TQM is an organizational philosophy and cannot deliver full benefits without complete organizational acceptance. In order to put the five pillars into perspective, Creech formulated 16 guidelines for the TQM process (Table 13-3).

Figure 13-2 shows that organization is the central pillar of the five. How the organization is perceived and what its cultural orientation is will have an impact on the implementation and consequences of TQM. Also, whereas centralization has been the traditional management approach, decentralization appears to be better suited to TQM. Consequently, multidisciplinary teams play an important role. As Figure 13-2 shows, one of the pillars is leadership.

**Table 13-3   Creech Guidelines for Five-Pillars TQM**

1. Build your TQM approach, and its principles, on five system pillars.
2. Firmly establish the character and culture of your organization.
3. Use a decentralized, interactive system that integrates all levels.
4. Organization is the central pillar—it influences everything else.
5. Base the structural building blocks on small teams and not big functions.
6. Orient employees' focus and activity to their product, not their job.
7. Place the prime leadership focus on the outputs, not the inputs.
8. Keep score, assess, and provide timely feedback to one and all.
9. Know your marketplace inside out and create strong customer linkage.
10. Provide a climate of quality that promotes pride and professionalism.
11. Base any and all decisions on the inseparability of cost and value.
12. Provide detailed, focused training to employees at every level.
13. Give high priority and pay great attention to the communication flow.
14. Work unceasingly to instill common purpose from the bottom to the top.
15. Build the commitment through genuine ownership and shared success.
16. Build your TQM on all five pillars.

*Source:* From *The Five Pillars of TQM* by Bill Creech. Copyright © 1994 by W. L. Creech. Used by permission of Dutton, a division of Penguin Putnam Inc.

**FIGURE 13-2   TQM: The Need, the Issues, the Shape It Must Take**
*Source:* From *The Five Pillars of TQM* by Bill Creech, copyright © 1994 by W. L. Creech. Used by permission of Dutton, a division of Penguin Putnam Inc.

As indicated by the comment about decentralization, the leaders of the organization must be willing to share their power.

Organizational commitment to quality needs to occur at the border between the organization and its environment. If the frontline workers do not buy the quality message, TQM will be doomed to failure. In fact, everyone in the organization needs to make a commitment to quality.

### The CQI Toolkit

CQI makes use of a number of tools, including various kinds of charts and diagrams. Traditional tools include:

- control charts (for showing the results of statistical process activities)
- Pareto charts (for graphically showing defects or problems over time)
- fishbone diagrams (for tracing cause-and-effect relationships)
- run charts (for displaying trends over time)
- histograms (for showing service patterns at given time periods)
- scatter diagrams (for showing relationships between two factors)
- flowcharts (for showing input-output relationships)[36]

Seven new tools of use in CQI are shown in Figure 13-3 and described below.[37] The first is the affinity diagram, which allows a team to organize ideas and problems into general categories. The team would first sort the items into categories, then list the items in each category in a separate column. Affinity diagrams could be used for clarifying values; for constructing the organization's vision, the mission, and the goals and objectives; and for action and strategic planning. The affinity diagram process, like any group process, is affected by how well the team members get along.

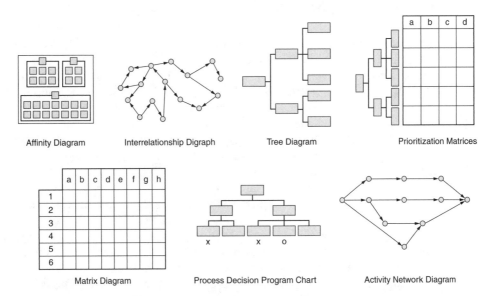

**FIGURE 13-3   Seven Management and Planning Tools**
*Source:* Reprinted with permission from M. Brassard, *The Memory Jogger,* © 1989, Goal and QPC.

The interrelationship digraph shows the interconnection between ideas, problems, actions, or other types of items. The arrows between the items show the direction of their relationship (e.g., cause to effect). Once a digraph is developed, it can be reworked to show new ways to relate the items. The team will want to simplify the digraph by looking for converging or diverging clusters of arrows. Constructing a digraph is especially useful for deciding on goals and objectives and during the action planning phase.

The third tool, the tree diagram, can be used in many leadership activities. For instance, a tree diagram could be used by the leadership team of a public health agency to map out how the agency's mission is to be fulfilled. The team might start by stating the mission, which, say, is to promote the health of the public and prevent disease. The next step would be to determine the goals and objectives needed to fulfill this mission, and the third step would be to decide on the tasks that must be performed to achieve the chosen goals and objectives. In CQI, the leadership team might use tree diagrams in developing quality improvement plans. In general, the process of creating a tree diagram begins with stating an overall goal (e.g., the agency's mission or an important subsidiary goal) and then breaking the process of achieving the goal into individual steps or tasks.

Prioritization matrices allow the leadership team to prioritize tasks, service activities, community activities, and so on. A prioritization matrix can be used in conjunction with a tree diagram to rank the tasks and responsibilities identified during the tree diagram process. If six activities are projected, the diagram allows the team to see what will happen if any two activities occur together. The team is able to calculate a score for each cell, and where the score falls in relation to the other scores determines the degree of importance of the conjunction of activities.

Brassard suggested that the prioritization process should encompass three steps.[38] The first step is to list and then rank the criteria that will be used in prioritizing the items (e.g., activities). Such criteria might include the speed of possible implementation, the likely degree of acceptance by staff, the impact on other parts of the agency, the cost, and the technology needed. Once the criteria are chosen, each should be assigned a percentage that reflects its perceived importance (the total of percentages should of course equal 100%). In step 2, each item is given a score in relation to each criterion. Finally, the total scores for all the items are calculated, and the results determine the priority ranking of the items.

The fifth tool is the matrix diagram, which allows the leadership team to compare two or more sets of items and explore the strength of the relationship between them.

Process decision program charts allow the leadership team to show probable events and contingencies that might occur as the action plan is implemented. For example, suppose the public health agency director wants to plan how the community will perform health assessment activities. The director might create a chart that shows how the community advisory board is to be selected, when the various activities will occur and how much time they will take, and how they will be carried out. Process decision program charts, like the other tools described here, can also be used to explore options.

The last tool, the activity network diagram, exhibits the schedule for the completion of tasks. This tool is also known as an arrow diagram. Exercise

13-2 provides an opportunity to practice applying the seven CQI tools just described.

CQI requires a total commitment by public health leaders and all their constituencies if it is to be successful. The professional staff of the public health agency must buy into the total quality approach. In order to get staff to do this, public health leaders must:

- develop a commitment to quality and best practices
- incorporate CQI into a systems framework
- become educated about CQI
- master the seven CQI tools
- educate the public about CQI
- inspire staff and others to see the value of the CQI approach
- train the public health workforce
- integrate strategic-planning techniques and CQI techniques

## Six Sigma

Many businesses interested in quality improvement methodologies have explored the new techniques of Six Sigma, which was developed and trademarked by Motorola. Six Sigma involves continuous process improvement methods that are oriented to improving the work processes of an organization to near perfect.[39] The issue of variation and monitoring the effects of variation are part of the methodology. The issue of variation is also applied to not only what goes on inside the organization but to the variance issues associated with customers outside the organization. The overall goal of Six Sigma is to cut the variation as much as possible. Data drive the process in that managers and leaders will use the data to make better decisions. Five stages define the process, which has the acronym DMAIC:[40]

1. Define the problem.
2. Measure defects in the process.
3. Analyze data to determine causes of problems.
4. Improve work processes to remove the causes of problems.
5. Control events so that the causes of problems do not recur.

A leadership dimension is part of Six Sigma, which involves training.[41] There is a Black Belt training for project managers that takes several weeks. Master Black Belts are generally leaders who are responsible for the training and coaching of others. Green Belts are people who are trained for specific roles in the process and also carry on other roles in the organization. Yellow Belts are individuals involved in the process but who did not go through specific training.[42] Other partners include the Executive Sponsor, who makes sure that the process is followed.[43] This person does not run the Six Sigma protocols but supports the activities related to the process. This may be the head of the organization. There will also be Department or Project Champions.

There have been many variations to the Six Sigma approach. Tools from inductive statistics, systems tools, CQI tools, and many other techniques have been adapted for use in Six Sigma. Although many of these tools are also used in public health, the application of Six Sigma methodology to public health has been limited. The development of the National Public Health Performance Standards, which utilize both a systems and a CQI approach, does begin to look at the way public health professionals work to carry out the essential public health services. The impact of performance improvement has yet to be tied to health outcomes.

Jacquescoley believes that Six Sigma may provide useful tools and methods to public health.[44] The Six Sigma framework does explore the impact of defects or program limitations on the process, operation, and practice of public health work. The definition of defects in public health is less clear. Are these defects specific health issues or lack of understanding of how to address these issues that are the relevant factors? How to transfer the idea of process in a business to process in the human services arena is a major challenge to the use of Six Sigma approaches. As leaders, we look at all possible methods and tools to better improve the way we work in public health.

## Re-engineering

Sometimes an organization cannot be fixed in its present form. If this is the case, the organization must be restructured so that it can make use of new approaches to problem solving and decision making. The restructuring of an organization is often referred to as re-engineering. Manganelli and Klein defined re-engineering as "the rapid and radical redesign of strategic, value-added business processes—and the systems, policies, and organizational structures that support them—to optimize the work flows and productivity in an organization."[45(pp.7-8)]

Imagine that a public health agency wants to incorporate bioterrorism interventions into the range of services it is capable of providing. If no new funding is currently available for the project, the agency leadership will look for methods to reorganize the agency and reassign staff to carry out the project. The leaders might not only phase out programs of less relevance but also re-educate the staff to work in different organizational units. This is not as easy a task as it might seem. Barriers to public health re-engineering include objections to the changes by a public employee union or by the board of health.

As Drucker pointed out, knowledge-intensive organizations require continual re-engineering.[46] Therefore, because the 21st century, like the 20th, will undoubtedly be a century of technological advances and new public health concerns, public health agencies will have to redefine and re-engineer themselves on an ongoing basis. Public health leaders will play an essential role in re-engineering projects, for, as pointed out repeatedly, they define their organization's vision and motivate others to share the vision.

To get stakeholders, including governing board members, involved in and committed to re-engineering, leaders must win their trust. Staff members are often wedded to the status quo and will have to be reassured that they will not lose their jobs as a result of the reorganization.[47] Another way to build trust is to include people from all parts of the organization on the re-engineering team. In the case of a local health department, the leaders might recruit community leaders and members of the local board of health to be on the team.

Several additional guidelines should be kept in mind when considering embarking on a re-engineering project. First, the leaders of an agency need to determine the agency's mission and how the re-engineering will increase its chances of fulfilling its mission.[48] If a local public health department is committed to the promotion of health but its activities are hindered by a cumbersome bureaucracy, it should explore re-engineering. Again, unless the legislature, city council, and board of health buy into the process, it will likely be unsuccessful.

Second, the leaders must recognize that the re-engineering process changes the culture as well as the job responsibilities of the staff. Third, they will need to develop new measures to evaluate staff performance and monitor the change process. Fourth, they should mobilize the staff for change and provide staff members with the tools they will need to carry out their re-engineering responsibilities. Fifth, they should define the goals and objectives of re-engineering. Sixth, they should ensure that communication channels exist between all those involved in the re-engineering process.

The leaders who are best qualified to oversee re-engineering projects tend to have a process orientation and a holistic perspective (Table 13-4) and to be comfortable with strategic thinking.[49] They are also creative, find the status quo boring, tend to be enthusiastic and able to motivate others, are persistent and tactful, and are excellent communicators who support teamwork and good interpersonal relations. In reviewing the best practices of organizations that underwent re-engineering, Carr and Johansson searched for the lessons to be learned.[50] The rules they discovered are listed in Table 13-5.

Manganelli and Klein presented a five-stage model for rapid re-engineering (Figure 13-4).[51] In the first stage, the leaders recognize there is a need for organizational change, foster a consensus among staff that such a need exists, clarify the mission of the organization, select and train a re-engineering team, and develop a plan to guide the re-engineering process (action plan).

### Table 13-4   Characteristics of a Re-engineering Leader

1. A process-oriented and holistic cognitive style: a facility for seeing the big picture, for distinguishing trees from forests, for understanding how tasks fit together to form a process and how process designs and organizational designs fit together to form a business.

2. Design skills: the facility both to envision a new way of doing things and then to flesh it out, turning it from a concept into something that can actually be implemented.

3. An inclination toward change that borders on restlessness: a congenital inability to accept things as they are, and a determination to find what lies over the rainbow.

4. Enthusiasm and optimism: the internal fortitude to keep going despite the slings and arrows of outraged constituencies and despite the fact that it often seems as though the light at the end of the tunnel is an oncoming train.

5. Persistence and tact: the ability to keep pushing despite the fact that people are pushing back at you and eventually to wear them down and convert them to your point of view.

6. Interpersonal, teamwork, and communication skills: the ability to work as part of a tightly woven team; the patience to listen to the needs, fears, and concerns of everyone who will be affected by reengineering; and the talent to craft messages that will induce them to accept unpalatable truths and their consequences.

*Source:* From *The Reengineering Revolution* by Michael Hammer p. 58. Copyright © 1995 by Hammer and Company. Reprinted with permission of HarperCollins Publishers, Inc.

**Table 13-5   Re-engineering Principles**

1. Recognize and articulate an "extremely compelling" need to change.
2. Start with and maintain executive-level support.
3. Understand the organization's "readiness to change."
4. Communicate effectively to create buy-in. Then communicate more.
5. Instill in the organization a "readiness and commitment" to sustained change.
6. Stay actively involved.
7. Create top-notch teams.
8. Use a structure framework.
9. Use consultants effectively.
10. Pay attention to what has worked.
11. Link goals to corporate strategy.
12. Listen to the "voice of the customer."
13. Select the right processes for re-engineering.
14. Maintain focus: don't try to reengineer too many processes.
15. Create an explicit vision of each process to be re-engineered.
16. Maintain teams as the key vehicle for change.
17. Quickly come to an as-is understanding of the processes to be re-engineered.
18. Choose and use the right metrics.
19. Create an environment conducive to creativity and innovation.
20. Take advantage of modeling and simulation tools.
21. Understand the risks and develop contingency plans.
22. Have plans for continuous improvement.
23. Align the infrastructure.
24. Position IT as an enabler, even if the extent of the IT change necessary is great.

*Source:* Reprinted with permission from D. K. Carr and H. J, Johansson, *Best Practices in Reengineering*, pp. 209–210. © 1995, McGraw Hill, Inc.

In stage 2, the leaders create a consumer-focused model for the organization, determine who the stakeholders are, and involve them in the re-engineering process. In stage 3, the leaders develop a realistic vision based on current process performance activities and on projections of where the organization is headed. In stage 4, a re-engineering plan tied to the vision is developed. Technical design issues are addressed in the first part (stage 4A), and social design issues are addressed in the second (stage 4B). Finally, the implementation of the new organizational model occurs during stage 5.

Public health leaders must be committed to restructuring the agency if substantial changes are necessary for it to carry out its mission. They must, therefore:

- learn to distinguish re-engineering, strategic planning, continuous quality improvement, and Six Sigma methodologies
- master new approaches to organizational improvement
- improve relationships with key stakeholders
- work closely with the re-engineering team
- master the five-stage rapid re-engineering model

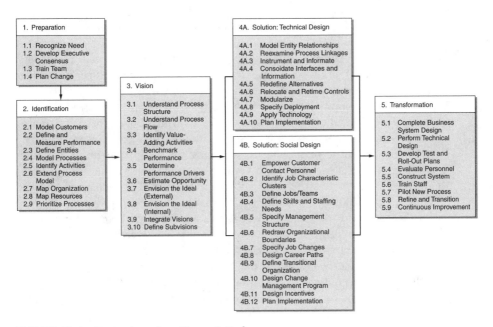

**FIGURE 13-4    Re-engineering: Stages & Tasks**
*Source:* Reprinted from *The Reengineering Handbook.* Copyright © 1994 Raymond L.
Manganelli et al. Reprinted by permission of AMACOM, a division of American
Management Association International, New York, NY. All rights reserved.
http://www.amanet.org.

## Reinventing Government

Since the 1990s, we have seen an increase in public discussions about the
structure and function of government. Some have argued that the old ways of
governing do not work any longer[52] and that the public sector must keep open
the option of employing entrepreneurial techniques from the business sector.
"Reinvention" is the term used to describe the use of entrepreneurial techniques by those in the public sector. Osborne and Plastrik defined reinvention
as "the fundamental transformation of public systems and organizations to
create dramatic increases in their effectiveness, efficiency, adaptability, and
capacity to innovate. This transformation is accomplished by changing their
purpose, incentives, accountability, power structure, and culture."[53(pp.13–14)]

Reinvention of government became more common during the 1990s and
was seen as less radical than originally believed.[54] Reinventing government
involves strategies such as tying rewards to performance, listening to and
being accountable to community consumers, making organizations less hierarchical and more decentralized, and empowering staff to make decisions and
influence work processes. Discussions on reinventing government have been
quieter since the terrorist events of September 11, 2001.

For reinvention to work, it needs to be seen as more than a patching operation. It must involve a significant restructuring of organizations, a re-
thinking of the activities and mission of the organization, and an
abandonment of old models that no longer work. Also necessary is the refor-
mation of the relationship between government entities and community-

based organizations.[55] For one thing, bureaucracy seems to get in the way of reinvention activities.

As for reinvention in the public health arena, we have seen this happen since September 11, 2001, where the preparedness model has been superimposed on public health's core functions and essential public health services paradigm. This new orientation with many new community partners has led to the development of innovative programs capable of being funded. Funding itself is an issue that may motivate reinvention efforts. The decrease in money available for local public health agencies for nonpreparedness activities means that the agencies have to become more efficient. Public health agencies also seem to be struggling with their identity. The general public and many public health professionals think that public health programs are only for the poor, and traditional public health activities are being taken over by the private managed care sector or community health center sector.

Other traditional public health activities are being transferred to other types of agencies. For example, most maternal and child health programs in Indiana have been outsourced through grants and contracts to local hospitals and agencies and out of local health departments. Despite these types of happenings, public health leaders seem reticent to lobby for the public health agenda.

Public health leaders must act as advocates for public health in the debate over the appropriate roles for government agencies. They have the responsibility to ensure that public health is practiced in schools, managed care organizations, community health centers, and other venues in the public and private sectors. The real goal of public health reinvention should be to create in each community an integrated health care system that increases access to health-related services so that no one is prevented from getting needed services.

> **Leadership Tips**
>
> *Live your values.*

According to Bacon, reinvention of government should encompass capacity building, workforce training, performance monitoring, and public and private collaboration.[56] Table 13-6 contains lists of recommended ingredients for reinvented government culled from three sources (the fourth list is a synthesis of the other three lists).

During the early 1990s, Vice President Gore headed a national performance review whose mission was to find out how to make government agencies more effective and less expensive. Every office and agency of the federal government was examined. Table 13-7 presents the principles that guided the review.[57] The goals were to cut spending while serving customers better and empowering employees and communities. The means to achieve these goals, listed in the second part of the table, included creating a clear sense of mission, delegating authority and responsibility, replacing regulations with incentives, and fostering competition. Although performance reviews still occur, they have played a much more minor role in recent years.

Local public health departments, too, need to be creative in their utilization of resources. For example, some local agencies, required to perform state nursing home inspections, have been burdened with additional responsibilities. A reinvention process could address the drain on resources caused by inspections through innovative techniques and collaboration among agencies.

**Table 13-6    Recommended Ingredients for More Effective and Efficient Government**

| Osborne/Gaebler* | NCSLPS† | Thompson‡ | Synthesis |
|---|---|---|---|
| Catalytic | Strong executive leadership | Leadership | Capacity building |
| Community-owned | Lean, responsive | Productive workforce | High performance |
| Competitive | High-performance workforce | Information management | Leadership |
| Mission-driven | Citizen involvement | Public/private networks | Public/private cooperation |
| Results-oriented | Fiscal stability | Fiscal reform | Fiscal stability |
| Enterprising | | | |
| Anticipatory | | | |
| Decentralized | | | |
| Market-oriented | | | |

*Source:* Data from
*D. Osborne and T. Gaebler, *Reinventing Government: How the Entrepreneurial Spirit Is Transforming the Public Sector* (Reading, MA: Addison-Wesley, 1992).
†The National Commission on the State and Local Public Service, *Hard Truths/Tough Choices: An Agenda for State and Local Reform* (Albany, NY: Nelson A. Rockefeller Institute of Government, 1993).
‡F. J. Thompson, ed., *Revitalizing State and Local Public Service: Strengthening Performance, Accountability and Citizen Confidence* (San Francisco: Jossey-Bass, 1993).

**Table 13-7    Principles of the National Performance Review**

We will invent a government that puts people first, by:
• Cutting unnecessary spending.
• Serving its customers.
• Empowering its employees.
• Helping communities solve their own problems.
• Fostering excellence.

Here's how. We will:
• Create a clear sense of mission.
• Steer more, row less.
• Delegate authority and responsibility.
• Replace regulations with incentives.
• Develop budgets based on outcomes.
• Expose federal operations to competition.
• Search for market, not administrative, solutions.
• Measure our success by customer satisfaction.

*Source:* Reprinted from A. Gore, *The Report of the National Performance Review*, 1993, Government Printing Office.

Reinvention should not be confused with internal reform or downsizing.[58] Its goal is change in the social and organizational fabric of a community, and its methods are entrepreneurial and self-renewing. Osborne and Plastrik likened the changes brought about by reinvention to changes in the DNA of government. They suggested there were five key strategies to reinventing government, the five C's, as they called them: the core strategy, the consequences strategy, the customer strategy, the control strategy, and the culture strategy (Table 13-8).[59] Note that a cookbook approach to reinvention is not really possible because each community and each government agency is different.

**Table 13-8    The Five C's: Changing Government's DNA**

| Lever | Strategy | Approaches |
|---|---|---|
| Purpose | Core strategy | Clarity of purpose<br>Clarity of role<br>Clarity of direction |
| Incentives | Consequences strategy | Managed competition<br>Enterprise management<br>Performance management |
| Accountability | Customer strategy | Customer choice<br>Competitive choice<br>Customer quality assurance |
| Power | Control strategy | Organizational empowerment<br>Employee empowerment<br>Community empowerment |
| Culture | Culture strategy | Breaking habits<br>Touching hearts<br>Winning minds |

*Source:* From "Banishing Bureaucracy: The Five Strategies for Reinventing Government" by David Osborne and Peter Plastrik. Reprinted by permission.

It is increasingly clear that traditional concepts of community are no longer relevant. As a consequence, community must be reinvented. In any actual community, community values must be clarified and redefined, key community stakeholders must be identified and empowered, and social structures and organizations that are consistent with the new values must be put into place. Once a community knows its values and its assets, it can tackle its problems, and thus a community assessment directed toward documenting community assets is another essential element of the reinvention process.

Public health agencies are not the only organizations that will address the public health needs of the community. Community reinvention should include creation of a partnership among all health care and public health stakeholders–a partnership in which all players are equal. In addition, the partners must work with other community stakeholders to ensure that public health needs are met. Thus, reinvention demands strategy and communication at many levels if it is to work.

Reinvention calls for new concepts of leadership. First, leadership must be shared among members of community teams. Second, community stakeholders must be empowered. With empowerment, people become free to influence their own future. Yet, for empowerment to occur, people need to be informed about their options and be provided with the skills needed to exercise these options. In particular, community stakeholders need to be educated about public health and have their leadership skills developed through continuous learning opportunities.

There is more to reinventing community and government than meets the eye. Reinvention provides an opportunity to make constructive changes. The danger is that it can be used to justify funding cuts and downsizing rather than as a means of strengthening the community and the public health system. Strategic planning and CQI methods can be combined with reinvention techniques as a way of improving the reinvention process and increasing the chance of success. In a sense, reinvention is a form of strategy, because it involves major medium- and long-term changes in the structure of the community for the improvement of community life.

Public health leaders must:

- be prepared to move from a traditional hierarchical organizational structure to an entrepreneurial one (which may still be hierarchical in form)
- use public funds and grants in new ways that increase productivity and efficiency
- create coalitions that support change
- understand the realities of the information age and how they can affect organizational change
- utilize reinvention techniques not only for organizational change but for system change as well
- see reinvention as necessary at the local, state, and federal levels
- empower staff and community partners to share leadership and responsibility for changes that occur
- practice the five C's strategy

## Public-Private Partnerships

A public health agency, although it must lead the way, cannot carry out all the public health activities needed to protect and improve the health of a community. Consequently, it must foster new types of alliances and partnerships, including joint ventures, research sharing, community-based projects and programs, and semi-structured alliances.[60] For example, a local public health agency might contract with a local federally qualified health center to provide childhood immunizations at a price that the local health department cannot match—an interesting example of what the business community calls outsourcing.

Because trust is a critical component of any partnership, the public health agency must know both its agenda and the agendas of its partners, whether from the public or private sector. Possible partners include businesses, hospitals and managed care organizations, community health centers, private health care providers, local community organizations, local community clubs, churches and synagogues, schools, and police and firefighter groups, among others.

A local health leader told the author that a good way to involve the private sector in public health is for public health leaders to become involved in local organizations, such as the Kiwanis or the local chamber of commerce, which will create opportunities for them to network with other leaders on community issues. Public health leaders need to become known in the community if they are to gain credibility. Their goal should be to create an integrated system of care that will provide every resident of the community with the care they need and at the same time promote a healthy lifestyle among the residents in order to prevent disease.

Public health leaders must:

- develop public and private relationships to improve the local community public health system
- share power and responsibility with other community members who have an interest in improving the community's health
- become involved in the activities of the community
- join local community groups and organizations
- act to gain the trust of the community

## Summary

The needs of the public are constantly changing, and public health agencies need to respond to the changes. The first step in responding adequately is to develop a plan of action, which is the subject of this chapter.

Leaders learn that creating a vision is not enough; the vision will remain just that without a strategy for making it a reality. Strategic planning, CQI, Six Sigma, re-engineering, and reinventing government are all useful, individually or jointly, for turning a vision into programs and services. For example, the tools of CQI can be used to monitor the strategic-planning process, and the CQI goal of improved customer service could be a guiding principle. Also, since the methods overlap, public health leaders can create a customized planning methodology that includes pieces from all of them.

Public and private alliances and partnerships are needed at the planning stage as well as at the implementation stage. Developing and maintaining collaborative relationships require leadership skills, and public health leaders must master these skills and the planning skills necessary to formulate strategies for improving the community's health.

## Discussion Questions

1. What is strategic planning?
2. What is the relationship between strategies and tactics?
3. What is the relationship between strategies and goals?
4. What roles do an organization's mission and vision play in strategic planning?
5. What are the five pillars of TQM?
6. What is Six Sigma, and can it be utilized in public health?
7. What steps are necessary for implementing a CQI process in a local health agency?
8. What are some of the tools used in TQM?
9. What distinguishes re-engineering from other forms of organizational reform?
10. What are the principles of reinventing government?
11. What are some ways to open the door to public-private partnerships?

### Exercise 13-1:   Training Course Development

*Purpose:* to use strategic thinking in developing a community education program and in creating a conducive environment for putting together a public health coalition

*Key concepts:* coalition building, community education plan, empowerment, leadership style, strategic thinking

*Procedure:* As a homework assignment, each student is given the task of devising a 10-step plan for implementing a community education program. The student is to imagine that he or she has been hired as a consultant by the Burchfield County Health Department. The health department has struggled unsuccessfully to create a coalition to promote public health in the county, which has few residents but many health-related problems. The head of the department, Dr. Hanson, has hired the consultant to devise a 10-step plan for implementing a program intended to educate the public on the advantages of community coalitions and empowerment.

All the students bring in the homework assignment on a designated day. The class is divided into groups of 8 to 10 members. One group member is assigned the role of the consultant; another, the role of Dr. Hanson, director of the county health department; a third, the role of Professor Alexander, a faculty member at the local university who has applied for a grant to train county residents in the techniques of empowerment; and a fourth, the role of Dr. Cassidy, prospective head of a wellness institute with a strong community education component that Western Health Alliance, an HMO servicing the county, plans to locate in the county. Dr. Hanson invites the consultant, Professor Alexander, and Dr. Cassidy to a 30-minute staff meeting to present and defend the community education plan the consultant has developed. The students playing Dr. Hanson, Professor Alexander, and Dr. Cassidy, since they have all created their own 10-step plans, should be able to offer insightful criticisms of the consultant's plan or make helpful recommendations to improve it. Following the review of the plan, the group should then discuss strategic thinking and its role in devising the plan.

### Exercise 13-2:   Planning Tools in Action

*Purpose:* to explore ways to combine strategic planning tools and continuous quality improvement tools

*Key concepts:* activity network diagram, affinity diagram, continuous quality improvement, interrelationship diagraph, matrix diagram, prioritization matrix, process decision, progress chart, strategic planning, tree diagram

*Procedure:* Each team should re-examine the community action plan developed in Exercise 10-1, identifying areas where one or more of the seven planning tools discussed in this chapter could be used to enhance the plan and its acceptance by the community. Discuss the relative advantages and disadvantages of using each planning tool in the creation of the plan. After 30 minutes of discussion, each team should reach consensus on the specific tools to be used in improving the plan and on how these tools are to be applied. A representative from each team should present the rationale and conclusions reached to the full class.

## References

1. B. J. Turnock, *Public Health: What It Is and How It Works*, 4th ed. (Sudbury, MA: Jones and Bartlett, 2008).
2. J. M. Bryson and B. C. Crosby, *Leadership for the Common Good* (San Francisco: Jossey-Bass, 1992).
3. G. Pickett and J. J. Hanlon, *Public Health: Administration and Practice*, 9th ed. (St. Louis: Times Mirror and Mosby College Publishing, 1990).
4. J. E. Rohrer, *Planning for Community-oriented Health Systems* (Washington, DC: American Public Health Association, 1996).
5. Rohrer, *Planning for Community-oriented Health Systems.*
6. Rohrer, *Planning for Community-oriented Health Systems.*
7. A. Ross, *Cornerstones of Leadership for Health Services Executives* (Ann Arbor, MI: American College of Healthcare Executives, 1992).
8. J. M. Bryson, *Strategic Planning for Public and Nonprofit Organizations*, 3rd ed. (San Francisco: Jossey-Bass, 2004).
9. L. Goodstein et al., *Applied Strategic Planning: A Comprehensive Guide* (New York: McGraw-Hill, 1993).
10. P. R. Scholtes, *The Leader's Handbook* (New York: McGraw-Hill, 1998).
11. Bryson, *Strategic Planning for Public and Nonprofit Organizations.*
12. Bryson, *Strategic Planning for Public and Nonprofit Organizations.*
13. Goodstein et al., *Applied Strategic Planning.*
14. H. Mintzberg, *The Rise and Fall of Strategic Planning* (New York: The Free Press, 1994).
15. Bryson, *Strategic Planning for Public and Nonprofit Organizations.*
16. Goodstein et al., *Applied Strategic Planning.*
17. C. A. Montgomery, "Putting Leadership Back into Strategy, *Harvard Business Review* 86, no. 1 (2008): 54–60.
18. E. A. Scutchfield et al., "The Presence of Total Quality Management and Continuous Quality Improvement Processes in California Public Health Clinics," *Journal of Public Health Management and Practice* 3, no. 3 (1997): 57–60.
19. Scutchfield et al., "The Presence of Total Quality Management and Continuous Quality Improvement Processes in California Public Health Clinics."
20. G. P. Mays et al., "CQI in Public Health Organizations," in *Continuous Quality Improvement in Health Care*, eds. C. P. McLaughlin and A. D. Kaluzny, 2nd ed. (Gaithersburg, MD: Aspen Publishers, 1999).
21. C. P. McLaughlin and A. D. Kaluzny, "Defining Quality Improvement: Past, Present, and Future," in *Continuous Quality Improvement in Health Care*, eds. C. P. McLaughlin and A. D. Kaluzny, 2nd ed. (Gaithersburg, MD: Aspen Publishers, 1999).
22. H. V. Roberts and B. F. Sergesketter, *Quality Is Personal* (New York: Free Press, 1993).
23. McLaughlin and Kaluzny, "Defining Quality Improvement."
24. A. V. Feigenbaum, *Total Quality Control* (New York: McGraw-Hill, 1961).
25. M. Sashkin and K. J. Kiser, *Putting Total Quality Management to Work* (San Francisco: Berrett-Koehler Publishers, 1993).
26. W. A. Shewhart, *Statistical Method from the Viewpoint of Quality Control* (Mineola, NY: Dover, 1986).
27. W. E. Deming, *Out of the Crisis* (Cambridge, MA: Massachusetts Institute of Technology, 1986).
28. M. Walton, *Deming Management at Work* (New York: Pedigree Books, 1991).

29. P. B. Crosby, *Quality Without Tears* (New York: Penguin Plume, 1984).
30. P. B. Crosby, *Completeness* (New York: Penguin Dutton, 1992).
31. P. B. Crosby, *Quality Is Free* (New York: McGraw-Hill, 1989).
32. P. B. Crosby, *Let's Talk Quality* (New York: Penguin Plume, 1990).
33. J. M. Juran, *Juran on Leadership for Quality: An Executive Handbook* (New York: The Free Press, 1989).
34. Feigenbaum, *Total Quality Control.*
35. B. Creech, *The Five Pillars of TQM* (New York: Truman Talley Books and Dutton, 1994).
36. Sashkin and Kiser, *Putting Total Quality Management to Work.*
37. M. Brassard, *The Memory Jogger+* (Methuen, MA: Goal and QPC, 1989).
38. Brassard, *The Memory Jogger+.*
39. M. D. Nichols and R. D. Collins, "Six Sigma," in *The Executive Guide to Improvement and Change,* G. D. Beecroft, G. L. Duffy, and J. W. Moran, eds. (Milwaukee, WI: ASQ Quality Press, 2003).
40. P. S. Pandi, R. P. Neuman, and R. R. Cavanagh, *The Six Sigma Way: Team Fieldbook* (New York: McGraw Hill, 2002).
41. Nichols and Collins, "Six Sigma."
42. http://en.wikipedia.org/wiki/Six Sigma
43. Nichols and Collins, "Six Sigma."
44. E. Jacquescoley, "Can Six Sigma Methods Meet the Demanding Rigors of Local Public Health Practice," *Helium* http://www.helium.com/200858/intoductionit-quality-drives-innovation
45. R. L. Manganelli and M. M. Klein, *The Reengineering Handbook* (New York: AMACOM [American Management Association], 1994).
46. P. P. Drucker, "Really Reinventing Government," *Atlantic Monthly* 275, no. 2 (1995): 49–61.
47. S. P. Robbins and M. Coulter, *Management,* 6th ed. (Upper Saddle River, NJ: Prentice-Hall, 1999).
48. J. Champy, *Reengineering Management* (New York: Harper Business, 1995).
49. M. Hammer, *The Reengineering Revolution* (New York: Harper-Collins, 1995).
50. D. K. Carr and H. J. Johansson, *Best Practices in Reengineering* (New York: McGraw-Hill, 1995).
51. Manganelli and Klein, *The Reengineering Handbook.*
52. D. Osborne and T. Gaebler, *Reinventing Government: How the Entrepreneurial Spirit Is Transforming the Public Sector* (Reading, MA: Addison-Wesley, 1992).
53. D. Osborne and P. Plastrik, *Banishing Bureaucracy* (Reading, MA: Addison-Wesley, 1997).
54. D. Osborne, "The State of the Revolution: An Interview," *Leader to Leader* 6 (1997): 43–49.
55. Osborne, "The State of the Revolution."
56. J. M. Bacon, "Reinventing Government for Public Health Improvement," *Leadership in Public Health* 3, no. 3 (1994): 1–5.
57. A. Gore, *The Report of the National Performance Review* (Washington, DC: Government Printing Office, 1993).
58. Osborne and Plastrik, *Banishing Bureaucracy.*
59. Osborne and Plastrik, *Banishing Bureaucracy.*
60. P. P. Drucker, *Managing in a Time of Great Change* (New York: Truman Talley Books and Dutton, 1995).

# CHAPTER 14

# LEADERSHIP, DECISION MAKING, CONFLICT, AND NEGOTIATION

Once a decision was made, I did not worry about it afterward.

Harry S. Truman, *Memoirs*

Leading involves decision making, and decision making involves taking risks. Public health leaders often confront disagreement or discontent with their decisions. They need to be aware of this possibility and that leadership and risk go together.[1] Risk taking is a prerequisite for "challenging the process" and being innovative.[2] As part of the decision-making process, public health leaders need to evaluate the costs and benefits of their decisions—the expenditures necessary to carry out their decisions and the consequences, good and bad, for the functioning of the public health agency—and also consider the ethical implications of their decisions.

Public health leaders, like all decision makers, will make mistakes and will learn from their mistakes.[3] Taking risks, after all, means opening oneself to the possibility of making mistakes. One way public health leaders can reduce the burden of the bad consequences of their decisions is to develop power-sharing arrangements with community partners. If different partners take responsibility for different pieces of a project, for example, the costs associated with problems that occur (or even the failure of the project) will be borne by more than one entity.

Our mental models will create boundaries for the way we view situations. This "bounded awareness" means that leaders will ignore information that does not fit into their conceptual orientations.[4] Leaders will need to expand their views of the world in order to increase their decision choices and decision-making accuracy. It becomes critical that leaders increase their perceptions by not only looking for information as if they were outsiders. They also need to look for information that is contradictory. Using information of different kinds for decision making is also important. Finally, sharing information with others may expand the information available to guide decisions.

Decisions will come about through other skills as well. Consequently, leaders will need to develop, in addition to decision-making skills, conflict resolution skills and negotiation skills. Although problem solving requires specialized skills, decision making as discussed below is different and requires different skills. Problem solving involves the resolution of conflicts and negotiation activities. Decision making is the end of the problem-solving process. This chapter discusses what can be done when decision making gets complicated by conflict. As should be obvious in decision making by leaders and managers, conflict resolution, negotiation, and communication skills are absolutely essential to ensure that all voices are heard before a decision is made. Case Study 14-A demonstrates a complex combination of relationships at different levels of the public health system that relate to problem solving, communication, conflict, and decision making.

---

### Case Study 14-A
### Lumps in the System: A Mumps Outbreak Story

*Diane Christen, Kelli Jones, Jan Klawitter, Debbie Konitzer, Jackie Ove, Kitty Rahl, and RoAnn Warden*

#### Abstract

In December 2005, two college students in the Midwest were diagnosed with mumps—the first two cases in what would become the largest mumps outbreak in the United States since 1991. By October 2006, 45 states and the District of Columbia reported 5,783 cases of mumps, with 54% of cases classified as confirmed, 45% as probable, and 1% unknown (*MMWR Weekly,* Oct. 27, 2006 [55(42); 1152–1153]).

The mumps virus spread from its epicenter in the Midwest state of Maize to surrounding states, including the state of Fromage, which had its first confirmed mumps case on March 20, 2006. By mid-May 2006, the Fromage State Health Laboratory (FSHL) would suspend its serological mumps testing because of concern about testing accuracy.

This factual and fictional case study examines the evolution of the mumps outbreak in the state of "Fromage" in the context of the core function of assessment and its essential public health services of "monitoring health status to identify community health problems" and "diagnosing and investigating health problems and health hazards in the community." The time frame will focus primarily on the March–May 2006 period, which saw the highest level of mumps activity in Fromage. The case study will focus on how decisions made and information distributed at the state level both helped and hindered the ability of local health departments around the state of Fromage to serve their communities. And it will tell the story of what happens when a disease that's rarely seen shows up in a highly vaccinated population and needs to be diagnosed by a test that's rarely performed.

#### Case Study

*Background*

In December 2005, two students at Northeastern Maize State University went to the student health center complaining of fever, head and muscle aches, and general malaise. The chief physician at the health center also noticed that the students had swelling in their parotid salivary glands causing their cheeks to swell near their jawlines. The physician collected parotid duct swab samples from the students and sent the samples off to the Maize Public Health Laboratory for viral culture. Test results came back positive for mumps virus. Little did the physician know that the outbreak had begun.

Since 2001, the United States has averaged a reported 265 mumps cases a year (range: 231–293) (*MMWR Dispatch,* March 30, 2006 [55(13);366–368]). College campuses are a perfect breeding ground for viruses such as mumps, which are spread by respiratory and oral secretions due to the communal living, dining, study-ing, and recreational areas. As college students mix with community members, travel home, visit friends at other schools, etc., the virus can spread far beyond the site of the original infection.

The vaccination requirements of colleges and universities vary. One dose of the MMR (measles-mumps-rubella) vaccine can prevent approximately 80% of mumps cases, while two doses can prevent about 90% of cases (CDC National Immun-ization Program Mumps Web site: http://www.cdc.gov/nip/diseases/mumps/faqs-outbreak.htm). So even if a school requires two doses of the MMR vaccine, the virus can still occur and spread—just not as widely. This is true of the general population as well. It's also speculated that the vaccine might be less effective in preventing asymptomatic infection than the classic parotitis mumps. Persons with asympto-matic mumps are capable of spreading the infection to others (*MMWR Dispatch,* May 18, 2006 [55(Dispatch);1-5]).

Adding to the difficulty of tracking and containing mumps outbreaks is the fact that the disease is so rarely seen. Many physicians, nurses, and public health profession-als have never seen a case of mumps and might dismiss the diagnosis in a vaccinated person. Also, up to 30% of persons infected with mumps never show signs of paroti-tis and can have nonspecific symptoms similar to many other respiratory infections. Laboratory serological testing for a disease in a highly vaccinated population like the United States is also problematic. A vaccinated person may not produce antibodies that indicate a recent mumps infection even though they have the disease. Hence, serological mumps testing cannot be used to rule out a case of mumps. It's clear that the health care and public health sectors have their work cut out for them.

*The Outbreak in Fromage*

Although the mumps outbreak was beginning to ramp up in Maize, it didn't really hit Fromage until March 2006. Staff at local health departments had been following the outbreak in Maize via the news media. Some sent alerts to their local health care providers offering information on mumps from the Maize State Health Department Web site. On March 20, 2006, the FSHL would report the first positive test result for mumps.

In early April 2006, the Fromage State Health Department (which is separate from the FSHL) sent local health departments a mumps frequently asked questions (FAQs) sheet along with information on collecting patient blood for IgM serologic testing at the FSHL. Wanting to err on the side of not missing cases and realizing that only 30% of mumps cases actually have the characteristic swelling, the Fromage State Health Department defined a suspect case as anyone with an upper respiratory in-fection. This meant that health care providers sent a large number of specimens to the FSHL for testing and many of these patients did not have mumps. This resulted in the probability of obtaining a "true" positive test result to be much less.

In late April the State Health Department issued a news release about the mumps situation in Fromage and recommended vaccinations for those unvaccinated for mumps. In early May, the State Health Department updated the FAQs and contin-ued to post to its Web site information related to Fromage's outbreak with national recommendations.

It became clear that there were four major issue areas in the Fromage mumps out-break: laboratory testing, schools/daycare centers, physicians/infection control prac-titioners, and the media.

*(continues)*

**Case Study 14-A** *continued*

*Laboratory Testing*

Just as mumps is a disease rarely seen by health care providers, the mumps IgM test is rarely performed by laboratories. Also, there is no standard mumps serological test that has been well validated, so different state laboratories use different test kits. The National Public Health Laboratory performs a test created in-house by its scientists. This lack of test uniformity and validation, combined with the lack of baseline data on the true prevalence of mumps in the population because it is so rarely seen, makes it difficult to track outbreaks and determine true case numbers.

FSHL began receiving specimens for mumps testing in March 2006, with its first positive mumps result on March 20, 2006. The initial testing algorithm called for health care providers to submit urine specimens and buccal (inside cheek) swabs for culture testing. Although culture is the gold standard for mumps testing, its diagnostic sensitivity is only 30%.

For this reason, health care providers were encouraged to also submit blood serum specimens for IgM and IgG testing. In mid-April 2006, FSHL brought online a DNA-based real-time PCR test for mumps. This molecular test provides results in hours rather than days. PCR testing is more sensitive than either culture or IgM testing. The downside is that it's a more expensive test to perform. However, the rapid results and increased sensitivity allow for better control and management of outbreaks.

Many health care providers submitted specimens for culture/PCR and IgM testing for each patient. In the first week of May 2006, Fromage State Lab scientists noticed a worrisome trend in the test data. Of specimens from patients submitted, only three patients were positive for mumps by culture/PCR testing, but 177 patients were positive by IgM testing. Because the culture/PCR testing combination should be detecting more than 30% of infected individuals, the scientists were worried that more people were being called "positive" for mumps than actually were. They asked the Fromage State Health Department to correlate the IgM results with patients' clinical data received from the patients' physicians. The positive IgM test results and the clinical data *appeared* to correlate based on the information the State Health Department was receiving. However, FSHL scientists still had their suspicions.

Also during the first week of May, the FSHL received calls from a few physicians suggesting there might have been false positive IgM test results reported for their elderly patients because the patients had no symptoms of and no exposure to mumps.

FSHL began an investigation. Scientists tested 30 serum specimens collected during the summer of 2005 (when no mumps was present in Fromage) from patients suspected of having a mosquito-borne virus. Nineteen of the 30 specimens tested positive for mumps by IgM testing. It was clear—the IgM test could not be trusted. The FSHL also contacted the National Public Health Laboratory to alert them to the issue and ask for assistance in the investigation.

The FSHL consulted with the State Health Department, and scientific leaders at the two agencies agreed that the State Lab should suspend its IgM serology testing due to a concern about false positive test results. The State Health Department sent a memo to all local health officers and infection-control practitioners explaining that the Fromage State Lab was suspending IgM serology testing for mumps, but that patient specimens should still be submitted for PCR and culture testing, which are reliable test methods. The State Lab also sent the memo to all hospital and clinic laboratories in the state. The memo was also posted on Fromage's password-protected Health Alert Web site.

In their conversations with mumps experts at the National Public Health Laboratory, scientists from the Fromage State Lab were told that the National Lab was hearing from other state labs that they were also seeing false positive tests results from their IgM testing (although no state other than Fromage had suspended this form of testing yet). After deciding to suspend the IgM testing, FSHL sent a number of its IgM-positive mumps specimens to the National Lab for further testing. The National Lab found that less than half of the Fromage specimens were positive for mumps by the National Lab's in-house test method. The National Lab was also conducting follow-up testing on specimens from other states that had expressed concerns about false positive test results. The National Lab verbally acknowledged that there were discrepancies between the number of positive test results derived from those states' test methods and the National Lab's method. The problem in Fromage was being experienced in other states, too. This investigation continues.

### Schools/Daycare Centers

With the first positively diagnosed case of mumps in Fromage, the local public health departments responded by assessing the at-risk populations of daycare and school attendees and staff. The impact that this vaccine-preventable disease could have on a daycare or school is great given the incubation period, communicability of the disease, and that 30% of the population can be infected and be asymptomatic. Thus, not only were local health departments concerned with the vaccinated population, but of greater concern were those that had not been vaccinated at all or had not been adequately vaccinated, because isolation and quarantine could occur up to 25 days post exposure.

Public Health Nurses assessed vaccination records of daycare attendees and students of public and parochial schools. Staff at these facilities were asked to report history of disease or vaccination status also. In accordance with Fromage Administrative Code HFS 145 Control of Communicable Disease, a letter was drafted and sent home with attendees and staff of all daycares and schools explaining the disease, the incubation period, signs and symptoms, and especially the need for vaccination of susceptibles if the child or adult had been previously unvaccinated. This letter also explained the procedure for isolation and quarantine if persons not adequately protected were exposed to a suspect, probable, or confirmed case, and for close contacts to a case.

Local health department staff reinforced to key personnel, school attendance secretaries, school principals, and daycare directors the importance of reporting suspected or possible cases to the health department.

### Physicians/Infection Control Practitioners

As medical and infection control practitioners became aware that mumps was in the neighboring state of Maize during March 2006, the assessment process began within the local communities. Individuals who were coming into the clinics and emergency departments with signs and symptoms of mumps were being tested for mumps with IgM and IgG serological tests and instructed by their health care provider to remain isolated. In addition they were told that someone from their local health department would be contacting them with more information. Infection control practitioners (ICP) and health care providers started collecting the necessary patient information for the mumps worksheet or communicable disease reporting form and then forwarded this information to the health departments. Local health departments proceeded to follow up on the suspect mumps cases reported.

*(continues)*

**Case Study 14-A** *continued*

As new information was coming from the Fromage State Health Department in late April and May 2006 regarding mumps testing recommendations, isolation/quarantine, and revaccinating, it was passed on to the local health care providers. Many ICPs and physicians were invited and tuned into the mumps teleconference updates put on by the Fromage State Health Department. Local health officers routinely forwarded to local health care providers and ICPs the e-mails and correspondence from the state health department as well as checking the Health Alert Web site for new information that covered the mumps outbreak. Physicians primarily wanted to know what tests they should run and where they should send the samples for the testing. ICPs relied on the state and local health departments for getting this needed information out to their physicians and facilities.

ICPs and physicians were not as confident in their understanding of the state's and the National Public Health Department's recommendations on who should be vaccinated or revaccinated for health care workers and teachers. The recommendations from the national level were different than those of the Fromage State Health Department. In the past, ICPs could accept the employee's word if the individual knew whether he or she had ever had mumps. Now employees were being required to have lab work done to determine their immune status for mumps if they were not adequately immunized or if they were born before 1957.

On May 11, 2006, the Fromage State Health Department announced that the FSHL was suspending the IgM and IgG serology testing for mumps because of concern over testing accuracy. The announcement came with very clear and concise recommendations for health care providers and ICPs to follow.

Billing issues also arose in some areas because some insurance companies would not cover the cost of specimen collection for patients who were being screened for mumps. Patients were being billed for the uncovered charges even though the laboratory testing was being done on the recommendation of the State Health Department.

*Media*
Within five days of receiving the initial notice of the Maize outbreak, Clear Water County in west central Fromage received its first media inquiry about local mumps status and implications for the community. The health officer provided a television news interview on April 11, 2006, to report there had been no case of mumps locally and to provide information about mumps disease, signs and symptoms, and vaccination as a preventive measure.

Nine days later, the Southern Big City Health Department recommended that all colleges and universities in the Southern Big City metro area set up special mumps vaccination clinics to update vaccinations for all college students. The action was reported in the *Southern Big City Gazette*. This was followed a day later by a Fromage State Health Department news release regarding the Midwest mumps outbreak.

In Clear Water County, these stories raised concerns among students at the University of Fromage–Clear Water campus. A campus newspaper reporter contacted the local health department for information. The health officer provided information about the disease, signs and symptoms, and the importance of updated vaccination and referred the reporter also to the director of the local student health services. The story headlines were *"Mumps Mayhem in Midwest: Disease is making appearances even among vaccinated."* The health officer and the student health services director coordinated media messages on an ongoing basis.

By May 5, 2006, Clear Water County received reports of two laboratory-confirmed cases of mumps in the county. The health officer provided interviews to television and newspaper reporters. The local newspaper's front-page headline that evening boldly stated, *"Mumps Confirmed: Infectious Disease Spreads to Clear Water County."* The media messages emphasized and accurately reported were that (1) the cases were not related and their sources of exposure were unknown; (2) the county health department was working closely with all health care providers; and (3) up-to-date immunization is an important protection.

On May 6, 2006, a campus newspaper reporter again approached the health department for information for a follow-up story to educate concerned students. The published article was entitled *"Experts Say Mumps No Reason for Alarm: Viral Disease reaches area for first time since '90s."* The article identified the emergence of mumps as a concern but not a reason for alarm. Key points included the importance of vaccination, respiratory hygiene, and seeking medical care if symptomatic.

Community and media interest subsided when case counts remained at two over a two-week period. No further cases were identified in Clear Water County. The local media did not pursue stories about suspension of mumps IgM testing.

### Conclusions/Areas for Improvement

Based on the experiences related in this case study:

1. The identification and required reporting of communicable disease is a very effective assessment/surveillance system when health care providers and ICPs are informed in a timely manner with up-to-date recommendations and guidelines from the health departments (state and local). In order for public health to do their job of assessment and "monitor health status to identify community health problems" and "diagnosis and investigate health problems and health hazards in the community," it is critical that they have a good partnership/relationship with their clinics and ICPs. Having an established contact person, like an ICP, within the clinics and hospitals who can act as a conduit for the sharing of information back and forth was very effective in this mumps outbreak.

2. Local health departments need clarification for payer source for specimen collection if the testing is being done for screening/epidemiological purposes. Testing can be done at the State Laboratory fee-exempt, but who covers the costs of specimen collection? As noted in *Healthiest Fromage 2010*, one of the core principles and values that support the transformation of Fromage's public health system is "All Fromage residents deserve a basic level of health services. Improved individual and community health will happen when basic health services are affordable for all and access does not depend on race, cultural heritage or geographic location."

3. The authority for the control of communicable disease comes from Fromage Administrative Code HFS 145 Control of Communicable Disease; however, there is confusion surrounding the health officer's ability to isolate and quarantine an unvaccinated or inadequately vaccinated individual. A clear answer as to the authority to follow through on that process was never established from the State Health Department and continues to be an unanswered question for local health officers.

4. Local health departments rely on the State Health Department to provide clear, consistent, and timely information about the situation. Delay on the part of the

*(continues)*

state can force local health departments to take independent action and release their messages and intervention recommendations before the state.

5. When it became clear that other states were also experiencing problems with their mumps IgM testing, federal-level leadership was needed to address the issue.

## Decision Making

Any organization's vision and mission need to be tied to the real world.[5] A vision without substance is pointless. The challenge for the leaders of an organization is to figure out what strategies will be most effective in realizing its vision, make the hard decisions required to implement these strategies, and get others in the organization to accept the decisions and commit themselves to carrying out the strategies.[6] Decisions involve the making of choices from alternative possible solutions. Decision making is also about the taking of risks by the decision maker. Leaders need to be aware that a decision itself does not change an organization; rather the actions resulting from the decision are what bring about change.[7]

Decision making is an essential outcome step in problem solving. Leaders need to address problems as they arise and modify operations in light of the factors introduced by the problems. One strategy is to appoint a task force to develop potential solutions to a problem and then decide what to do based on recommendations of the task force or the information provided by it. For example, a public health administrator in a suburb adjoining an urban neighborhood with a high crime rate might appoint a community task force consisting of professionals from the health department and the police department to determine how the community could prevent gang violence.

Problem solving can sometimes assume a cyclic form.[8] Suppose the leaders of an organization discover a serious problem that demands action. They determine the nature of the problem, come up with solutions, and begin to implement them. The problem, as it begins to be addressed, becomes less serious and of less concern to the leaders and others in the organization. One result might well be that the implementation of the solutions is not carried through to its conclusion, allowing the problem to intensify again and eventually causing the leaders to restart the problem-solving process. Organizations that concentrate on putting out fires do not advance much but instead struggle constantly with maintaining the status quo. Figure 14-1 graphically shows this process.

Leadership style, leadership practices, and governing paradigms affect the process of making decisions and the outcomes of the decisions. Also affecting the process and outcomes are the kind and quality of the information that is available. In particular, public health leaders depend on epidemiological assessment data, among other types of information, for making decisions about community health programs. The Cynefin framework addresses the important issue of context as a critical dimension of decisions.[9] Contexts can be simple, complicated, complex, or chaotic. Leaders need to learn to shift their

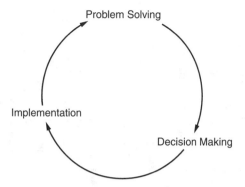

**FIGURE 14-1    Decision-making Cycle**

decision-making strategies to address the public health context in which the decision needs to be made. Table 14-1 presents a guide on these four contexts for leaders.

### Decision-Making Roles and Styles

Mintzberg identified four decisional roles that leaders assume.[10] First, leaders take on an entrepreneurial role when making decisions that expand the parameters of the organization. As pointed out previously, leaders of public health agencies need to look for resources from the private and public sectors if they want to fulfill the overall public health mission—improving health and preventing disease.[11] Approaching businesses for funds to support public health programs is a form of entrepreneurism. Second, leaders are occasionally confronted with work disturbances that require administrative decisions for their resolution.[12] Third, leaders must act as resource allocators and determine where the limited human and financial resources of the agency could best be applied to implement or operate agency programs. Finally, leaders must occasionally act as negotiators.

There are three conditions that affect the decision-making style of a leader.[13] If all the potential outcomes are known, this brings some evidence of certainty and accuracy to the decision. Fear of risk is one of the main barriers to the making of rational decisions. Effective leaders constantly take risks and do not avoid them. A strategy of incremental change will weaken an organization if substantial reforms are necessary. By giving into caution, leaders pass up the chance of being creative. Such leaders also tend to ignore negative feedback, which can lead to disaster. The third condition is one of almost complete uncertainty and the possibility that the decision will not be applicable. These conditions will clearly affect the decision and be affected by the decision style of the leader.

In contrast to Mintzberg, Robbins and Coulter have a four-category model for decision styles.[14] Decision making can be rational or intuitive, and it can also exhibit a high or low degree of tolerance for ambiguity.[15,16] As

**Table 14-1 Decisions in Multiple Contexts: A Leader's Guide**

| | The Context's Characteristics | The Leader's Job | Danger Signals | Response to Danger Signals |
|---|---|---|---|---|
| **Simple** | Repeating patterns and consistent events<br>Clear cause-and-effect relationships evident to everyone; right answer exists<br>Known knowns<br>Fact-based management | Sense, categorize, respond<br>Ensure that proper processes are in place<br>Delegate<br>Use best practices<br>Communicate in clear, direct ways<br>Understand that extensive interactive communication may not be necessary | Complacency and comfort<br>Desire to make complex problems simple<br>Entrained thinking<br>No challenge of received wisdom<br>Overreliance on best practice if context shifts | Create communication channels to challenge orthodoxy<br>Stay connected without micromanaging<br>Don't assume things are simple<br>Recognize both the value and the limitations of best practice |
| **Complicated** | Expert diagnosis required<br>Cause-and-effect relationships discoverable but not immediately apparent to everyone; more than one right answer possible<br>Known unknowns<br>Fact-based management | Sense, analyze, respond<br>Create panels of experts<br>Listen to conflicting advice | Experts overconfident in their own solutions or in the efficacy of past solutions<br>Analysis paralysis<br>Expert panels<br>Viewpoints of nonexperts excluded | Encourage external and internal stakeholders to challenge expert opinions to combat entrained thinking<br>Use experiments and games to force people to think outside the familiar |
| **Complex** | Flux and unpredictability<br>No right answers; emergent instructive patterns<br>Unknown unknowns | Probe, sense, respond<br>Create environments and experiments that allow patterns to emerge<br>Increase levels of | Temptation to fall back into habitual, command-and-control mode<br>Temptation to look for facts rather than allowing patterns to emerge | Be patient and allow time for reflection<br>Use approaches that encourage interaction so patterns can emerge |

| | | | |
|---|---|---|---|
| Many competing ideas<br>A need for creative and innovative approaches<br>Pattern-based leadership | interaction and communication<br>Use methods that can help generate ideas: open up discussion (as through large group methods); set barriers; stimulate attractors; encourage dissent and diversity; and manage starting conditions and monitor for emergence | Desire for accelerated resolution of problems or exploitation of opportunities | |
| **Chaotic**<br>High turbulence<br>No clear cause-and-effect relationships, so no point in looking for right answers<br>Unknowables<br>Many decisions to make and no time to think<br>High tension<br>Pattern-based leadership | Act, sense, respond<br>Look for what works instead of seeking right answers<br>Take immediate action to reestablish order (command and control)<br>Provide clear, direct communication | Applying a command-and-control approach longer than needed<br>"Cult of the leader"<br>Missed opportunity for innovation<br>Chaos unabated | Set up mechanisms (such as parallel teams) to take advantage of opportunities afforded by a chaotic environment<br>Encourage advisers to challenge your point of view once the crisis has abated<br>Work to shift the context from chaotic to complex |

*Source:* From D. J. Snowden and M. E. Boone, "A Leader's Framework for Decision Making," *Harvard Business Review, 85*, 11 (2007): 68–76.

shown in Figure 14-2, an analytical style of decision making is rational and exhibits a high degree of tolerance for ambiguity. Analytical decision makers base their decisions on information. A directive style is characterized by a high degree of rationality but a low degree of tolerance for ambiguity. Directive decision makers are logical and tend to make decisions quickly and for the short term. Directive decision making is a style favored by managers. Conceptual decision making is intuitive and exhibits a low degree of tolerance for ambiguity. Conceptual decision makers tend to concentrate on the future and its possibilities, and they also tend to be very creative. The behavioral style of decision making is intuitive and shows a low degree of tolerance for ambiguity. Decision makers who use this style concentrate on people relationships and tend to accept information from other staff before making a decision. Exercise 14-1 will give you a chance to test the two decision-style models as they relate to you and others.

Decisions require implementation, and the implementation process is often complex and hard to complete.[17] Leaders must determine the sequence of implementation steps and the interactions that are likely to occur at each step. Further, they must understand that the implementation process has important decision points—places where critical decisions must be made. At these decision points, the leaders review the implementation process in order to determine if modifications are necessary and if the objectives of the implementation are being achieved.

## Shared Decision Making

Decision making may be a shared activity. Much public health work occurs in teams, coalitions, and other groups, and if power is shared, decision making would likely be shared as well. There are at least four advantages to

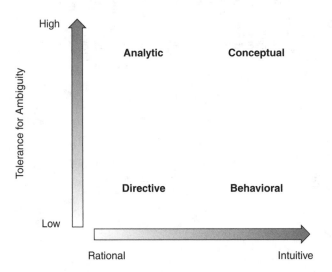

**FIGURE 14-2  Decision Making Styles by Ways of Thinking and Tolerance for Ambiguity**
*Source:* S. P. Robbins and D. A. DeCenzo, *Supervision Today,* 5th ed. © 2007, p. 193. (Upper Saddle River, NJ: Prentice Hall). Reprinted by permission of Pearson Education, Inc.

shared decision making.[18] First, each party brings to the group new information, a diversity of experience, different professional credentials, and a different perspective. Second, a group is likely to come up with more options than an individual. Third, there is likely to be more acceptance of a decision if more people are involved in making the decision. A group-made decision is a decision with a ready-made consensus. Finally, the involvement of others increases the legitimacy of the decision.

There are also four disadvantages to shared decision making, whether in a team, coalition, or other group.[19] First, the process can consume a great amount of time. In decision making, reaching a quick decision is often critical, and delays can prevent a solution from being fully effective. Second, a strong minority will sometimes try to dominate the whole process—and will sometimes succeed. Third, the appearance of agreement or consensus may disguise the fact that there really is no agreement. Finally, shared decision making and the shared sense of responsibility that goes with it can lead to a situation where no one feels responsible for negative outcomes related to the decisions.

### Decision-making Models

Table 14-2 presents an outline of three decision-making models. As can be seen, the basic decision-making process is similar in all three. Each model starts with a problem, utilizes information to evaluate the problem, and eventually leads to a decision.

In the first model, designed by Liebler and colleagues, the first step is to set an agenda, which includes recognizing that a problem or challenge to the status quo has arisen and collecting information to validate the problem or challenge.[20] Searching for alternative solutions is the second step. The leaders need to be objective and to listen to possible scenarios presented by their colleagues. The third step is the evaluation of the alternative solutions to determine which one is the most promising. The task in the fourth stage is to get a commitment to the chosen solution from participants in the decision-making process. The solution is then pilot tested, and if the results are positive, the leaders devise an implementation plan. The final step involves

**Table 14-2  Three Contrasting Approaches to Decision Making**

| Liebler and McConnell* | Robbins and Coulter† | Systems Approach |
|---|---|---|
| Build agenda. | Identify problems. | Set goals and objectives. |
| Search for alternatives. | Identify decision criteria. | Engage in action planning. |
| Evaluate alternatives. | Allocate weights to criteria. | Implement action plans. |
| Commit to chosen alternatives. | Develop alternatives. | Evaluate implementation of plans. |
| Continually assess decisions. | Select alternative. Implement alternative. Evaluate effectiveness of implementation. | |

*Source:* *Data from J. G. Liebler and C. R. McConnell, *Management Principles for Health Professionals,* 4th ed., pp. 235–236. © 2004, Jones and Bartlett, Publishers.
†S. P. Robbins and M. Coulter, *Management,* 8th ed. (New York: Prentice Hall, 2005).

assessing the results of the chosen solution during the implementation, including the results of decisions made as part of the implementation process.

The second model, designed by Robbins and Coulter, begins with roughly the same first step as the model described above, that is, problem identification.[21] The problem identified might be related to legal mandates, budget restrictions, lack of information, or lack of support from the local board or from community constituencies. The next two steps are to identify decision criteria and attach weights to them (so that relatively unimportant criteria do not influence the decision to the same degree as important criteria). Then alternative solutions are developed and analyzed. The best solution (or the one that seems the best) is chosen and implemented. Finally, as in the preceding model, the results of the implementation are evaluated.

In the third model, the first step is to identify goals and objectives based on the organization's mission and vision. The next step is to embark on the task of devising action plans to achieve the goals and objectives. The plans are then implemented and the implementation process is evaluated, as in the other two models. This model follows the Leadership Wheel paradigm presented in Chapter 7.

To be effective decision makers, public health leaders must:

- learn that making decisions involves risk taking
- learn the differences between problem solving and decision making
- build decision-making strategies into implementation plans
- empower employees and community partners to take an active role in decision making
- identify their style of leadership and understand how to use it in decision making
- tie decisions to the goals and objectives of the organization

## Conflict Resolution

### The Dangers of Conflict

Life and leadership are full of twists and turns, and there are always individuals who disagree with any position taken on an issue. This is partially explained by the multicultural nature of our society and partially by the wide spectrum of political positions held by policy makers.

Conflict over a decision needs to be resolved if the decision is to be effective. As pointed out above, decision making does not occur in a vacuum and is usually a group process. Even when conflict appears to be absent or to have been resolved, there is no guarantee of full acceptance of the solution.[22] Moreover, the main disagreement may be not over the solution, but over how to implement the solution.[23]

Conflict, although based in the facts of a given situation, is often partly the result of differences in ideology,[24] and there are typically mythologies that support the positions of the partners to a conflict. Ideology, information, and key players change over time, and thus the techniques needed to resolve conflicts also change.

Conflict is the reverse of cooperation.[25] When it permeates an entire organization, it needs to be addressed immediately. Conflict entails negativity and opposition to decisions.[26] In addition, people fear conflict and suffer stress as a result of conflict, another serious consequence of a situation in which conflict remains rampant.[27]

Yet, life without conflict is not a possibility, especially in our complex society.[28,29] In fact, conflict has, if anything, become more prevalent in the 21st century. Therefore, leaders must learn how to handle conflict. Exercise 14-2 allows students to explore the meaning of conflict and to experience ways in which conflict may be resolved.

Conflict within an organization can have diverse causes, including the culture and atmosphere of the organization, its structure, the needs of the leadership and the organization, and the solutions to past conflict.[30] Major sources of conflict and obstacles to conflict resolution include the following:[31]

- Conflict arises when different leaders assert their authority and engage in a power struggle. In the U.S. Congress, power struggles are common causes of gridlock (the inability to pass major legislation).
- The assignment of the wrong people to a team or task force can lead to conflict. It is unfortunately common to see an executive appointed to a major task force either not attend most of the meetings or send as a proxy someone without the power to make decisions.
- Conflict will naturally arise in a meeting run by someone who lacks respect for the attendees, communicates poorly, or hides the reason for the meeting.

Having a clear mission and vision and basing the discussion of issues on these is essential for conflict avoidance. Conflict will inevitably occur in a team, for example, if the members are unclear as to the team's mission.

It is important not to spend time revisiting conflicts that have been resolved unless the solutions did not win real agreement. Some groups continually return to conflicts that have already been worked out, thereby wasting time and often generating frustration.

Conflict resolution by a group requires that the group be given full authority to resolve the conflict. If the group doesn't have adequate authority, it will spend fruitless hours discussing issues that are beyond its power to do anything about.

Conflicts use up much of the leader's time. For example, if a public health leader is spending 20% or more of the workday resolving conflicts, he or she should look at ways to reduce that amount. And time is not the only issue. As noted above, conflict creates stress, and the leader must not allow his or her personal health to be jeopardized as a result of managing conflict.

A third danger is the potential for sabotage by employees who have become disaffected because of the prevalence of conflict.[32] Conflict can also increase workplace violence. For example, if employees who are members of a union come in conflict with employees who are not members, the difference in perspective between these two groups could lead to a buildup of tension and eventually to actual violence.

## Dealing with Conflict

A preliminary step in resolving conflict is to select an appropriate strategy or style. Which conflict resolution style is best will depend on the nature of the conflict and the situation in which the conflict occurs.[33] Rahim defined five styles that a leader might use to deal with conflict between him- or herself and other parties.[34] Figure 14-3 arranges these styles based on the degree of concern for self and degree of concern for others exhibited by the leader. The integrating style, which involves collecting pertinent facts as part of the conflict resolution process, is oriented toward finding an innovative solution that satisfies both parties. The leader who uses this style exhibits a concern both for self and others.

An obliging style would be typical of a leader who showed great concern for others but little concern for self. The leader would tend to go along with whatever the other party to the conflict wanted, perhaps out of a worry that he or she lacked the expertise necessary to resolve the conflict in any other way. This style is diametrically opposite to the dominating style, in which the leader exhibits great concern for self but little for others. The leader acts in an authoritarian manner and basically lays down what the resolution is going to be.

One way to deal with conflict is to avoid it, and the avoiding style is often used by leaders who exhibit a low degree of concern for self and for others. The goal is to protect the status quo, and the conflict-avoiding leader stays in the background and lets others deal with the conflict and its ramifications.

The compromising style is the middle-of-the-road style, and the compromising leader shows average concern for self and others. Compromise involves reciprocity, which means that each party to the conflict gets something. This style is very useful for resolving conflict between individuals engaged in a partnership, because the partners are treated as they expect to be—with equal respect. Collaboration is difficult if not impossible if conflict exists or is not resolved. The major advantage of resolving conflict is that each party to the discussion has his or her position stated and the resolution will often create the buy-in to the eventual decision.

Conflict may be planned or unplanned (Figure 14-4). Conflict stimulation is sometimes needed if change is to occur. It can be a method of ending grid-

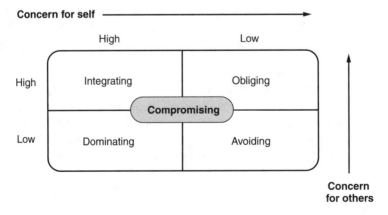

**FIGURE 14-3** **Five Conflict Management Styles**
*Source:* Reprinted with permission. From W. Hendricks, How to Manage Conflict, p. 33, National Press Publications, 1-800-255-4436.

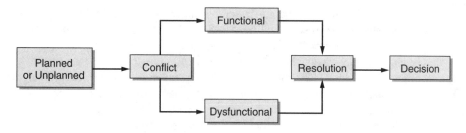

**FIGURE 14-4    Elements of Resolution of Conflict**

lock and breaking through barriers protecting the status quo. Leaders need to know not only when to stimulate conflict for the good of the organization but also how to deal with it once it occurs.

Robbins and Coulter make a distinction between functional and dysfunctional conflicts.[35] Functional conflicts contribute to the attainment of goals and objectives, whereas dysfunctional conflicts hinder their achievement. The former, of course, are conflicts of the kind that leaders would want to stimulate if they were not occurring in the natural order of things.

The end result of all these activities is a regimen of activities that leads to the favorable or unfavorable resolution of the conflict. The resolution of the conflict is not sufficient. The leader still needs to make a decision and put the solution into action.

### A Conflict Resolution Process

Weeks devised a process for dealing with conflict.[36] The steps are as follows:

1. Create an effective atmosphere.
2. Clarify perceptions.
3. Focus on individual and shared needs.
4. Build shared positive power.
5. Lead to the future, then learn from the past.
6. Generate options.
7. Develop doables.
8. Make mutually beneficial agreements.

There are at least two sides to every conflict. Each party enters the conflict situation with an agenda based on personal, organizational, or community concerns and values and possibly goals and objectives. Emotions get involved. Out of this mix a consensus of some kind needs to be forged. To achieve a consensus, the leader needs to create an environment conducive to working on a resolution to the conflict (step 1 in the conflict resolution process outlined above). For instance, the leader must try to create the right atmosphere for meetings between the parties and make sure that the times and locations of meetings are agreeable to everyone. A neutral meeting place is often the best choice. The leader, in preparation for the first meeting, might develop several possible scenarios for starting the conflict resolution process. The choice of the right scenario might have to happen at a moment's notice.

People's perceptions are affected by many factors, including past experiences as well as present realities. In step 2, the leader needs to determine whether the conflict is tied to personal, organizational, community, or professional concerns. Is the conflict related to values or needs? Are goals and objectives driving the process? Finally, the leader must examine the components of the conflict and develop strategies based on his or her analysis.

In step 3, each party to the conflict identifies his or her personal needs. The leader then helps the parties to identify needs that they share. The process of looking at their needs often helps the parties to discover needs, values, and perceptions they unknowingly possess.

The goal in step 4 is to develop the power (means) to resolve the conflict and get the parties to share in this power. For power sharing to occur, the parties must come to share a clear mission and vision, be willing to settle for realistic goals and objectives, and view resolution of the conflict as in everyone's best interest.

Step 5 requires the leader to evaluate how past decisions influence the present conflict and prepare the way for a less conflictive future. The parties need to be careful not to let past experiences keep them from building a better future.

In step 6, the parties identify and explore options for resolving the conflict. These options can help the parties to see the issues more clearly and be less governed by previous perspectives. This step requires the parties to be creative and to use imaging techniques to examine the likely consequences of the various options. The use of the dialogue technique described in Chapter 9 might be beneficial here. Dialogue allows each party to present his or her position and possible solutions to the conflict without interruption and comment. When the parties move into the discussion phase, the agenda of each party will be helpfully on the table.

> **Leadership Tip**
>
> *Fit your personal talents, knowledge, and skills to the tasks to be accomplished.*

In step 7, the parties need to develop a set of "doables," which are small actions that are easy to complete and that will improve the relationship between the parties.

As their relationship improves, they will be better able, in step 8, to agree on a final resolution to the conflict. This resolution, like the doables, must be realistic and mutually beneficial. Otherwise the process will fail.

Conflict resolution is best achieved through a fairly flexible series of activities that are modified to address the unique issues associated with the particular conflict. The model presented above allows flexibility in each of the eight steps so that the different perspectives of the parties can be accommodated. Guidelines for conflict resolution are listed below. To reduce the number and intensity of conflicts and resolve them when they occur, public health leaders must:

- utilize conflict resolution techniques to define disagreements between colleagues or external partners
- define whether a conflict enhances or hinders the ability of the organization to fulfill its mission, vision, goals, and objectives

- monitor power struggles between colleagues or external partners
- decrease (if possible) the percentage of time allocated to conflict resolution
- select the best method of conflict resolution to use based on their personal leadership styles and the core functions of public health
- implement a protocol that colleagues or partners agree upon in order to resolve conflicts
- put solutions to conflict into action as quickly as possible after a decision is made
- identify the mutual benefits to be obtained by conflict resolution

## Negotiation

Conflict can be resolved through coercion (the threat or exercise of physical force), adjudication (legal proceedings), mediation, arbitration, or negotiation.[37] Negotiation, the topic of this section, is also used in bargaining (e.g., when two parties are engaged in working out an exchange of goods and services) and in forming partnerships and other types of alliances.

In negotiation, two or more parties are involved in trying to reach an agreement (or resolve a conflict); each is represented by a negotiator, whose role is to help make the agreement satisfactory to all parties. Mediation occurs when a neutral third party takes on the role of honest broker and tries to get the interested parties to reach an agreement. Both negotiation and mediation are covered in this section.

Every person is continually involved in informal negotiations throughout life.[38] Negotiation skills can be used to resolve personal, organizational, community, and professional issues and problems. Most people use what might be called soft negotiation techniques. In soft negotiation, each party wants a decision reached or a problem resolved with as little fuss as possible and without antagonizing the other parties. Hard negotiation is favored by those who love the challenge of the negotiation game and tend to shoot for more than they can easily get.

Principled negotiation occurs when the parties attempt to resolve a conflict based on merit rather than on their personal agendas.[39] In a sense, the relationship between the parties becomes more important than the conflict. In some cases, this type of negotiation is not applicable, because objective criteria needed to reach a "fair" or defensible resolution may be lacking. Each party simply possesses a given agenda, the agendas are inconsistent with each other, and there is no right or wrong conclusion to the process.

Table 14-3 lists 16 skills and abilities that a leader-negotiator (or leader-mediator) needs in order to be successful.[40] Negotiation skills are applicable to a range of types of negotiation, from union negotiations to bargaining over salary and position title to negotiations with the local health board regarding the distribution of funds for specific activities.

Negotiation is both an art and a science.[41] It is a science inasmuch as negotiation models exist that lay out procedures for reaching agreements and resolving conflicts. It is an art inasmuch as effective negotiations require flexibility and an intuitive ability to choose the appropriate skills and apply them expertly and at the right time.

**Table 14-3 Interpersonal Skills for the Negotiator**

1. Being in control of oneself
2. The ability to elicit the needs, interests, and goals of those on whose behalf the negotiator is acting
3. The ability to properly counsel those persons regarding the realities of the situation
4. Obtaining clear authority from the appropriate decision maker
5. Understanding and being able to utilize the full range of effective strategies and tactics
6. Planning efficiently
7. Being credible
8. Perceptively analyzing the other party and its negotiator
9. Being able to tolerate conflict and ambiguity
10. Knowing or learning the relevant market factors
11. Disclosing information selectively and persuasively
12. Obtaining necessary information
13. Listening to and perceiving the real information being conveyed
14. Making changes in strategy and tactics or counseling those for whom the negotiator is acting regarding terms, as appropriate during the negotiation
15. Being both patient and tireless
16. Knowing when and how to either close the negotiation with an agreement or to terminate it because a desirable agreement cannot be reached

*Source:* Reprinted with permission from M. K. Shoenfield and R. M. Shoenfield, *The McGraw-Hill 36-Hour Negotiating Course,* p. 10, © 1991.

### Prenegotiation

Negotiators must deal with a number of issues before the actual negotiations begin.[42] First, they must determine how many individuals or group representatives will be involved in the process. The more might not be the merrier. They must also consider whether the organizations being represented are monolithic or made up of diverse components each with its own perspective. In a complex, multiperspective organization, an agreement reached through the efforts of a single representative might not be perceived as acceptable by certain components within the organization.

The negotiator for each organization should find out if the other organizations involved in the negotiations spend large amounts of time in bargaining situations. If they do, the process may become more important than the outcome, and the negotiator should be forewarned of this possibility.

Another issue is whether there is a connection between the outcome of the negotiations at hand and the outcomes of other negotiations. If there is, this will complicate the current negotiations. Other issues include whether an agreement must be reached, whether ratification is required, and whether agreement between the parties creates a binding contract. The negotiators need to know if there are any internal or external threats to the negotiation process. They also need to determine whether the negotiations are to be open or closed.

### Negotiation Barriers

Negotiations, like any human activity, face many obstacles in the way of their completion.[43] First, the process might become more expensive, in time and money, than expected. Second, people are often resistant to change and will fight for maintenance of the status quo. Third, negotiators sometimes view the issues at stake in the negotiations as making up a "fixed pie" and assume that their role is to ensure that their slice is as big as or bigger than it was before. They seem not to realize that negotiations can result in a bigger piece of pie for everyone.

Another obstacle is that negotiators occasionally hold on to old opinions or keep bringing up issues that were settled early in the negotiations. In addition, they may present information to the other negotiators in a way that leads to the disintegration of the whole process. A sixth obstacle is that important information is sometimes unavailable, and an agreement reached on the basis of partial information may not be the best agreement for one or more of the parties.

There is also the "winner's curse."[44] The "winner" in a negotiation may wish that the process would continue and may be depressed about its closure. Further, the negotiators must not allow overconfidence to thwart the process, nor should they make the mistake of treating disagreement among the parties as more important than the relationship that is being forged between them.[45]

Negotiation has unique characteristics that differentiate it from other types of conflict resolution. Two processes, with feedback loops connecting them, are going on at the same time: the planning process and the actual negotiations. Public health leaders in negotiations receive feedback from the community, they receive feedback from colleagues in the public health agency, and they and the other negotiating parties give and receive feedback from each other.

### Getting to Yes

There are many approaches to prenegotiation and negotiation activities. We will look at two of them. First, Fisher and colleagues developed the "Getting to Yes" model.[46] This model, which is intended to be user friendly, allows great flexibility. The steps are as follows:

1. Determine interests.
2. Identify options.
3. Determine alternatives.
4. Review the legitimacy of the process.
5. Choose appropriate communication strategies.
6. Strengthen relationships.
7. Promote commitment.

The first step is to determine the interests of the parties to the negotiation. These interests are more important than the official position held by each party. The negotiators must try to clarify the issues involved. The second step is to identify options for resolving the conflict. The parties should be aware that they all could gain from the resolution of the conflict although no party is likely to get everything desired.[47] The third step is to determine alternatives. The fourth step is to review the legitimacy of the process. Because complete agreement between the parties is not likely to occur, they must accept the legitimacy of the process and its outcome. The fifth step is to choose an appropriate communication strategy. Two-way communication is essential if the negotiations are to proceed smoothly. For one thing, the re-framing of issues may be a continuous activity. In step 6, the negotiators try to strengthen their relationship. It is important in this step to separate substance from relationship. The promotion of commitment to the agreed solution occurs in the final step. This commitment is critical to the success of the whole process.

The "Getting to Yes" model has been criticized as unrealistic.[48] Nonetheless, the model seems to work and has been used successfully in teacher-college administration contract negotiations. Public health leaders may find the model easier to use if the proper coalition development has occurred, because then the parties to the negotiations will have already established a working relationship.

### The Schoenfield and Schoenfield Negotiation Model

Schoenfield and Schoenfield developed a 14-step model that incorporates major steps from other negotiation models.[49] The model comprises both prenegotiation and negotiation steps.

Prenegotiation:

1. prenegotiation information gathering
2. determining goals
3. identifying issues
4. analyzing the market
5. assessing strengths and weaknesses
6. estimating the other party's bottom line and opening position
7. considering win-win outcomes

Negotiation:

8. setting the opening position
9. setting the bottom line
10. choosing strategies and tactics
11. considering concessions and trade-offs
12. determining an agenda
13. analyzing timing
14. choosing the modes of communication

The first seven steps of this model overlap the steps of the "Getting to Yes" model, although the Schoenfield and Schoenfield model is more specific. Its higher degree of specificity can be both an advantage (because it provides detailed guidance) and a disadvantage (because it decreases flexibility and increases the burden placed on the negotiators). One of its faults is that it does not take into account the feedback loops that need to exist if the negotiations are to be as effective as possible and lead to agreements that the parties can commit to.

In the first step, each negotiator collects needed data. For public health issues, data from community assessments will have to be gathered. The parties should identify information gaps and make plans to search for the missing data or knowingly proceed with the negotiations under the current data limitations. (Note that public health negotiations often involve more than two parties,[50] but for ease of exposition this account of the model assumes there are just two parties.)

Step two involves setting goals for the planning process. These goals will include short- and long-term goals and also essential and merely desirable goals. The last task in this step is to prioritize the goals.

In step 3, the parties identify the issues that will be the focus of the negotiations and begin to discuss concessions and trade-offs.

The purpose of step 4 is to look at the market (or the community, in the case of public health) and identify the market factors that might influence the negotiations. Public health leaders, in their negotiations, must keep in mind that the public might have an agenda that diverges from the agenda of each negotiating party. They should also review the culture and norms of the specific population that will be directly affected by the outcome of the negotiations. In general, they have an obligation to look after the needs of the community during the negotiation process.

In planning step 5, each party looks at its own strengths and weaknesses and, to the extent possible, those of the other party. The problem here is that each party assesses strengths and weaknesses based on its own worldview. During this step, each party also considers settlement alternatives and determines what, in its view, would be the "best alternative to a negotiated agreement" (BATNA).[51]

In step 6, each party estimates the other party's bottom line and likely opening position. This step aids in identifying areas of agreement as well as difference. The negotiators also need to determine if personal values could interfere with the process.

The final step in the prenegotiation phase is the consideration of win-win scenarios—outcomes that represent net gains for each of the negotiating parties. This step is essential, because win-win outcomes are the ones that both parties are liable to accept eventually. Each party should understand going into the negotiations that it is not going to get everything it wants but can get some of what it wants if it is willing to compromise and allow the other party to win something as well.

The eighth step is the opening step in the negotiations themselves. Here the parties put forth their opening positions. In the ninth step, each party sets the bottom line—the minimum it will accept. In other words, each party lets the other know what its particular BATNA is. The discussion in this step helps to determine if a negotiated agreement is possible or not.

At any stage in the negotiation process, one or both parties may return to an earlier step and redo it in the interests of arriving at a better outcome. For example, the negotiators may want to re-evaluate information collected earlier in order to determine whether their current bottom line is justified or needs to be revised.

Negotiation strategies and tactics are chosen in step 10. The negotiators might use the strategy of expressing upfront their desire to achieve a win-win outcome and or they might take a no-concessions stance. Each strategy has several tactics associated with it. Examples of tactics include the setting of deadlines and methods for dealing with a deadlock.

In step 11, the negotiators consider concessions and possible trade-offs. Planned concessions and trade-offs are needed for a successful outcome.[52] Negotiations in which there are more than two parties provide extra opportunities for trade-offs, because deals can be struck between some of the parties but not all. During this step especially, the parties need to make an effort to act respectfully toward each other and build trust among themselves. The best strategy is to focus on the issues at the heart of the negotiations and not on the personalities of the people at the table.

Also, the beginning positions set forth by the negotiators need to be open to revision. If they are not, the result will be inaction and a breakdown in the negotiations. The best strategy is to focus on the interests that lie behind the stated positions rather than the positions themselves. In addition, the development of options should be separated from the decision making, and objective criteria should be used in the decision-making process, because they provide the parties with a template for action and make concessions and trade-offs easier to navigate.

Agenda setting occurs in step 12. The main task is to determine the actions that are going to have to be completed, such as the identification of issues and the making of concessions. The parties need to agree on the agenda, and if they are unable to reach an agreement, they may have to return to an earlier step and work through the process again.

The agenda identifies the actions; the schedule, to be devised in step 13, lays down time frames in which the actions are to occur. The task of creating a schedule is complicated by the fact that the parties to a negotiation often have hidden agendas (and even hidden deadlines) that only become apparent over time.

The model's final step is to choose the modes of communication that are most appropriate to the situation (see Chapter 11 for a discussion of communication skills and strategies). Of course, resolution of the negotiation issues and obtainment of an agreement are yet to come, and they might be considered to compose the fifteenth step.

## Negotiation Strategies

The two models of negotiation described above cover the major steps that parties to a negotiation need to go through. A separate issue is the strategies that are available for use during these steps. Following is a list of strategies that negotiators can use to reach an outcome satisfactory to them (strategies 1–9 are described in Fuller[53] and 10–16 are described in Schoenfield and Schoenfield):[54]

1. win-win
2. stonewalling
3. good Samaritan
4. finessing the process
5. splitting the difference
6. nickel and dime tactics
7. controlling the action

8. ambiguity
9. defensive techniques
10. no concessions
11. deadlock-breaking techniques
12. high realistic expectations with small systematic concessions
13. concede first
14. problem solving
15. extraneous goals
16. closure strategies

Several of these strategies can undermine the negotiation process. Therefore, they must be used cautiously. Also, note that for every strategy, there is a counterstrategy.

As pointed out, each party to a negotiation wants to gain something as a result of the negotiation. A commitment to try to win and let the other party win too—the essence of a win-win strategy—increases the chances that the negotiation will continue until a final agreement is reached. A win-win strategy, although it seems to make good sense, is not always easy to follow, because negotiators tend to be protective of their interests and do not want to lose anything. For some negotiators, the goal is to prevent losses rather than accumulate gains, and this goal is usually inconsistent with a win-win strategy, because it is rare that both parties can win without cost.

Stonewalling is used to slow down the negotiation process. Some negotiators look for bargain solutions and practice stonewalling to wait for the bargains to appear. Negotiators need to learn how to break through stone walls and get the negotiation process moving again. One useful tactic is to set deadlines for decisions.

Some negotiators present themselves as good Samaritans and try to convince the other parties of their beneficent motives. This kind of behavior should send up a warning signal. Most "good Samaritan" negotiators are dishonest and their protestations of good intentions are a sham. To counteract this strategy, the other parties need to refocus on the facts and get away from considering motives.

A good example of finessing the process is to engage in a form of brinkmanship and confront the other parties with a stark choice: accept the terms of agreement currently on offer or watch the negotiation process disintegrate. This strategy can sometime scare parties into accepting terms they otherwise wouldn't have agreed to, but it runs the risk of causing a lose-lose situation—that is, if the negotiations really end without an agreement.

Some negotiators and partners are committed to compromise and are willing to split the differences in order to come to a solution. The negative side of this strategy may be a half win-win situation with losses involved for all partners. The selection of this strategy must be weighed carefully to determine its relevance to a specific set of negotiations.

There are also strategies that micromanage the process and are so detail-based that very little seems to be done. The nickel and dime strategy is a very slow one where each element is evaluated piece by piece. The advantage of this strategy is that it lessens the disagreements of the parties to the negotiation. On the negative side, it often seems that a final agreement is not reached.

Most people feel more secure on their own turf, and negotiators who demand that the negotiation talks take place in their work environment are trying to control the action. If any of the negotiators feel uncomfortable with a potential meeting location, neutral territory should be found.

Language is not a perfect tool, and there is likely to be some unclarity of meaning and some vagueness to any agreement no matter how long and carefully the negotiators work on it. What have to be watched out for are cases of intentional ambiguity, where one of the negotiators tries to keep the language so loose that the agreement doesn't adequately resolve the pertinent issues but merely seems to. Of course, the negotiators may allow some loose ends to remain untied in order to permit flexibility in the interpretation of the agreement, but they should do this with their eyes open and not be fooled into doing it.

Because some negotiating strategies are deceitful, negotiators need to learn defensive techniques to combat these strategies. Public health leaders acting as negotiators must thoroughly understand the negotiation process and the major impediments to a successful completion of the process.

Sometimes a negotiator will decide that a point in the negotiations has been reached beyond which no further concessions will even be entertained.[55] Though dangerous, because it can cause the negotiations to break down entirely, this strategy has the potential to force the parties to come to some kind of agreement.

Some strategies, including stonewalling and the no-concessions strategy just mentioned, can cause negotiations to become deadlocked. Because a deadlock is an impasse, negotiators should have on hand strategies to break deadlocks. One strategy is a return to one of the prenegotiation steps in order to clarify issues and goals and thereby get the negotiations back on track.

The twelfth strategy listed is abbreviated as HRESSC (high realistic expectations with small systematic concessions).[56] Negotiators who use this strategy maintain expectations that are high but can be met. They also realize they will have to make some concessions in order to keep the negotiation process headed toward completion. Because the expectations are high, the concessions and trade-offs tend to be small.

Some negotiators start the negotiating process by making concessions immediately. This strategy can disarm the other party and actually lead to a better outcome for the party using the strategy. It is best employed from a position of strength. If the party doing the conceding is perceived as weak, the other party will view the strategy as a further sign of weakness and may try to push its own agenda as far as it can, defeating the purpose of the strategy.

The next strategy involves a focus on problem solving. The strategy demonstrates that there is confusion between conflict resolution strategies oriented to the long term and problem solving, which tends to be more short-term in effect. Many factors and interests enter into negotiation.

One delaying tactic used by negotiators is to direct attention to goals or issues that are peripheral to the main goals or issues. This may seem to be a counterproductive strategy, but in some situations it can in fact clarify the major interests involved, prevent a breakdown in the negotiation process, allow important information to be discovered, and influence the other parties to come to a resolution more quickly.

Finally, negotiators make use of closure strategies to get an agreement written and accepted by all parties. Once this is done, closure can occur. However, a decision may be made to review progress in a specified period of time.

Every negotiation is unique, and negotiators often combine standard strategies or create new ones to deal with the specifics of the individual case. Exercise 14-2, adapted from a case study by Jurkowski and Neuberger,[57] presents a scenario in which the students have the opportunity to carry out a negotiation regarding a critical public health problem. The students can either use some of the strategies described above or create their own strategies.

Negotiation is a complex type of process that has many potential pitfalls. It is related to the other types of process described in this chapter, and indeed decision making, problem solving, and conflict resolution can all play a role in typical negotiations. Public health leaders must:

- learn to resolve conflict through negotiation, adjudication, mediation, and arbitration
- learn various methods for carrying out negotiations
- use well-trained and experienced negotiators for negotiating with other parties
- make sure that the negotiators have skills and abilities described in this section
- learn to use the "Getting to Yes" and the Schoenfield and Schoenfield negotiation models
- master the steps of the negotiation process
- learn the standard negotiation strategies and tactics

## Summary

This chapter has presented new tools to add to the public health leadership toolkit. Public health leadership, like other kinds of leadership, encompasses the essential activities of decision making, conflict resolution, and negotiation. Public health leaders who lack the skills needed to perform these activities will fail, at least partially, to live up to their responsibility as leaders.

Further, to develop these skills, they must open up the public health leadership toolkit and work with the tools, even if they are less adept at using them than more experienced colleagues.

Learning new skills is difficult and requires dedication and a willingness to take risks. Leaders who put in the time and effort, however, will soon master the skills and become expert at making decisions, resolving conflicts, and negotiating agreements that are beneficial to their organizations.

### Discussion Questions

1. Why is risk taking an important part of public health leadership?
2. What are three examples in which you have taken a leadership risk during the last year?
3. What are the differences and similarities between decision making and problem solving?

4. What are some effective conflict resolution strategies?
5. Is intraorganizational conflict always to be avoided? Explain.
6. What are some usual obstacles to successful negotiation?
7. What is the difference between mediation and negotiation?
8. What are the key elements in the prenegotiation phase and the negotiation phase?
9. What are some common negotiation strategies?

## Exercise 14-1: Decision-making Styles

*Purpose:* to explore two models of decision-making styles

*Key concepts:* decision-making styles

*Procedure:* Divide the class or training group into groups of five to seven people. Each group discusses what is involved in being a good decision maker. Discuss your personal experience in making decisions with your group. For example, how did you make a decision to either take this class or come to this training workshop? Pick a decision that you made at work and one you made at home. Did your style shift in the two different situations? Using the Mintzberg and the Robbins and Coulter models of decision-making styles, do you fit in one or more categories in the two models. Compare and contrast the two models. Does your style change in a team situation where you are the sole decision maker? What are the leadership issues in your decision-making style?

## Exercise 14-2: The Meaning of Conflict

*Purpose:* to recognize the causes of conflict and how to resolve conflict

*Key concepts:* conflict, conflict resolution

*Procedure:* The class should break into groups of 8 to 10 members. First, each group member offers one word in reaction to the term "conflict." The words are put on a large sheet of paper and discussed by the group. The group then divides into two subgroups, one of which assumes the role of a team from the local health department, the second of which assumes the role of a management team from a local health maintenance organization (HMO). The HMO wants to build a major new medical center on land owned by the city, but the public health department wants the land for a new substance abuse clinic. Each team explains its position, and together they try to resolve the conflict between them.

## Exercise 14-3: Negotiation and HIV Prevention Case

*Purpose:* to explore the use of negotiation techniques to address a major community health problem

*Key concepts:* coalition building, negotiation, prenegotiation, win-win strategy

*Scenario:* The Benton County HIV Prevention Council has experienced internal disagreements about how to allocate federal funds for human immunodeficiency virus (HIV)/acquired immune deficiency syndrome (AIDS) community programs. Some members of the council adamantly reject needle exchange programs whereas others are strongly in favor of them. Because the conflict between the council representatives has lasted more than two years, the council has agreed to implement a negotiation process to build an agenda and protocol to guide the allocation of financial resources for HIV/AIDS prevention and treatment. The key players include a variety of stakeholders and constituency groups from the local department of health (located in Hamilton, the largest city in the county), the Benton County Health Department, and the community at large. Substance abuse is a major problem in Hamilton, and the number of reported HIV/AIDS cases has doubled in the last five years. HIV/AIDS cases are also increasing in the rural areas of the county. The Benton County Board of Health has hired a professional negotiator to work with the Benton County HIV Prevention Council. The county has also been informed that it will receive a million dollars from the federal government to fund the protocol that is developed.

*Procedure:* The class should divide into groups of eight. Seven of the group act as members of the Benton County HIV/AIDS Prevention Council, taking a specific role and position as discussed in the group before starting the exercise. For example, one person can be a conservative minister. One individual becomes the negotiator. The group should spend an hour negotiating an end to the conflict using the Fisher et al. model and another hour using the 14 steps of the Schoenfield and Schoenfield model, if possible. If both models are used, the group should discuss the similarities and differences between the two models. Once all groups have completed their comparison of the two models, a representative from each group should present a five-minute talk to other groups about the negotiation process, and then all groups should engage in a discussion about the negotiation strategies that were used.

Benton County Cast of Characters

| | |
|---|---|
| Connie Sultan | Professional Negotiator |
| I. M. Leader | Director of the Benton County Health Department |
| Rev. Smith | Minister of the Benton County Methodist Church |
| Sally Justice | Social Worker, Hamilton AIDS Foundation |
| Tom Driver | Chief executive officer of Benton County Admiral Motors Company |
| Guy Brown | President, Benton County Gay and Lesbian Alliance |
| Vera Straight | President, Hamilton Parent Teachers Assembly |
| Berry Organized | Hamilton City Manager |

*Source:* Adapted from E. Jurkowski and B. Neuberger, *Negotiation Skills for Community Resource Planning,* 1995, the Centers for Disease Control and Prevention, Illinois Public Health Leadership Institute.

# References

1. M. DePree, "The Leaders Legacy," in *Leader to Leader,* eds. F. Hesselbein and P. M. Cohen (San Francisco: Jossey-Bass, 1999).

2. J. M. Kouzes and B. Z. Posner, *The Leadership Challenge,* 4th ed. (San Francisco: Jossey-Bass, 2007).

3. N. L. Frigon and J. K. Jackson Jr., *The Leader* (New York: AMACOM [American Management Association], 1996).

4. M. H. Bazerman and D. Chugh, "Decisions Without Blinders," *Harvard Business Review* 84, no. 1 (2006): 88–97.

5. R. Fritz, *Corporate Tides* (San Francisco: Berrett-Koehler, 1996).

6. P. Hersey et al., *Management of Organizational Behavior,* 9th ed. (Upper Saddle River, NJ: Prentice Hall, 2007).

7. J. Pfeffer, *Managing with Power* (Boston: Harvard Business School Press, 1992).

8. Fritz, *Corporate Tides.*

9. D. J. Snowden and M. E. Boone, "A Leader's Framework for Decision Making," *Harvard Business Review* 85, no. 11 (2007): 68–76.

10. H. Mintzberg, *Mintzberg on Management* (New York: The Free Press, 1989).

11. D. Osborne and T. Gaebler, *Reinventing Government: How the Entrepreneurial Spirit Is Transforming the Public Sector* (Reading, MA: Addison-Wesley, 1992).

12. Mintzberg, *Mintzberg on Management.*

13. S. P. Robbins and M. Coulter, *Management,* 8th ed. (Upper Saddle River, NJ: Prentice Hall, 2005).

14. Robbins and Coulter, *Management.*

15. S. P. Robbins and D. A. DeCenzo, *Supervision Today,* 2nd ed. (Upper Saddle River, NJ: Prentice Hall, 1997).

16. Robbins and Coulter, *Management.*

17. J. L. Pressman and A. Wildavsky, *Implementation,* 3rd ed. (Berkeley, CA: University of California Press, 1984).

18. Robbins and Coulter, *Management.*

19. Robbins and Coulter, *Management.*

20. J. G. Liebler and C. R. McConnell, *Management Principles for Health Professionals,* 4th ed. (Sudbury, MA: Jones and Bartlett, 2004).

21. Robbins and Coulter, *Management.*

22. B. Wall et al., *The Visionary Leader* (Rocklin, CA: Prima Publishing & Communication, 1992).

23. A. J. DuBrin, *The Complete Idiot's Guide to Leadership* (New York: Alpha Books, 1998).

24. J. A. Schellenberg, *Conflict Resolution: Theory, Research, and Practice* (Albany, NY: State University of New York Press, 1996).

25. Liebler and McConnell, *Management Principles for Health Professionals.*

26. Robbins and Coulter, *Management.*

27. P. C. Nutt, *Making Tough Choices* (San Francisco: Jossey-Bass, 1989).

28. W. Hendricks, *How to Manage Conflict* (Shawnee Mission, KS: National Press Publications, 1991).

29. D. Weeks, *The Eight Essential Steps to Conflict Resolution* (New York: Jeremy P. Tarcher and Putnam Books, 1994).

30. Liebler and McConnell, *Management Principles for Health Professionals.*

31. M. Winer and K. Ray, *Collaboration Handbook* (St. Paul, MN: Amherst H. Wilder Foundation, 1994).

32. DuBrin, *The Complete Idiot's Guide to Leadership.*

33. Robbins and Coulter, *Management.*

34. A. Rahim, *Organizational Conflict Inventories* (Palo Alto, CA: Consulting Psychologists Press, 1983).

35. Robbins and Coulter, *Management.*

36. Weeks, *The Eight Essential Steps to Conflict Resolution.*

37. Schellenberg, *Conflict Resolution.*

38. R. Fisher et al., *Getting to Yes,* 2nd ed. (New York: Penguin Books, 1991).

39. F. E. Jandt, *Win-Win Negotiating* (New York: Wiley and Paul Gillett Books, 1985).

40. M. K. Schoenfield and R. M. Schoenfield, *The McGraw-Hill 36-Hour Negotiating Course* (New York: McGraw-Hill, 1991).
41. H. Raiffa, *The Art and Science of Negotiation* (Cambridge, MA: Harvard University Press, 1982).
42. Raiffa, *The Art and Science of Negotiation.*
43. Robbins and Coulter, *Management.*
44. Robbins and Coulter, *Management.*
45. Jandt, *Win-Win Negotiating.*
46. Fisher et al., *Getting to Yes.*
47. Jandt, *Win-Win Negotiating.*
48. Jandt, *Win-Win Negotiating.*
49. Schoenfield and Schoenfield, *The McGraw-Hill 36-Hour Negotiating Course.*
50. E. Jurkowski and B. Neuberger, *Negotiation Skills for Community Resource Planning* (Chicago: Illinois Public Health Leadership Institute, 1995).
51. R. Fisher and D. Ertel, *Getting Ready to Negotiate* (New York: Penguin Books, 1995).
52. Schoenfield and Schoenfield, *The McGraw-Hill 36-Hour Negotiating Course.*
53. G. Fuller, *The Negotiator's Handbook* (Paramus, NJ: Prentice Hall, 1991).
54. Schoenfield and Schoenfield, *The McGraw-Hill 36-Hour Negotiating Course.*
55. Schoenfield and Schoenfield, *The McGraw-Hill 36-Hour Negotiating Course.*
56. Schoenfield and Schoenfield, *The McGraw-Hill 36-Hour Negotiating Course.*
57. Jurkowski and Neuberger, *Negotiation Skills for Community Resource Planning.*

# CHAPTER 15

# CULTURAL COMPETENCY

> Only by venturing into the unknown do we enable
> new ideas to take shape, and those shapes are different
> for each voyager.
>
> Margaret Wheatley, *Leadership and the New Science*

By the year 2030, racial and ethnic minorities are expected to total 40% of the U.S. population (Figure 15-1), up from 25% at the start of the new century.[1] In 2000, African-Americans represented about 12.3% of the population, Hispanic or Latino about 12.5%, Asians about 3.6%, and other groups at about 8% (Table 15-1).[2] As a result, the professions, like the general population, will include a steadily increasing percentage of ethnically diverse populations as members. The growth in minority representation will bring both challenge and promise.

A recent federal report on the public health workforce in the 21st century stated that it would be in the best interests of the American public to be served by a workforce that is ethnically and culturally diverse.[3] Furthermore, a study of middle-class Americans found that these Americans generally support multiculturalism.[4] However, they also generally believe that all immigrants should learn English and become integrated into American society—a point of view referred to as "benign multiculturalism."[5] Many immigrants and native-born people think that the emphasis on integration into the mainstream is a form of disrespect toward and denigration of the cultural values of the diverse minority groups that make up a large portion of the U.S. population. In short, it seems as if recent attempts to value the full range of diverse population groups have been a failure.[6] Some of these issues are explored in Case Study 15-A, which explores the issue of racism in a small rural city undergoing demographic change.

**Racial and Ethnic Distribution of the Population, Actual and Projected Percent**

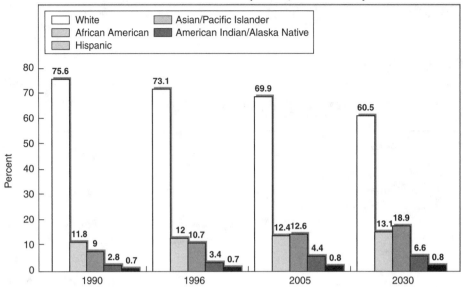

**FIGURE 15-1   Diversity in the United States. Minority (African American, Hispanic, Asian/Pacific Islander, American Indian/Alaska Native) Representation in the U.S. Population is expected to exceed 30 percent within the decade and climb to nearly 40 percent by 2030.**
*Source:* Reprinted from Statistical Abstract of the U.S., 1997 MidProjection Series, Bureau of the Census.

**Table 15-1   Population by Race and Hispanic Origin for the United States: 2000**

| Race and Hispanic or Latino | Number (in thousands) | Percent of Total Population |
|---|---|---|
| RACE | | |
| Total Population | 281,421 | 100.0 |
| One race | 274,595 | 97.6 |
| White | 211,460 | 75.1 |
| Black or African-American | 34,658 | 12.3 |
| American Indian and Alaska Native | 2,475 | 0.9 |
| Asian | 10,242 | 3.6 |
| Native Hawaiian and Other Pacific Islander | 399 | 0.1 |
| Some other race | 15,359 | 5.5 |
| Two or more races | 6,826 | 2.4 |
| HISPANIC OR LATINO | | |
| Total population | 281,421 | 100.0 |
| Hispanic or Latino | 35,305 | 12.5 |
| Not Hispanic or Latino | 246,116 | 87.5 |

*Source:* U.S. Census Bureau, Census 2000. In *Population Profile of the United States: 2000* (Internet Release).

---

## Case Study 15-A
## Racism: A Mental Health Issue

*D. Clemons, J. A. Janssen, K. Pakieser-Reed, J. Pitzer, and S. Strachniak*

### Background

A Mexican-American male (father of two children, married, intact family) was accused of molesting a young "white" girl. The incident occurred in Harvest City. The allegation was publicized in the local paper. A group of Anglo males gathered outside the Mexican-American's home and stoned it. Two Anglos were arrested for ethnic intimidation. The charge against the Mexican-American male was dropped as a false charge, without publicity.

The local newspaper's editorial declared the incident was racist in nature and stated that the community cannot "sweep [it] under the carpet." Local church leaders offered (1) to facilitate the process of cultural awareness by the majority population of the minority population, (2) to increase awareness of racism in the community, and (3) to increase understanding among people.

The Harvest City Council established a human relations committee in the fall of 1991 and hired Mr. George as a consultant to help define the committee's role. As a result of George's actions, the city forwarded a survey to the local schools for distribution to all parents and high school seniors. The survey focused on identifying the perceived community needs as determined by the parents and seniors. The committee's actions would then be directed by the survey results. In the spring of 1992, tension continued to grow, and some fighting occurred between Anglos and Hispanics in the Harvest community.

The human relations committee sponsored "Fiesta Days" to increase cultural awareness in a fun atmosphere in the summer of 1992. The celebration was a success!

### Case Study Chronology

*Fall 1992*

Tension increased between Anglo and Hispanic students at Harvest High School. The Harvest City Council Human Relations Committee met with the dean of students to discuss the problem. They determined that this was not a gang problem but did have some "ganglike" aspects. The school hired George to serve as a consultant and to develop plans to deflate the racial tension. The Harvest police chief said that the problems were the responsibility of the parents and that the parents needed to be involved in the solutions.

Fistfights broke out among the Anglo and Hispanic students at Harvest High School and Junior High School. Both Anglo and Hispanic students were suspended. School officials believed that the fights were racially motivated. (About 10% of the high school students were Hispanic.) Additional fights between Anglos and Hispanics were reported at various locations within the community.

The Temporary Farmers Association approached the Macmillian County Mental Health Board with a request for funding a mental health advocate position (Hispanic liaison) that would be "bilingual and bicultural and dedicated to improving the

*(continues)*

**Case Study 15-A** *continued*

accessibility and quality of mental health and social services for the Hispanic residents of Macmillian County." The association stated that a growing number of residents in the county were Hispanic, spoke only Spanish, and were becoming an "at-risk" population due to little or no access to services that would improve their lives. The board denied the request and recommended formation of a task force to study the issue.

In a separate request, the Temporary Farmers Association requested funding from the Macmillian County Mental Health Board for a six-month study of racism in the county and its effects on the mental health of Hispanic residents. This project was funded.

As a result of the Mental Health Board's recommendation, an Hispanic connection task force was developed, primarily through the efforts of the association. The task force represented almost all of the social service, law enforcement, and religious organizations within the county. In its first meeting, the task force discussed the difficulties of providing services to the Hispanic population. The task force concluded that each member organization would benefit from the services of a countywide Hispanic liaison. They also decided that a "needs assessment should be done to determine county resources and needs regarding Hispanics."

The task force met a second time to design the needs assessment survey and to identify who should receive it. The task force also discussed the Hispanic liaison position: what should be the focus, where would the position be "housed," and how would it be funded? The members agreed that the position should be within the Temporary Farmers Association because the association was the "only agency within the county that has an ongoing and committed relationship with the county's Hispanic population." They also agreed that it must be apparent that all of the task force's member agencies endorsed and supported the liaison role and that the task force would actively support and coach the person chosen as liaison.

In an unrelated action, the Harvest City Council Human Relations Committee requested from the Macmillian County Mental Health Board funding for and/or assistance with the creation of workplace cultural diversity training programs to build bridges between people (Anglos and Hispanics). The project was not funded because it did not directly relate to the provision of mental health services.

*Winter 1992–1993*
The Hispanic Connection Task Force forwarded a survey to social service and mental health agencies to "better assess available county resources and needs related to our Hispanic population."

A second survey, one for the Hispanic community, was developed by the Hispanic Connection Task Force and distributed to the population through member agencies of the task force. Survey results were slow coming in, partially due to the length of the survey. The task force extended the time for the survey to receive sufficient responses to make a conclusion.

After summarizing results from both needs assessments, the task force developed and forwarded a resolution to government and social service agencies countywide. The resolution acknowledged the value of ethnic and cultural diversity and showed the organizations' support of the Hispanic liaison position. Sixty organizations signed the resolution, including churches, libraries, and mental health and health organizations as well as the county board.

The Macmillian County Board voted 19–2 in support of the liaison position. However, some board members felt that all non-English-speaking residents should have liaison services available to them and that the position as proposed was providing Hispanics with special status. No funding decision was made with this vote.

Following the passing of the resolution, the Macmillian County Mental Health Board approved partial funding for a Hispanic liaison position as presented by the Temporary Farmers Association. They forwarded information about the position and a request for the second half of the salary (up to $20,000) to the Macmillian County Mental Health Board and Human Services Committee. The mental health board felt that the liaison position would help the Hispanic population of 11,000 people access mental health, school, social service, and government programs and enhance their functioning within the county as a whole. The mental health board felt that prevention and lessening of barriers would decrease the likelihood of more intensive (and expensive) mental health interventions in the future. The liaison would also be responsible for community coordination between Latino and non-Latino organizations.

*Spring 1993*

Two agencies that did not originally sign the resolution altered their positions to a more positive stance regarding the liaison position. The All Faith Church wrote a letter to the Macmillian County Mental Health Board in full support of the liaison position. Charitable Services signed the resolution with qualifications noted.

The Macmillian County Board and Human Services Committee voted in favor of funding the liaison position to "bridge the cultural gap between Hispanics and county officials in delivering services." Prior to the vote, one member of the committee raised the question of the appropriateness of mental health funds being allocated for a Hispanic liaison position that was developed in response to racist actions. Members of the committee who voted for the position felt that racism was a mental health issue. The committee forwarded the position and funding request to the Macmillian County Board Finance Committee for final recommendation to the county board.

A week after the health and human services committee voted in favor of the liaison position, Charitable Services stated that it had been providing liaison services for the past three and a half years in Harvest and Stone Lake. The county board chairperson, Ms. Ace, stated that she would investigate to see if the new liaison services were needed and would determine if it was appropriate for the county board to fund the position. The mental health board president, Mr. Jones, stated that the proposed liaison position was much broader in scope than the newly discovered social service position.

The county board chairperson decided to not recommend funding to the finance committee of the county board for the proposed liaison position until the Temporary Farmers Association and Charitable Services met, discussed the proposed position, and resolved funding issues. (By now, both groups wanted to be considered for the total of $40,000 salary funds.) The groups agreed to meet with the mental health board executive director, Mr. Jones, and come to a resolution.

Mr. Jones and Ms. Hope, Temporary Farmers Association director, kept a scheduled meeting with the Macmillian County Board Finance Committee to discuss the position. The committee then voted 4–3 against funding the position but agreed to discuss the position again in two months after further study.

*(continues)*

**Case Study 15-A** *continued*

The Charitable Services and Temporary Farmers Association directors met and clarified the roles of the two liaison positions. A letter was sent to the county board chairperson noting the clarification and joint support of the new position as proposed.

In the meantime, the mental health board voted to fund the proposed liaison position on a full-time basis for six months. The board felt that the issue was too important to wait for a final funding vote by the county board. The Temporary Farmers Association had to make a decision whether to take the risk and hire a full-time liaison or wait for the county board's funding decision.

The Temporary Farmers Association filled the position; Mr. George gave up his SASS position to become the liaison through November with the hope that additional funds would be approved by the county board.

Two months later, after a positive recommendation from Ms. Ace, the Macmillian County Board Finance Committee met again and unanimously recommended funding of the position through FY 93. The next month, the finance committee's recommendation for funding went to the full county board. The vote was 20–4 in favor of funding the position.

Since 1993, the position has continued to be funded jointly by the county board and the mental health board and has been responsible for the development of five community human relations councils and hundreds of interventions with the Latino and non-Latino communities on individual and organizational levels.

**Conclusion**

Racism is a topic that many people would rather not address, as evidenced by the population described at the beginning of the case study. When racism finally reaches a level that cannot easily be ignored, ownership of the resolution process can be difficult to determine.

Racism can be evidenced by property and personal damages. Wouldn't the proper "owner of the problem" be the legal and law enforcement authorities? When the symptoms lead to physical harm that requires medical attention, then wouldn't the "owner" be the health care institution? If the symptoms are acts of disregard for the human spirit, then isn't the rightful "owner" the church membership? What symptoms need to be exhibited for the problem of racism to fall under the ownership of mental health?

Using the core values of public health as a guideline, answers to these questions can be achieved, as well as a perspective on how racism becomes a public health problem falling within the purview of mental health.

---

Public health leaders, to function effectively in a more culturally diverse environment, will have to confront their personal prejudices and stereotypes and take measures to overcome them. They also should try to understand the nature of the challenges presented by increased cultural diversity at the organizational and community levels.[7] First, many people want to maintain things as they are because they feel comfortable with the familiar. Second, some people are prejudiced against certain racial or ethnic groups because of how they were raised. Third, organizations often use impersonal hiring methods and favor people who fit the organizational mode, which usually means people like those who are already organizational members.

Affirmative action programs were instituted to address the fact that the makeup of many organizations did not reflect the makeup of the general population. Their goal is not to obliterate differences but rather to create an environment in which cultural diversity becomes a strength: having employees with a range of different backgrounds and cultural values can create synergy and lead to greater effectiveness. A synergistic system is not one in which individual differences are obliterated but rather one in which the parts work together harmoniously. Therefore, if public health leaders are to be successful in the 21st century, they need to deal with the issue of cultural diversity today and learn to appreciate the diversity that exists in our society.[8] In the past, leaders expected people to adjust to the existing organizational culture and suppress their unique characteristics. This expectation has ceased to be a reasonable one.

Moreover, no public health agency operates independently of other organizations, the community in which it is located, or, for that matter, other parts of the globe. Global health issues have a way of affecting local communities. Thus, local public health leaders may find themselves dealing with an extremely diverse range of colleagues from around the world, one more reason for these leaders to work at becoming culturally competent.

## Multiculturalism

Multiculturalism is tied to what has been called the "politics of recognition."[9] Each cultural group in an organization, community, or country strives for acceptance. If not accepted, the group feels demeaned or looked down upon. The politics of recognition are not new in the United States. Different cultural groups have repeatedly fought for public recognition.

The nature and degree of the public's commitment to multiculturalism are not easy to determine.[10] For instance, public health leaders and others argue in support of "multiculturalism" but typically expect different cultural groups to accept the dominant Western European culture. Public health organizations need to review, restudy, rethink, and reorganize their structure in order to truly become multicultural.[11] Differences based on culture and language should enhance the profession of public health community rather than create divisions within it. Yet divisiveness seems to be increasing.

Culturally competent leaders have the skills and attitudes needed to relate to people with different backgrounds and with different characteristics, including people of different races, genders, ages, sexual orientations, social classes, and lifestyles (see Table 15-2).[12] One way to develop these skills is to walk around the workplace and the community and talk to people regularly. Furthermore, talking directly to individuals defuses friction caused by cultural differences. The development of others is clearly an important role for leaders and managers. There are a number of multicultural principles to keep in mind when working with people with different backgrounds:[13]

1. Understand your own cultural background and respect the background of others.
2. Lessen individualism and promote the value of teams and working together.

**Table 15-2    Categories of Diversity**

Race

Sex

Religion

Age (young, middle-aged, old)

Ethnicity (country of origin)

Education

Job-relevant abilities

Mental disabilities (attention deficit disorder)

Physical disabilities (hearing impairment, wheelchair use)

Values and motivation

Sexual orientation (heterosexual, homosexual, bisexual)

Marital status (married, single, cohabiting, widow, widower)

Family status (children, no children, two-parent family, single parent, grandparent)

Personality traits (introverted, extroverted, conscientious)

Functional background (area of specialization)

Technology interest (high-tech, low-tech, technophobe)

Weight (average, obese, underweight, anorexic)

Hair (full head of hair, bald, wild hair, tame hair, long hair, short hair)

Tobacco use (smoker versus nonsmoker, chewer versus nonchewer)

Gum use (chewer versus nonchewer)

Styles of clothing and appearance (dress up, dress down, professional appearance, casual appearance)

*Source:* Reprinted with the permission of Alpha Books, an imprint of Macmillan USA, a division of Pearson Education, from *The Complete Idiot's Guide to Leadership,* by Andrew Dubrin. Copyright © 1998.

3. Demonstrate an empathy for others.
4. Share leadership.
5. Promote social justice and health equity.
6. Make servant leadership your goal.
7. Develop a shared vision with the community.
8. Utilize culturally appropriate language.
9. Treat people like family.
10. Promote "gratitude, hope, and forgiveness."

Public health leaders must get to know not only their workforce but also their community. Getting out of the office and meeting with different cultural groups helps leaders define the public health needs of the community better and also presents the public health agency in a better light. The agency might hold an open house to allow the community to get a better sense of what a public health agency does. An agency leader might invite residents from a range of backgrounds to his or her home for a party. By eating at local ethnic restaurants, leaders can learn about different cultural groups and reach out to those groups at the same time. Public health practitioners in general should be encouraged to learn languages, because being able to speak the native language of a community group will enhance the public health agency's credibility.

Although most cross-border alliances are business related, public health leaders may be involved in the creation of a cross-border alliance or partnership, in which case they need to engage in assessing and understanding the cultural differences that exist as one of the preliminary steps.[14] Further, they must continue to address cultural factors even when they seem to have become less important. Management of cultural differences should be a part of any cross-cultural relationship.

To increase their cultural competency and act with cultural sensitivity, leaders should follow these five guidelines:

1. They need to be aware of their own strengths and weaknesses as well as their own prejudices. Without this kind of self-awareness, they will not be able to address effectively the cultural issues that arise in their organization.
2. They need to be alert for opportunities to receive feedback. Feedback, in this area as well as others, is an important information source.
3. They need to become lifelong learners always on the lookout for new knowledge and skill development opportunities.
4. They need to integrate work life with personal life and to maintain a multicultural perspective in both.
5. They also need to learn to respect the differences between people. Out of existing differences can come strength.

Multicultural issues need to be addressed early in the formulation of a multicultural team, coalition, or partnership.[15] Exercise 15-1 was developed by Rosenthal to gauge the effectiveness of a group in addressing multicultural issues. To deal with multicultural issues, public health leaders must:

- learn how to analyze demographic data
- study social, economic, and political trends
- increase the number of minority public health staff so that the agency's makeup reflects the community's makeup
- consult with community leaders with different cultural backgrounds to guarantee that the programs developed fit the needs of the relevant cultural groups
- use feedback to monitor communication with cultural groups
- evaluate the workplace using the inclusivity checklist (see Exercise 15-1)

## Cultural Diversity

Cultural diversity programs are distinct from affirmative action programs. Affirmative action programs are generally intended to guarantee access to jobs by minority groups. Cultural diversity programs address the differences between people and try to ensure that people from different cultural backgrounds respect each other and are able to work together in harmony. They teach people to look beyond race, gender, and sexual orientation, for example, and treat each individual with the full respect due a human being. Diversity issues need to be incorporated into the strategic thinking activities of leaders. One interesting program was developed at IBM where it was thought that the needs of different groups might require different approaches.[16] With diversity as a strategic goal, IBM developed eight tasks forces to deal with these issues, including a group on Asian issues, African-American issues, issues of people with disabilities, white males issues, women issues, issues related to sexual orientation, Hispanic and Latino concerns, and issues of Native Americans. In Exercise 15-2, students explore the cultural diversity that exists among themselves with the purpose of gaining greater cultural understanding.

It is imperative that leaders view multicultural differences from a positive perspective rather than a negative one. Negativism undermines the communication process and obstructs the positive effects of building community partnerships. It is worth pointing out here the essential role that communication plays in dealing with cultural diversity. Little progress can be made unless everyone understands each other. Note that communication encompasses vocal inflections, hand gestures, and other types of nonverbal communication.

The two major ways in which diversity has been viewed in the workplace are limiting in perspective.[17] The first diversity paradigm has been defined as the discrimination and fairness model. With an awareness that discrimination and segregation are a reality, this model posits the negative aspects of discrimination, and fairness is required in recruitment, hiring, and retention of employees from different gender, racial, and ethnic groups. The second model is an access and legitimacy model. Here agencies will attempt to hire people that fit the demographic profile of the community that is being served. Thomas and Ely find this model lacking in that people hired under this model feel marginalized.[18] A third paradigm is emerging in which the values and perspectives of diverse people are incorporated into the mission, vision, and work of the organization. In order to shift to this new paradigm, leaders in the organization must understand the value of diversity as well as the learning opportunities that become available. High performance standards will be required of all staff. Training programs are important as well.

> **Leadership Tip**
>
> *Having friends at work keeps you more committed to your organization.*

Public health leaders must keep track of trends that have the potential to affect the extent and nature of the cultural diversity confronting them, such as the globalization of business, changing community demographics, and the ways of dealing with cultural diversity, such as new types of programs. Public health leaders must be devoted to promoting the health of everyone in the community, including members of diverse minority populations. The special health needs of these populations and their lack of access to programs and services must be addressed. Noncommonality of language is sometimes an obstacle in the way of residents receiving needed services, and public health leaders need to ensure that individuals who do not speak English will still get the care or services they require.

A report of the President's Initiative on Race cited major health findings regarding culturally diverse populations.[19] For example, the infant mortality rate is two and a half times higher for African-Americans and one and a half times higher for Native Americans than for whites. In 1995, the age-adjusted rate of death attributable to heart disease for African-Americans was 147 deaths per 100,000 people, compared with 105 deaths per 100,000 for whites and 108 deaths per 100,000 overall. The number of new acquired immune deficiency syndrome cases among African-Americans is now greater than the number of new cases among whites. The prevalence of diabetes is 70% higher among African-Americans than among whites, and the prevalence among Hispanics is nearly double the prevalence among whites. As for national immunization rates, 79% of white children less than two years of age have the full series of vaccinations, whereas only 74% of African-American youngsters and 71% of Hispanic youngsters do. There are inequities in access to health care as well. For example, minority mothers are less likely than white mothers to get prenatal care. Access seems to be directly related to income level, which partly explains why certain minority groups have low rates of service use. Another access-related issue is whether a cultural group favors using traditional healers rather than medical school–trained physicians.

Figure 15-2 presents an interactionist model showing how diversity influences the careers of leaders and the effectiveness of their organizations.[20] As can be seen in column one, cultural diversity can have an impact at the individual, team, and agency levels (and, as noted above, it can also influence relations between a public health agency and the community in which it is located). The next two columns list possible effects on the individual and the organization. To get a fix on the diversity climate in an agency or a community, agency leaders can answer the questions in Table 15-3.

If you are trying to develop a diversity training and coaching programs, it is necessary to include several dimensions in the content. Some of these dimensions are:[21]

1. Information and skill development to work with people with diverse backgrounds
2. Use of surveys and personal interviews to address any potential problems
3. Promoting accountability that the agency's diversity goals are being implemented throughout the organization

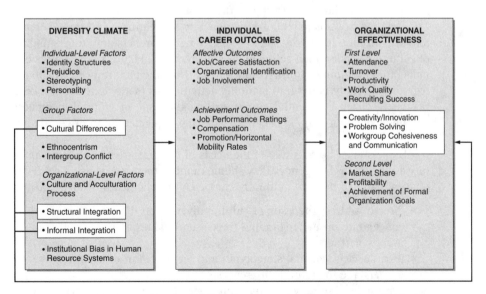

**FIGURE 15-2    An International Model of the Impact of Diversity on Individual Career Outcomes and Organizational Effectiveness**
*Source:* Reprinted with permission of the publisher. From *Cultural Diversity in Organizations,* copyright © 1993 by T. Cox, Jr., Berrett-Koehler Publishers, Inc., San Francisco, CA. All rights reserved. 1-800-929-2929.

**Table 15-3  Diversity Climate Index**

1. Identify personal stereotypes and prejudices.
2. Do these stereotypes affect my job performance?
3. Does the staff in my agency judge others by standards different from community standards?
4. How is intergroup conflict resolved?
5. Within the agency, does the composition of the workforce reflect the community diversity?
6. Are culturally diverse people in the upper echelons of the organization?
7. How do agency personnel interact with the community?
8. How does the community relate to the agency?
9. Does the agency address the key health issues of concern to the community?
10. Have community partnerships been developed?

*Source:* Reprinted with permission of the publisher. From *Cultural Diversity in Organizations,* copyright © 1993 by T. Cox, Jr., Berrett-Koehler Publishers, Inc., San Francisco, CA. All rights reserved. 1-800-929-2929.

4. Work with employees and work teams to make sure diversity is part of the composition of these groups
5. Provide assistance when special needs are apparent
6. Communication strategies related to the organization's commitment to diversity
7. Mentoring and coaching of employees

People with different backgrounds need to be involved in the planning related to any training initiative. It is also important that top leadership and management in the agency support these activities.

The road from merely managing diversity to creating a culturally competent organization has many steps.[22] First comes awareness and understanding of cultural diversity; then action plans are developed. Figure 15-3 presents one model for developing cultural competency.[23] Note the importance given to integrating diversity issues into planning activities. As in any extended process, regular feedback is essential, and revisiting the issue of cultural awareness and understanding may be beneficial after the implementation of certain action steps.

Leaders must be sensitive to the needs of cultural groups in the community as well as in the agency. They should monitor these needs using epidemiological data. To be fully culturally competent, public health leaders must:

- directly address the issue of cultural diversity in the workplace
- concentrate on understanding the cultural values and norms of community partners
- learn to face personal stereotypes and prejudices in order to remove barriers due to cultural differences
- learn to be culturally sensitive and empathic to those they interact with
- evaluate the work environment to determine the positive and negative effects of a diverse workforce
- learn epidemiological techniques for analyzing the health needs of the community

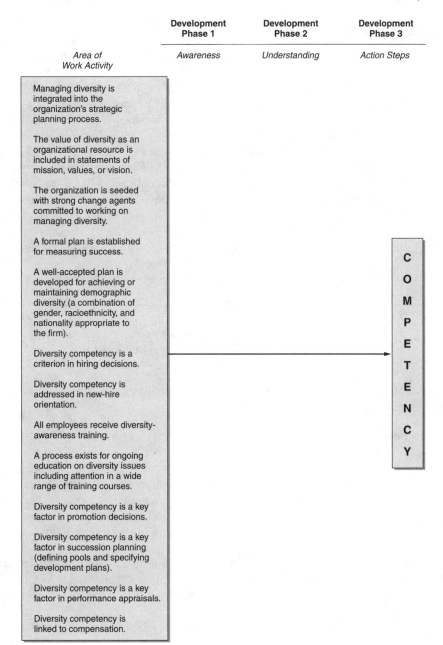

| | Development Phase 1 | Development Phase 2 | Development Phase 3 |
|---|---|---|---|
| *Area of Work Activity* | *Awareness* | *Understanding* | *Action Steps* |

**FIGURE 15-3   Diversity Competency Model of Organizations**
*Source:* Reprinted with permission of the publisher. From *Developing Competency To Manage Diversity,* copyright © 1997 by T. Cox, Jr. and R. L. Beale, Berrett-Koehler Publishers, Inc., San Francisco, CA. All rights reserved. 1-800-929-2929.

- analyze diversity issues at each step in the leadership process
- develop a cultural diversity training program for all employees
- develop a workplace policy statement on cultural differences

Exercise 15-3 provides an opportunity to explore the way in which cultural diversity affects public leadership activities.

## Cultural Competency Skills

Cultural competency includes the willingness and ability to develop programs and services for people of different cultures. As the report of the President's Initiative on Race states, "By understanding, valuing, and incorporating the cultural differences of America's diverse population and examining one's own health-related values and beliefs, health providers deliver more effective and cost-efficient care."[24(p.17)]

Further, public health leaders need to ensure that all agency staff act in a culturally sensitive way by setting and publicizing appropriate policies and procedures. A lack of concern for the needs of culturally diverse populations can have legal consequences. Case Study 15-B involves a discrimination complaint made to an Office for Civil Rights. (This case study was written by a team of public health leaders based on their personal experiences.) Another important set of issues involves a local public health agency and undocumented immigrants. (This case was also written by a team of public health leaders.) Some of these issues are discussed in Case Study 15-C.

---

### Case Study 15-B
### Gold County Health Department:
### A Case of Discrimination Requiring Assessment,
### Policy Development, and Assurance Practices

*Nancy Bluhm, Valerie L. Webb, Ann Rodriguez, Robert Brewster, and Dale W. Galassie*

#### Introduction

The Gold County Health Department received a discrimination complaint from the Office for Civil Rights (OCR) necessitating identification (assessment practices), development of policies and plans (policy development practices), and management of organizational resources (assurance practices) to adequately address the complaint, which claimed a lack of adequate interpreter services. Approximately 46% of this large urban health department's budget was funded by grants or reimbursables now placed at risk due to the discrimination complaint.

The landmark document *Healthy People 2000: National Health Promotion and Disease Prevention Objectives* noted that by the year 2000 the racial and ethnic composition of the American population would differ significantly. Whites will decline in population from 76% to 72% of the population. The Hispanic population could rise from 8% to 11.3%. Blacks could increase their proportion from 12.4% to 13.1%. In addition, other groups are projected to increase from 3.4% to 4.3%. The coloring of the American workforce is clearly evident by these statistics. That information further grounded the need for the Gold County Health Department to offer adequate interpreter services to meet the needs of its constituency.

#### Statement of Facts

The OCR received a complaint filed against the Gold County Health Department on October 8, 1992. The complainant, Mr. Peter Citizen, who filed on behalf of himself and non-English- and limited-English-speaking people, alleged a violation of Title VI of the Civil Rights Act of 1964 and its implementing regulation, 45 CRF Part 80. Specifically, the complainant alleged that the Gold County Health Department discriminated against non-English- and limited-English-speaking people on the basis of national origin by denying and delaying services, requiring them to provide their own interpreters, and treating them in a discriminatory manner, as evidenced by negative comments and a hostile attitude and by assigning them to Spanish-speaking clinics.

The behavior cited in the allegation would constitute a violation of Title VI and its implementing regulation. OCR has jurisdiction over complaints alleging discrimination on the basis of race, color, and national origin by recipients of federal financial assistance. The Gold County Health Department is a recipient of substantial federal financial assistance and is, therefore, subject to the provisions of Title VI, which prohibits such discrimination. The millions of federal dollars received by the agency are for the Alcohol, Drug Abuse, and Mental Health Block Grant, Medicare, and Medicaid programs.

A prompt investigation to determine whether a violation occurred was scheduled by OCR (within 30 days). During the course of the investigation, the OCR representatives advised they would investigate all allegations in the complaint, interview the complainant, contact and develop information from the Gold County Health Department, and interview any witnesses having information or material relevant to the alleged discrimination.

If a violation had occurred, OCR would attempt to bring the affected institution into voluntary compliance through negotiations. If such corrective action was not secured, OCR would initiate formal enforcement action and perhaps freeze future funding.

The OCR Office notified the Gold County Health Department of the following request prior to the investigation scheduled for November 20, 1992:

1. Copies of policies and procedures relating to the provision of translators for people who are non-English- or limited-English-speaking and how this information is disseminated to staff, persons seeking services, and relevant community organizations
2. A description of staff training on how and when to offer and use a translator
3. A list of bilingual staff (or other translators available to the recipient) showing:
   a. Name
   b. Position, unit in which employed or name of outside organization, if appropriate, and telephone number
   c. Language spoken and level of fluency
   d. Hours of availability
   e. For each outside organization used, a copy of any agreement or a description of the nature of the arrangement
4. Copies of brochures, forms, and other information in each language in which they are available
5. An explanation of how written information, policies, consents for treatments, etc. are provided to persons not fluent in English
6. A copy of the complainant's job description
7. Copies of the complainant's past and current work evaluations

### Background

Racial, cultural, and linguistic minorities comprise a rapidly increasing percentage of the county population. The number of Hispanics, for example, increased by 83.1% since 1980.

*(continues)*

**Case Study 15-B** *continued*

**Exhibit 15-B-1    Gold County 1990 Census**

|                              | Total    | Hispanic |
|------------------------------|----------|----------|
| County population            | 516,418  | 38,570   |
| White                        | 450,666  | 20,100   |
| Black                        | 34,771   | 1,035    |
| Asian and Pacific Islander   | 12,588   | 453      |
| American Indian              | 1,198    | 189      |
| Other                        | 17,195   | 16,793   |

**Hispanic Population 1980–90 Change**

| 1980   | 1990   | Number   | Percent |
|--------|--------|----------|---------|
| 21,064 | 38,570 | +17,506  | +83.1%  |

**Hispanic Origins (1990)**

| Mexican         | 27,220 | 5.3%                        |
|-----------------|--------|-----------------------------|
| Puerto Rican    | 4,829  | 0.9%                        |
| Cuban           | 539    | 0.1%                        |
| Other Hispanics | 5,976  | 1.2%                        |
| Hispanic origin | 38,570 | 7.5% of county population   |

The Gold County Health Department, as a major provider of preventive and primary health and mental health services, experienced serious difficulties in meeting the needs of non-English-speaking clients. During 1992, for example, the ambulatory primary health care clinics alone delivered 23,649 patient visits. Hispanics now account for nearly 30% of the visits, with nearly half requiring assistance from bilingual staff.

Other linguistic minorities are also served. In Gold County, the number of major languages spoken at home is representative of the challenges faced by federally funded primary care providers throughout the country.

**Table 15-B-1    Language Spoken at Home (Gold County Census Data)**

| Language | Number of Persons |
|----------|-------------------|
| Spanish  | 30,759            |
| German   | 5,000             |
| Polish   | 3,348             |
| Italian  | 3,041             |
| French   | 2,599             |
| Tagalog  | 2,402             |
| Chinese  | 1,635             |
| Indic    | 1,397             |
| Korean   | 1,248             |
| Slavic   | 1,050             |
| Greek    | 1,028             |

Despite Gold County Health Department's having spent considerable resources to meet multicultural needs through the development of Hispanic clinics, bilingual brochures, and recruitment of minority staff, the OCR investigation directly advised the Gold County Health Department that, effective immediately, Hispanic clinics must be abolished and clients must be served in their primary language.

OCR requested that Gold County Health Department compile and forward the requested information to its office within 20 days of the date of the written request. These data would be retained by the reviewer as partial documentation of the findings.

The Gold County Health Department was in the midst of an administrative transition as well. The executive officer had resigned only two and a half months earlier, and the health board appointed an interim director. The recruitment process for the executive officer occurred at the same time as the complaint investigation.

The breadth of the discrimination complaint required that all clinic facilities countywide be audited for multicultural sensitivity and the ability to meet non-English-speaking clients' needs. In addition, the health board recently had approved a hiring freeze to be implemented on December 1, which would inhibit increasing the current staff to address the need for interpreters.

An on-site investigation was scheduled for November 20, 1992.

---

## Case Study 15-C
## Two Countries/Two Names/Broken Policies

*Lisa Crane, RN, BSN, Laura M. Hurt, RN, BSN, Nohora Keener, BA, Beth Morris, LCSW, MSW, Mary Ellen Nelson, BA, and Petra Shepard, PhD 2005–2006 Mid-America Regional Public Health Leadership Institute*

**Introduction**

The increasing diversity in many areas of the United States has posed both challenges and opportunities for health care providers. These challenges can be especially salient in rural areas that have been largely homogeneous until the last five to eight years, and that may not have the dual language support materials, people, and processes in place to respond to an influx of non-English speakers.

Maria Guadalupe Gom, age 22 and married, was five months pregnant with her first baby in January 2006 when she walked into Clinica Medica, the Hispanic health clinic in a rural area of southern Indiana. She had been in the United States for five years, immigrating from near Puebla, Mexico. She and her husband were living with her sister's family, which included her sister's husband and two children. Although previously a patient at Clinica Medica, which sees only uninsured patients, she had not needed clinic services since she had become employed full time at a local factory that provided her with health insurance benefits. Catherine Z. Jones, the registered nurse who serves as the clinic coordinator at Clinica Medica, was surprised when Maria nervously signaled her in the crowded waiting room indicating a need to speak with her. Catherine could sense, upon seeing Maria's demeanor, that her former patient was especially agitated about something.

Inviting her into a quiet corner of the exceedingly busy clinic, she inquired, "Did you need to speak with me?"

"Sí. I hope you can sign paper for me, yes?"

"Well, I am happy to help you if I can. What paper is it?"

*(continues)*

**Case Study 15-C** *continued*

"Just a paper for my employer so that I can have my job back after my baby is born." She presented Catherine with a Family Medical Leave Act (FMLA) form, nearly 10 pages long.

It took several minutes of conversation for Catherine to understand what Maria was asking. Maria's face and neck turned bright red and she lowered her voice as she explained. Since getting pregnant, Maria had been receiving prenatal services at a federally qualified health clinic (FQHC) in another county without telling clinic officials that she had insurance. She had chosen this route because her employer knew her by one name, the name on her purchased social security card. But she wanted her baby born with *her* name, not the false name known to her employer. She dared not tell her employer of her correct name. Nor did she want the clinic where she received prenatal care to know she was insured or she believed she would be compelled to use the false name. Not really understanding how the U.S. system worked, Maria had decided to tell her employer she would be going to Mexico to have her baby and would return following the birth. Although she actually had no intention of going to Mexico for the birth, she thought that this falsehood would explain why she was not using her insurance, should her employer ever become curious about their pregnant employee. Although not fully understanding the rules and expectations of her new home, Maria did know she wanted to keep her job at all costs following the birth of her child. She showed great anxiety and embarrassment in sharing all of this with Catherine, clearly uncomfortable with the position she was in yet not seeing any way out that did not involve additional deception.

Maria insisted that she simply needed a signature on the form. When she presented it to Catherine, Catherine saw it was an FMLA application and knew she would not be able to complete it. She encouraged Maria to take it to the physician at the FQHC that was providing her prenatal care. However, she knew from Maria's reaction that Maria was in a very difficult situation. Should she take the FMLA form to her physician, they would know she had misrepresented her insurance status. At the same time, failing to have it signed could mean the loss of a stable income, her reason for coming to the United States in the first place. She had approached Catherine as a trusted community professional whom, she hoped, would have a solution for this dilemma. Instead, needing to follow the law as well as the ethics of the nursing profession, Catherine could only encourage Maria to take the form to the prenatal clinic for completion. It tugged at Catherine's heart to see, once again, the stress on Mexican immigrants of our failed immigration and health policies and the knotty dilemmas often faced by people like Maria, who are existing as second-class citizens in a foreign country while displaced by their own because of the lack of opportunities. How many other Marias were out there, struggling with similar issues that put them in no-win situations where a lie of one kind or another seemed to them to be the only way to cope? How many immigrants were forgoing health care so as to avoid interacting with a system they did not understand or trust? The stress of living day to day under these circumstances seemed exhausting and, in fact, Catherine had seen many symptoms of post-traumatic stress syndrome in her immigrant patients.

**Case**

Catherine had no crisis of conscience regarding her refusal to sign Maria's FMLA form; it would only be ethical to sign such a form if Catherine's clinic had currently been providing care for Maria and her unborn child. But Catherine was nevertheless very unsettled by the circumstances that led Maria to make such a request.

Numerous times this bicultural nurse, who was also born in Mexico, had seen her fellow countrymen arrive in this country not only for the chance to better their lives but also to meet a real economic need in her adopted country.

A town of 35,000, Catherine's adopted home had changed dramatically in the last six years. She had been among a handful of Latin-American immigrants who had married United States citizens and had become naturalized themselves 20 years ago or so. This small, closely knit bicultural community ballooned in the late 1990s as economic circumstances led to labor shortages in the manufacturing and service sectors of her town (see Figure 15-4).

In fact, Catherine had heard the human resource director not only at Maria's factory but also at other local factories say that if it had not been for the Mexican laborers who came to fill jobs at the factory, they would have had to move the entire operation offshore or else close down. Undocumented immigrant labor had provided important support for economic development in the community in recent years. Employers and community leaders seemed all too willing to keep their collective heads in the sand regarding the true legal status of their workforce. As long as prospective employees presented the required social security card, employers appeared to have little interest in discovering the vast underground economy that had sprung up to provide false cards to willing Mexican laborers who come to this country without documents, or to understand the compounding problems that these laborers experience outside of their work environment.

As Emily Friedman recently wrote, "projected patterns of demographic change [in the United States] are more complex than they were historically, and the implications for the health care system are profound . . . Furthermore, the presence of minorities is being felt more in communities that historically have not been very diverse. Both native-born and immigrant minority Americans are moving to areas in New England and the Midwest, which traditionally were far less diverse than the South, the West, and the industrial Northeast" (Friedman, 2006).

Maria's story was truly remarkable for the persistence she had demonstrated and the strength of character she had needed to navigate from her home country to the United States. Maria was the oldest child and lived with her parents, four brothers,

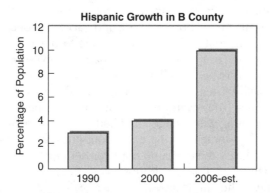

**FIGURE 15-4    Hispanic Growth in B County, Indiana from 1990 Through 2006 (estimated)**
*Source:* Lisa Crane, RN, BSN, Laura M. Hurt, RN, BSN, Nohora Keener, BA, Beth Morris, LCSW, MSW, Mary Ellen Nelson, BA, and Petra Shepard, PhD.

*(continues)*

**Case Study 15-C** *continued*

and three sisters in a two-room house. They had no electricity and no running water. When Maria was little, both her mother and father had to work to survive. They would leave the young children alone all day. Maria, being the oldest (eight years old at this point in time), cared for her brothers and sisters while her parents worked. On good days her mother and father would earn $10. (Dad made belts and Mom cleaned in various places.) Some days there was very little food. Maria and her brother often sold gum on the street corners to earn extra money. Other times, they would wash car windows for people stopping on the streets. Maria went to school until sixth grade. She loved school and wanted to continue but her parents could not afford to buy the uniforms and supplies that were needed to go to school. Maria had to quit to allow the rest of her brothers and sisters to go.

When Maria was 17, her Dad was suffering with diabetes and needed medical care. Her mother also had various medical problems. Maria had heard that if she went "north" she would be able to earn money and send enough back to help her parents and brothers and sisters. She had a cousin Luis who was anxious to go, too.

Maria and Luis made plans to go to the United States. They needed a lot of money, $1,500 each for a "coyote" who would take them across the border. They were able to collect money from many different family members and were ready to go. The coyote led them through the desert. During the day it was very, very hot. They had nothing to eat or drink. They had not been told to bring anything with them and nothing was provided. At night they would walk through the desert not being able to see where they were going and hearing all kinds of animals. One night they were left with a group of people in a shack. It was filthy. It was evident that this place was used often. There was no place to go to the bathroom, no food or water. In the desert it can get very cold at night. After sweating all day in the heat, they froze at night. The five people that were left in the shack had to huddle together to keep warm. They could hear real coyotes howling just outside. The coyote (person bringing them to the border) left them there for three days. They were very frightened and felt if they left the shack they would be caught by immigration. They didn't know what to do. Finally on the third night the coyote returned to take them on their way. They finally made their way to the *frontera* (border). The scariest part of the trip was at the border. In Mexico there are many dangerous people preying on the people leaving. It is almost like the Mafia on the border. Maria and Luis were robbed three times and beaten. There were areas that had electrical fencing to prevent people from crossing. Tunnels had been dug in the ground. They had to crawl down in the ground to get through. The holes were very small and it was very dark and scary. After six days, three days walking with blisters and swollen feet and three days spent in the shack, they crossed the border. They were terrified at not knowing what would happen next. Someone was waiting with a large van filled with other people to take them to where they were going—Indiana—where someone they knew from Mexico lived. Maria was scared but knew there was no hope for her or her family in Mexico. She was very sad and depressed to leave all those she loved, but she had a responsibility to help and this was the only way.

Catherine knew Maria's story and dozens of others, too. Her concerns and commitment to this growing population had led her to exert leadership in the community to create a more welcoming environment for Hispanic workers. She was proud of the Hispanic clinic she had helped to form and for which she was responsible for recruiting volunteer physicians, nurses, and interpreters. No other community in southern Indiana had been as proactive in responding to and welcoming the workers who were keeping local services going. Thank goodness the faith community had also joined in these efforts, allowing Maria to get free prenatal vitamins through Mary's Chapel, a local, ecumenical food pantry with aid for prescriptions.

## Closing

It is clear to Catherine and to other leaders in her community that there is a growing number of people with challenging emotional problems due to the situations they face where their behavior is at odds with their values. The anxiety, depression, and stress-related illnesses seen at Clinica Medica are seen at many other sites serving the undocumented workers who are keeping many Midwestern communities alive. It seems inhumane, yet there is no solution in sight. Interested, concerned people feel unable to help as our state and country's laws become more and more strict. Growing numbers of immigrants are driving without licenses or insurance, living with the fear of being sent back to extreme poverty in their home countries, living without loved family members whom they are supporting with checks sent home, and so on. The history of first-generation immigrants in the United States is fraught with challenges and continues unabated to this day.

## References

Friedman, E. (2006). Tapestry. *Hospitals and Health Networks Online,* February 9, 2006. Accessed February 27, 2006 at http://members.aol.com/emilyafriedman/columns/2006-02-tapestry.html.

Tienda, M. & Mitchell, F., eds. (2006). *Multiple Origins, Uncertain Destinies: Hispanics and the American Future.* Washington, DC: The National Academies Press.

United States Census Bureau (2005). Accessed February 8, 2006 at http://quickfacts.census.gov/qfd/states/18/18005.html.

---

It is through language that we express our culture and our personal needs. Words have power.[25] In American society, most people view English as the language of choice. The assumption that only English should be spoken in public venues, such as a health care clinic, constitutes a denigration of other languages and leads to a resistance to helping people who do not speak English or speak English peppered with words from their native language. Public health leaders and organizations have to address the issue of bilingualism in their community if they are to maintain credibility.

As pointed out, it is necessary to go through a series of stages—awareness, understanding, and action—before cultural competency is attained.[26] Of course, this analysis of the process of achieving cultural competency is very general, and the process can be broken down further, as in the following model:[27]

1. Cultural destructiveness occurs when cultural groups are discriminated against.
2. If the public health system is biased and culturally incompetent, it will be unable to facilitate change in health behaviors of culturally diverse groups.
3. Cultural incompetency may in part be a result of cultural blindness on the part of public health leaders, including a lack of awareness of the cultural factors in health and disease.
4. The fourth stage is reached when public health leaders and other practitioners begin to achieve cultural sensitivity. They become aware of

**438** Chapter 15 Cultural Competency

cultural differences and attempt to develop special programs to address the needs of different cultural groups.

5. Cultural competency is achieved when the leaders develop programs tied to different cultural groups.

6. If the programs are successful in meeting the special needs of different cultural groups, the public health leaders can be said to have become culturally proficient.

Exercise 15-4, based on Case Study 15-B, allows the students to develop an action plan based on the cultural competency models presented previously.

Cultural competency must start at the individual level, but it also must be present at the organizational and community levels (Figure 15-5).[28] Each individual in an organization has the responsibility of becoming culturally competent, and the organization's leaders need to support cultural competency by developing a written policy on cultural competency and providing awareness training to staff. They themselves need to be trained in demographic analysis, at least to the extent of being able to understand the demographic changes in the community and in the health status of culturally diverse populations.[29] The achievement of organization-wide cultural competency will likely result in changes in recruitment programs, staff orientation, performance appraisals, compensation packages, and promotion rules.

It is important to reinforce culturally competent staff behavior[30] and to recognize the value of cultural competency and the value of protecting diverse viewpoints. Public health leaders need to celebrate diversity in the community by holding, for example, an annual diversity and health fair. Leaders should also honor individuals involved in innovative diversity programs and publicize the positive results of these programs.

Cultural competency confers many benefits (Figure 15-6).[31] For one thing, community residents want to feel that the programs of the

**FIGURE 15-5  Multidisciplinary Aspects of Cultural Competency**
*Source:* Adapted from T. Cox Jr. and R. L. Beale, *Developing Competency to Manage Diversity* (San Francisco: Berrett-Koehler, 1997).

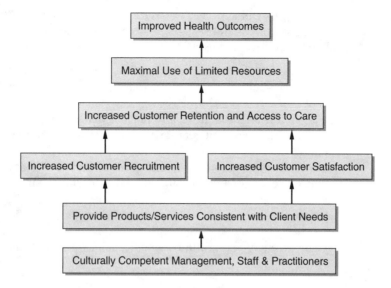

**FIGURE 15-6    Benefits of Cultural Competence in Health Care**
*Source:* Adapted with permission from Minority Managerial Programs, © 1997, American Association of Health Plans.

**Table 15-4    Positive Effects of Cultural Competency in Health Agencies**

- It allows the provider to obtain more specific and complete information to make a more appropriate diagnosis.
- It facilitates the development of treatment plans that are followed by the patient and supported by the family.
- It reduces delays in seeking care and allows for more use of health services.
- It enhances overall communication and the clinical interaction between provider and patient.
- It enhances the compatibility between Western health practices and traditional cultural health practices.

*Source:* Reprinted from President's Initiative on Race, *Health Care RX: Access for All,* 1998, Health Resources and Services Administration, U.S. Department of Health and Human Services.

local public health agency are oriented toward them and will be more satisfied with programs that are culturally competent. Such programs will increase access to care by culturally diverse groups. Table 15-4 lists five of the benefits of cultural competency that accrue to health agencies and the recipients of their services.

It is true that money is always an issue. Leaders will need to make choices as to how many resources to devote to creating a culturally competent organization. They will also need to ensure that the resources assigned to improving the level of cultural sensitivity are used as efficiently as possible.

Public health leaders must:

- lead the agency at all times with cultural diversity in mind
- monitor the appropriateness of programs and services for multicultural groups
- put cultural diversity policies into practice and live the policies
- develop cultural awareness programs and foster intercultural understanding
- understand the stages necessary to make cultural proficiency a reality
- evaluate agency progress toward cultural competency on an ongoing basis
- celebrate the accomplishments of others in the area of cultural competency
- develop diversity and health community fairs with community partners

## Summary

People do not feel that many social programs work. There is a critical need to concentrate on what works rather than what does not work. It is up to the public health system and its leadership to help find solutions for problems related to our cultural diversity. The task will not be easy and yet it is necessary. The trend toward greater cultural diversity will not stop. Public health leaders need to be at the forefront of attempts to get rid of our stereotypes, correct inaccurate cultural assumptions, build solid relationships with cultural neighbors, and empower all Americans.

### Discussion Questions

1. How would you as a public health leader deal with the alleged ethnic discrimination described in Case Study 15-A?
2. How would you set about helping the local high school develop a cultural diversity training program?
3. What are the guidelines for dealing with cultural diversity in the community and in the public health agency workforce?
4. What are the steps that someone needs to go through to reach cultural competency?
5. What are some strategies for creating a cultural competent staff?

### Exercise 15-1:   Rosenthal Inclusivity Checklist

*Purpose:* to learn how to build multicultural teams and coalitions and evaluate inclusivity issues

*Key concepts:* inclusivity, multiculturalism, team performance

*Procedure:* The class should divide into teams of seven or eight members. Each team then fills out the Rosenthal inclusivity checklist and discusses how the team might function in a multicultural environment. The discussion should focus on those items on the checklist that are not checked and the implications for team functioning and performance. As part of the discussion, team members should also consider the types of environments in which the team would be likely to perform well and the types of environments in which the team would perform poorly. Representatives from each team should then summarize their results and conclusions for the class as a whole.

**Table 15-5   Inclusivity Checklist**

*Instructions:*

*Use this Inclusivity Checklist to measure how prepared your coalition is for multicultural work and to identify areas for improvement. Place a check mark in the box next to each statement that applies to your group. If you cannot put a check in the box, this may indicate an area for change.*

☐   The leadership of our coalition is multiracial and multicultural.

☐   We make special efforts to cultivate new leaders, particularly women and people of color.

☐   Our mission, operations, and products reflect the contributions of diverse cultural and social groups.

☐   We are committed to fighting social oppression within the coalition and in our work with the community.

☐   Members of diverse cultural and social groups are full participants in all aspects of our coalition's work.

☐   Meetings are not dominated by speakers from any one group.

☐   All segments of our community are represented in decision making.

☐   There is sensitivity and awareness regarding different religious and cultural holidays, customs, recreation, and food preferences.

☐   We communicate clearly, and people of different cultures feel comfortable sharing their opinions and participating in meetings.

☐   We prohibit the use of stereotypes and prejudicial comments.

☐   Ethnic, racial, and sexual slurs or jokes are not welcome.

*Source:* Reprinted from T. Wolff and G. Kaye, eds., *From the Ground Up: A Workbook on Coalition Building and Community Development,* pp. 54–55, 69. © 1995 AHEC/Community Partners, by permission of the editors.

### Exercise 15-2:   Cultural Understanding

*Purpose:* to explore the issue of diversity and the best means of increasing cultural understanding

*Key concepts:* cultural diversity, cultural understanding, personal characteristics

*Procedure:* Each student is given a "Quest for Diversity" form and, for each category, tries to find the person in the class who best represents that category. When the student succeeds in identifying a person for a category, the student then talks to that person about one of his or her personal characteristics. Students should be careful to avoid cultural stereotyping and similar barriers to understanding. Students who find representatives for the most categories and for the least categories should be selected to present their findings to the class as a whole. The class should discuss the merits and limitations of each student's approach to diversity categorization.

**Table 15-6 Quest for Diversity Form**

| Diversity Categories | Found People | Personal Characteristics |
|---|---|---|
| professional woman/ homemaker | | |
| oldest grandparent | | |
| youngest parent | | |
| Native American background | | |
| Asian-American background | | |
| African-American background | | |
| in public health at least 30 years | | |
| parent was a migrant worker | | |
| parent who was an immigrant | | |
| largest number of siblings | | |
| first in family with college degree | | |
| Latino background | | |
| Russian or Polish background | | |
| an elected official | | |
| most children | | |
| man who is homemaker | | |
| rural dweller | | |
| world traveler | | |
| person with a disability | | |
| speaks five languages | | |

### Exercise 15-3 Leadership and Cultural Diversity

*Purpose:* to explore how diversity influences the way in which public health leaders carry out their responsibilities

*Key concepts:* cultural diversity, leadership system activities

*Procedure:* The class or training group should divide into groups of seven or eight members. Each group explores the ways in which diversity affects team building; values clarification; the development of a mission, a vision, goals and objectives, and action plans; the implementation of program interventions; and the evaluation of programs. After the discussion, each group prepares a five-minute presentation based on the discussion and shares its findings with the other groups.

**Exercise 15-4:    Cultural Competency in Gold County**

*Purpose:* to develop a personnel recruitment action plan to diversify the public health agency workforce

*Key concepts:* action planning, cultural competency, cultural sensitivity, personnel recruitment

*Procedure:* Case Study 15-B presents the demographics for Gold County. An analysis of the ethnic and racial makeup of the county health department indicates that 80% of the staff are white, 15% are African-American, and 5% are Hispanic. The class should divide into teams, and each team should discuss the action steps needed to ensure that the health department is culturally competent. One area of focus should be the development of a personnel recruitment plan to ensure that the health department's workforce is capable of understanding and responding appropriately to cultural issues within the community it serves. An issue that needs to be decided is whether the best approach is to attempt to recruit a workforce that mirrors the demographic composition of the community.

# References

1. Bureau of the Census, *Statistical Abstract of the United States* (Washington, DC: Bureau of the Census, 1997).
2. Bureau of the Census, *Population Profile of the United States: 2000 Internet Release* (Washington, DC: Bureau of the Census, 2000).
3. Public Health Service, *Public Health Workforce: An Agenda for the 21st Century* (Washington, DC: U.S. Department of Health and Human Services, 1997).
4. A. Wolf, *One Nation, After All* (New York: Viking Penguin Books, 1998).
5. Wolf, *One Nation, After All.*
6. T. Wicker, *Tragic Failure* (New York: Morrow, 1996).
7. W. J. Paul and A. A. Schnidman, "Valuing Differences: The Challenges of Personal Prejudice and Organizational Preference," in *The Promise of Diversity*, eds. E. Y. Cross et al. (Burr Ridge, IL: Irwin Professional Publishing, 1994).
8. A. M. Schlesinger Jr., *The Disuniting of America* (New York: Norton, 1992).
9. C. Taylor, ed., *Multiculturalism* (Princeton, NJ: Princeton University Press, 1994).
10. R. Bernstein, *Dictatorship of Virtue* (New York: Knopf, 1994).
11. E. Y. Cross et al., eds., *The Promise of Diversity* (Burr Ridge, IL: Irwin Professional Publishing, 1994).
12. A. J. DuBrin, *The Complete Idiot's Guide to Leadership* (New York: Alpha Books, 1998).
13. J. Bordas, "How Salsa, Soul, and Spirit Strengthen Leadership," *Leader to Leader* 46, no. 46 (2007): 35–41.
14. L. Segil, "Managing Culture in Cross-Cultural Alliances," *Leader to Leader* 6 (Fall 1997): 12–14.
15. B. Rosenthal, "Inclusivity Checklist," in *From the Ground Up: A Workbook on Coalition-Building and Community Development*, eds. T. Wolff and G. Kaye (Amherst, MA: AHEC Community Partners, 1995).

16. D. A. Thomas, "Diversity as Strategy," *Harvard Business Review* 82, no. 9 (2004): 88–107.

17. D. A. Thomas and R. J. Ely, "Making Differences Matter: A New Paradigm for Managing Diversity," *Harvard Business Review* 74, no. 5 (1996): 79–90.

18. Thomas and Ely, "Making Differences Matter."

19. President's Initiative on Race, *Health Care Rx: Access for All* (Washington, DC: U.S. Department of Health and Human Services, Health Resources and Services Administration, 1998).

20. T. Cox Jr., *Cultural Diversity in Organizations* (San Francisco: Berrett-Koehler, 1993).

21. C. R. O'Connell, *Umiker's Management Skills,* 4th ed. (Sudbury, MA: Jones and Bartlett, 2006).

22. T. Cox Jr. and R. L. Beale, *Developing Competency to Manage Diversity* (San Francisco: Berrett-Koehler, 1997).

23. Cox and Beale, *Developing Competency to Manage Diversity.*

24. President's Initiative on Race, *Health Care Rx: Access for All.*

25. C. Lemert, ed., *Social Theory: The Multicultural and Classic Readings* (Boulder, CO: Westview Press, 1993).

26. Cox and Beale, *Developing Competency to Manage Diversity.*

27. J. L. Rorie et al., "Primary Care for Women: Cultural Competence in Primary Care Services," *Journal of Nurse Midwifery* 41, no. 2 (1996): 92–100.

28. Cox and Beale, *Developing Competency to Manage Diversity.*

29. T. H. Cox and S. Blake, "Managing Cultural Diversity: Implications for Organizational Competitiveness," *The Executive* 5, no. 3 (1991): 45–56.

30. S. P. Robbins and M. Coulter, *Management,* 8th ed. (Upper Saddle River, NJ: Prentice Hall, 2005).

31. American Association of Health Plans, *Minority Managerial Programs* (Washington, DC: American Association of Health Plans, 1997).

# CHAPTER 16

# MENTORING, COACHING, AND TRAINING IN PUBLIC HEALTH

> My experiences as a mentor were first rate. Just say yes, if you're asked to serve as a mentor.
>
> S. F. Randolph, "The Mentoring Experience"

Mentoring and coaching are critical leadership activities. Leadership development depends on experienced leaders acting as role models for novice leaders. Leader-mentors and coaches need to understand leadership and promote the development of leadership skills by others.[1] Mentoring and coaching novice and experienced leaders has become even more important in the last few years than in the century past. An important aspect of the increase of interest in mentoring, coaching, and training is the lifelong learning acceptance by leaders and managers as well as young public health professionals. As leaders, we plan our actions as a key aspect of our work and nonwork lives. We often plan life projects related to family, work, recreation, creative activities, and social action and our contributions to our social justice values.[2] Life projects give us direction and motivation.

In general, mentoring is a form of one-to-one teaching, to be contrasted with training, which involves instructing more than one person. Public health leaders do engage in training as well, such as in team building.[3] A public health leader might facilitate the team-building process by presenting guidelines to the team as a whole and also act as a mentor for each team member. (Peer mentoring is also possible in a team situation.) Mentors generally do not give formal instruction but instead teach by example.[4] They understand how public health works and can explain the written and unwritten laws to their mentees.[5]

Some authors use the term "coaching"[6] rather than "mentoring." This has become confusing. Coaching is more about how to do a specific job more effectively, and mentoring is more about career and career choices.[7] Leadership development is important in both mentoring and coaching situations. The relationship between the mentor and the mentee or the coach and the coached are true partnerships, and each involved individual should gain something from it (in other words, it should be a win-win relationship). It should also be contractual, which means that the needs and expectations of both parties should be addressed when the relationship is first established.

Mentors can help in the training of a team by guiding the learning of each team member in leadership. The challenge for the mentor in formal training situations is to help the team become a learning community. The mentor must be committed to the goals of the team and facilitate the learning process for the team members, including through direct one-on-one interaction related to the professional needs of a given member. It may be beneficial to also help the trainee address job-related issues, which means that a modified coaching relationship will be established in addition to the mentoring one. Thus, the boundary between mentoring and coaching becomes blurry.

The learning contract model has been utilized by both coaches and mentors to guide their development process with their protégés.[8] The learning contract has evolved from the literature on adult learning. In 1970, Knowles utilized the concept of andragogy to discuss the four assumptions of learning by adults.[9,10] The major assumption is that adult learners tend to move from a dependency model where they are passive learners to an approach that is more active and self-directed. Adult learning is also experiential in that adults incorporate their experiences into the learning process. Third, adults tend to accept that learning will be a part of all new jobs and activities in which they engage. Finally, adults learn new knowledge as required by new tasks. Leaders who accept adult learning approaches tend to become ecological leaders who tie their learning experiences to the contexts in which they work and play.

In developing a learning contract, several steps are followed:[11]

1. Diagnose personal learning needs.
2. Specify learning objectives.
3. Designate learning resources and strategies.
4. Determine target dates for completion.
5. Specify ways to determine objectives are met.
6. Determine how evidence will be judged.
7. Review the contract personally and also with your mentor or coach.
8. Carry out the goals of the contract.
9. Monitor the process.
10. Evaluate the contract.

One way to translate these steps into a usable form is to create a chart with the objectives (step 2) on one axis and the remaining steps on the other axis as columns. Step 1 can be listed separately.

Experiment with a learning contract in Exercise 16-1.

The remainder of this chapter explores the nature of mentoring, coaching, and training, and their role in leadership development. As will be seen in the following discussion, friendship is an important element in mentoring and coaching as is trust in a training situation. In discussing the importance of having vital friendships at work that are relationships benefitting both parties, Rath defined eight types of friendship roles: builder, champion, collaborator, companion, connector, energizer, mind opener, and navigator.[12] A friend at work may have a combination of the behaviors associated with each role. Mentors and coaches tend to be builders who are friends and who support your personal growth and are not threatened by your progress. When you appear valued by your organization, you enjoy the work more and become more committed to the work of the organization.

# Mentoring

## The Benefits of Mentoring

Mentoring offers a number of benefits.[13] First, mentoring young professionals in a given field expands the network of professionals working in that field. This is especially important in public health, where practitioners come from many different disciplines. The mentees also gain the knowledge and tools needed to develop leadership skills. (Note that mentors give tools to their mentees, but the tools need to be translated into action for leadership skills to begin to evolve.) In addition, mentoring usually increases the mentees' chances for promotion.[14]

If a mentor is impressed by a mentee, the mentee may be assigned more challenging tasks. The mentor helps the mentee not only solve problems but make decisions as well. The mentee can acquire cutting-edge information that will aid the mentee in providing technical assistance to others in the future. The mentor can help the mentee navigate through tough choices. The mentee learns the ropes and will know, during his or her tenure as a leader, how to change the ropes as they fray.

For the mentor, the relationship can be extremely positive. Being a role model increases the self-esteem of the mentor and adds to the mentor's legacy.[15] To be looked upon as a person who has knowledge to impart also is important for the mentor. Mentors are usually among the senior members of an organization, and having the sense of being needed by younger members is a clear benefit for them.[16] In general, mentoring is a renewal process for mentors, who may feel rejuvenated. Case Study 16-A reports on the experiences of a mentor.

---

### Case Study 16-A
### The Mentoring Experience: What Is a Mentor?

*Shirley F. Randolph for University of Illinois School of Public Health, Illinois Public Health Leadership Institute*

The literature defines a mentor in a number of ways, none of which fulfills the mission of mentors as envisioned by the Illinois Public Health Leadership Institute. So, those of us who enjoyed the privilege of being in the original group of five mentors developed a definition to fit that vision.

The definition agreed on by the mentors has two parts. Part one covered the mentors' role during the three-day conference with the initial group of 25 Fellows. The mentors determined that their role for the conference would be one of facilitator and "coach."

Part two of our definition of "mentor" refers to the mentoring role following the conference. The mentors defined their role for that portion of their year-long responsibility to be one of teacher, counselor, friend, and "encourager."

The mentoring experiences that are described herein relate to part one: facilitator and "coach" during the three-day conference.

The most critical experience—not only for me as a mentor but also, I think, for the five fellows assigned to my group—was to be part of a small cadre of public health professionals, all of whom are leaders in their agencies, who developed a sharing, caring, and trusting relationship with all members of the group. There was plenty of

*(continues)*

**Case Study 16-A** *continued*

"give and take" and exchange of viewpoints and information as we moved through the three-day agenda.

My responsibility as a facilitator turned out to be easily fulfilled due to the professional approach taken by each of "my" Fellows and the fact that each had prepared by reviewing materials in advance of the conference.

The role of "coach" turned out to be exciting, rewarding, and fun as the conference progressed. It was a challenge to be "coach" to five bright, well-prepared individuals. It was also a tad "scary" because being a mentor to a group of public health practitioners was a role I had never performed prior to the conference.

The challenge was to direct attention to new concepts, to encourage the group to examine issues from a different perspective, and to delve into certain aspects of the issues presented in the case studies we dissected. That meant that I, as a mentor, had to stretch my personal limits in order to be an effective coach!

In my attempts to be effective as a coach, I uncovered a truism that constitutes another critical experience: mentoring is not a mystery. It goes beyond the sharing of information and guidance from a more experienced person to one with less experience, the traditional mentoring role. Mentoring is the giving of time and thought. It is caring coupled with gentle guidance.

I discovered that being a mentor also requires patience and a willingness to listen carefully. Some of the choice discussions in our group evolved from pertinent issues and personal experiences brought up and shared with the group by the Fellows as opposed to discussions stimulated by the content of the more formal sessions.

One of the unexpected experiences of being a mentor occurred when I realized that maybe one of my most important contributions as a mentor could be just being available when needed, to be someone who could reinforce an idea, or affirm a reaction, or lend credence to a different approach.

I experienced many other, less subtle "happenings" during the first annual conference of the Illinois Public Health Leadership Institute. Such as:

- the harried feeling of being pushed to cover as much ground and to "cram in" as much information as possible in short three days
- the pressure to excel and to make the initial conference a "showpiece"
- the lack of time to relax and socialize more with the entire group of Fellows
- the excitement that comes with learning something new
- the mental and physical exhaustion following an intense, 12-hour—or longer—day
- the joy of sharing time and thoughts with longtime public health colleagues
- the excitement of making new public health friends
- the eagerness and anticipation for each new session on the agenda
- the nostalgia that came with spending time on a university campus
- the satisfaction of "seeing a plan come together"
- the pleasure in knowing that the vision for the Institute was "right-on target" judging from the response of the Fellows
- the intellectual stimulation that occurs when listening to ideas presented by noted public health leaders
- the annoyance that comes with not doing well playing parlor games

That about sums it up. Bottom line: my experiences as a mentor were first rate. Just say yes, if you're asked to serve as a mentor, whether it be for the Illinois Public Health Leadership Institute, in a more traditional role within your community, or for the agency in which you work. You will be richly rewarded!

Mentoring is increasing in many organizations as the value of mentoring and coaching becomes recognized.[17] A key factor about mentoring is that age is not the critical issue but rather knowledge, skills, and experience in the field. Mentoring is also not about forever relationships. Mentoring occurs when it is needed. Either the potential mentor or mentee can begin the relationship, which is usually a volunteer one. An important fact is that individuals need to understand when they need coaching and when they need mentoring. In addition, different mentors may be needed for different concerns. I may need a mentor to guide and help me better understand public health and a different mentor to help my leadership development. All parties to a mentoring situation gain from the relationship.

The organization also gains from mentoring.[18] Often both the mentor and the mentee become more productive as a result of their relationship. Working together, they are able to assess problems and find solutions better than when working solo. Because mentoring leads to leadership development, the mentee is soon able to take over leadership activities. The mentoring relationship may also lead to the discovery and nurturing of hidden talents possessed by the mentee and can help the mentee hone his or her rough edges. Mentored professionals tend to stay in organizations for longer periods and also move up in the organizational hierarchy more easily.[19] Mentoring can occur anywhere in the organization. What is needed is an organizational commitment to mentoring. As one author put it, professionals need "mentorcentives."[20]

Table 16-1 lists qualities that mentors should possess and roles they should play.[21] At various times in the mentoring process different qualities and roles will predominate, partly because the influence of the mentor decreases over time as the mentee begins to develop the skills that the relationship is intended to foster.[22] Indeed, mentoring needs to be time limited; it should not result in long-term dependency.

Professionals want mentors who will give advice, support, and assistance, such as with the task of setting career goals.[23] The mentee has a responsibility to allocate time and effort to improving skills and competence.[24] Because not all leaders are good mentors, mentees should be careful in choosing whom to establish a mentoring relationship with. Mentoring can be formal, with each new employee assigned to a mentor for a period of time, or informal, where professionals who want a mentor seek one who will understand their professional aspirations. In general, it is preferable for mentees to choose their own mentors.

**Table 16-1    Mentor Qualities and Roles**

| Role Model | Trusted Counselor | Observes Confidentiality |
|---|---|---|
| Guide | Leader | Interested |
| Willing to be a mentor | Friend | Shows mutual respect |
| Supporter | Listener | Shows affection |
| Experienced | Knowledgeable | Accessible |
| Adviser | Shares resources | Networker |

*Source:* Reprinted with permission from J. Curruthers, "The Principles and Practices of Mentoring," in *The Return of the Mentor: Strategies for Workplace Learning,* B. J. Caldwell and E. M. A. Carter, eds., p. 20. © 1993, The Falmer Press, Taylor & Francis, Inc.

## Developing a Mentoring Relationship

Public health professionals may look for mentors outside of their agency. For example, a community leader or board of health member may help a public health professional better understand how the community works. It is possible to have more than one mentor at a given time, but the more usual scenario is to have several mentors sequentially. Exercise 16-2 allows students to explore their personal mentoring history.

As mentioned above, in some organizations mentees are assigned to mentors. Whether a mentor is assigned or freely chosen, there is no guarantee mentor and mentee will be right for each other. To increase the chance that they will be, a potential mentee can go through a selection process such as the one presented in Table 16-2.[25] As can be seen, the mentee needs to determine the things that he or she wants to accomplish and then select at least one goal to attain. The process is complex, for the mentee must first engage in personal values clarification and develop a personal vision as steps on the way toward developing personal goals, and then determine if there is anyone in the organization who has accomplished similar goals. The best strategy is to identify several possible mentors and do research on them. Table 16-3 presents a contrasting set of selection criteria.

After a mentor is selected, the mentor and mentee go through a series of steps as part of the development of the mentoring relationship. They need to set meeting goals, make appointments, and set an agenda. Early on, the mentor should tell his or her personal story, and together the mentor and mentee will discuss possible goals for the relationship and set a timetable for achieving the goals they choose. The deadlines should be flexible, however, and the timetable can be revised if both parties approve. During the entire relationship, mentor and mentee will need to negotiate with each other and discuss results on a regular basis. Another view of mentoring is provided by the 16 laws listed in Table 16-4.[26]

For mentoring to be successful, whether within an agency or within a community, the environment must nurture the mentoring relationship. In addition, the focus should be on developing the mentee's character as well as on the sharing of information. Finally, the mentoring relationship should

### Table 16-2 The 21 Steps to Choosing Your Mentor

| | |
|---|---|
| 1. Brainstorm desires. | 12. Ask for suggestions. |
| 2. Set goal. | 13. End trial. |
| 3. Identify achievers. | 14. Send thank-you note, gift. |
| 4. Select top candidates. | 15. Evaluate information. |
| 5. Research backgrounds. | 16. Take action on mentor suggestions. |
| 6. Set goals for meeting. | 17. Call mentor with activity results. |
| 7. Write letter to mentor prospect. | 18. Evaluate prospect's response. |
| 8. Call to set appointment. | 19. Request second appointment. |
| 9. Prepare 10 questions. | 20. Propose a mentoring relationship. |
| 10. Ask to hear life story. | 21. Commit to the 16 Laws of Mentoring |
| 11. State goals, and ask questions. | (see Table 16-4). |

*Source:* Reprinted with permission from F. Wickman and T. Sjodin, *Mentoring*, p. 70. © 1996, The McGraw-Hill Companies.

**Table 16-3   Criteria for Selection of Mentors**

1. Must be an accomplished, recognized leader in the health and public health arena
2. Must be willing to work for one year as a mentor to five fellows, providing consultation and assistance as appropriate
3. Must be able to participate in orientation/training; the three-day Institute; the two-day, six-month follow-up meeting; the one-day, 12-month follow-up meeting; and four to six meetings with the assigned fellows' group
4. Must have the skills to provide insights to fellows during discussion of case studies
5. Must be able to facilitate small-group discussions and guide group to consider most important factors in case studies and readings
6. Must be willing to provide ongoing support to fellows in their professional growth and implementation of successful leadership practices following the formal training program
7. Must be supported by employer (i.e., time off from regular duties to serve as mentor)
8. Must have held a leadership position in public health for at least 10 years
9. Should have national leadership credentials as well as state/local recognition
10. Must have demonstrated skills in administering and directing the three core governmental functions: needs assessment, policy development, and assurance
11. Must have considerable experience in working successfully with subordinates

*Source:* Reprinted, with permission, from *Criteria for the Selection of Mentors,* University of Illinois School of Public Health, Illinois Public Health Leadership Institute.

**Table 16-4   The 16 Laws of Mentoring**

1. The law of positive environment
2. The law of developing character
3. The law of independence
4. The law of limited responsibility
5. The law of shared mistakes
6. The law of planned objectives
7. The law of inspection
8. The law of tough love
9. The law of small successes
10. The law of direction
11. The law of risks
12. The law of mutual protection
13. The law of communication
14. The law of extended commitment
15. The law of life transition
16. The law of fun

*Source:* Reprinted with permission from F. Wickman and T. Sjodin, *Mentoring,* p. 70. © 1996, The McGraw-Hill Companies.

have as its ultimate goal independence for the mentee. Good mentoring will make the mentee feel so comfortable with change that his or her reliance on the mentor eventually disappears.

The mentee shares the responsibility for the relationship and its direction. The mentor and mentee are partners who together choose goals for the relationship, make plans to achieve the goals, and implement the plans. They will regularly study options and scenarios. If the mentee becomes overly dependent on the mentor, the latter may have to exhibit a little tough love. The mentoring process usually consists of a series of small changes that accumulate; massive sudden changes are rare. The relationship also carries with it some risk. A mentee can adversely affect the reputation of the mentor. In addition, the mentor's advice may not work in some situations. These caveats aside, the mentoring relationship tends to be mutually beneficial.

The mentoring relationship is mainly a working-hours relationship unless the two partners define it differently. The mentor guides the mentee in learning how to be effective on the job, not how to deal with his or her personal life. One secret of mentoring is that it should be fun as well as exciting. Another is that the best mentoring relationships are mismatches rather than pairings of similar individuals.

### Mentoring and Cultural Diversity

As pointed out in the last chapter, cultural diversity issues may affect many relationships in an organization. Mentor and mentee should respect each other as human beings and not let race, ethnicity, or gender get in the way of the relationship. Currently, men often mentor women, partly because men still predominate in the higher levels of most organizations. Cross-sex mentoring must include rules for the relationship that preclude sexual involvement of any kind, coerced or not.[27] Whereas sex can be an issue in cross-sex mentoring, the dearth of women in some organizations can cause women at the top to feel threatened by women poised to move upward, and the feeling of threat can prevent same-sex mentoring relationships from being effective. Note that women make up a large proportion of the public health workforce and that women in the upper echelons of public health often serve as mentors to both men and women.

Mentoring by women, according to one author, is "more about commitment than about chemistry. It's about personal growth and development rather than about promotions and plums. And it's more about learning than power."[28(p.188)] Many of the old approaches to mentoring have been revised by women. Female mentees tend to get mentoring from several different mentors on different issues.

### Mentoring Guidelines

Figure 16-1 presents a mentoring model that includes mentoring functions and activities.[29] The mentoring relationship is based on role modeling, nurturing, and caregiving. There are many functions associated with mentoring related to teaching: sponsorship, encouragement, counseling, and friendship. The purpose of the relationship is to get the mentee to put the lessons learned into action. Table 16-5 presents a list of 10 rules that apply to mentoring.[30]

Public health leaders should research mentoring and develop a mentoring program within their agencies. Guidance is needed if the core public

**Mentoring Model**

**FIGURE 16-1    Anderson and Shannon Mentoring Model**
*Source:* From E. M. Anderson and A. L. Shannon, Toward a Conceptualization of Mentoring, *Journal of Teacher Education,* pp. 38–42, copyright © 1988 by American Association of Colleges for Teacher Education. Reprinted by permission of Sage Publications, Inc.

health functions model, the organizational practices model, the essential services model, or some combination model is to be implemented successfully in a public health organization. Public health leaders must:

- adopt a formal agency mentoring program
- devise "mentorcentives" to increase the number of mentoring relationships
- develop a mentoring contract for use by mentors and mentees
- integrate leadership skills with core public health functions in the mentoring relationship
- support and guide the long-term personal growth of the mentee; the relationship needs to be consensual
- mentee is responsible for putting the learning into action
- mentors need to maintain objectivity through the mentoring process

**Table 16-5 The Ten Commandments of Mentoring**

1. Don't be afraid to be a mentor. Many people, especially women, underestimate the amount of knowledge that they have about . . . their organization, the contacts they have, and the avenues they can use to help someone else. A person does not have to be at the absolute top of his or her profession or discipline to be a mentor.

2. Remember that you don't have to fulfill every possible function of a mentor to be effective, but let your mentees know where you are willing to help and what kind of information or support you can give that you believe will be particularly helpful.

3. Clarify your expectations about how much time and guidance you are prepared to offer.

4. Let mentees know if they are asking for too much or too little of your time.

5. Be sure to give criticism, as well as praise, when warranted, but present it with specific suggestions for improvement. Do it in a private and nonthreatening context.

6. Where appropriate, "talk up" your mentees' accomplishments to others in your department and institution, as well as at conferences and other meetings.

7. Include mentees in informal activities whenever possible.

8. Teach mentees how to seek other career help whenever possible, such as money to attend workshops or release time for special projects.

9. Work within your institution to develop formal and informal mentoring programs and to encourage social networks as well.

10. Be willing to provide support for people different from yourself. "It is far easier for women than it is for many men to cross boundaries such as race, color, ethnicity, class, and religion in working with others. But we all need to practice this skill and avoid the temptation to assist only those with whom we feel the most comfortable, those who are the closest to being clones of ourselves."

*Source:* Reprinted with permission from B. R. Sandler, "Women as Mentors: Myths and Commandments," *Chronicle of Higher Education.* © 1993.

# Coaching

Coaching and mentoring are leadership partners. Most of the information in Tables 16-1 to 16-5 is also applicable to coaching. Coaching is about improving performance on the job.[31] The coaching process is one way to close the gap between present performance and improved performance. Executive coaching involves the hiring of a professional coach to counsel the leaders and managers in an organization.[32,33] As stated several times throughout this book, it is important to look at performance from the vantage point of an individual's talents, knowledge, and skills. An individual's emotional response is also a critical dimension of the coaching relationship. In structuring the coaching process, several steps are important:[34,35]

1. coach needs to observe coachee in action
2. discuss issues and process
3. determination of performance goals
4. specify active coaching methodology with defined times to meet
5. analyzing present performance
6. options or strategies to reach new goals
7. timetable for actions

8. implementation of actions
9. feedback and follow-up

Coaching fosters skill development based on talents and knowledge acquisition. Coaching thus involves the learning of new information and finding its fit with preexisting information. The individual who is being coached needs to tie the new knowledge to the vision, mission, goals, and values of the home organization. Action applications are important. A manager needs to see how his or her new skill applications fit the agency, and the leader needs to tie his or her new knowledge to work both inside and outside the agency. As seen above, the feedback mechanism is very

> **Leadership Tips**
>
> *Act positively even when you do not feel like it.*

important in coaching. Objectivity is important, and the feedback and response will concentrate on performance improvement and the future rather than the past, be given in a timely fashion, focus on behavior and how to change it, be specific in recommendations, give criticism in a positive way, and be realistic about what is possible.[36] O'Neill has stated that coaches do have emotional reactions to what they observe but need to keep their emotions in check.

Goldsmith has argued for the use of the concept of "feedforward" rather than feedback.[37] The new concept emphasizes the future rather than the past. It also emphasizes the concept of progress rather than dwelling on the mistakes of the past. Successful people tend to be visionary and concentrate on where they want their organizations to go. Feedforward also creates a climate in which support comes not only from the coach but also from colleagues. This new concept tends to be oriented to the goals of the organization and less to the personality of the leader.

Successful coaching has several benefits:[38]

1. It aids in improving performance of managers and leaders.
2. It helps all employees gather new knowledge and skills based on talents.
3. Productivity improves in positive work environments.
4. Coaching increases promotion opportunities and career choices.
5. Retention rates improve.
6. Coaching shows that employees are valued.

Executive coaches need to utilize both the skills of a coach and the skills of a mentor. They need to observe both on-the-job behavior in the day-to-day activities of the leader and manager inside the agency and for the leader inside and outside the agency. Executive coaches also need to explore present job issues with the professional and long-term career goals of their clients. These two sets of skills related to job and career can affect present job performance or affect future effectiveness. Successful coaches will utilize their own backgrounds and work with other clients while always protecting the privacy of other clients in order to guide their present clients.

There are a number of keys to creating a successful executive coaching relationship. The underlying dimension of coaching is that the relationship needs to be reciprocal. Both parties need to contribute to the relationship. At the meeting level, regular meetings need to be scheduled at least monthly and more often if necessary. Executive coaches will sometimes request that the client take a battery of tests similar to some of the ones discussed in Chapter 17. The results of these tests need to be discussed and used to explain how the client leader or manager is carrying out leadership activities in the agency or in the community. The coach will also observe the leader or manager in action. This technique, which is sometimes called shadowing, gives much relevant information to both the coach and the client. Books and journals will also be used to expand the knowledge of the leader and manager. The learning contract will be discussed and monitored throughout the coaching experience. Coaches in the guise of a mentor will examine professional goals as they relate to the future of the leader's agency. Exercise 16-3 will give you the opportunity to try shadowing.

Coaching is important for successful leadership and management of an organization. There will be times in the tenure of an individual when coaching may be needed. The leader will:

- utilize a coach when necessary
- develop a learning contract with the coach
- schedule regular meetings
- take leadership profiles to evaluate personal leadership characteristics
- read articles and books on leadership and management to expand resources and knowledge

## Training

Business leaders have known for a long time that an educated workforce will increase the effectiveness and efficiency of a company. They view the cost for training as low in comparison with the long-term benefits. In the government sector, on the other hand, training has been seen as a luxury that often cannot be justified. The result for public health has been a learning gap that has kept public health practitioners from promoting public health in their communities in an effective manner. There is increasing fear that public health agencies may not have a future. The challenge is to train public health leaders for the 21st century. Many public health leaders lack an adequate background in public health, have had limited exposure to academic public health content, are ignorant of advanced information technology, and have had limited leadership training.

### A Strategy for Training the Public Health Workforce

In a report of the Public Health Functions Project of the U.S. Department of Health and Human Services (DHHS), a five-pronged strategy was laid out for training the public health workforce for the 21st century. The report also included a series of steps for achieving training-related goals.[39]

The first prong concerns the development of a national public health leadership (Table 16-6).[40] The suggested federal role is to provide standards and guidelines, promote and conduct research, disseminate the results, guarantee equity across states, and develop priorities for the nation every 10 years.

The second prong concerns leadership at the state and local levels (Table 16-7).[41] Each state is different, and public health leaders, in applying any public health model, need to be guided by the unique characteristics of their state or locality. Training should include leadership development initiatives created in partnership with academia. Local and state public health leaders need to let the national leadership know about the day-to-day realities of public health practice.

The training process includes monitoring the public health workforce and acting to ensure that its composition reflects the ethnic and racial diversity of the society at large (Table 16-8).[42] The first step is to define the public health workforce. The DHHS report defined the workforce as all professionals who are responsible for providing essential public health services regardless of the organization for which they work. One of the next steps is to classify and count the public health professionals, and the final step is to identify and implement plans to ensure that the workforce is ethnically and culturally diverse.

The fourth prong of the strategy is to develop a curriculum based on the competencies needed for public health practice (Tables 16-9 and 16-10).[43] Public health leaders need to determine the skills, abilities, and knowledge bases that the public health workforce will need in the 21st century. Included

---

**Table 16-6    Proposed Action Steps for National Public Health Leadership**

A. Organize a national forum of key stakeholders from both the public and private sectors to examine human resource allocation and trends in public health. Potential forum participants in addition to the Public Health Functions Steering Committee members include the American Association of Health Plans, Health Care and Financing Administration, state Medicaid directors, social workers, substance abuse and mental health professionals, nurses, professional organizations, and the business community in general.

B. Develop and implement modules for Leadership Training Institutes that enable public health leaders to better assess their roles in providing public health services in a changing environment.

C. Involve frontline public health practitioners from all types of organizations in the efforts to enumerate, plan for, and educate the public health workforce.

*Source:* Reprinted from Public Health Service, *Public Health Workforce: An Agenda for the 21st Century,* pp. 11–12, 1997, U.S. Department of Health and Human Services.

---

**Table 16-7    Proposed Action Steps for State and Local Public Health Leaders**

A. Ensure that workforce planning takes place in all appropriate jurisdictions. Allocation of human resources should be determined by state and local governments or on a regional basis when appropriate due to resources, geography, or other factors.

B. Within each jurisdiction encourage the participation of medical care delivery systems and others with public health responsibilities to achieve mutual goals in workforce development.

C. Develop a partnership with states to quantify the supply and demand of personnel providing essential public health services at the state, local, and private sector levels.

*Source:* Reprinted from Public Health Service, *Public Health Workforce: An Agenda for the 21st Century,* p. 12, 1997, U.S. Department of Health and Human Services.

**Table 16-8  Proposed Action Steps Related to Workforce Composition**

A.  Identify a lead agency or organization to provide leadership in continuing efforts to assess the size, composition, and distribution of the workforce as related to essential services of public health.

B.  Examine methods used by professional organizations such as the American Nurses Association, American Medical Association, American Psychological Association, American Dental Association, and National Environmental Health Association to classify their respective workforces and incorporate where helpful.

C.  Develop a standard taxonomy based on the 10 essential public health services to qualitatively characterize the public health workforce. This classification scheme must be derived through collaboration and consensus of the entire public health community.

D.  Use the SOC System of the workforce and data from the Bureau of Labor Statistics and census surveys to track shifts in the staffing mix of personnel among the governmental, private, and voluntary sectors.

E.  Identify and take action steps to ensure that the public health workforce is ethnically and culturally diverse.

F.  Work with the Office of Management and Budget to include appropriate public health entries in the SOC System to facilitate identification of public health worksites, such as local health departments and other organizations providing essential public health services.

*Source:* Reprinted from Public Health Service, *Public Health Workforce: An Agenda for the 21st Century,* p. 12, 1997, U.S. Department of Health and Human Services.

**Table 16-9  Proposed Action Steps for Competency Development**

A.  Verify that identified competencies are indeed necessary for efficient and effective practice of public health. Validations of these competencies should be provided by a panel of practice-based experts who are in public health organizations, including employers.

B.  Identify competencies critical to all public health practitioners and those critical to successful practice in specific organizational settings. The competencies should be viewed as "organizational" competencies, those required for the entire workforce deployed within a given public health setting. (Although all public health practitioners should be familiar with the essential services of public health, few, if any, individuals will be equally competent in all areas.) Categorizing competencies should be conducted by a review panel of experts including practitioners and employers from all practice settings.

C.  Improve long-range planning. Public health competencies are evolutionary. They are affected by changes in responsibilities and the practice of public health. There must be a formal mechanism to update competencies to reflect changing demands. A mechanism for assuring current and accurate competencies may take the form of an institute, task force, or other entity supported by government, foundations, and/or the academic community. Responsibilities will include monitoring trends in the demand for public health services and interpreting those demands in terms of the skill and knowledge needed to provide the 10 essential services of public health.

*Source:* Reprinted from Public Health Service, *Public Health Workforce: An Agenda for the 21st Century,* p. 13, 1997, U.S. Department of Health and Human Services.

among these are the following: analytical skills, communication skills, policy and development and program planning skills, cultural competency, and basic public health sciences knowledge. Once public health leaders determine the appropriate competencies, they should help develop training initiatives to foster these competencies. Linkages between academics and practicing professionals are critical for ensuring the proper education of the public health workforce.

**Table 16-10    Proposed Action Steps for Curriculum Development**

A.  Ensure that the practice community has a substantial role in the curriculum development process. Examine existing models that link the academic and practice communities as a first step in facilitating practitioner involvement and target efforts and resources in their replication.

B.  Determine the current status of "competency" of the workforce. Develop and implement a methodology (survey, direct observation, etc.) to assess the current level of proficiency in the practice of the competencies. This research effort will include an evaluation of how the competencies have been acquired (on-the-job training, formal education, mentoring, continuing education, etc.) and the perceived adequacy of these approaches in the context of the communities being served.

C.  Develop measurable performance indicators for identified competencies.

D.  Survey public health training/education institutions to assess the extent to which competencies are currently being employed to structure the curriculum.

E.  Conduct an analysis of the competency statements and make revisions for their most effective use in curriculum development. Education and training specialists should conduct this analysis.

F.  Identify gaps between high-priority competencies that are needed and those competencies already present in the workforce. The competencies proposed by the Competency-Based Curriculum Workgroup incorporate projections of competencies needed now and in the future (five years hence). After additional review, these projections can serve as a baseline. Identification and prioritization between the actual and the needed profile of competencies may best be accomplished by a panel composed of practice association representatives, academic institutions, and federal agencies.

G.  Translate competencies into discrete didactic and field-based learning experiences and activities.

H.  Create a matrix of addressed and unaddressed competencies based on public health organizational needs with the results of the instructional provider survey (data collected during the needs assessment activity) by cross-referencing each element in the competency listing.

I.  Support a curriculum development process that is sensitive to the needs of local communities in order to be responsive to the local priorities of each agency, state, or local community relating to the essential services of public health.

J.  Recommend to the Council for Education in Public Health and other organizations within the accreditation community that competency-based approaches be incorporated into the standards for educational institution accreditation and into the standards for professional certification and/or licensure.

K.  Develop criteria for identifying providers of public health training and education that are "models of excellence" and support these providers through grants and other forms of support.

L.  Implement the operation of a "clearinghouse" to promote sharing of exemplary teaching approaches among institutions.

*Source:* Reprinted from Public Health Service, *Public Health Workforce: An Agenda for the 21st Century,* pp. 14–15, 1997, U.S. Department of Health and Human Services.

The fifth prong is to prepare for the increased use of distance learning that will occur in the new century (Table 16-11).[44] The point is not to demean face-to-face learning but to foster other learning options for public health professionals. Distance learning technologies are constantly evolving, and each technology will be especially effective in some applications and ineffective in others. Public health professionals seem to opt for on-site training because of the obvious fact that public health practitioners practice their craft face to face with clients. However, distance learning can be integrated into the overall education system without reducing the ability of practitioners to handle actual encounters with clients.

## Using Education and Collaboration to Heal the Division Between Public Health and Medicine

The last few decades have seen the rise of divisiveness between medicine and public health.[45] Many of the physicians chosen to head health departments

**Table 16-11  Proposed Action Steps for Distance Learning**

A. Establish a formal structure to advocate for the integration of distance learning techniques into practice and academic entities involved in public health strategies for training, education, and communication. Actions necessary for this to proceed include:

- Evaluate previous studies that document distance learning resources among partners.
- Develop a strategy for participant registration that is compatible across agencies and that is supported by a technology that allows for orders of magnitude expansion and comparability of data.
- Establish a standard practice and methodology for stakeholder's evaluation of distance learning results.
- Institute a common practice for program promotion and marketing.
- Develop a strategy to facilitate sharing resources across organizational lines (e.g., interagency agreements, cooperative agreements, grants, memorandums of understanding).
- Initiate standards for distance learning technology that permit system integration across agencies.
- Encourage and support the use of public/private assignments to promote collaboration in training.
- Share innovative and effective procurement mechanisms for distance learning services (e.g., task order contracts and other procurement mechanisms).
- Assist in identifying and developing distance learning faculty and subject matter experts and establishing incentives for their support.
- Provide grant assistance for development of distance learning programs at regional and local levels.

B. Directly link distance learning systems and program development priorities to the information generated by the Workgroups on Workforce Composition and Competency-based Curriculum.

C. Routinely gather input from key partners regarding training needs and technological capabilities.

D. Develop agency expertise in distance learning; participate in relevant organizations such as the United States Distance Learning Association (USDLA) and Government Alliance for Training and Education (GATE).

E. Provide access to information about public health distance learning programs and resources through mechanisms such as FedWorld Training Mall and the Public Health Training Network Web site.

F. Organize a mechanism for pooling and accessing resources and expertise on distance learning across all of public health.

*Source:* Reprinted from Public Health Service, *Public Health Workforce: An Agenda for the 21st Century,* p. 16, 1997, U.S. Department of Health and Human Services.

whose statutes require a physician at the helm had little knowledge of public health. In fact, public health seemed artificially separated from primary care. In many countries, primary care and public health are seen as one. Several years ago, I traveled to Armenia to teach a group of public health professionals about public health leadership. The experience led me to make two important observations. First, clinical activities supported at a countrywide level define the official public health policy. Primary care is public health. Second, independent public health leadership is generally not possible in a country where the nationalized system of health care is politically controlled. Administrators have the responsibility to maintain the status quo. The 21st century will see renewed collaboration between medicine and public health in the United States. This type of collaboration has been called cross-sectoral.[46]

Four actions are necessary for the relationship between medicine and public health to improve.[47] First, both physicians and public health professionals must be educated about strategies for fostering cross-sectoral collaboration. Second, each group must legitimize the process. Third, physicians and public health professionals must develop tools to promote the collaboration approach. Finally, they must examine barriers to collaboration and program options and create policies to support collaboration. All four of these actions have a strong training component. Public health leaders need the skills to carry out collaboration and need to train staff to support collaborative efforts. In other words, they must understand both the culture of medicine and the culture of public health.

Table 16-12 presents goals and strategies (under the headings "Synergy" and "Models") for medicine-public health collaboration.[48] The use of "synergy" is intended to indicate that the results of collaboration are greater than would occur if the activities were performed separately.

Training raises important concerns for public health leaders. These leaders need to make a commitment to continuing their own education and to supporting the continued learning of others, including community partners. Training for practitioners needs to be experientially based so that the skills acquired can be put into practice. As regards training, public health leaders must:

- be lifelong learners
- master emerging information technologies
- share information
- mentor and coach others
- support training initiatives
- train their partners
- orient training toward the future of public health
- make training programs experientially based

## Training Through Mentoring

In public health, training can be enhanced by incorporating mentoring as one of the components. The Illinois Public Health Leadership Institute (now the Mid-America Regional Public Health Leadership Institute) used mentoring to create the foundation for leadership development in its one-year training program. Four different types of mentors were and are included in the training

**Table 16-12  Models of Medicine and Public Health Collaboration**

| Synergy | Models |
|---------|--------|
| I  Improving health care by coordinating services for individuals | A. Bring new personnel and services to existing practice sites<br>B. Establish "one-stop" centers<br>C. Coordinate services provided at different sites |
| II  Improving access to care by establishing frameworks to provide care for the uninsured | A. Establish free clinics<br>B. Establish referral networks<br>C. Enhance clinical staffing at public health facilities<br>D. Shift indigent patients to mainstream medical settings |
| III  Improving the quality and cost-effectiveness of care by applying a population perspective to medical practice | A. Use population-based information to enhance clinical decision-making<br>B. Use population-based strategies to "funnel" patients to medical care<br>C. Use population-based analytic tools to enhance practice management |
| IV  Using clinical practice to identify and address community health problems | A. Use clinical encounters to build community-wide databases<br>B. Use clinical opportunities to identify and address underlying causes of health problems<br>C. Collaborate to achieve clinically oriented community health objectives |
| V  Strengthening health promotion and health protection by mobilizing community campaigns | A. Conduct community health assessments<br>B. Mount health education campaigns<br>C. Advocate health-related laws and regulations<br>D. Engage in community-wide campaigns to achieve health promotion objectives<br>E. Launch "Healthy Communities" initiatives |
| VI  Shaping the future direction of the health system by collaborating around policy, training, and research | A. Influence health system policy<br>B. Engage in cross-sectoral education and training<br>C. Conduct cross-sectoral research |

*Source:* Reprinted, with permission from the New York Academy of Medicine, from *Medicine & Public Health: The Power of Collaboration* by Roz D. Lasker and the Committee on Medicine and Public Health (Chicago: Health Administration Press, 1997).

(Figure 16-2). First, a mentor advocate—a public health leader with 10 years of experience who usually has graduated from the national or a state or regional public health leadership institute—is assigned the responsibility of facilitating the training experiences of a team of public health leaders. The mentor advocate helps each team member network with an experienced pub-

**FIGURE 16-2    Leadership Development Mentoring System**
*Source:* Adapted from S. F. Randolph, *Mentoring and the Illinois Public Health Leadership Institute,* 1993, University of Illinois School of Public Health, Illinois Public Health Leadership Institute.

lic health professional, helps team members deal with concerns and questions, and assists in the development of the team's training projects. The mentor advocate is available to the trainees throughout the year.

In order to explore new skills in the work setting, each leadership trainee selects an agency mentor and coach to help solve work-related problems. Whatever the problem, the solution needs to involve the application of leadership skills and the placement of the problem in a public health core functions context. The trainee has the responsibility of giving the mentor agency advisor readings or case studies that explain or demonstrate the conceptual approaches included in the leadership development training. The trainee and advisor can also explore ways to use leadership skills in the public health agency.

The third mentor is the trainee's "buddy," a person who has gone through the leadership development program a year or more ago. The buddy offers the new trainee insights about the leadership training approaches. He or she can provide friendship, can help the trainee interpret the program's readings and case studies, and can strengthen the public health leadership networking activities. The buddy relationship puts the responsibility for the development of these activities clearly in the hands of the buddy and the trainee. This relationship tends to be an informal one usually determined by the trainee and the leadership graduate.

Finally, a fourth mentor type has emerged in leadership development programs. Trainees develop mentoring relationships with their peers. A training team creates opportunities for the team members to interact, and individual members can look to other members for guidance. Peer mentoring clearly enhances the learning experiences of the trainees by enriching their understanding of readings and presentations and allowing them to get more out of experientially based projects.

The Illinois Public Health Leadership Institute, founded in 1991, was the first state leadership institute funded by the Centers for Disease Control and Prevention (CDC). In 1999, it was renamed the Mid-America Regional Public Health Leadership Institute, and it now trains public health leaders from Illinois, Indiana, Wisconsin, and Michigan. Teams have also participated from North Dakota, Arkansas, and the Canadian province of Quebec. Public health leaders in all 50 states currently have access to state or regional public health leadership development programs. There has been increasing recognition of the importance of the training they provide. Owing to the expansion of leadership development programs, the CDC has encouraged the development of the National Public Health Leadership Development Network Conference to address the common concerns of public health leadership programs.

Public health leaders will be both mentees and coached individuals and mentors and coaches at various stages in their careers. In particular, they should consider:

- volunteering to mentor a leadership development team
- serving as an mentor and coach agency advisor to public health professionals confronted with local or state public health issues
- increasing networking between graduates of public health leadership programs
- utilizing peer mentoring as a way to spread the use of effective conflict resolution and decision-making strategies
- encouraging the development of state and regional leadership programs

## A Leadership Ladder of Learning

Learning needs to be a lifelong process. Public health leaders live in a constantly changing environment, and the public health agenda is partly unpredictable. As stated above, public health leaders will need different training opportunities at different times in their professional lives, but it is clear that mentoring adds to virtually any learning experience. Figure 16-3 presents a lifelong learning agenda for leaders. As leaders move up the ladder, they begin to focus more on national or even global public health concerns rather than local ones and also to become aware of the abstract aspects of leadership and develop conceptual models to guide their leadership activities.

On the first step of the ladder, where public health professionals initially take on supervisory or other administrative roles, they need to learn how to utilize basic management and leadership tools. They need training in planning, organizing, monitoring, and administering.[49] They also need to learn to distinguish clinical activities from management activities and to learn leadership skills that will help them advance to a more creative leadership role in the organization. There are numerous courses and training materials available for new leader-administrators. The foundation skills are fairly concrete and less conceptual than at the higher levels of leadership.

Entry-level leadership development can occur through involvement with a profession-specific group or a multidisciplinary group. After three to five years in an organizational leadership position, leaders will benefit from training at a state or regional public health leadership institute. Such training is intended to integrate leadership concepts and public health governing paradigms.

National public health leadership institutes, such as the CDC-funded Public Health Leadership Institute, are useful for leaders in key state positions. Top-level leaders may also gain from specialized training programs that stress some major leadership functions. For example, the International Center for Health Leadership Development at the University of Illinois at Chicago has developed a series of weeklong training programs on partnering, coalition building, and policy development for public health partners.

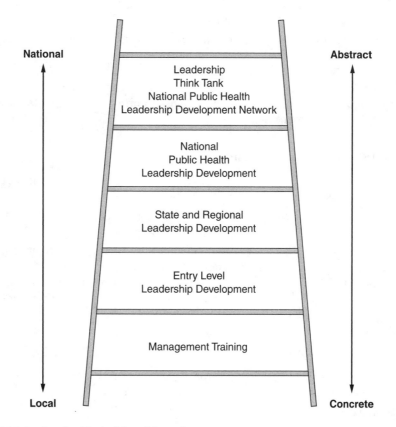

**FIGURE 16-3   Leadership Ladder of Learning**
*Source:* Reprinted from Public Health Practice Program Office, 1999, the Centers for Disease Control and Prevention.

At the highest step on the ladder, public health leaders can become involved in a think tank in order to explore public health issues with graduates of national leadership development programs and state and local public health leadership institutes. Public health think tanks are in the business of producing policy papers to guide public health action.

## Summary

This chapter has emphasized the importance of mentoring, coaching, and training public health leaders. Mentoring in all its guises enhances leadership development. A combination of mentoring, coaching, and training facilitates the learning of leadership skills. Therefore, experienced leaders must be willing to mentor novice leaders, who, of course, must be willing to be mentored. In addition, public health leaders who head agencies and health departments must find ways to foster mentoring within their organizations.

### Discussion Questions

1. What are the benefits of mentoring and coaching for the mentee or coachee?

2. What are the benefits for the mentor or a coach?
3. What examples of mentoring have you experienced, either as mentee or mentor?
4. How are personal mentoring and team mentoring related?
5. What skills are needed for someone to become a mentor?
6. What strategies would you propose to bring medicine and public health closer together in your community?

### Exercise 16-1:   The Learning Contract

*Purpose:* to utilize the learning contract to structure a training or educational experience

*Key Concepts:* adult learning, mentoring, coaching, learning contract

*Procedure:* Following the general procedure for devoping a learning contract, write out such a contract related to either this course or this training program. Create dyads in the class or training program. Each person in the dyad takes the role of a coach or mentor and discusses how to use this educational or training experience to guide your future or present work as a manager or leader in public health.

### Exercise 16-2:   Mentoring

*Purpose:* to explore both sides of a mentoring relationship and to evaluate the experience of being a mentor and a mentee

*Key concepts:* mentee, mentor

*Procedure:* As a homework assignment, each student or trainee writes two one-page stories, the first about a situation in which the student or trainee was mentored, the second about a situation in which the student or trainee acted as a mentor. The stories are read to the class or training group and discussed. (If the group is large, it should divide into smaller groups, and each group will listen to and discuss the stories of those in that particular group.)

### Exercise 16-3:   Shadowing

*Purpose:* to follow a leader for several hours or a day to see how a leader works in the real world

*Key concepts:* shadowing, leadership

*Procedure:* Choose a leader of your choice in government or a health organization. Arrange to follow him or her for a designated amount of time. Discuss the experience with the leader you chose. Share the experience with your class or training group.

## References

1. C. R. Bell, *Managing as Mentors,* 2nd ed. (San Francisco: Berrett-Koehler, 2002).
2. T. Fields, *Planning Life's Projects* (Tucson, AZ: Hats Off Books, 2001).
3. F. Wickman and T. Sjodin, *Mentoring* (Chicago: Irwin Professional Publishing, 1996).

4. Bell, *Managing as Mentors.*
5. B. Nelson and P. Economy, *Managing for Dummies* (Foster City, CA: IDG Books Worldwide, 1996).
6. T. Peters and N. Austin, *A Passion for Excellence* (New York: Random House, 1985).
7. Harvard Business Essentials, *Coaching and Mentoring* (Boston: Harvard Business School Press, 2004).
8. M. S. Knowles, *Using Learning Contracts* (San-Francisco: Jossey-Bass, 1986).
9. M. S. Knowles, *The Modern Practice of Adult Education,* revised and updated (Chicago: Follett Publishing Co., 1980).
10. M. S. Knowles, E. F. Holton III, and R. A. Swanson, *The Adult Learner,* 6th ed. (New York: Butterworth-Heinemann, 2005)
11. R. Hiemstra, http??home.twcnv.rr.com/hiemstra/contract.html
12. T. Rath, *Vital Friends* (New York: Gallup Press, 2006).
13. J. Carruthers, "The Principles and Practices of Mentoring," in *The Return of the Mentor: Strategies for Workplace Learning,* eds. B. J. Caldwell and E. M. A. Carter (London: The Falmer Press, 1993).
14. Carruthers, "The Principles and Practices of Mentoring."
15. Wickman and Sjodin, *Mentoring.*
16. Wickman and Sjodin, *Mentoring.*
17. L. Phillips-Jones, *The New Mentors and Proteges* (Grass Valley, CA: Coalition of Counseling Centers, 2001).
18. E. Alleman, "Two Planned Mentoring Programs That Worked," *Mentoring International* 3, no. 1 (1989): 6–12.
19. Alleman, "Two Planned Mentoring Programs That Worked."
20. C. Dahle, "Women's Ways of Mentoring," *Fast Company* 17 (1998): 187–195.
21. Carruthers, "The Principles and Practices of Mentoring."
22. W. A. Gray, "Situational Mentoring: Custom Designing Planned Mentoring Programs," *International Journal of Mentoring* 3, no. 1 (1989): 19–28.
23. S. P. Robbins and M. Coulter, *Management,* 8th ed. (Upper Saddle River, NJ: Prentice-Hall, 2005).
24. J. G. Liebler and C. R. McConnell., *Management Principles for Health Professionals,* 4th ed. (Sudbury, MA: Jones and Bartlett, 2004).
25. Wickman and Sjodin, *Mentoring.*
26. Wickman and Sjodin, *Mentoring.*
27. Carruthers, "The Principles and Practices of Mentoring."
28. C. Dahle, "Women's Ways of Mentoring."
29. E. M. Anderson and A. L. Shannon, "Toward a Conceptualization of Mentoring," *Journal of Teacher Education* 39 (1988): 38–42.
30. B. R. Sandler, "Women as Mentors: Myths and Commandments," *Chronicle of Higher Education,* March 10, 1993, B3.
31. J. Eaton and R. Johnson, *Coaching Successfully* (New York: Dorling Kindersley Books, 2000).
32. Eaton and Johnson, *Coaching Successfully.*
33. M. B. O'Neill, *Executive Coaching with Backbone and Heart* (San Francisco, Jossey-Bass, 2000).
34. Eaton and Johnson, *Coaching Successfully.*
35. O'Neill, *Executive Coaching with Backbone and Heart.*
36. Harvard Business Essentials, *Coaching and Mentoring.*
37. M. Goldsmith, "Try Feedforward Instead of Feedback," in *Coaching for Leadership,* 2nd ed., eds. M. Goldsmith and L. Lyons (San Francisco: Pfeiffer, 2006).

38. Harvard Business Essentials, *Coaching and Mentoring.*

39. Public Health Service, *Public Health Workforce: An Agenda for the 21st Century* (Washington, DC: U.S. Department of Health and Human Services, 1997).

40. Public Health Service, *Public Health Workforce.*

41. Public Health Service, *Public Health Workforce.*

42. Public Health Service, *Public Health Workforce.*

43. Public Health Service, *Public Health Workforce.*

44. Public Health Service, *Public Health Workforce.*

45. R. D. Lasker, *Medicine and Public Health: The Power of Collaboration* (New York: New York Academy of Medicine, 1997).

46. Lasker, *Medicine and Public Health.*

47. Lasker, *Medicine and Public Health.*

48. Lasker, *Medicine and Public Health.*

49. Robbins and Coulter, *Management.*

# PART IV

# Leadership, Evaluation, and Research

# CHAPTER 17

# MEASURING THE LEADER

> Work experience, hardship, opportunity, education, role
> models, and mentors all go together to craft a leader.
>
> J. A. Conger, *Learning to Lead*

Leadership is multidisciplinary as well as multilayered, and no single measure of leadership exists. Most quantitative evaluation instruments do not have specific public health leadership dimensions and are quite general to begin with. Case studies, interviews, and stories, of course, provide qualitative information. The quantitative and qualitative information that is available can be used to evaluate the development of leadership skills and determine whether leadership development programs lead to changes in behavior.

The purpose of this chapter is not to review all the leadership assessment instruments on the market but rather to describe several instruments currently used in various public health leadership development programs. This chapter will also explore the concept of 360-degree feedback and consider recent arguments for and against credentialing public health administrators.

## A Leadership Competencies Framework

The late 1990s saw a renewal of interest in training the public health workforce, including public health leaders. The issue of leadership training was addressed by the Public Health Functions Project, which was coordinated by the Assistant Secretary of Health and the Surgeon General.[1] Table 17-1 presents the 10 tasks this project undertook. A project subcommittee was appointed to:

> Provide a profile of the current public health workforce and make projections regarding the workforce of the 21st century. The subcommittee should also address training and education issues, including curriculum development, to ensure a competent workforce to perform the essential services of public health now and in the future. Minority representation should be analyzed and the programs to increase representation should be evaluated. Distance learning should be explored. The subcommittee should examine the financing mechanisms for curriculum development and for strengthening the training and education infrastructure.[2(p.v)]

One of the subcommittee's tasks was to look at the feasibility of a competency-based curriculum. In the past, learning objectives were used to evaluate educational attainment. A competency-based system is intended to

**Table 17-1 Public Health Functions Project**

The following tasks will be undertaken as part of the Public Health Functions Project:

1. Develop a taxonomy of the essential services of public health that can be readily understood and widely accepted for use by the public health community.

2. Using the taxonomy developed, assess the public health infrastructure and document the federal, state, and local expenditures on essential services of public health.

3. Propose a mechanism to ensure accountability for outcomes related to the delivery of essential public health services at the state and local levels, in return for greater flexibility in administration of federal grants to support public health.

4. Develop a strategy for communicating to the general public and key policy makers the nature and impact of essential public health services.

5. Document and publish analyses of the health and economic returns on investments in essential public health services.

6. Identify the key categories of public health personnel necessary to carry out the essential services of public health, assess the nation's current capacity and shortfalls, and establish a mechanism for ongoing monitoring of workforce strength and capability.

7. Develop and publish a full set of evidence-based guidelines for sound public health practice.

8. Collaborate with the PHS Data Policy Committee to identify the information and data needs for the effective implementation of the essential services of public health and develop a strategy for the interface between the personal services and population-wide systems, ensuring the availability of information necessary to both.

9. Develop a process to ensure the appropriate collaboration of the public health community and adequate inclusion of public health perspectives in the development of national health goals and objectives for the year 2010.

10. Develop a strategy for regular communication among interested parties at the national, state, and local levels on progress related to these activities.

*Source:* Reprinted from Public Health Service, *Public Health Workforce: An Agenda for the 21st Century,* 1997, U.S. Department of Health and Human Services.

be more oriented toward outcomes. Both learning objectives and competency-based outcomes can be useful for gauging a student's or trainee's mastery of new skills and abilities. Learning objectives define the key topics of the course or curriculum in a general way, whereas competencies define what a student or trainee is supposed to master over the long run. The critical issue is how to measure progress toward achieving the competencies and objectives.

The project subcommittee reported on six priority areas for a competency-based curriculum: cultural competency, health promotion skills, leadership development, program management, data analysis, and community organization. It identified a number of action steps for acquiring the competencies.

The development of competencies is a complex process. At the 1995 annual meeting of National Public Health Leadership Development Network (then under a different name), a project was undertaken to develop a series of leadership competencies for use in the creation and evaluation of state and regional public health leadership programs. The task groups formed at the meeting named four core categories for the competency exercise: transformational leadership skills, political competencies, transorganizational skills, and team-building skills. Over the course of 1996, the framework evolved. With the advent of a concern for competencies for leaders in a public health preparedness environment, Dr. Kate Wright and the Heartland Center for Public Health Preparedness have modified the framework to include these new competencies. Appendix 17-A presents this modified framework.[3]

Transformational leadership skills are needed by public health leaders because leaders are change agents. Leaders need to have a mission and vision and need to motivate and manage change effectively. As for political competencies, leaders need to understand how the political process works, how to negotiate, how to build alliances, and how to market public health and educate the community about public health issues. Because so much public health activity occurs between organizations, public health leaders need transorganizational competencies, including an understanding of organizational dynamics, interorganizational collaboration mechanisms, and social forecasting and marketing. The team-building skills they require include the ability to develop team-oriented structures for purposes of planning and implementing objectives and evaluating progress toward the objectives, the ability to facilitate team development, and the ability to mediate when a conflict occurs.

The framework presented in Appendix 17-A provides a template for learning and for making sense of the multidimensional aspects of public health leadership. No framework should be etched in stone. It must be allowed to evolve. Data need to be collected to determine if the identified competencies can be taught and put into practice. For example, Discovery Learning has developed a 360-degree public health Leadership Profile based on the framework that will provide these data in the future.[4] The profile is based on evaluation of such skills as innovation, client service, mentoring, collaboration, team skills, and conflict and negotiation skills.

The main problem with most competency frameworks is that the competencies are not defined with sufficient specificity to permit their measurement. Take, for example, the competency "Identify, articulate and model professional values and ethics," which is obviously very general and difficult to gauge. The solution is to break down each competency into specific components that can be measured. Discovery Learning has attempted to do this. In addition, there must be an applied research strategy to evaluate the leadership competencies routinely and revise them as necessary. None of this is to imply that the leadership competency framework is useless. The process of refining the framework has just begun and will probably take several years to complete. The end result is hoped to be a performance standards system capable of evaluating leadership outcomes.

## Credentialing and Accreditation

The credentialing of public health professionals became a live issue in the 1990s. In 1971, the U.S. Department of Health, Education, and Welfare defined credentialing as "the process by which a nongovernmental agency or association grants recognition to an individual who has met certain predetermined qualifications specified by that agency or association. Such qualifications may include: (a) graduation from an accredited or approved program; (b) acceptable performance on a qualifying examination or series of examinations; and/or (c) completion of a given amount of work experience."[5]

The supporters of credentialing argue that it will increase the credibility of public health professionals in the political arena as well as with the public at large. Professional standards will be developed that will guide public health programs. Some supporters want to tie credentialing to licensure. The critics argue that no credentialing system is possible because of the multidisciplinary background of public health professionals. Despite this criticism, a credentialing examination for graduates of accredited schools of public health and public health programs was given for the first time in the summer of 2008 and supervised by a recently created National Board of Public Health Examiners.

Schools of public health point out that they go through an accreditation process overseen by the Council on Education in Public Health. Accreditation would be prima facie evidence that graduating students have the necessary competence to practice public health, and a master's degree in public health from an accredited school of public health should preclude the necessity of further testing. On the other hand, many public health practitioners have not been trained in public health and thus don't have the stamp of approval conferred by graduation from a school of public health. In addition, there is a question whether schools of public health are teaching the skills that practitioners need to have. For example, leadership courses do not exist in some schools of public health.

A report to the U.S. Health Resources and Services Administration defined accreditation as follows: "Accreditation is generally used to refer to the evaluation of academic programs which prepare individuals for professional practice and to determine whether such programs meet predetermined standards. Accreditation may be carried out by public and private agencies or associations."[6(p.9)]

Licensure, credentialing, and accreditation are related, although proponents of credentialing may argue that accreditation is not a guarantee that the credentialed public health professional has acquired the desired knowledge or the ability to translate this knowledge into practice. Credentialing proponents point out that a process of evaluating professional knowledge helps develop standards for professional performance whereas accreditation is tied to an organization rather than a specific individual.

A report prepared for the Association of Schools of Public Health discussed factors that need to be included in any sound credentialing system.[7] First, role delineation that distinguishes between professionals who have different skills and levels of knowledge is a requisite. Because the role of public health administrators would be distinguished from that of other practitioners in the field, the credentialing of public health leaders could occur. Second, the credentialing system must specify the knowledge and skills required to carry out the duties of a credentialed professional and public health leader. Third, the system must determine the education, training, or experience necessary to generate the required competencies. Fourth, a testing procedure or other form of assessment must be devised to determine when a practitioner has achieved entry-level competency levels as well as more advanced levels of ability and knowledge. Finally, the system must include a process for recertification and require certified practitioners to undergo recertification periodically. Because leadership tools and skills change over time, the recertification process would encourage advanced training.

In the early 1990s, the American Public Health Association looked at the issue of professional credentialing.[8] The committee assigned to the task found very little information in the literature related to credentialing. To further its understanding of the issue, the committee conducted interviews with leaders in the field and with credentialing experts and also surveyed these two groups. The committee found that public health leaders generally did not support the development of a credentialing system. The leaders recognized that a credentialing system would need to be multifaceted and be able to accommodate a number of subspecialties and different education levels. The reaction of the credentialing experts was similar. The committee concluded that, despite the obvious benefits of credentialing, there was no consensus on the form credentialing should take.

One successful credentialing system was developed by the Society for Public Health Education (SOPHE) for undergraduate health educators.[9] The National Commission for Health Education Credentialing (NCHEC) was organized to carry out the certification of health educators. Since 1988, over 2,000 individuals have become certified health education specialists. The certification process, which is based on what NCHEC has determined are necessary educational and professional experiences, is voluntary. A health educator cannot take the examination unless he or she has a college degree from an accredited institution. A candidate also must have a minimum of 25 college semester hours in health education.

At the present time, there are more than 100 sites in the United States where the examination is given twice a year. Those people who pass the certification examination are seen as having met the minimal health education requirements. New criteria were introduced in 2006.[10] A three-tiered model for credentialing was developed for health education practice at the entry level and two advanced levels. SOPHE also became concerned with leadership and developed a leadership program for its members.

Questions have been raised about the qualifications of local health officers. During the 1990s, the Health Resources and Services Administration gave a three-year grant to the School of Public Health at the University of Illinois at Chicago to develop procedures for credentialing health administrators. A voluntary credentialing program was developed. It is too early to evaluate the experiment, but the experience of public health management and leadership programs around the country indicates that public health leaders gain from the management and leadership development process. What they gain, on the other hand, is difficult to determine in other than a general way. The National Public Health Leadership Development Network will begin to discuss the issue of credentialing for public health leaders in 2008.

## 360-degree Leadership Assessment and Feedback

We all have perceptions of ourselves that others around us may not share. Leaders are no exception. They may view themselves one way and be viewed by their colleagues in quite a different way. Therefore, the assessment of a leader needs to include a self-evaluation as well as evaluations by colleagues. In other words, it should be a 360-degree assessment.

The 360-degree assessment process involves a multilevel evaluation that focuses on whether the leader's style of leadership supports or obstructs achievement of the mission and goals of the organization. In a comprehensive 360-degree assessment, all key stakeholders have a voice in evaluating the leader and assessing the direction in which the organization is moving.[11]

Requirements of a 360-degree assessment include the following:[12] First, the leaders of the organization must determine whether sufficient enthusiasm for and commitment to the process exists in the organization and whether they are willing to institute changes based on the results of the assessment. Second, they must collect high-quality assessment data. Finally, they must identify possible responses to the results, such as the development of leadership training programs or formal mentoring programs.

There is a much utilized 360-degree leadership assessment instrument, the Leadership Practices Inventory (LPI), which evaluates leaders based on their performance of best leadership practices.[13] The five practices in the initial LPI were selected on the basis of interviews with senior and midlevel administrators and on leadership case studies. These five practices still are the major emphasis of the LPI. The practices are (1) modeling the way, (2) inspiring a shared vision, (3) challenging the way, (4) enabling others to act, and (5) encouraging the heart.

The third edition of the LPI has 30 leadership practice items, and for each item there are 10 possible responses, from "almost never" to "almost always." (In the first edition, there were only five choices for each item, from "rarely" to "very frequent.") The score for a given practice therefore can range from a low of 6 to a high of 60. One version of the LPI is used for self-evaluation, and a second version is used for evaluation by observers (colleagues and stakeholders). The LPI can be used at different times to determine whether the leader has made progress in performing the five leadership practices.

Using the original LPI, data on 43,000 leaders from around the world were collected, and means, standard deviations, and internal reliability measures were computed.[14] Most of the leaders were from the business sector but some were from academia and the public sector. The reliability rates fell between 0.81 and 0.91. Enabling others to act was seen by leaders and their observers as the most common practice, followed by challenging the process, modeling the way, encouraging the heart, and, in last place, inspiring a shared vision.

In a pilot study using the LPI, baseline leadership information was collected from 163 public health leaders selected as fellows by the Illinois Public Health Leadership Institute between 1992 and 1997. There may be a self-selection bias built into the study, because fellows are likely to have identified themselves as leaders before embarking on the leadership program and to be committed to leadership development to enhance their skills. Thus far, public health leaders have not specifically been studied. Comparisons of public health leader self-evaluations and observer evaluations have not been done thus far. Some preliminary data indicate that observers rate their leaders higher than the leaders rate themselves.

Mean scores for business leaders and public health leaders are presented in Table 17-2. The scores for public health leaders are consistently higher, but a confounder is the fact that the sample of business leaders includes academics and human service professionals. The scores for the two groups were not

**Table 17-2    Means and Standard Deviations for Public Health and Business Leaders**

| Leadership Practice Item | Business Leaders (N = 43,889) | | Public Health Leaders (N = 166) | | Significant Difference |
|---|---|---|---|---|---|
| | Mean | SD | Mean | SD | |
| Challenging the process | 22.38 | 4.17 | 23.4 | 3.46 | None |
| Inspiring a shared vision | 20.48 | 4.90 | 21.6 | 3.98 | None |
| Enabling others to act | 20.48 | 4.37 | 25.3 | 2.46 | $p \leq .0015$ |
| Modeling the way | 22.89 | 4.16 | 23.8 | 3.24 | $p \leq .001$ |
| Encouraging the heart | 21.89 | 5.22 | 23.6 | 3.59 | $p \leq .001$ |

*Note:* This study was done with Elanine Jurkowski.

significantly different on the practice "challenging the process," an indicator of orientation to change, nor on the practice "inspiring a shared vision" (both groups scored relatively low). The public health leaders scored significantly higher than the business leaders on the other three practices, all of which are associated with the quality of work-related relationships.

One of the difficulties of using the LPI in studies of leadership is that the main purpose of the instrument is to assess individual leaders through self-evaluation and observer evaluation. The aggregation of LPI data should hide the characteristics of individual leaders, but nonetheless they need to be informed of the fact that their evaluations may be used for research. The instrument also may create biases in the responses because it is tied to a conceptual model that the developers promote. Not every leader supports this model.

Another instrument used in several public health leadership programs is the Skillscope 360-degree assessment developed by the Center for Creative Leadership.[15] This instrument assesses information skills, decision-making skills, interpersonal skills, personal resources, and effective use of self. The instrument is flexible to use and can be used for individual assessments tied to coaching as well as a part of a structured leadership program. On a group level, the Skillscope can help to establish a group profile related to the strengths of the group and areas that need work. Another instrument developed by the Center for Creative Leadership is the 360-degree Benchmarks profile, which is one of the leadership instruments used in the National Public Health Leadership Institute.[16] Benchmarks is a comprehensive tool that measures 16 success skills and five career derailers. The 16 skills fall into the four categories of meeting job challenges, respect yourself and others, leading people, and potential for derailment.

On the negative side, a 360-degree assessment is often expensive and time consuming.[17] Not only must the measurement instruments be bought, but staff need to be trained to interpret the results. Another issue is whether leaders are willing to reveal self-perceived weaknesses to their colleagues and whether subordinates feel comfortable rating their leaders. This issue is of special concern in smaller organizations. If anonymity is not maintained and the observer evaluations are negative, animosity may occur between leaders and their professional colleagues. Finally, there is the question whether the process will make any difference.[18]

Despite these issues, the process can result in important information. If the leadership data are linked to organizational needs, organizational efficiency and effectiveness can be improved. The results need to be communicated to the entire workforce, but with a sensitivity for the possible impact on the person who was evaluated. On the whole, the 360-degree approach offers individuals and the organization information that can improve the services provided by the organization.

## Qualitative Leadership Assessment

Public health programming is driven by population-based statistics, including mortality and morbidity rates. The problem is that the vitality of public health as an approach and perspective can get lost in the numbers, with the result that public health loses credibility among community residents.[19] As a consequence, public health leaders need to acquire qualitative information to help them evaluate their performance and to publicize public health as a way of enhancing their credibility.

Qualitative information often comes in the form of stories, which were discussed in Chapter 11 and in case studies. The case studies of interest to us here describe public health practitioners in action and present conclusions about what was done right and what could have been done better. As we will use the term, "case" refers to whatever is the subject of a case study (usually a single event or a series of events).

Case studies, for our purposes, can be divided into four classes: (1) specific empirical studies, (2) general empirical studies, (3) specific theoretical studies, and (4) general theoretical studies. Empirical case studies describe actual cases, whereas theoretical case studies are constructed specifically to illustrate some point. Specific case studies have definable boundaries, and general case studies are examples already available that can be used to demonstrate a perspective.

The cases chosen for research inquiry are typically different from those chosen for training purposes. In this section, we are interested in the latter, especially their potential to clarify the application of leadership principles in the real world of public health practice. Training case studies describe how professionals handle problems and thus can serve as guides to future action. Leaders can develop their own case studies in order to analyze public health community activities and evaluate their own leadership skills.

Public health case studies are used for three main purposes.[20] First, they can be used to offer insights into how a public health agency carries out its activities. Second, they can be used to help public health leaders explore different scenarios as part of a problem-solving process. Table 17-3, for instance, presents a number of public health scenarios helpful for defining outcomes that might occur if a public health agency instituted a certain policy or embarked in a certain direction. Third, case studies can be used to illuminate why events unfolded in a certain way and to explore better ways to handle an emergency situation, for instance.

As regards the last two uses, the role of leadership and the causal consequences of actions need to be interpreted carefully. It is always difficult to tease out the causal factors in a complex set of relationships and happenings.

**Table 17-3    Public Health Scenarios Based on Schwartz Categories**

**Scenario 1: Winners and Losers**
A health reform plan passes Congress. The plan presents a system redesign that is state based and involves local health alliances. The health plans incorporate most of the direct service functions of local health departments. Block grant funds that remain are given directly to the health alliances for distribution. This scenario initially positions the local health department as a loser.

**Scenario 2: Challenge and Response**
The American Public Health Association creates a strong lobbying coalition that includes representatives from all the major public health interest groups and organizations. As Congress reviews changes in the financing of health services, the public health community is able to affect legislation so that CDC and state public health agencies become responsible for collecting all data related to health care, are responsible for oversight of all health programs, become the lead agency for all government-sponsored primary prevention programs, are directly funded for health-related community programs by a block grant, and so on. Public health meets every challenge and wins.

**Scenario 3: Evolution**
There is a major change in the economy of the state. Several new biotechnology companies move to the state, and many new jobs are created. The state unemployment rate drops to 3%. With the increase in employment, the number of people on welfare drops significantly. With new jobs, the teenage pregnancy rate drops, as does the incidence of gang-related violence, because gang members get jobs.

**Scenario 4: Revolution**
Congress passes a major piece of legislation. The government decides to get out of the public health business. All public health activities are transferred to the private health care system.

**Scenario 5: Cycle**
Five years after the evolution scenario above takes place, the American economy collapses. A major depression occurs. People lose their jobs. Gang warfare increases. The teenage pregnancy rate expands significantly.

**Scenario 6: Infinite Possibilities**
A health reform package passes that provides universal coverage.

**Scenario 7: The Lone Ranger**
Through the efforts of public health professionals and researchers, a cure for AIDS is found, a chemical substance that purifies all water is discovered, and a vaccine that prevents Alzheimer's disease is developed. Because of these breakthroughs, the American public unequivocally supports all public health initiatives.

**Scenario 8: My Generation**
The early years of the 21st century see a major increase in births in the United States.

The above scenarios can be looked at individually or can be combined to form more complex scenarios.
*Source:* Adapted from *The Art of the Long View* by Peter Schwartz. Copyright © 1991 by Peter Schwartz. Used by permission of Doubleday, a division of Random House, Inc.

In addition, the events that make up a case rarely repeat themselves in exactly the same way.

Some case studies are merely free-flowing stories about examples of leadership, for instance. These stories nonetheless must have a message intended for a well-defined audience.[21] There are three main types of leadership stories. One is the "Who am I?" story. The second is the "Who are we?" story. The third is a story of the realization of a vision. It is possible to add a fourth category consisting of "What I learned on my summer vacation" stories. These stories describe what a leader learned from other leaders or from workshops on leadership. As discussed in Chapter 11, other story formats are available as well.

Case study stories have plots intended to elucidate ideas or values. They should be tested before being released to the public to make sure that their messages are clear. One variant of the personal story is the biographical portrait.[22] A portrait of a historical or present-day leader, such as C. Edward Koop or Paul Farmer, can be employed for the same purposes as a personal story. Another variant is to focus on a leader whose values stand in contrast to those of a typical public health leader, such as a senator from a tobacco state.

An interview can also make up the content of a case study. Questions serve as the mechanism for getting information. For example, the author interviewed more than 130 public health leaders in four countries in order to explore their understanding of the meaning of public health, their vision of the future, and the changing characteristics of leaders. (Table 17-4 consists of a guide for interviewing public health leaders.)

An interesting variation on the interview is the focus group, in which leaders, for example, might answer questions as a team. A conversation is another variation—a variation explored in Exercise 17-l.

A case study protocol for public health practice narratives was developed for public health practitioners in a leadership development program under the assumption that structured case studies provide trainees and other lifelong learners with models of public health practice.[23] Case studies can also be used to explore cutting-edge issues in public health that are in need of resolution. In other words, case studies can be based on completed events or on situations in progress.

**Table 17-4  Interview Guide for Public Health Leaders**

1. What are the reasons that you decided on a career in public health?
2. How would you define public health?
3. What is your definition of leadership?
4. What are the necessary leadership practices and skills that a public health leader needs to use?
5. Are these practices and skills different from the practices and skills of business leaders?
6. What elements of public health's organizational system enhance or create barriers to leadership?
7. What is the role of public health in carrying out the core functions of assessment, policy development, and assurance?
8. What is your vision for public health in the 21st century? What are the three most important systems issues for the future, and what are the key health issues for the future?
9. How successful is the system in promoting community coalitions to address the health of the community?
10. Are public-private partnerships that address public health concerns possible? What is public health's role in managed care?
11. Does the public understand public health? If not, what can you do to change this situation?
12. Should public health be integrated into the general health sector or should public health be maintained as part of a separate governmental office?
13. What distinguishes a practitioner, a manager, and a leader?
14. Is the mentoring of future leaders important? What type of mentoring program do you recommend?
15. What is the role of politics in public health?

Each case has a unique character.[24] For example, even similar cases will differ in historical background, setting, or economic, political, legal, social, or cultural aspects. They also can have a different slant depending on the reason they were written.

Case studies, as stories, have characters, a plot, and a setting. Their purpose is to give insight into leadership styles and practices, personality concerns, power concerns, organizational intrigues, politics in action, media involvement, and so on. They can be effective mentoring tools; the mentor can assign a case study for the mentee to read, and then the two can discuss the issues raised in the case study. A problem-based case study can present a possible vision of the future.

The best case studies are built on real experiences. Whereas ideal cases can be constructed, most people seem to relate better to real-life situations that seem real in their unfolding. That is one of the reasons that every case study in this book is factually based, although names and places have sometimes been changed to protect the actual participants.

Most case studies are written as narratives and have a beginning, middle, and end[25] (Table 17-5). The opening should present the issue that the case is intended to illustrate and describe the setting and key characters. The middle, or the body of the case study, describes the events that make up the case. If this is done properly, then the lesson of the case becomes clear. In some instances, elements of the setting and key characters may be described in more

---

**Table 17-5   Case Study Development Protocol**

**Opening (first few paragraphs)**
Name and title of responsible professional
Date: month and year (fix the case in time)
Synopsis of decision required or problem setting or issues presented, keeping in the forefront the core functions of health departments

**Case body (no more than four to five pages)**
Department/agency history, if pertinent
Environmental setting, if pertinent
Political concerns
Expanded description of the decision or problem situation
Human interaction facts, etc.
Human element
Personality impact
Public relations factor
Presence/absence of vision/enthusiasm
Organizational relationships
Other case characters or entities
Program and process
Financial concerns, where pertinent

**Closing (last paragraph or two)**

**Conclusion of the case**

**Suggested methods**
Setting the scene to establish a sense of urgency about the problem or decision
Setting out a range of decision options

---

*Source:* Reprinted with permission from J. Munson, *Case Study Development: Guidelines and Protocols for Case Study Development,* 2nd Ed., 2003. © 1994, University of Illinois School of Public Health, Mid-American Regional Public Health Leadership Institute.

detail than was provided in the opening. Political factors that affected the outcome may be critically examined.

Many case studies include all sorts of supplemental documentation to elucidate the circumstances. The closing reviews the issue in light of the events described and analyzes the decisions made by the key characters.[26] It may explore possible options that might have led to an outcome different from the one that actually occurred. (Some case studies are intended to deal with multiple issues and use a slightly different organization to address the issues in a coherent manner.)

Case Study 17-A has the classic organization described here. It deals with the issues of privatization of laboratory services and the lack of involvement by public health laboratory directors in public health policy issues. It is also based on variations of real-life situations.

---

## Case Study 17-A
## Organization of Public Health and Clinical Laboratory Services in a Reformed Health Service Delivery System

*Jon Counts*

### Introduction
In 2009 the U.S. Congress passed comprehensive legislation that would establish universal health care coverage by the year 2012. Congress mandated that each state would develop a strategic plan that would integrate and restructure the public and private health care programs. The commissioner of health, Dr. Strangelove, has designated you, Dr. Vision, to develop a plan to define the role of hospital, commercial, public health, and academic laboratories as part of the state of Innovation's strategy for a reformed health system.

### Case Body
The result of three decades of heavy clinical laboratory utilization has been the development of a fractured, duplicative, and costly laboratory system in the state of Innovation. The laboratory network in this state fits the general description of the current health system: a patchwork of private and public programs, with goals and objectives as varied as the groups and organizations represented in the system. Clinical laboratories represent a significant component of the rapidly increasing costs of health care. The Health Care Financing Administration estimates that spending on laboratory services comprises 4.5% of all national health care expenditures.

Clinical laboratories, like the rest of the health care community, have been significantly affected by the nation's health reform legislation, the Health Services Act of 1993. The primary vehicle for the implementation of the legislation is the new Health Services Commission. The Health Services Act will enable each state to control spending by:

1. shifting the state toward a system of "managed" health care
2. defining a uniform benefit package and developing standards of certified health plans through which the uniform benefits package will be provided
3. setting the maximum rate a certified health plan may charge for the uniform benefit package
4. establishing a maximum health care inflation rate and lowering the rate until it matches the rate of general inflation

5. setting rules for fair competition among certified health plans
6. minimizing malpractice and its costs
7. simplifying the administration of claims, billing, and information
8. promoting the use of cost-effective health care practices and services
9. defining the role and function of public health agencies

Dr. Vision realizes that the task ahead of him will be a challenge and very controversial.

1. First, the development of any coalition among laboratory organizations, physicians, pathologists, laboratory managers, hospital and commercial laboratories, and government will be exceedingly difficult to achieve.
   a. There will be opposition to a government agency leading the discussion about the role of laboratories in a reformed system. There will be suspicion, lack of trust, and concern about the regulatory approach that government agencies might mandate.
   b. For the most part there has been little or no historical interaction among individuals/organizations who will be involved in the coalition; therefore, the plan must be carefully developed and staged, ensuring that a process for developing consensus has been established.
   c. The activities of coalition will be monitored closely; therefore, there cannot be any secrecy and they must be open to the public, outside review, and scrutiny. There must be a system for dissemination of information and recommendations to the laboratory and medical community.
   d. There will be strong opposition to the possibility that the plan will lead to the re-engineering and downsizing of commercial and hospital laboratory staff.
   e. The issue of competition between public health laboratories and private sector facilities will be raised as well as the need to consider the privatization of diagnostic services provided by government laboratories. This obviously will be a contentious point because Dr. Vision will have a vested interest in the outcome.
2. The nature of health problems has changed dramatically during the 20th century; chronic conditions have become predominant as well as new and re-emerging infectious diseases.
3. The utilization of managed care plans and capitation to control costs and share the risk with providers has increased dramatically. The march of managed care, new technologies, and alternative treatment settings will prompt a 34% decrease in inpatient hospital days over the five years from 2003 to 2008. Ambulatory facilities will eliminate many surgical inpatient days, use of birthing centers will increase, mental health care will be delivered more often in residential settings such as halfway houses, and home care will be the most dramatic and fastest growing segment of the health care industry. These changes will have a significant impact upon diagnostic laboratory testing. Hospital laboratories will undergo significant reduction in routine and inpatient testing, vertical integration will occur, and regional delivery systems will consolidate and centralize laboratory testing. Large national commercial laboratories will capture the vast majority of testing.

*(continues)*

**Case Study 17-A** *continued*

4. The role of laboratory medicine will be expanded into promoting health and preventing disease. Home testing will increase, as will the need to promote direct public access to preventive and screening testing. Genetic testing obviously is going to expand. Hospital and commercial laboratories will play a much more active role in the nation's disease surveillance, promoting the need for a statewide electronic network between private clinical laboratories and the public health systems. Other anticipated changes in the future laboratory system include:

- active management of laboratory utilization, elimination of unnecessary testing, and utilization of practice guidelines
- standardization of lab instrumentation and testing methodology and increasing automation
- utilization of clinical patient outcome measures of laboratory quality

*Proposal Solution*

The implementation of health reform makes strategic planning imperative for all components of the health system. Historically there have been few efforts to draw the clinical laboratory community together into cooperative efforts toward long-range planning except in the area of laboratory regulation and the credentialing of laboratory personnel. This initiative has been developed to assist the leadership of the clinical laboratory community in the state of Innovation in assessing the impact of health reform and in developing recommendations for integrating the diverse segments of the existing laboratory system into a more cost-effective and -efficient structure. The process will include creation of a steering committee to provide recommendations to Dr. Vision for the guidance, direction, and oversight of the initiative. The steering committee may also appoint technical advisory work groups to study and develop specific recommendations on such issues as the following:

- structure and integration of delivery system
- utilization of clinical laboratories in medical decisions or development of practice parameters
- laboratory regulations
- impact of malpractice tort reform on laboratory utilization
- utilization of new technology in laboratories
- personnel resource training and credentialing
- utilization of out-of-state laboratories
- reimbursement policies
- direct billing
- laboratory information systems—collection, analysis, integration, and dissemination of data
- surveillance of emerging infectious diseases
- point-of-care testing
- home testing
- public access to laboratory testing

The steering committee will consolidate its recommendations into a report to be submitted to the commissioner of health, Dr. Strangelove, for his consideration in establishing public policy.

Dr. Vision must first establish a process to identify and appoint members from the department and community to the steering committee, individuals who are experts in laboratory science, strategic planning, public policy, development of community constituencies, and consensus building and who are representatives of medical specialties.

Next, the steering committee must establish a strategic-planning process, including identification and prioritization of major components and issues. In order to address those issues listed, it is essential that a mechanism be developed to collect and evaluate health-related data to determine the need for diagnostic laboratory services. Finally, it must be determined by the steering committee how it will solicit public input.

---

Exercise 17-2 provides the opportunity to write a case study. The work of researching and writing the case study, which may take several weeks, is done using teams. The case studies presented in this text can serve as models.

---

## Quantitative Leadership Assessment Techniques

Leadership assessment comes in more than one variety. Part of the explanation is that the standard leadership assessment instruments grow out of different theories of leadership. Another part of the explanation is that there are at least five levels of leadership and different traits and behaviors that are needed for each level. Most leadership assessment techniques are oriented toward the personal level, but leadership can also be evaluated at the team, agency, community, and professional levels.

Because it is usually the individual who fills out the leadership assessment instrument, most leadership assessment relates to personal traits and behavior, and these traits and behaviors, unsurprisingly, are stressed by psychometricians. One of the best-known personality assessment tools has been adopted by a number of public health leadership programs.

> **Leadership Tips**
>
> *Serve refreshments at meetings.*
>
> *It reduces absenteeism.*

The Myers-Briggs Type Indicator (MBTI), based on Jung's theory of psychological types, measures personality along four dimensions.[27] The first is the extroversion (E) and introversion (I) dimension. Where someone falls along this dimension is determined by whether he or she relates more to the external world or more to his or her inner world. The second dimension, defined by the contrast between sensing perceptions (S) and intuitive perceptions (N), measures whether a person focuses on the here and now or on future possibilities and abstract theory and symbols. The next dimension, defined by the contrast between thinking (T) and feeling (F), measures whether a person responds to situations rationally or emotionally. The fourth dimension, defined by the contrast between judgment (J) and perception (P), measures whether the person tends naturally to engage in organizing, planning, and decision making or instead tends to want to keep options open.

The MBTI instrument is quite comprehensive[28] and requires the person being tested to answer numerous forced-choice questions. After completing the questionnaire, the person receives a report on his or her profile. The author, who filled out the questionnaire in order to gain a better understanding of how it is used, was found to be an ENTJ. The report said that the author tends to be decisive and frank, quick to take charge of people and projects, applies logic and analysis, prefers action to contemplation, and often pays more attention to tasks than to the people.

To discover how leaders in the public sector would score, researchers tested and compared five groups of leaders in local, state, and federal government.[29] The first group included 1,394 senior federal government administrators tested from 1983 to 1986. The next three groups, tested in the early 1980s, consisted of managers attending special government institutes at the University of North Carolina. The fifth group consisted of about 100 social service administrators from Nebraska. Figure 17-1 shows how these groups scored on the four dimensions. The point to note is that leaders do not score in a uniform way. Different patterns emerge. Leaders with different styles engage in different leadership practices.

The Leader Behavior Analysis II instrument differs substantially from the MBTI.[30] It presents the person being tested with 20 typical job situations that involve a leader and one or more staff members. After reading each scenario, the person, putting him- or herself in the position of the leader, selects one of four possible actions. The instrument, which can be self-scored, investigates three dimensions. The first is flexibility (whether the person tends to try to be directive or be supportive). There are four score categories for this dimension:

| S1: high directive, low supportive behavior |
| S2: high directive, high supportive behavior |
| S3: high supportive, low directive behavior |
| S4: low supportive, low directive behavior |

The responses to the pertinent scenarios are used to compute a style flexibility score between 0 and 30. The higher the score, the greater the flexibility. The second dimension is leadership effectiveness, and the third is diagnosis.

Scores for these dimensions are computed in roughly the same way as for the first dimension. There is also a form for others to fill out, which allows for a 360-degree personal leadership evaluation.

A study of an earlier version of this instrument found that leadership assessment tools help leaders evaluate their leadership styles and compare their self-perceptions with the perceptions of colleagues.[31] The sample included evaluations of 20,000 leaders from 14 cultures (each evaluation comprised a self-assessment and assessments by others). About 2,000 leaders from industry and education were interviewed, and about 500 in-depth interviews were done. The situational leadership model was supported by the data collected.

There is a Team Leadership Practices Inventory that is basically similar to the LPI developed for leaders and colleagues.[32] The Team LPI is based on the same five leadership practices used in the initial version of the LPI: challenging the process, inspiring a shared vision, enabling others to act, modeling the way, and encouraging the heart. Because the use of teams has increased in most organizations, evaluating how teams function is essential. Each team member fills out the Team LPI, which has 30 items. The scores for each practice are totaled and then averaged. By using the Team LPI, a team can deter-

| | ISTJ | ISFJ | INFJ | INTJ |
|---|---|---|---|---|
| Federal A Senior | 26.3 + | 2.7 | 1.8 | 14.9 |
| State–City B Top Level | 30.7 + | 6.2 | 2.0 | 7.4 |
| C Midlevel | 17.9 | 9.7 | 0.7 | 5.9 |
| D Public | 26.4 + | 5.5 | 1.5 | 5.5 |
| E Soc Serv | 16.8 | 19.8 | 1.0 | 2.0 |

| | ISTP | ISFP | INFP | INTP |
|---|---|---|---|---|
| Federal A Senior | 5.4 | 0.4 | 2.4 | 9.1 |
| State–City B Top Level | 4.7 | 1.6 | 1.2 | 3.9 |
| C Midlevel | 3.1 | 3.1 | 1.7 | 2.1 |
| D Public | 4.8 | 1.9 | 1.5 | 2.9 |
| E Soc Serv | 5.0 | 3.0 | 2.0 | 4.0 |

| | ESTP | ESFP | ENFP | ENTP |
|---|---|---|---|---|
| Federal A Senior | 2.0 | 0.6 | 2.4 | 5.8 |
| State–City B Top Level | 1.6 | 1.6 | 2.0 | 1.6 |
| C Midlevel | 5.5 | 2.1 | 2.4 | 3.8 |
| D Public | 2.7 | 1.9 | 3.4 | 2.7 |
| E Soc Serv | 3.0 | 2.0 | 1.0 | 2.0 |

| | ESTJ | ESFJ | ENFJ | ENTJ |
|---|---|---|---|---|
| Federal A Senior | 12.3 | 1.4 | 1.9 | 10.6 |
| State–City B Top Level | 22.2 + | 3.9 | 2.7 | 7.0 |
| C Midlevel | 24.1 + | 6.2 | 3.1 | 8.6 |
| D Public | 22.8 + | 7.1 | 2.5 | 6.9 |
| E Soc Serv | 19.8 | 10.9 | 5.0 | 3.0 |

**FIGURE 17-1** **Myers-Brigg Type Indicator Percentages for Managers in Federal, State, and Local Government**
*Source:* Reprinted with permission from M. H. McCaulley, The Myers-Briggs Type Indicator and Leadership, in *Measures of Leadership,* K. E. Clark and M. B. Clark, eds., p. 389, © 1990, Leadership Library of America, Center for Creative Leadership.

mine its strengths as well as the practices that need improvement. The LPI is highly correlated with the Team LPI. Both instruments are less concerned about leadership style than about the practices of leadership.

There has been growing interest in leadership skills and practices at the organizational level. In 1984, a study of effective organizational leadership was undertaken,[33] and it led to the development of the Leader Behavior Questionnaire (LBQ). The LBQ consists of 50 questions. It is intended to measure focused leadership (listening ability), communication abilities, trust leadership, respectful leadership (how leaders treat others), risk leadership, bottom-line leadership (the belief of leaders that they can make a difference), empowered leadership (sharing power), long-term leadership (visionary leadership), organizational leadership, and cultural leadership (leadership based on the values of the organization). An important underlying assumption of the LBQ is that leadership is multidimensional and that each of its dimensions must be evaluated.

An important assessment-related breakthrough occurred in the mid-1990s. The health care sector became more interested in the measurement of outcomes as a way of evaluating effectiveness.[34] Performance measurement encompasses the measurement of program inputs, intermediate outcomes (process issues), and end outcomes.[35] One goal of performance measurement is to determine whether changes in public health expenditures affect the outputs of public health agencies and the final outcomes for the community.

Two important new instruments give added clarity to the way talents affect leadership and also thinking and behavioral preferences. The Gallup Organization has been studying managers and leaders for over 40 years. From its work has come an instrument called Strength Finder (now Strength Finder 2.0).[36] This instrument measures the strengths of an individual as tied to 34 talent themes (see Table 2-4). Rath has pointed out that it is important to build on individual talents to create strengths at work and not concentrate on individual weaknesses. This instrument is easy to take and is not costly. A leader buys the book, which has a unique access code to the Gallup Organization Web site. The recipient will receive a profile of the top five strengths.

> **Leadership Tips**
>
> *Read your mail or answer e-mails*
>
> *when your energy level is low.*
>
> *Do important tasks when your*
>
> *energy levels tend to be high.*

The Emergenetics instrument gives the individual a profile in color of his or her thinking preferences and behavioral attributes (see Figure 3-1).[37] This instrument has also been tested on individuals throughout the world. The instrument relates to four major thinking preferences of people: analytical, structural, conceptual, and social. Most individuals have profiles that show some mixture of all four preferences, but they tend to have dominance in one, two, three, or four thinking domains. The three behavioral attributes are expressiveness, assertiveness, and flexibility.

An Institute of Medicine report presented a framework for improving the health of community residents. The community health improvement process is shown in Figure 17-2.[38] It encompasses the identification and analysis of health issues, the development and implementation of strategies to resolve the issues, and the monitoring of the implementation process and outcomes. One of the steps is to develop an indicator set that links the implementation of strategies with their outcomes so that the effectiveness of the strategies can be determined, which is the essence of performance measurement. Figure 17-3 presents a performance measurement model consisting of six steps.[39] Despite the existence of this model, public state and local agencies have been slow in adopting the performance measurement approach.[40] This is beginning to change as mentioned below.

Performance monitoring is related to evidence-based public health.[41] Evidence-based public health promotes the use of traditional biostatistics measures, epidemiology, healthy communities assessment, and continuous quality improvement methods. Public health agencies and their leaders have

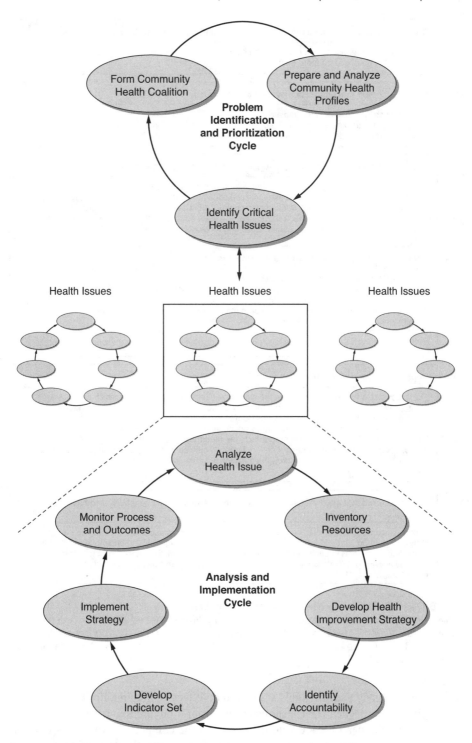

**FIGURE 17-2    The Community Health Improvement Process (CHIP)**
*Source:* Reprinted with permission from *Improving Health in the Community: A Role for Performance Monitoring,* p. 6. Copyright 1997 by the National Academy of Sciences. Courtesy of the National Academy Press, Washington, DC.

| STEP 1 | **Relate the performance measure to an important national, state, or local priority area.** |
|---|---|
| | Maryland has undertaken work related to the national health objective to reduce coronary heart disease deaths to no more than 100 per 100,000 people. |

| STEP 2 | **Measure a result that can be achieved in 5 years or less.** |
|---|---|
| | Maryland has identified an achievable result that is linked scientifically to the Healthy People 2000 Heart Disease and Stroke priority area: Increase the proportion of people who engage in light to moderate physical activity to at least 30 percent of the population. |

| STEP 3 | **Ensure that the result is meaningful to a wide audience of stakeholders.** |
|---|---|
| | Target stakeholders are essentially all Marylanders, with an emphasis on school-age children and people at high risk for diseases and medical conditions associated with physical inactivity (for example, persons with hypertension and high cholesterol). Stakeholders include principals, teachers, students, parent-teacher associations, the state education department, state and local health and recreational agencies, public health and medical professionals, and others. |

| STEP 4 | **Define the strategy that will be used to reach a result.** |
|---|---|
| | The State of Maryland has selected four strategies: 1. Implement a combination of strategies that include consumer education and skills development, health assessment, professional training, and environmental changes. 2. Reinforce risk reduction messages and promote programs and policies in schools, worksites, faith communities, and other settings. 3. Focus on youth and families so that healthy habits are started early and nurtured in the family. 4. Use a health promotion approach tailored to reach diverse ethnic and socioeconomic groups. |

| STEP 5 | **Define the accountable entities.** |
|---|---|
| | The accountable entities depend upon the strategies selected and the way in which a particular community is organized. For Maryland's Strategy 2, these entities include schools, worksites, and community centers. For example, the Cecil County Public Schools have agreed to be accountable for specific tasks related to Strategy 2 and are working in partnership with the Cecil County Health Department to offer health lifestyle programs to elementary school children. The programs, such as the **Heart Challenge Course**, bring teachers and food service workers together to promote healthy eating habits and physical fitness through educational games, classroom projects, and other activities that appeal to children. |

| STEP 6 | **Draft measures that meet statistical requirements of validity and reliability and have an existing source of data.** |
|---|---|
| | In consultation with biostaticians and epidemiologists, organizations can draft measures that are statistically sound. One of Maryland's performance measures might be "Increase to 30 percent the proportion of students in each Cecil County elementary school who engage in light to moderate physical activity for 30 minutes or longer every school day by participating in school physical fitness activities." |

**FIGURE 17-3 Performance Measurement Step-by-Step**
*Source:* Based on example of State of Maryland's *Healthy Maryland 2000.* Reprinted from *Improving the Nation's Health with Performance Measurement, Prevention Report,* Vol. 12, No. 1, p. 3, 1997, Office of Disease Prevention and Health Services, U.S. Department of Health and Human Services.

not routinely used the tools at hand in an effective manner, nor have they routinely approached their responsibilities from a population-based perspective.

Public health leaders need to develop the competencies to carry out performance monitoring. Currently, they often assign the task of performance monitoring to other staff members. They also need to ensure that performance measurement is accepted by agency staff and that the information gained is used by the staff to improve operations. In fact, performance measures for evaluating the activities of public health leaders and their community partners utilizing a systems perspective and the essential public health services in the performance process have been developed in the National Public Health Performance Standards Program discussed in Part II of this book. The use of performance measurement by leaders will become more prevalent with the accreditation of local health departments beginning in 2011.

## Summary

Evaluation plays a multifaceted role in public health. Evaluation techniques are used for uncovering the public health problems that exist in a given community and for assessing the implementation of the programs intended to deal with such problems. They can also be used to assess the level of a leader's skills and abilities.

The chapter began with a description of the leadership competencies framework and listed some of the competencies that public health leaders need to have. It then discussed the question of whether a system should be put in place for credentialing public health leaders—a question over which public health leaders are divided.

Quantitative leadership evaluations are problematic at best. Each instrument incorporates a conceptual model on which the instrument is based. The organization in which the leader works often is conceptually different from the model used in the instrument. One alternative is to do a qualitative evaluation using case studies and other qualitative techniques and a battery of several quantitative tools. No matter what type of evaluation is done, however, the evaluation should include the opinions of both the leader being evaluated and the opinions of colleagues. In short, it should be a 360-degree evaluation. Furthermore, the evaluation should cover the leader's performance at the agency level and also at the community level.

### Discussion Questions

1. What is one of the problems with using competencies as a means of evaluating leadership?
2. What are the pros and cons of credentialing leaders?
3. What are five personal leadership lessons you learned during the last year?
4. What is a 360-degree assessment?
5. What are some difficulties associated with performing a 360-degree assessment?
6. What is a qualitative leadership assessment and what are some techniques for performing such an assessment?

### Exercise 17-1:    Conversations with Leaders

*Purpose:* to learn how peers view public health and what they think about current public health leadership issues

*Key concepts:* core functions, evaluation of leadership, focus group, interviewing skills, leadership skills

*Procedure:* It is possible to learn many things from peers. The class should divide into focus groups of six to eight members. Each group engages in a discussion of leadership using the interview questions in the text as a guide (Table 17-4). The discussion should last at least an hour, although it is not necessary to go through all the questions. The group should allow the discussion to go in any direction it naturally moves. The class can repeat the exercise several times, each time concentrating on a different set of issues.

**Exercise 17-2:  Development of a Public Health Case Study**

*Purpose:* to develop a public health case study to examine how leaders address public health issues

*Key concepts:* case study, core functions, essential services, leadership, team learning

*Procedure:* The class should divide into teams of five to eight members. Each team will be responsible for writing a case study using the Munson protocol (Table 17-5). Much of the work will take place outside of class. Follow these steps: (1) Select a facilitator to monitor each phase of the project. (2) Identify a public health case worthy of being written about. (3) Investigate the case and collect information for writing up the case. (4) Analyze the case from a policy development perspective. (5) Identify leadership issues involved in the case. (6) Write up the case (the study should be five to ten pages). (7) Give an oral report on the case to the other teams.

# References

1. Public Health Service, *The Public Health Workforce: An Agenda for the 21st Century* (Washington, DC: U.S. Department of Health and Human Services, 1997).
2. Public Health Service, *The Public Health Workforce.*
3. National Public Health Leadership Development Network and the Heartland Center for Public Health Preparedness (Dr. K. Wright, Director).
4. Discovery Learning. http://www.discoverylearning.com/products/profile-public-health.aspx
5. U.S. Department of Health, Education, and Welfare, *Report on Licensure and Related Health Personnel Credentialing* (Washington, DC: U.S. Department of Health, Education, and Welfare, 1971).
6. A. C. Gielen et al., *Health Education in the 21st Century: A White Paper*, report prepared for Health Resources and Services Administration (Washington, DC: Health Resources and Services Administration, 1997).
7. E. Carpenter, *Proposed Credentialing System for Public Health Professionals: What Would It Mean for Schools of Public Health* (Washington, DC: Association of Schools of Public Health, 1990).
8. W. C. Livingood et al., *Perceived Feasibility and Desirability of Public Health Credentialing: Final Report* (Washington, DC: American Public Health Association, 1993).
9. Gielen et al., *Health Education in the 21st Century.*
10. http://www.nchec.org
11. M. R. Edwards and A. J. Ewen, *360° Feedback* (New York: ANACOM, 1996).
12. R. Lepsinger and A. D. Lucia, *The Art and Science of 360° Feedback* (San Francisco: Jossey-Bass, 1997).

13. J. M. Kouzes and B. Z. Posner, *Leadership Practices Inventory (LPI): Facilitators Guide*, 3rd ed. (San Francisco: Jossey-Bass, 2003).
14. J. M. Kouzes and B. Z. Posner, *The Leadership Challenge*, 4th ed. (San Francisco: Jossey-Bass, 2007).
15. www.ccl.org
16. www.ccl.org
17. Lepsinger and Lucia, *The Art and Science of 360° Feedback.*
18. Lepsinger and Lucia, *The Art and Science of 360° Feedback.*
19. J. M. Kouzes and B. Z. Posner, *Credibility* (San Francisco: Jossey-Bass, 1993).
20. H. C. White, "Cases Are for Identity, for Explanation, or for Control," in *What Is a Case? Exploring the Foundations of Social Inquiry*, eds. C. C. Ragin and H. S. Becker (Cambridge: Cambridge University Press, 1992).
21. N. M. Tichy, *The Leadership Engine* (New York: Harper Business, 1997).
22. G. Wills, *Certain Trumpets* (New York: Simon & Schuster, 1994).
23. J. Munson, *Case Study Manual: Guidelines and Protocol for Case Study Development*, 2nd ed., Leadership in Public Health Monograph 1 (Chicago: University of Illinois School of Public Health, Mid-America Regional Public Health Leadership Institute, 2003).
24. R. E. Stake, "Case Studies," in *Handbook of Qualitative Research*, eds. N. K. Denzin and Y. S. Lincoln (Thousand Oaks, CA: Sage Publications, 1994).
25. Munson, *Case Study Manual.*
26. Munson, *Case Study Manual.*
27. M. H. McCaulley, "The Myers-Briggs Type Indicator and Leadership," in *Measures of Leadership*, eds. K. E. Clark and M. B. Clark (West Orange, NJ: Leadership Library of America, 1990).
28. K. C. Briggs and L. B. Myers, Myers-Briggs Type Indicator Step II Booklet (Form K) (Palo Alto, CA: Consulting Psychologists Press, 1991).
29. McCaulley, "The Myers-Briggs Type Indicator and Leadership."
30. http://www.kenblanchard.com
31. P. Hersey et al., *Management of Organizational Behavior*, 9th ed. (Upper Saddle River, NJ: Prentice Hall, 2007).
32. J. M. Kouzes and B. Z. Posner, *The Team Leadership Practices Inventory* (San Francisco: Pfeiffer and Co., 1992).
33. W. G. Bennis, "The Four Competencies of Leadership," *Training and Development Journal* 38, no. 8 (1984): 15–18.
34. G. E. A. Dever, *Improving Outcomes in Public Health Practice* (Gaithersburg, MD: Aspen Publishers, 1997).
35. K. E. Newcomer, "Using Performance Measurement to Improve Programs," *New Directions for Evaluation* 75 (1997): 8–13.
36. T. Rath, *Strength Finder 2.0* (New York: Gallup Press, 2007).
37. G. Browning, *Emergenetics* (New York: Collins, 2006).
38. National Academy of Science, *Improving the Nation's Health with Performance Measurement* (Washington, DC: National Academy Press, 1997).
39. National Academy of Science, *Improving the Nation's Health with Performance Monitoring.*
40. H. P. Hatry, "Where the Rubber Meets the Road: Performance Measurement for State and Local Public Measurement," *New Directions for Evaluation* 75 (1997): 31–44.
41. Dever, *Improving Outcomes in Public Health Practice.*

# APPENDIX 17-A

Leadership Competency Framework: Public Health Leadership Competencies for State/Regional Programs

Adapted by the Heartland Center for Public Health Preparedness, St. Louis University School of Public Health, from K.S. Wright, et al., Competency Development in Public Health Leadership, 2000, *American Journal of Public Health, 90,*8(2000) 1202–1207.

I. CORE TRANSFORMATIONAL COMPETENCIES

A. Visionary Leadership

1. Articulates vision and scenarios for change
2. Facilitates development of vision
3. Encourages others to share the vision
4. Applies innovative methods for strategic decision making

B. Sense of Mission

1. Articulates and models professional values, beliefs, and ethics
2. Facilitates development of mission and purpose
3. Facilitates reassessment and adaptation of mission to vision
4. Facilitates development of strategies to achieve mission

C. Effective Change Agent

1. Facilitates development of a learning organization.
2. Creates systems and structures for transformational change
3. Creates evaluation systems for change strategies
4. Facilitates strategic and tactical assessment and planning
5. Facilitates identification of emerging and acute problems
6. Utilizes change theories and models in strategic development
7. Identifies emotional and rational elements in strategic planning
8. Creates critical dynamic tension within change strategies
9. Facilitates development of effective dialogue
10. Utilizes methods to empower others to take action
11. Models active learning and personal mastery
12. Models and facilitates cultural sensitivity and competence
13. Models utilization and application of systems thinking
14. Models critical thinking and analysis skills
15. Models appropriate risk taking behaviors
16. Models group process behaviors; listening, dialoging, negotiating, encouraging, and motivating
17. Models leadership traits; integrity, credibility, enthusiasm, commitment, honesty, caring, and trust

## II. POLITICAL COMPETENCIES[1]

### A. Political Processes

1. Directs mission driven strategic planning at policy and operational levels
2. Articulates political processes and variables operating at federal/state/local levels
3. Identifies and assesses critical political issues and related stakeholders
4. Identify policies and alternatives related to critical public health problems
5. Develops capability for advocacy, community education, and social marketing
6. Utilizes principles of media advocacy to support public policy change
7. Assesses political resources to address needs of diverse and under-served communities
8. Implements collaborative strategies to involve constituencies and stakeholders
9. Utilizes political action models for infrastructure development and capacity building
10. Collaborates to analyze needs and develop regulatory actions and legislative proposals
11. Facilitates analysis and development of legislative action on public health issues
12. Directs development of systems, programs, and services for policy implementation

### B. Negotiation and Mediation

1. Identifies emerging public health issues and guides, or mediates action to avoid crises
2. Guides and mediates the investigation and resolution of acute public health crises
3. Identifies key stakeholders and resources necessary for mediating, negotiating, and/or collective bargaining

### C. Ethics and Power

1. Models use of professional values and ethics
2. Models use of principles of integrity and high ethical standards
3. Creates collaborative systems using high ethical standards
4. Describes the role of public health law and public health practice
5. Describes the role of clinical/research ethics in public health practice
6. Develops power-based alliances with a values-based and ethical perspective
7. Utilizes transitional/conditional ethics when interpreting functions of power structures

### D. Marketing and Education

1. Communicates with target audiences utilizing principles of social marketing and health education

---

1. University of North Carolina School of Public Health Doctoral Program Leadership Competences were used adapted in part for use in this domain [sic].

2. Communicates with target audiences regarding needs, objectives, and accomplishments

III. TRANSORGANIZATIONAL COMPETENCIES

A. Organizational Capacity and Dynamics

1. Utilizes models to assess environment, needs, opportunities, threats, and resources
2. Utilizes models of new organizational development, behavior, and culture
3. Develop structures for workforce development and organizational capacity improvement
4. Implements structures and capability as need, opportunity, risk, or threat arises

B. Trans-Organizational Capacity and Collaboration

1. Identifies and includes power brokers and stakeholders in collaborative ventures
2. Implements and evaluates collaborative and partnering strategies
3. Facilitates networking and broad and diverse stakeholder participation
4. Facilitates change with a balance of critical tensions within collaborative systems
5. Develops and evaluates collaborative strategic action plans
6. Facilitates trans-organizational shared or complementary mission and vision
7. Creates transorganizational systems with an ethical and values-based approach

C. Social Forecasting and Marketing

1. Utilizes social forecasting methods and interprets emerging needs and trends
2. Creates and articulates predictions and potential scenarios
3. Communicates analysis and interpretation of information to partners and constituents
4. Utilizes social marketing for media, health, and risk communications, and community relations

IV. TEAM BUILDING COMPETENCIES

A. Team Structures and Systems

1. Develops structures for organizational learning and systems thinking
2. Creates systems for team development and evaluation
3. Creates incentive and reward systems
4. Facilitates strategic outcomes-based team activities
5. Develops team systems for customer service and quality improvement
6. Facilitates collaborative leadership and entrepreneurial spirit

B. Team Development

1. Facilitates development of shared vision, mission, and values
2. Facilitates development of clear goals and objectives
3. Facilitates group process and dynamics
4. Implements communication processes for team development

5. Develops problem solving, conflict resolution, and decision making skills
6. Communicates need to balance critical tensions for team development
7. Facilitates empowerment and motivation to accomplish objectives
8. Celebrates team culture and accomplishments
9. Facilitates development of cultural sensitivity and competence
10. Facilitates development of appropriate risk taking behavior
11. Develops servant leadership; selflessness, integrity, and perspective mastery
12. Facilitates development of personal mastery and team learning

C. Facilitation and Mediation

1. Establishes team member roles and responsibilities
2. Facilitates effective workgroup processes and relationships
3. Mediates in non-productive, dissident, or demoralized team situations
4. Facilitates problem-centered coaching
5. Utilizes negotiation to mediate disputes and resolve conflicts

V. CRISIS LEADERSHIP COMPETENCIES
A. Planning for the unthinkable[2]

1. Articulates the definition of crisis levels and its elements
2. Articulates the definition of crisis management
3. Articulates the definition of crisis leadership
4. Articulates the difference between crisis leadership and crisis management
5. Articulates the role of leaders before and during crisis events
6. Articulates the systemic nature of crisis leadership
7. Identifies the elements of crisis anticipation and its relevance to crisis leadership
8. Utilizes methods and processes for anticipatory thinking and "thinking the unthinkable" before and during crisis events
9. Identifies the difference between normal/abnormal accidents/events and natural disasters
10. Identifies the elements of crisis types and methods for signal detection
11. Identifies and analyzes elements of multiple, inter-related or non-related and unthinkable crises events
12. Analyzes problems partner organizations experience during multiple crises events
13. Articulates the full range of crises that can potentially affect the organization/systems
14. Articulates the range and scope of crisis for which the organization/system should prepare
15. Develops the competence and capability necessary to anticipate, prepare for, respond to and mitigate multiple crises
16. Develops a unified planning, capability, and resource system among partner organizations

---

2. Competency sets were developed by the Heartland Centers in collaboration with Dr. Ian Mitroff, Comprehensive Crisis Management, Inc.

    17. Develops an emergency management/unified command system prepared for multiple crises

B. Crisis Patterns and Key Elements[2]

    1. Utilizes the concept of technical and ethical uncertainties in a crisis event.

    2. Articulates the concept of objectivity as a "turnoff" during crises events

    3. Articulates the concept of the court of public opinion vs. the court of law during crisis events

    4. Articulates the importance of no secrets and complete transparency during crisis events

    5. Articulates the importance of the concept of lessons ignored and not learned during a crisis event

    6. Identifies the six phases of crisis leadership

    7. Identifies the set of different crisis types

    8. Identifies the impact of different crisis mechanisms

    9. Identifies the different crisis families

    10. Identifies different crisis stakeholders in relation to crisis types

C. Risk Assessment[2]

    1. Utilizes the four elements of the crisis framework to identify how organizations/systems responds to crisis events

    2. Applies the crisis framework to human-caused crises (normal/abnormal accidents) and natural disasters

    3. Recognizes the basic patterns of organizational/system response and what elements should be reinforced or changed

    4. Utilizes six phases of crisis leadership to redesign effective crisis systems

D. Command Capability and Improvement

    1. Develops and implements a unified chain of command for emergency response

    2. Demonstrates individual functional and leadership roles/responsibilities for emergency response

    3. Demonstrates ability to make critical decisions and take decisive actions during crisis events

    4. Facilitates development of key values and shared vision to guide decisions and actions during crisis events

    5. Implements a multi-year emergency preparedness education, training, and exercise system

    6. Implements a system for performance measurement, after action reviews and improvement planning

    7. Identifies, communicates, and retests performance and maturity levels

E. Ethics and Crisis/Emergency Response[3]

    1. Articulates the role of ethics in crisis leadership

    2. Utilizes methods to balance emotion and use of reason during crisis events

---

3. Competencies were developed by the Heartland Centers in collaboration with Dr. Shugg Yagel-McBay

3. Identifies historical incidence of leaders who faced moral challenges
4. Utilizes professional ethics in the context of community and society during crisis
5. Models ethical decision-making during emergencies/crisis
6. Utilizes ethical decision making to apply/alter use of emergency plan procedures
7. Describes the role of public health law during emergencies/crisis events
8. Describes ethical issues regarding public health challenges and emergency events
9. Describes principles of ethical leadership and caring competence during disasters

F. Personality and Emotional Intelligence[4]
*Personality Factors and Crisis Response*

1. Identifies personality styles of leaders and leadership teams during crisis events
2. Utilizes assessment methods to determine personality style/preferences and crisis
3. Analyzes the relationship of personality type/preferences to functioning during crisis
4. Analyzes the impact of leadership cognitive and emotional intelligence during crisis
5. Recognizes and reconciles rational and emotional elements during crisis events

*Emotions and Performance: Leaders*

1. Identifies critical emotional intelligence competencies during crisis events
2. Analyzes how feelings impact personal performance in stressful situations
3. Describes emotions that are aroused during crisis
4. Describes personal strengths and weaknesses associated with emotions and stress
5. Utilizes methods to resist acting or responding in impulses during high stress events
6. Utilizes methods to behave calmly in stressful or emergency situations
7. Utilizes methods to stay composed and positive during crisis events
8. Utilizes methods to calm others in stressful situations and emergency events
9. Utilizes methods to change ideas and perceptions under stressful situations
10. Utilizes methods to balance emotional and rational elements for decision making and decisive action during crisis
11. Utilizes methods to handle ambiguity and multiple demands associated with crisis
12. Utilizes methods to chronicle individual experience for after-action analysis

---

4. Comprehensive Crisis Management, Inc., as well as Therese Jacobs-Stewart, M.A., and materials from the HayGroup, Dr. Daniel Goleman, Harvard University

*Emotions and Performance: Others*

1. Utilizes assessment methods to identify personality style and the relation to performance others during crisis
2. Utilizes methods to identify moods, feelings, and non-verbal cues of others under stress
3. Analyzes underlying causes for feelings, behavior, or concerns of others under stress
4. Utilizes factual arguments (reason or data) to persuade/influence others under stress
5. Utilizes the support of influential parties to convince others in stressful situations
6. Utilizes methods to increase perception and perspectives of others during crisis
7. Utilizes methods for reducing stereotyping of and reactions to diverse populations
8. Utilizes methods for broad support for increasing persuasive impact during crisis
9. Utilizes methods to promote cooperation/collaboration in stressful situations
10. Utilizes methods to reduce conflict in crisis situations
11. Utilizes methods to chronicle experience of others to prepare for after-action analysis

G. Risk and Crisis Communication[5]

1. Identifies leadership role/responsibilities to develop a crisis communication plan
2. Utilizes theoretical methods for and stages of risk communication
3. Identifies primary obstacles for use of appropriate risk/crises communication in emergency situations
4. Utilizes basic elements of the concept of risk and factors associated with determining magnitude of risk
5. Articulates the Environmental Protection Agencyís seven rules of risk communication
6. Utilizes the 21 guidelines for effective communication by leaders during high anxiety, stress threat situations
7. Utilizes appropriate risk/crisis communication methods during crisis events
8. Utilizes problem solving, conflict resolution, and decision making skills using principles and methods for risk communication
9. Utilizes communication role and methods with team members during emergency events
10. Utilizes communication role and methods with partner organizations during emergency events
11. Utilizes communication role and methods with the media during emergency events
12. Utilizes communication role and methods with the public during emergency events

---

5. Competencies developed by the Heartland Centers in collaboration with Dr. Vincent Covello, http://centerforriskcommunication.com/home.htm

H. Cultural Competence and Crisis[6]

1. Defines cultural competencies
2. Describes the process of cultural competencies
3. Identifies the role of cultural, social, and behavioral factors in determining the delivering of public health services
4. Describes the relationship(s) between cultural and health
5. Explores and describes knowledge about worldviews, beliefs, practices, and/or ways of other cultural groups
6. Identifies and discusses differences within cultural groups as well as across cultural groups
7. Describes the dynamic forces contributing to cultural diversity
8. Interacts sensitively and effectively with persons from diverse (cultural, socioeconomic, educational, racial, ethnic, professional, age, lifestyle preferences) backgrounds in the practice setting and in crisis situations
9. Actively seeks ongoing education, consultation, and/or training experience to enhance understanding and effectiveness with culturally and ethnically diverse populations in both normal and crisis situations
10. Identifies own competence level when interacting with cultural/ ethnically diverse populations in normal and crisis situations
11. Identifies own stereotyping attitudes, preconceived notions, and feelings towards members of other ethinic/cultural groups
12. Participates in cultural/ethnic groups in practice and community settings
13. Develops and adapts approaches to problems and emergency/crisis situations that take into account cultural differences
14. Identifies institutional barriers that prevent cultural/ethnic groups from seeking public health services and assistance in emergency or crisis situations
15. Facilitates understanding of the importance of and methods to increase diversity in the public health workforce
16. Recognizes that communication and related actions are culturally bound

I. Legal Basis for Preparedness[7]

1. Identifies the source and scope of State and Federal powers to protect the public's health, safety, and welfare in the event of emergency events
2. Analyzes and applies how public health law contributes to emergency response
3. Identifies and applies the basic legal framework for public health preparation in emergency events and the roles of federal, state, and local governmental agencies
4. Identifies and applies basic provisions of the governmental unitís health code and regulations during public health emergencies

---

6. Competencies developed by the Heartland Centers in collaboration with Josepha Camphine-Bacote, PhD, and adapted from the *Core Competencies in Public Health,* Council on Linkages Between Public Health Practice and Academia, and the *Inventory for Assessing the Process of Cultural Competency Among Health Professionals.*

7. Competencies developed by the Heartland Centers in collaboration with Jason Sapsin, JD, MPH, the Johns Hopkins Center for Law and the Public's Health

# CHAPTER 18

# LEADERSHIP EVALUATION
# AND RESEARCH

> It requires a very unusual mind to undertake the analysis of
> the obvious.
>                           Alfred North Whitehead, *Science and the Modern World*

During the 1990s, the public health community realized the importance of developing public health leaders. A national Public Health Leadership Institute (PHLI) was created by a consortium of California universities through a grant from the Centers for Disease Control and Prevention (CDC). Since 2000, the national program has been housed at the University of North Carolina Institute for Public Health. In 1991, the first two state public health leadership institutes were founded in Illinois at the University of Illinois School of Public Health and in Missouri at the Saint Louis University School of Public Health. The Illinois program began with CDC support and the Missouri program with support from the state of Missouri. There are currently a number of public health regional and state leadership development programs covering 49 of the 50 states. Georgia (50th state) is in the process of developing a state-based program. As leadership programs have proliferated, there has grown a concern about the effectiveness of these programs in training leaders.

Leaders need information for making decisions. Ongoing program evaluation creates an atmosphere in which effective leadership and organizational learning can flourish.[1] Leaders need to show strong support for program evaluation and include evaluation as a part of the mission and vision of their agency. They also need to be involved in the evaluation process and work with other agency professionals to ensure that the process is successful. The organization will not achieve excellence without opportunities for continual learning provided by training and leadership development programs.

In 1999, the CDC reported on the deliberations of the CDC Evaluation Working Group regarding effective program evaluation.[2] The working group developed a framework for program evaluation in public health (see Figure 4-3). The top part of Table 18-1 lists the steps in the evaluation process, from engaging stakeholders in the process to ensuring that the lessons learned are applied. The bottom part of the table lists the four major standards of program evaluation: utility, feasibility, propriety, and accuracy.

The term "program" has a broad meaning.[3] Indeed, the CDC Evaluation Working Group listed 12 different program categories: direct service interventions, community mobilization efforts, research initiatives, surveillance

**Table 18-1 Narrative Steps and Standards of the CDC Evaluation Framework**

Engage stakeholders
Those involved, those affected, primary intended users
Describe the program
Need, expected effects, activities, resources, stage, context, logic model
Focus the evaluation design
Purpose, users, uses, questions, methods, agreements
Gather credible evidence
Indicators, sources, quality, quantity, logistics
Justify conclusions
Standards, analysis/synthesis, interpretation, judgment, recommendations
Ensure use and share lessons learned
Design, preparation, feedback, follow-up, dissemination
Utility
Serve the information needs of intended users
Feasibility
Be realistic, prudent, diplomatic, and frugal
Propriety
Behave legally, ethically, and with due regard for the welfare of those involved and those affected
Accuracy
Reveal and convey technically accurate information

*Source:* Reprinted from "Framework for Program Evaluation in Public Health," *Morbidity and Mortality Weekly Report,* Vol. 48, 1999, the Centers for Disease Control and Prevention.

systems, policy development activities, outbreak investigations, laboratory diagnostics, communication campaigns, infrastructure building projects, training and education services, administrative systems, and other programs. In this chapter, the focus is on the evaluation of leadership development programs.

## Evaluation of Training Programs

A training program must have a reason for being. If a training program is developed but no one registers for it, it obviously does not address a need. That is why the first step in the training process is to determine whether the proposed training program is required. The program planners should investigate the needs of the target population using focus groups, surveys, and interviews. The planners themselves will also have an agenda that should be built into the needs assessment. If the purpose of the assessment is to determine the need for training in governance, then the assessment must include questions about governance.

In a study of board of health members' understanding of public health, it was found that the members believed their most important role was in the area of policy development.[4] They believed they were least effective in the area of assessment. In addition, board members thought that they were not given appropriate training for their board activities and that the principles of governance were not clear. They were also concerned about the lack of funds for the running of the board, the lack of information about public health in general, and the lack of awareness of political priorities and statutory regulations. All of these findings can be translated into training objectives.

Once the training topics are determined, the program's objectives are set and the program is developed.[5] Among the things that need to be determined are procedures for the selection of participants, the times and places of the training, the best speakers for each topic, and methods for evaluating the program's outcomes.

The third step is to offer the training program itself. Measurements need to be done before or at the start of the training program and also at its conclusion in order to determine changes that occurred. Session and speaker evaluations also need to be done in order to assess the quality of the program. It is beneficial to tie the program evaluation to changes reported by the trainees. Research can be done on:

- the association between program elements and leadership change
- lessons learned from the training course (see Exercise 18-1)
- measurable and unmeasurable leadership competencies
- differences between new leaders and more established ones
- differences between trainees and colleagues who have not been trained
- differences between continuing education approaches and academic approaches
- 360-degree measures at the start and the conclusion of the training program

If trainees do not take new information and skills back to their agencies, the training course loses much of its effectiveness. One way to spread the benefits of training is for graduates of training, using what they learned, to develop a training workshop for colleagues who were unable to attend the training.

The last step in the training process involves following the trainees over time to determine what parts of the program work in practice. By taking the same measurements as were taken during the training, the planners can determine the changes that occurred over time and pinpoint areas in which skills deteriorated. The information gained can be used to develop follow-up programs and make the current program more effective in the future. A few public health leadership institutes have created annual update courses for graduates of their programs.

Evaluation itself can be divided into four components. First, the trainees' reactions to the program need to be assessed. There may be differences between reactions to in-house programs and reactions to programs outside the organization.

Second, the learning that occurred has to be evaluated. The hoped-for results of training include the acquiring of new skills and new knowledge.

Third, behavior changes due to the training need to be identified. The ultimate goal of all training programs is to alter the behavior of the trainees in ways that improve their effectiveness on the job. The expected behavior changes do not always occur, sometimes because leaders go to the training course with a personal agenda or believe that they already know everything about leadership that they need to. In addition, trainees who are primarily managers sometimes do not understand the difference between managing and leading. Finally, trainees often face community or organizational barriers to putting their new skills into action.

Fourth, the long-term effects of the training need to be studied. One leader who attended a state-based leadership program showed very little change of behavior at the end of the program but reported that he eventually used the skills learned two years later to improve the agency environment. This example shows the difficulty of evaluating results in a training program. Follow-up is clearly important, as is measuring behavior change in a control group that has not been through training.

The above model has been criticized for not going far enough. Performance evaluation needs to extend into the community.[6] In addition, the work environment must be analyzed to determine whether changes in behavior will be possible. It is important to keep in mind that behavior change is affected not only by the training but also by such factors as attitude and the reaction of others to proposed changes.[7]

## Evaluation of Leadership Development Programs

The Center for Creative Leadership (CCL) undertook a study of leadership programs for school superintendents in Florida.[8] The study focused on the outcomes of training, the influence of the curriculum on the outcomes, and the influence of other factors on the outcomes. Three general outcomes were discovered to have occurred. First, leaders became committed to continuous learning and believed that they had acquired continuous learning strategies and skills. Second, they acquired personal leadership skills and underwent personal changes. Third, they were able to perform their jobs more effectively.

With regard to factors affecting the outcomes, the trainees were influenced by their contact with facilitators, who appear to have taken a mentoring role. These facilitators helped the trainees to conceptualize their experientially based learning projects. The trainees also kept a journal during training, which helped document their learning experiences and contributed to the development of their leadership abilities.

The outcomes of training differ for different individuals.[9] Some leaders have much experience and use the new training to fine-tune their skills. Others struggle with self-control and self-esteem issues and have trouble maintaining flexibility. These leaders often do not benefit from leadership programs. A third group of leaders thrive in leadership programs and make substantial progress in developing their skills. For example, they often learn the importance of sharing power and how to create a better balance in their lives. Exercise 18-1 explores the expectations that students had starting the leadership program and the extent to which their expectations were met.

In their comprehensive approach to leadership program evaluation, the CCL made a distinction between leader development as discussed in the last chapter and leadership development.[10] Leader development evaluation refers to evaluation done on how individuals use their leadership development training to become more effective in carrying out their leadership activities.

Leadership development evaluation refers to how organizations and agencies increase their capacity to carry out the agency's work and also to carry out public health's work. In other words, training enhances the performance of leaders and has an important effect on increasing the capacity of the public health organization to carry out public health work collaboratively with internal and external stakeholders and public health clients.[11]

Evaluators have discussed the importance of strategic evaluation, which relates to a determination of the values of organization-based processes and interventions to see if the values that affect an agency are maintained by the changes promoted through leadership training or whether the training increases the capacity of the agency to do its work.[12] The purpose of strategic evaluation is to use training to add value for the leaders and their leadership partners over time. There are challenges that affect the successes of strategic evaluation. Because leadership development is sometimes used as a reward for public health professionals, there is a danger that this reward will benefit the individual and not the public health system if the training opportunity is not evaluated relative to the needs of the system. Another challenge relates to the fact that leadership development may not show an immediate return on investment.

> **Leadership Tips**
>
> *Hold meetings at a round table.*
>
> *It levels the playing field.*

This delay between leadership development and the development of strategic outcomes creates difficulties in determining the value of training programs. The costs of the training provide challenges for agencies with limited training resources. The cost of these leadership programs is often prohibitive for public health professionals. There is also a feasibility challenge related to information. Because there are privacy protection concerns to trainees, leadership development programs cannot relate the use of leadership behavior tools to action outcomes without the specific consent of the person going through the training. Another challenge relates to the lack of funding in public health leadership development for the evaluation function. There is also a lack of understanding about what evaluation is supposed to accomplish.

Despite some of these challenges, we still learn much about the benefits of evaluation when it does occur. This chapter presents two program evaluation case studies. The first, Case Study 18-A, describes the process of developing an evaluation program for the South Central Public Health Leadership Institute in the late 1990s. One of the themes is that funding concerns can have an impact on training programs. The project team recognized the importance of evaluation and the complexity of the leadership development process, and it explored the possibility of using observers to monitor the training process. However, the team decided that the leadership trainees would not accept this technique, and so it adopted a 360-degree self-evaluation and observer feedback procedure in which confidentiality was protected. The case study includes a postscript on what has happened since the evaluation.

Case Study 18-B describes the comprehensive evaluation of the PHLI from 1991 to 2006.[13] The retrospective evaluation explored what alumni were doing, what skills have been used, and what skills can be attributed to the training experience. Results from this evaluation are now available.

## Case Study 18-A
## Be Careful What You Ask For, You May Get It, with 2008 Postscript

*Sheila W. Chauvin* and *Ann Anderson*

*This case study was developed based on the experiences of the South Central Public Health Leadership Institute (SCPHLI), Tulane University School of Public Health and Tropical Medicine, and the development of an objectives- and performance-based 360-degree feedback process.*

*Issue:* How does one assess effective leadership and leadership development among public health professionals?

*Time Period:* May 1997–October 1999.

*Professionals involved:* Alata Angst, project director; Ben Thare, program coordinator; Helen Bach, evaluation consultant.

Alata sat at her desk feeling rather good about the progress of the new leadership development program. This first year had been really stressful, as is often the case with any new program. Alata had worried quite a bit about how the program would be perceived in the region, because participants were being drawn from practicing and experienced supervisors, managers, and leaders in the public health sector. She had just returned from the project team meeting for the SCPHLI, and from all indications the first year had been successful indeed. A good thing, because everyone had worked so hard. Participants in the first cohort had completed feedback forms at the end of each multiday session throughout the year, and their comments revealed high levels of satisfaction with most of the program offerings and activities. Of course, as always there were a few negative and pessimistic comments, and there were indeed areas for improvement and expansion that the project team agreed they would need to target in the future. However, for the most part everyone thought that the first year of development and implementation was a success. Ben Thare, the project coordinator, had raised an interesting issue during the meeting: is it sufficient to gauge the effectiveness of the institute based simply on participants' satisfaction with the sessions? Shouldn't the team base its judgments on the extent to which participants actually demonstrate new and enhanced leadership skills in everyday practice? That's the true test, isn't it? As he said, satisfaction and the "friendly factor" were not necessarily going to get people to participate in the second year.

Ben's comments were working their way to the surface as Alata sat contemplating the future of the SCPHLI. Ben's right. How do we really know if the institute is making a difference? Certainly this was going to be an issue, probably sooner than she or Ben or even the participants might realize. While they had funding for the institute now, Alata knew that she would need additional extramural funding to continue and enhance the institute in the future, especially if they were going to add more states to the group of participatory states. A visual reminder lay on her desk in the form of a request for proposals from the CDC. If the team was going to seek funding for the institute from the CDC, surely they would need a stronger evaluation plan than just session feedback forms asking participants to comment on what they liked and disliked. Ben was right. Even if she wasn't seeking additional funding, sooner or later officials in the various state agencies were going to want evidence that sending their public health leaders to multiday retreats and seminars was worth their investments of time, effort, and dollars. Sooner or later, state agency directors were going to expect visible evidence back "in the trenches."

But what could they do? What kind of evidence would they need? This was clearly out of Alata's comfort zone. Public health administration and microbiology were areas in which she could hold her own, even excel, but measuring the effectiveness of educational programs was clearly not part of her expertise. Certainly Alata had statistical support available in the school, but statisticians didn't know much about evaluating educational programs or things like leadership development, change facilitation, communication, conflict resolution, coalition building, coaching and mentoring skills, and so on. Now Alata was concerned! Who could help? Maybe the institute wasn't as successful as she had thought originally. Maybe it was just fluff, as had been suggested by a few of the negative and pessimistic comments that she was now reflecting on once again. As Alata continued to think about how the team could really know whether the institute was making a difference in participants' leadership development and practices, she got up and started to walk down the hall toward Ben's office. She thought, Ben should be back from the team meeting by now. He raised the question about effectiveness and evaluation, so maybe he has some ideas as to how to proceed? Yes, that's it, ask Ben.

**One Week Later**
Alata and Ben walked into the office of Helen Bach. They were meeting with Helen to discuss how they might examine the extent to which the SCPHLI participants develop and use key leadership concepts and skills in everyday practice. Luckily, Ben had met Helen earlier in the year at a conference, during which he learned about Helen's background in leadership development and change process and her expertise in instrument development and program evaluation. Lucky that Ben met her in the first place and doubly fortunate that she had the background that seemed ideally suited to meet their project needs. Alata knew about Helen and the medical education research office that she directed in the School of Medicine, but she hadn't realized that the unit might be a potential resource. In any case, they were glad the connection was made. With the CDC proposal deadlines looming near, they would not have had much time to search for an evaluation consultant, much less one with a leadership development background. As they waited in the reception area to meet with Helen, Alata and Ben reviewed the program goals and expectations that they planned to share with Helen.

**After the Meeting**
As Alata and Ben left Helen's office, they were feeling both drained and overwhelmed. They had no idea that evaluating the effectiveness of the leadership institute could be so complex. Going into the meeting, both Alata and Ben thought they could just administer some type of test or survey and have some of the staff or faculty in the biostatistics department "crunch the numbers" and give them the results. What Helen had suggested was more of a performance-based assessment. Direct observation by several trained assessors over several occasions would be an ideal approach, she had told them, but the associated costs and time constraints were formidable. In addition, potential difficulties and political and interpersonal considerations were at the top of the list for decision making. For example, who would assess, how would assessors be trained and monitored, who would own the data, and how would the data be used for programming decisions and for helping individuals improve their leadership abilities? These were some of the questions raised and scenarios discussed.

Ultimately, the results of any assessments must be used for decision making and

*(continues)*

**Case Study 18-A** *continued*

continuous improvement. Certainly, if the participants' direct supervisors were the ones doing the assessments, there might be little potential for collaborative reflection and professional development to occur, at least at first. For example, individuals might tend to view the assessments as yet another formal job evaluation rather than an opportunity to learn and develop new abilities. On the other hand, if peers were trained to do the observations, how would their assessor responsibilities affect day-to-day work relationships? Should the peer assessors be individuals who work with participants on a regular basis or should they be brought in from some other office, agency, or region to conduct "snapshot" observations and assessment reports? In what context should the assessments be explained and occur? And then there were all the instrument development, validity, and reliability issues that Helen raised for them to consider. How were they going to accomplish this? Alata and Ben had no idea what they had asked for. What they had was a task of elephantine proportions.

Alata and Ben felt like they should run—not walk—out of Helen's office. This was way too much work and complexity for their program. Participants would never agree to be observed and rated on behaviors, and after their discussion paper-and-pencil tests did not seem much better than session feedback forms. But they felt a ray of hope when Helen suggested that they limit the scope of work and take things one step at a time. Obviously she had noted the look of being overwhelmed on Ben and Alata's faces. She said, "Folks, this is an evolutionary process, not a revolution." Phew! Alata and Ben stayed in their seats and leaned forward with interest. Helen went on to describe several other options for their evaluation goals. She mentioned self-assessment and peer-assessment methods and told them about techniques that were currently being described as 360-degree feedback processes. Helen also discussed concepts such as self-efficacy and organizational context and explored the notion of assessment performance levels at the beginning of the institute and then again at the end (i.e., pre- and postassessments). By the end of the meeting, they had an action plan in place and a renewed sense of confidence about the tasks that lay ahead. As they left Helen's office, they thought about the last thing she said to them: "If you're going to eat an elephant, do so one bite at a time. Let's approach this as a team."

Over the next several months, Helen worked with Alata and Ben to review the goals and objectives of the SCPHLI to identify key leadership traits that were being addressed by the program. As she explained, it would be impossible to measure everything, so they should concentrate on the specifics of the program. They also began to work on a process that included pre- and postassessments and self- and peer-assessment components. Once again, ideal approaches were identified first, but then, once they figured out what their resources were, they settled for less than the ideal.

In the end, the SCPHLI had an observation-based questionnaire that included multiple descriptions of leadership behaviors grounded in the program goals and objectives. Participants completed a self-assessment form at the beginning and at the end of the institute. They identified five individuals in their work environment with whom they work regularly and who agreed to complete a confidential peer assessment form of the questionnaire, again before and after participation in the institute. A process was developed by which all data were submitted directly to Helen's office and voluntary and confidential assurances were established. Preassessment profiles and postassessment profiles were completed by the staff in Helen's office and mailed directly to each participant, with options for confidential and individualized consultation. Only group or cohort assessment data were available to the project team, and no individually identifiable data were shared. In essence, they were able to achieve many of the 360-degree feedback features and minimize the political and interpersonal threats that are often associated with on-the-job performance assessments.

## October 1999

Alata sat at her desk feeling rather good about the progress of the SCPHLI. She had just returned from the project team meeting. As another cohort containing participants from four states completed the institute, Ben shared in the meeting evidence that suggested another successful year indeed. A good thing, because everyone had worked so hard—not this year, but for the past several years. Alata thought about the first year that they implemented a pilot version of the self-assessment questionnaire and the anxiety it had raised among the participants and the large number of individuals who initially expressed their apprehension about peers completing a similar form. She remembered watching Ben manage the group discussions about the participants' concerns pertaining to confidentiality of assessment data. She thought, just hearing the word "evaluation" does tend to make the hair on the back of your neck stand on end. Now, two years later, most, if not all, participants embraced the pre- and postassessments for the 360-degree feedback process. At first individuals thought about evaluation as being done "to them"; now it seems evaluation is being done "with them." She looked out the window and chuckled to herself: guess we do need to be careful about what we ask for—we just might get it!

## Postscript: February 2008

The case study above was originally developed based on the early experiences of the SCPHLI, Tulane University School of Public Health and Tropical Medicine, and the development of an objectives- and performance-based 360-degree feedback process. Since 1999, the SCPHLI has continued and expanded. The leadership development resulting from the program and ongoing development of its project team members has contributed substantially to professional development of public health staff and formation of a strong and ever-expanding academic-practice partnership in the region. As was the case from the onset of the SCPHLI, formative and summative evaluation have been a core component and a driving force of the ongoing development of the South Central Public Health Partnership, as a regional consortium, and of the new centers and expanded curriculum and programs that have been achieved since 1999. This postscript provides a brief summary of some of the major accomplishments that have contributed to leadership development both through formal educational processes and on-the-job collaboration. In each instance, performance and overall program evaluation has been used from the onset to support ongoing monitoring, guide mid-course adjustments, and to regularly gauge progress toward achieving important goals and value-added impact.

For the SCPHLI, the continuation of the 360-degree assessment in the SCPHLI has continued to provide evidence of the effectiveness of its educational program. Statistically significant and positive gains have been observed in every year of the SCPHLI since the 360-degree assessment was implemented. The curriculum continues to offer substantial benefit and only minor modifications have been necessary (e.g., routine updates and refinements). In 2003–2004 further validation of the 360-degree assessment was completed, and 20 of the original 24 items continue to be retained on the instrument. Today, full participation of SCPHLI fellows is common and pre/post-SCPHLI 360-degree profiles continue to be used to provide individual and programmatic guidance. In 2006–2007 and with modest funding from the CDC,

*(continues)*

**Case Study 18-A** *continued*

a longitudinal and follow-up study of all SCPHLI graduates was completed using a mixed methods research design to further examine the impact of the program on its graduates and the supporting public health agencies. Based on quantitative and qualitative results, the SCPHLI is highly regarded by leaders, graduates, and public health professionals generally throughout the region. The SCPHLI is viewed by many as a substantial source for developing future public health leaders. Enrollment in the SCPHLI continues to be strong and individuals within the various practice partner agencies actually view participation (and then graduation) as an honor. When the region was devastated by Hurricane Katrina, the SCPHLI was interrupted, as was the case for most other things, and the opportunity for losing momentum was certainly present. However, there was strong support for resuming the program. In 2006, the SCPHLI was resumed and expanded to offer graduates additional learning opportunities through an Advanced Crisis Leadership course that has been well subscribed to for each offering. Finally, an SCPHLI Alumni Society continues to offer graduates opportunities for collaboration and ongoing professional development.

The SCPHLI has served as a foundation for additional program development, and through such efforts individuals have developed leadership skills on-the-job. For example, in 1999, the SCPHLI project team decided to invite colleagues from the University of Alabama–Birmingham School of Public Health to join with them. This expanded team of leaders and representatives of four public health agencies (Alabama, Arkansas, Louisiana, and Mississippi) and two academic institutions (Tulane and UAB) reorganized to form a steering committee for the regional partnership. In addition, with successful acquisition of funding from the Health Resources and Services Administration, the South Central Public Health Training Center (SCPHTC) was established in 2000 to develop and provide competency-based training courses and resources for public health professionals in the region. Grounded in the core functions and essential services endorsed for public health professions at the time, overall program evaluation (including systematic training needs assessments) was used to establish goals, provide focus and guidance, and maintain forward momentum. Achieving early success with the SCPHTC, the Partnership Steering Committee (of which many members were graduates of the SCPHLI) continued put into practice essential leadership competencies they had learned in their SCPHLI experiences (e.g., creating and sharing vision, obtaining resources, providing professional development and ongoing assistance, communicating effectively, and building coalitions).

In 2001, they sought additional resources from the CDC to establish a third center, the South Central Center for Public Health Preparedness (SCCPHP), to lead an effort in preparing the region's public health professionals in emergency and bioterrorism preparedness. Again, with a successful funding award from the CDC, the SCCPHP was established in 2002 and together with the SCPHLI and SCPHTC, a synergy of efforts and resources has since continued to expand.

Since 2000, an overall program evaluation model has been used to provide formative and summative input for the regional consortium (partnership) and for each of the three centers, with particular emphasis on goal achievement, consortium effectiveness, and value added to public health professional development. Each year, the overall program evaluation activities provide opportunities for direct input from all stakeholders. Quantitative and qualitative methods have been used to answer core questions across years, including longitudinal study of innovation and change process, and to address specific issues at hand within each year. Reports of ongoing evaluation are provided at least twice each year to provide external review of progress to goals and summative assessment of goal achievement, consortium effectiveness, and value-added impact.

Leadership development has been a core component of both formal and on-the-job educational opportunities affiliated with the partnership and each of its centers. A much expanded South Central Public Health Advisory Board has now replaced the Partnership Steering Committee and reflects a greater variety of agency and academic partners that interact with each other to support public health. Again, real-life experiences within the partnership have fostered leadership development and putting into practice the core leadership competencies that are reflected in the SCPHLI curriculum (e.g., shared visions, communication skills, coalition building, strategic planning, and change facilitation). So, as Alata reflected in the original case above, we have been careful about what we asked for and through the ongoing collaboration and development of individual and group leadership, we have achieved quite a lot.

---

### Case Study 18-B
### Evaluation of the National Public Health Leadership Institute 1991–2006

*Karl E. Umble, Sandra J. Diehl, and Susan Haws (2007). Developing Leaders, Building Networks: An Evaluation of the National Public Health Leadership Institute—1991–2006.* Chapel Hill, NC: North Carolina Institute for Public Health.

**Background**

The PHLI is a leadership development program in the United States sponsored by the CDC. The institute's mission is to strengthen the leadership competencies of senior public health leaders and to build a network of senior leaders who can work together and share knowledge on how to address public health challenges.

The CDC founded PHLI in 1990 and remains its sponsor. PHLI represented a significant CDC commitment to improve public health infrastructure following the influential 1988 Institute of Medicine report, *The Future of Public Health,* which called for major improvements in the practice of public health in the United States.

From 1991–2000, PHLI was offered under the continuous management of the Center for Health Leadership and Practice, which is part of the nonprofit Public Health Institute in Oakland, California. During this time, nine cohorts of about 50 scholars per year were developed. In 2000, the CDC selected a new partnership to offer PHLI, headed by the North Carolina Institute for Public Health at the University of North Carolina at Chapel Hill (UNC) School of Public Health. Other partners included the Kenan-Flagler Business School at UNC-Chapel Hill and the nonprofit CCL in Greensboro, North Carolina. This partnership developed an additional six cohorts of scholars through 2006. The total number of graduates was 806.

In 2006–2007, the CDC sponsored an evaluation of the program's first 15 years of operation. This report presents the results of that evaluation, which examined PHLI's influence on the following major domains:

Domain 1. Individual Leader Development

Domain 2. Leader Actions: Career-Related Outcomes and Voluntary Leadership Positions Taken

Domain 4. Network Actions: Public Health Systems and Infrastructure Development

*(continues)*

**Case Study 18-B** *continued*

In addition, the evaluation examined graduate and stakeholder perspectives on PHLI and the future direction of public health leadership development in the United States, which was Domain 5.

The evaluators developed those themes on the basis of interviews with CDC staff who were involved with the evaluation; present and past PHLI staff members; a few selected graduates of the program from city, state, and federal government; previous evaluations of PHLI; and literature from evaluations of other leadership development programs. This process reflected the first step in the CDC's evaluation framework, which is to "engage stakeholders." By giving us ideas of key outcomes to measure, these interviews also greatly helped us in developing our evaluation instruments.

*Methods*

Evaluators used quantitative and qualitative data from an online survey sent to all program graduates and qualitative data from telephone interviews with a subset of program graduates and with key informants.

*Survey*

The Web-based survey sought to ascertain whether the program achieved basic objectives and focused on key areas that most interested stakeholders. It included questions related to:

- Career patterns of graduates and voluntary service in public health
- Individual leader development, including the influence of PHLI on scholars' understanding, skills, interest in leadership service, confidence, courage, sense of belonging to the national cadre of leaders in public health, self-awareness, openness to the ideas of others, networks, and overall leadership
- Individual practices, including changes in involvement in local, state, and national leadership activities
- Specific results of PHLI and improved leadership, including changes in programs, organizations, policies, and systems

We took great care while developing these instruments to be sure they would capture the data requested by the CDC and other stakeholders, and went through many drafts and item formats over a period of six intensive weeks before finalizing the instruments. This stage included pilot tests with program graduates in several locations, and with our own staff and graduate students. When the survey was ready, we uploaded it into a Web-based survey tool. Using Internet search engines and key informant referrals, we located a working (nonbouncing) e-mail address for 80% (n=646) of the 806 graduates. To encourage participation, we sent a hard copy letter from the director of the North Carolina Institute for Public Health to all graduates, requesting participation in the survey, while the director of the PHLI alumni association also sent an e-mail encouraging participation. We then sent an e-mail to all graduates with a link to the survey, and approximately four additional e-mails to all graduates who had not yet responded to the survey over a period of about eight weeks. The final response rate was 61% (n=393) out of those 646 for whom we had working e-mail addresses.

*Interviews*

We interviewed 17 graduates on how PHLI influenced their leadership knowledge, attitudes, skills, practices, positions, and involvement in voluntary work, leadership networks, and collaborations. We also asked about changes at organizational and systems levels that they could attribute at least partially to PHLI. Of the 17, eight

(47%) were graduates of the California PHLI, and nine (53%) were graduates of the UNC program. We also conducted 18 interviews with key informants who had knowledge of the history, purpose, and results of PHLI. These interviews focused on national level trends and changes that they could trace to PHLI, plus recommendations for future leadership programming and related efforts.

Quantitative survey data were analyzed using SAS (SAS Institute, Cary, NC). Differences in means were analyzed using paired samples t-tests. Qualitative data from the open-ended survey questions were analyzed using content analysis methods. Interviews with program graduates and key informants were digitally recorded and transcribed. The two staff members who conducted the interviews conducted a content analysis (Patton, 1990) of the transcripts using across-case matrices derived from within case summaries (Miles and Huberman, 1994).

### Findings

Figure 18-1 summarizes study findings and their relationships to one another.

*Domain 1. Individual Leader Development*
We asked graduates to rate PHLI's long-term influence on their leadership; 36% chose "large," 43% chose "moderate," 18% chose "small," and 2% chose "no influence." The majority reported that PHLI had strengthened these constructs related to understanding and skills to a "moderate" or "large" degree:

- Understanding useful general principles of leadership (81%)
- Awareness of best practices and models for public health leadership (68%)
- Understanding of the breadth of the public health system and their role (56%)
- Openness to the ideas of others about how to address problems (75%)

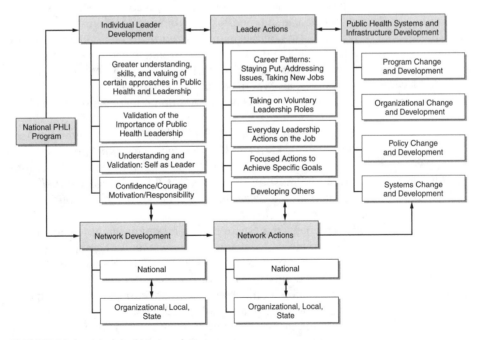

**FIGURE 18-1**    Model of National Outcomes.

*(continues)*

**Case Study 18-B** *continued*

- Skills in leading efforts that require the collaboration of many people or organizations (73%) and other specific leadership practices that are useful in public health (73%)

The majority reported that PHLI had strengthened their interest in the following possible involvements to a "moderate" or "great" extent:

- Interest in deepening their involvement with leadership efforts to improve their agency or community (78%)
- Interest in deepening their involvement with public health leadership efforts at the national level (59%) and at the state level (54%)
- Their commitment to staying in public health in their work (66%)

In addition, the majority reported that PHLI has strengthened these constructs to a "moderate" or "great" extent:

- Self-awareness as a leader: their strengths, liabilities, and how others view and receive their leadership (82%)
- Sense that as a public health leader, they are important and have a valuable role to play (77%) and belong to the national cadre of leaders in public health (68%)
- Professional network of people they can contact for ideas about how to handle their leadership (55%)
- Confidence to take on public health leadership responsibilities (75%)
- Courage to take the initiative and act to improve public health (75%)

Interview themes and hundreds of survey comments reinforced and explained scholars' improvements in understanding of leadership; improved understanding, skill, and valuing of collaborative leadership and systems thinking to address challenges; and other specific skills gained. Many also emphasized that PHLI connected them to a wide network of leaders with whom they could exchange valuable information. The network helped them feel that they "belonged" to a national network of public health leaders and were themselves "valid" leaders and increased their courage and confidence to "step up to the plate" and take on additional leadership responsibilities. One put it succinctly:

*PHLI helped to give me the requisite leadership skills, the support group to feel others in my position were making/could make a difference, gave me the confidence to step up to the plate, and impressed upon me the obligation to do so. PHLI was a very limited opportunity and almost all of us in it felt this privilege we had been given should be reciprocated for via active public health leadership in our respective work and personal spheres of influence.*

Although some of these benefits may seem "soft" and unimportant to some readers, they are directly related to more recent and holistic concepts of competence that are widely embraced today. "Competence is not to be synonymous with skill. A competence is defined as the ability to successfully meet complex demands in a particular context. Its manifestation, competent performance, depends on the mobilization of knowledge, cognitive and practical skills, and social and behavioral components such as attitudes, emotions, values, and motivations. This holistic notion of competence is not reducible to one cognitive dimension" (Hakkarainen et al., 2004, p. 16).

Put differently, these findings about scholars' perceptions of important gains from PHLI remind us that leaders are not "machines" in need only of new practical skills, but complex personalities in search of a role and mission, vision, courage and encouragement, validation and confidence, and companions for the journey.

*Domain 2. Leader Actions: Career-Related Outcomes and Voluntary Leadership Positions Taken*

The great majority—87%—of survey respondents were still working in public health. Seven percent were working in another closely related field. About 20% of all PHLI graduates have now retired, but nearly all of them had remained in public health until they retired.

Using the construct of "trained leader-years"—full-time employment years after PHLI graduation—we found that graduates had invested 1,210 trained leader-years in local government, 640 years in state government, and 314 in federal government. In addition, scholars had spent 366 years in academic work, and 3 years working in health care.

Main foci for graduates' daily work after graduation included general organizational leadership in governmental agencies, community public health development, bioterrorism and preparedness, policy development and advocacy, and workforce development (both general and leadership development). Other fairly common foci included nonprofit leadership, epidemiology, chronic disease, health care leadership, and infectious disease.

About 52% had stayed in the same organization and position since graduation—which interviewees attributed to commitment to a place rather than any form of stagnation.

About 19% said that PHLI had helped them attain new jobs by increasing their skills, confidence, interest, and networks, or by impressing the employer that the scholar had attended. Jobs that PHLI helped scholars attain often included federal bureau or division chief and state or local health officer, deputy, or division chief.

About 81% had taken on additional "voluntary" leadership roles that were not required by their jobs, such as task forces, boards, professional associations, and informal advocacy; 54% had taken on such roles *and* responded that PHLI had played some role in their doing so, mainly by increasing their confidence, interest in the work, skills, and networks.

Examples of voluntary roles scholars had taken on with PHLI's influence included, at the national level, serving on boards and committees with NACCHO, ASTHO, NLN, PHLS, APHA, and other associations. At the state level, roles commonly included helping with or serving on boards with a state public health association or state association of county and city health officials. At the local level, many worked with community-level task forces and boards. The great majority of scholars responded that PHLI had made "some" or a "great" contribution to the leadership actions that they took when they assumed these voluntary roles.

*I was appointed shortly after I graduated [from PHLI] to the board of the Massachusetts Public Health Association, the nation's largest APHA affiliate, and successfully implemented at MPHA a statewide initiative called the Coalition for Local Public Health, which is finally before the Legislature dealing with reform of a fragmented . . . local health structure . . . taking on a reform of local public health structure . . . has taken almost 10 years of steady development to arrive now at active dialogue with the state legislature. Without PHLI, I would never have conceptualized developing a statewide local public health coalition comprising five major public health associations to achieve a reorganization of the antiquated Massachusetts local health department structure.*

*(continues)*

**Case Study 18-B** *continued*

*Domain 3. Public Health Leadership Network Development and Network Actions*
When asked to "explain in some detail one of the most important influences that PHLI has had on your leadership," over 80 scholars (24% of the respondents who answered this question) cited gaining improved and valuable network connections.

The most commonly cited benefits of these connections included enhanced overall understanding of public health leadership's roles and goals; long-term professional knowledge-sharing; social support for taking action—such as ideas, encouragement, and good examples set by others; and being introduced to opportunities for formal collaborative work, such as with NACCHO or a state public health association. In addition, many described how these collaborations had led to specific improvements in organizations, programs, policies, and "systems" at organizational, community, and state levels.

Forty-five percent had sought "wise counsel" from another PHLI graduate in the past two years, while 55% had collaborated with other PHLI graduates on projects or activities. Formal network activities that emerged from PHLI included the PHLS, the NLN, and state and regional PHLI's. These comments were typical about the value of network development:

*Being part of a national cadre of very outstanding leaders, developing good relationships within that network, had a significant impact on me and my work. It continues to affect how I think, what I ask about, and how I approach many challenging situations.*

*Through PHLI, I met other public health leaders across the country and have maintained friendships with them since 1997. This network of accomplished leaders has been an invaluable source of advice, best practices, referrals, and support. I have held leadership positions at the local (health officer) and state (deputy health secretary) level for almost 12 years, and have found that a leadership network has been essential in my career.*

*Domain 4. Public Health Systems and Infrastructure Development*
We wanted to know if PHLI had wide influences on programs, organizations, relationships, and policies. We operationalized these concepts by asking the question in this way:

Can you think of an *organizational change* that PHLI graduates influenced directly or indirectly? (e.g., revised mission, process, positions, expansion, reorganization, funding, or other)

Can you think of a *program change* that PHLI graduates influenced directly or indirectly? (e.g., new, expanded, improved, better-funded program)

Can you think of a *systems change* that PHLI graduates influenced directly or indirectly? (e.g., a partnership, collaboration, new cross-organizational system or method for improving practice)

Can you think of a *policy (law) change* that PHLI graduates influenced directly or indirectly?

For each question, the response options were "Yes," "No," and "Not sure." The results were as follows:

- 40% reported having observed a *policy (law) change* that PHLI graduates influenced directly or indirectly
- 60% reported having observed a *program change* that PHLI graduates influenced directly or indirectly
- 66% reported having observed an *organizational change* that PHLI graduates influenced directly or indirectly

- 67% reported having observed a *systems change* that PHLI graduates influenced directly or indirectly

We asked graduates to pick *one* such change and "(a) describe in some detail the change that was made, (b) explain how PHLI contributed to it, and (c) tell us why you view the change as important." We received nearly 300 responses, many of them extensive paragraphs, with these general themes:

- 96 described improved collaborations, partnerships, coalitions, and relationships at the national (n=525), state (n=542), or local (n=526) levels.
- 76 described developing or implementing specific methods and tools for improving organizational and system performance, such as Essential Services, Performance Standards, accreditation systems for public health agencies, the National Code of Ethics, Mobilizing for Action Through Planning and Partnerships (MAPP), and Assessment Protocol for Excellence in Public Health (APEX*PH*). Others described substantial restructuring and improvements in local health services on a statewide basis, and other more specific state and local efforts in such domains as immunization and Medicaid fraud prevention.
- 31 described new policies passed at the national (n=4), state (n=23), and local levels (n=4) in domains such as preparedness, tobacco control, injury control, public health systems funding, and health insurance for preventive care.
- 94 described organizational changes including reorganizations (n=26), developing and adopting new approaches to planning for organizational or community public health improvement (n=15), adopting stakeholder and community engagement as a fundamental way of leading an agency (n=10), new (n=8), installation of performance management and improvement tools (n=7), quality improvements (n=6), and other diverse improvements.
- 68 described improved or new programs at national (n=14), state (n=39), and local/organizational levels (n=15) including workforce and leadership development, human immunodeficiency virus testing, worksite wellness, dental public health, and other diverse areas.

Many scholars described specific changes they *personally* had initiated, or which their team had initiated through the *applied team project* component of the program.

A large number of others explained that a *group* or *critical mass* of PHLI graduates had accumulated over time within a state or federal agency, jurisdiction, or association (such as NACCHO) and collaborated to shape a new initiative.

Very frequently, graduates collaborated *with one another* to lead *others* through a collaborative process that led to infrastructure and systems improvements—such as leading a community public health system through a MAPP process, or leading an organization through a participatory strategic planning process that engaged a wider group of stakeholders than had previously been included.

A general historical pattern emerged from the data: a group of thought leaders met at PHLI and worked together to reconceptualize how public health systems should be structured and should function, and also how public health leaders should work to improve them. This highly influential group of graduates worked with others in senior positions nationally, and through associations such as NACCHO, ASTHO, PHLS, and National Association of Local Boards of Health, to devise and disseminate new tools to help state and local governments define and improve public health infrastructure and systems. These tools included but were not limited to the Essential Services,

*(continues)*

**Case Study 18-B** *continued*

Performance Standards, agency accreditation systems, APEX*PH* and MAPP, the Code of Ethics, and state and regional public health leadership development institutes.

Many PHLI graduates working at national, state, and local levels followed the lead of the early thought leaders by further refining these tools and ideas, and leading national, state, and local implementation of them.

These quotations were typical of many we received describing these developments:

*[A] reconceptualization of the public health system following [the 1988] IOM Future of Public Health report. Early graduates and subsequent graduates have been the "thought leaders" advancing the reconceptualization. [This is important because it] has helped a whole new generation of public health officials rethink their work.*

*Relating to "systems" change, several key PHLI graduates were directly responsible for the exploration of a new national accreditation program for state and local public health agencies. This was effective and visionary leadership at its best. PHLI contributed in two ways, first, by developing the sense of shared leadership among top public health professionals as the "standard" for how we would achieve advances in public health practice, and second, and importantly, PHLI brought public health leaders together to share experiences, become true colleagues, and create a common ideal for WHAT public health could become. I do not believe we would have pushed public health in the direction of creating a national accreditation system to assess and improve public health agencies across the nation without the efforts and vision of PHLI graduates.*

*[PHLI influenced] the growth of local health departments in Nebraska in 2001. Prior to a local-statewide initiative, there were 16 local health departments covering 22 counties in the state. After the intervention, there were 32 health departments covering the ENTIRE state (all 94 counties). Several PHLI alums were involved, along with public health leaders that had participated in the state-level PLHI. These folks served as change-agents and were leaders that help guide and got the process passed. This change was HUGE in that an entire state went from part-time to full-time coverage of public health services. Health status change-measures are now in place to evaluate and affirm the positive impact that local public coverage DOES make.*

*Domain 5. PHLI and the Future Direction of Public Health Leadership Development in the United States*

Graduates and key informants made these observations:

- Individual leader development and network development are important synergistic efforts that have helped to create a common public health framework and a fertile ground for diffusion of innovation.
- Adequate and ongoing funding is needed in order to support innovative programming and to enhance the existing leadership development foundation.

Graduates and key informants offered these recommendations:

- Offer a continuum of "cutting-edge" or forward-looking development opportunities, including a national institute as well as continuing education and informal development activities to build a culture of lifelong learning and to sustain vibrant networks.
- Consider how to support a more integrated and coordinated system of leadership development at the national and state levels.
- Consider strategies to strengthen networks beyond the current methods, including enhanced connections to support succession planning and to facilitate opportunities to work on issues of national importance.

- Build in an ongoing evaluation system, focusing on both process and out-come measures.

## Discussion

### Leader Development and Network Development: Warp and Woof

In PHLI, leader and network development were simultaneous, mutually supportive, and parts of one another. We might say that they were "warp and woof," essential parts of the same woven cloth, or a virtual cycle. Either one without the other would have been less effective.

All of the personal gains that leaders made in PHLI helped them become interested, knowledgeable, skilled, and confident network members. Likewise, being part of a network of trusted colleagues at the vanguard of public health leadership promoted confidence and courage, inspired graduates to imitate their peers and network colleagues, and taught them much more than they could learn in a classroom setting.

This study's observations of the complementary but distinct roles of leader development and leadership network development reflect wider discussions in the leadership literature. For example, some writers recently have used "leader development" to refer to initiatives designed primarily to develop individual leaders' capabilities, and reserve "leadership development" for efforts to develop networks of leaders who can work together (Day, 2003). That conception of leadership development is becoming more prominent as the concepts of collaborative or shared leadership have gained favor for use in complex multiparty settings (Chrislip and Larson, 1994).

This understanding of leader and network development as warp and woof also fits very closely with models of collective expertise being discussed in scientific literature about networks (Cross, 2004), competence, expertise, professional development and communities of practice (Wenger, 2002), and professional performance. "The expertise needed in the knowledge society cannot be understood by referring only to a sum of individual cognitive competencies, but also to joint or shared competence manifest in the dynamic functioning of communities and networks of experts and professionals as well as supporting tools and instruments" (Hakkarainen et al., 2004, p. 8).

### Visions for the Future Direction of Public Health Leadership Development in the United States

The data and recommendations from graduates and key informants summarized above endorse the program's historic emphases on both leader and network development, and offer ways to strengthen both. Future versions of PHLI should integrate leader development and leadership network development tightly with one another and with applied leadership work on issues of importance to agencies and systems. Such applied work can be quite valuable for both leadership learning and network development during the program itself. In addition, the long-term collaborations that emerge from PHLI can and should be nurtured. This study found that they can have significant impacts.

## Evaluation Case Study Summary

This study benefited from sufficient resources to hire a lead program evaluator and several graduate research assistants to assist with all phases. Keys to success were taking great care to design the study to meet stakeholders' information needs; spending

*(continues)*

**Case Study 18-B** *continued*

a great deal of time developing the survey and interview guides and basing them on preliminary interviews and pilot tests with graduates; and taking several months to carefully analyze and interpret the data. We also learned to allot enough time for data analysis, and were reminded of the importance of limiting data collected to amounts that one will have time to analyze thoroughly. The full study and the instruments used are available at www.phli.org/evalreports

## Appendix 18-B References

Chrislip, D.D., & Larson, C.E. (1994). *Collaborative leadership: How citizens and civic leaders can make a difference.* San Francisco, CA: Jossey-Bass.

Cross, R., & Cummings, J.N. (2004). Tie and network correlates of individual performance in knowledge-intensive work. *Academy of Management Journal,* 47(6), 928-937.

Day, D. (2003). "Leadership development: A review in context." *Leadership Quarterly,* Vol No 4, pp. 581-613.

Hakkarainen, K., Palonen, T., Paavola, S., & Lehtinen, E. (2004). *Communities of networked expertise.* Oxford, UK: Elsevier Ltd.

Miles, M. B., & Huberman, A.M. (1994). *Qualitative data analysis* (2nd ed.). Thousand Oaks, CA: Sage Publications.

Patton, M.Q. (1990). *Qualitative research and evaluation methods.* Thousand Oaks, CA: Sage Publications.

Wenger, E., McDermott, R., & Snyder, W. (2002). *Cultivating communities of practice: A guide to managing knowledge.* Boston: Harvard Business School Press.

## Summary

This chapter looked at the issue of evaluation of training programs, specifically leadership development programs. A number of research questions were raised for future leadership investigations. The chapter's case studies concern program evaluation at a regional and a national public health leadership institute. They document the complexity of leadership development and the concerns of trainers regarding how to assess leadership training and make it more effective.

## Discussion Questions

1. Why is leadership program evaluation important?
2. What is one difficulty in evaluating leadership programs?
3. How do leadership development programs differ from other training or educational programs?
4. What leadership issues do you think should be the focus of research?
5. Would are some benefits to be gained by keeping a leadership journal?

## Exercise 18-1:   Great Expectations

*Purpose:* to investigate the relationship between personal expectations and training experiences

*Key concepts:* evaluation, leadership development, leadership expectations, lessons learned

*Procedure:* In Exercise 1-1, each student or trainee wrote down five expectations he or she had regarding the course. Each student or trainee should now review those expectations, indicate to what degree each was met, and whether he or she learned things that were not anticipated. The class or training groups should then divide into groups of five to ten members and discuss the expectations and their fulfillment or lack of fulfillment.

# References

1. S. T. Gray, *Leadership Is: Evaluation with Power* (Washington, DC: Independent Sector, 1995).
2. Centers for Disease Control and Prevention, "Framework for Program Evaluation in Public Health," *MMWR* 48 (1999): RR11.
3. Centers for Disease Control and Prevention, "Framework for Program Evaluation in Public Health."
4. E. Jurkowski et al., "The Core Functions and the Role of Governance Within the Public Health Arena: A Perspective from Board of Health Members" (submitted for publication).
5. D. L. Kirkpatrick, *Evaluating Training Programs: The Four Levels,* 2nd ed. (San Francisco: Berrett-Koehler, 1998).
6. J. Hale, "Evaluation: It's Time to Go Beyond Levels 1, 2, 3, and 4," in *The 1999 ASTD Training and Performance Yearbook,* eds. J. A. Woods and J. W. Cortada (New York: McGraw-Hill, 1999).
7. M. L. Lanigan, "New Theory and Measures for Training Evaluation," in *The 1999 ASTD Training and Performance Yearbook,* eds. J. A. Woods and J. W. Cortada (New York: McGraw-Hill, 1999).
8. C. D. McCauley and M. W. Hughes-James, *An Evaluation of the Outcomes of a Leadership Development Program* (Greensboro, NC: Center for Creative Leadership, 1994).
9. McCauley and Hughes-James, *An Evaluation of the Outcomes of a Leadership Development Program.*
10. C. D. McCauley and E. Van Velsor (eds.), *The Center for Creative Leadership Handbook of Leadership Development,* 2nd ed. (San Francisco: Jossey-Bass, 2004).
11. J. W. Martineau, K. M. Hannum, and C. Reinelt, "Introduction," in *The Handbook of Leadership Development Evaluation,* K. M. Hannum, J. W. Martineau, and C. Reinelt, eds. (San Francisco: Jossey-Bass, 2007).
12. E. J. Davidson and J. W. Martineau, "Strategic Uses of Evaluation," in *The Handbook of Leadership Development Evaluation,* K. M. Hannum, J. W. Martineeau, and C. Reinelt, eds. (San Francisco: Jossey-Bass, 2007).
13. K. E. Umble, S. J. Diehl, A. Gunn, and S. Haws, *Developing Leaders, Building Networks: An Evaluation of the National Public Health Leadership Institute—1991-2006* (Chapel Hill: North Carolina Institute for Public Health, 2007).

PART V

# The Future

# CHAPTER 19

# LEADERSHIP FOR THE 21ST CENTURY

*"Everyone overrates the significance of his own era. . . .*
*Things change."*

*Robert Stone, Damascus Gate*

The purpose to this book is to explore public health leadership in depth and suggest ways in which leadership knowledge can be translated into practice, especially in the coming years. American society is changing, and old leadership approaches are no longer working. Change did not stop with the new millennium, neither in society in general, nor in the area of public health. Therefore, public health leaders have to be trained to work in an environment of constant change. Chapter 20 will deal with the issue of leadership in traditional public health agencies and the demands for crisis leaders in a preparedness environment.

American social life does not seem to be governed by natural laws.[1] Because different eras bring forth different social circumstances, different types of leaders are needed at different times. It is clear that leaders will guide social developments whatever the social climate is.

Many organizational practices now in use are out of date. Drucker identified seven organizational assumptions that no longer hold true.[2] He also identified seven realities of contemporary management. The seven realities entail that no cookie-cutter approach to the development of organizations is feasible. People cannot be managed all in the same way. Everybody is different. Each organization has multilevel activities and services, and no one service drives the organization. New technologies, such as communication via the Internet, are constantly being created. Complexity rules. In addition, the command and control approaches of the past will no longer be acceptable. Finally, global concerns will drive the organizations of the future.

## Leadership Challenges in the 21st Century[3]

Public health leaders face 13 strategic challenges as we near the close of the first decade of the 21st century (Table 19-1). When I first talked with Lenihan for the first edition of this book, the challenges were more categorical in nature. Now his challenges are systemic and more strategic in nature. Lenihan now posits that leadership challenges necessitate an adaptive response of a whole agency or an entire community and not just a technical response to a single public health initiative or program. With increasing complexity in

**Table 19-1 Public Health Strategic Challenges: A Baker's Dozen**

1) Changing scope of public health
2) Greater accountability and performance
3) Growing competition for roles and resources
4) A focus on the public health system
5) Shifting demographic composition
6) Alternative organizational arrangements
7) The chronic disease epidemic
8) Emerging and reemerging threats
9) Invisibility and search for public support
10) A strained health care system and growing number of uninsured
11) Stagnant revenues
12) The technology revolution: information and biological
13) Devolution of federal responsibilities to the state and local level

*Source:* Courtesy of D. Patrick Lenihan.

public health as in life generally, all these challenges are interrelated. With changes occurring every day in our environment, these changes cannot help but affect the daily operations of our public health agencies. In addition, public health agencies are being asked to do work on many new areas of concern and often with limited financial resources. An important consideration is a determination of whether our agencies should do the work, whether our partners should do it, or whether some form of collaboration can be developed to do it.

The first challenge relates to this changing and evolving scope of public health. In the past, public health agencies concentrated much of their work on communicable disease control. Now our agencies are involved in public health preparedness, regulation of health care providers, and providing health care services to the poor and uninsured as a provider of last resort. Those public health professionals with a strong social justice orientation seem to be unable to say no as more programs are added to our agency portfolios.

The second challenge is an expectation of greater accountability and performance. It seems that the public and our elected officials are requiring more and more service for each tax dollar spent. These expectations also require that public health leaders demonstrate how the money was spent and how the expenditures improved the health of the public. This is further complicated by local governments and agencies being more accountable for public health than the state or federal level. As discussed throughout this book and especially in Chapter 8, many new instruments have been developed to show how public health works and performs. For example, the Mobilizing for Action Through Planning and Partnerships assessment process and the National Public Health Performance Standards are two sets of tools that have been developed to demonstrate accountability and quality improvement.

The third challenge involves the issue of growing competition for roles and resources. Competition is something that the business community understands and something that public health professionals have difficulty understanding because we are collaborative in our orientation. However, public health leaders still have difficulty in demonstrating the value of our work. We still struggle to carry out the mission of public health as our resources dwindle and our work is being done by other organizations in the health care sector. The boundaries between the public, private, and not-for profit sectors in health seem to be dissolving. We see this especially in the area of emergency preparedness and response and the emphasis on meta-leadership skills and strategies, which were discussed in Chapter 3.

The fourth strategic challenge involves systems thinking and the focus on the public health system. There has been a shift from a public health agency focus to a community-based public health focus. The core functions and essential public health services model emphasizes community partnerships to carry out the public health enterprise. Many of the leadership tools discussed in this book and other books provide a toolkit for leaders engaged in community and systems work.[4] As discussed in several chapters in this book, public health leaders will need to become navigators who steer and guide public health work rather than only reacting to today's crisis. Collaboration with partners is a system-level involvement. Public health leaders need to increase their skills in policy formulation and development.

Shifting demographic composition is the next strategic challenge. Our population is aging, and this will require that public health be more involved in chronic disease and aging issues. The increasing diversity of our population and the erosion of the middle class bring the potential for increasing our public health involvement in health care issues such as access to service and to health disparities concerns. The global economy and the increase in illegal immigration raises important policy and health service delivery issues because our health and public health system are already overburdened.

> **Leadership Tip**
>
> *Leaders know the primary importance of family and community.*

The next challenge involves alternative organizational arrangements. Over the last two decades, we have seen the reorganization of the governmental service sector. We now have super-agencies trying to integrate a complex array of services and programs to residents. We are seeing some hospital systems now running county health departments with oversight from a county board of health. Regionalization will be an issue in the future when smaller health departments need to work together and share resources. This may lead, as it has in a number of areas of the United States, to regional health departments. Thus, we seem to be more open to exploring alternative organizational arrangements than in the past.

As discussed above on the challenge of shifting demographics, the challenge of chronic disease epidemics needs to be addressed. Chronic diseases are the major cause of death (over 70%) for the U.S. population. Although chronic diseases have been monitored and addressed by public health for many years, it seems that these diseases have taken a backseat to emergency preparedness and response agendas. Smoking bans have been one mechanism by which public health issues have been addressed by elected officials and public health professionals in recent years. The increased incidence of diabetes is also being addressed even though limited financial resources are available. Continuing need to address coronary heart disease and stroke through preventive mechanisms such as improved nutrition and exercise has been promoted. Improved lifestyle changes are more about education than treatment.

The next challenge relates to emerging and reemerging threats and the increased concern about such infectious diseases as severe acute respiratory syndrome, pandemic influenza, drug-resistant tuberculosis, and bioterrorism. As I have pointed out elsewhere, many reports have argued that we still have low levels of readiness, although there is some evidence of improvement to address these potential health problems.[5] We have developed critical skills related to emergency planning and response although work needs to occur on the issues of mitigation and recovery, as will be discussed in Chapter 20. The challenge for public health agencies is to be in a constant state of readiness in the future. This is difficult without financial support from our elected officials or interest from the public. An important question involves the impact of a preparedness agenda on the day-to-day activities of our local health departments.

The ninth strategic challenge involves the issue of public health's invisibility and the need for public health leaders to search for public support. Public health leaders tend not to promote their good deeds. Public health leaders monitor the health of the public, push prevention agendas, work collaboratively with their community partners, alert the public to potential health threats, give service when other health providers do not, push a preparedness agenda, and foster many other health-enhancing activities. We do not get recognition for most of these activities. We tend to be shy about our accomplishments. Perhaps we need to develop a "Brag About Public Health Week" that coincides with our annual Public Health Week. We need to make friends with our elected officials and our media representatives. Leaders need to create more public value for our activities. Part of this public health visibility is to demonstrate how a health department plays a role in these public health accomplishments.

Another strategic challenge that has been partially addressed above is the reality of a strained health care system and a growing uninsured population. In Dr. Malecki's comments in Chapter 10, she talked of the need for public health agencies to take a more visible role in community health care because she believes that the medical care system in our society is in disarray. Managed care organizations still address high costs and the difficulty of the uninsured having appropriate access to health care. Catastrophic illness has led to personal bankruptcies. Health disparities still exist. Local public health agencies no longer have the resources to provide direct health care services to our residents. We have not figured out our relationships to community health centers or to the clinics in drugstores and large retail stores like Wal-Mart. It is critical for public health to redefine its role in the public health activities in communities.

Stagnant revenues are our next strategic challenge. Since the terrorist acts of September 11, 2001, the federal budget for domestic programs has been decreasing as our government has had to put more funds into the Iraq war, other military activities, and strengthening our military. Public health agencies received funds after 2001 for preparedness activities as funding for other programs declined. Now we are seeing the decline in preparedness funding as well. Retirements of public health professionals is occurring without people being rehired when retirees leave. The public health workforce is shrinking at a time when more demands are being made on local health departments to increase their work in new areas. Future growth of public health will not happen without investment in the enterprise.

New technologies are creating another strategic challenge. Advances in information technology and the developing field of informatics, biotechnology, and research applications tied to our increasing knowledge of genomics will greatly change the public health agency of the future. The negative issue related to these changes involves such issues as invasions of privacy of individuals and ethical concerns in public health practice. Biotechnology concerns will become visible with more concentration on genetic profiling and discrimination. These new technologies will also be expensive and difficult to fund from our present tax base.

The final strategic challenge will have significant effects on the work of public health leaders and other professionals with possible devolution of federal responsibilites to the state and local level. This has been occurring since the 1980s. Of course, the scenario can change if political parties in the White House and Congress change their attitudes and funding priorities to strengthen the national public health system, increase support for state and local public health, pass universal health care programs, and continue to support training the public health workforce. The chances for this turnaround seem slight at this time, and an increasing federal role in public health does not seem on the horizon.

These strategic challenges will clearly affect the public health system of the future and increase the pressure on public health leaders to protect the health of people and the environment. Public health leaders need to be more proactive and not follow the crowd. They need, in other words, to both navigate and steer the course of public health program change rather than be among the rowers. They have the leadership skills to move public health organizations forward, and they need to apply these skills to this task. Public health leaders have an obligation to develop a set of ethical standards pertaining to public health and to use these standards for guiding the public health process.

## Public Health During the Third Wave

In Chapter 6, the third-wave theory was discussed.[6] Table 19-2 lists 12 third-wave public health issues. The third wave began with the transition from industrial forms of organization (which are characteristic of the second wave) to information-based forms of organization. The last two decades of the 20th century saw major changes in technology and the emergence of knowledge as an important commodity.

Table 19-3 compares certain elements of the second wave with corresponding elements of the third wave. Some of the changes have already

**Table 19-2 Public Health in the Third Wave**

1. Expanded models of public health
2. Team-based problem solving
3. Community health coalitions based on partnership
4. Privatization of assurance activities
5. Decentralization of responsibilities across the community
6. Community-wide governance
7. Value generation
8. A new political structure
9. Third-wave leadership
10. Integration between individuals' needs and the community's needs
11. Complete community empowerment
12. Universal access to a multitude of services to improve quality of life

**Table 19-3 The Second and Third Waves Compared**

| Second-Wave Civilization | Third-Wave Civilization |
| --- | --- |
| Nuclear family | Alternate families |
| Mass education | Individual education |
| Giant corporations | Small specialty organizations |
| Centralized nation-state | New democracy |
| Mass trade unions | Demassification |
| Hand work | Mind work |

*Source:* Data from "Products of the Third Wave," in *The Third Wave* by Alvin Toffler. Copyright © 1980 by Alvin Toffler. Reprinted by permission of HarperCollins Publishers, Inc.

occurred. For example, many alternative family approaches were already common in the 1990s, the use of educational vouchers to allow parents to select public or private schools for their children is under discussion, and some parents educate their children at home utilizing computers and educational software.

On the other hand, the large-organization model still prevails, and mergers are making big organizations bigger. It is true that there has been an increase in small specialty organizations, but this has been going on for a long time. Also, national struggles have continued to plague the world, and whether democracy will finally triumph as the one viable political system is open to question. In fact, the meaning and direction of our democratic society has come under increasing scrutiny. Trade unions have lost their strength, and many professionals are redefining the workplace. Thus, the year 2000 found American society still tied to the second wave, although clear examples of third-wave realities are disrupting society.

Table 19-4 lists 10 products that reflect the transition between the second wave and the third wave. Many of the products will have an impact on public health whether or not the third-wave theory is valid. For instance, public health leaders will require more information to do their jobs well. The

**Table 19-4    Products of the Third Wave**

1.  Information and innovation
2.  Management strategies
3.  Culture and pop culture
4.  Advanced technology
5.  Software
6.  Education
7.  Training
8.  Medical care through the private sector
9.  Financial services
10. Military protection

*Source:* Data from "Products of the Third Wave," in *The Third Wave* by Alvin Toffler. Copyright © 1980 by Alvin Toffler. Reprinted by permission of HarperCollins Publishers, Inc.

human genome project is changing our understanding of how diseases work and is leading to new techniques for helping people. Innovation will be the order of the day. Strategies for running organizations will be based on the leadership model rather than the management model. The old ways and the old methods will have to be modified.

Public health leaders and their human services colleagues will have to make public health a community-based activity through partnering with community leaders and community residents generally. Citizens of the 21st century will have to assume responsibility for improving their personal health and fitness. If it appears that technology is advanced now, wait 20 years. Think of the changes that have occurred since 1980. Desktop computers became as powerful as the massive computers of the past. The Internet grew from nothing into a whole new means of communicating, transferring information, and doing business.

The American educational system will have to change. The educational process will be different for each individual. The challenge will be to determine how to use our educational tools to meet the needs and wants of people committed to lifelong learning. The expansion of distancing-learning programs will be part of the answer. Training opportunities, including mentoring opportunities, will need to grow if public health professionals are to keep up with the changes in their field.

The medical care sector is already changing. Community health centers are only one approach. One major trend will be the creation of integrated systems of care. Another will be the development of public-private partnerships. Possibilities for the development of some procedures for a universal health care system are increasing. New financial services will also evolve. Finally, national and international military protection will require the continued development and production of more advanced weapon systems.

During the third wave, leaders who integrate their leadership skills and their management skills will be the ones who are most successful. In short, leadership and management will become united.

Following are 10 key leadership issues for the information age:

1. Leaders will need strategies oriented toward growth rather than retrenchment. They will also have to engage in strategic thinking rather than merely tactical thinking.
2. Customer- and community-focused activities will become more prominent.
3. More and more knowledge sources will appear. For example, the Internet will expand the professional horizons of public health practitioners.
4. The information age is also the age of teams, coalitions, and partnerships. Networking will be the preferred method of operation.
5. Public agencies will discover that they cannot serve all segments of the population. The service sector will need to be shared by both public and private entities. An integrated health care system will evolve, with public health agencies as lead partners. Each partner in the integrated system will serve specific client sectors.
6. Accounting systems will become more relevant to public health activities. Public health agencies will need to budget on the basis of core functions, organizational practices, and/or essential services rather than traditional public health service activities.
7. All partners in an enterprise will need to be empowered. Empowerment must be balanced against control.
8. Shared values will change. Leaders will have to review shared values regularly because changes in values have an impact on the program effectiveness of public health agencies.
9. Leaders must honor the best practices and the most effective individuals.
10. Leaders must work to transform a second-wave organization into a third-wave one.

Leaders need guidance in how to motivate and manage change to facilitate the transformation to the third wave or the modification of the present system.[7] Leadership commitment to the transformation is also a major factor. Figure 19-1 presents a model of transformation for health care organizations. One critical task to address before starting a transformation is to make certain that a real need for change exists. If change is inevitable, then the leaders need to restructure teams and coalitions so as to bring about the change with as little difficulty as possible.

A successful transformation requires that all the steps shown in Figure 19-1 be followed. Leaders will need to adopt strategic planning, total quality process, re-engineering, and reinvention methods, among others, to expedite the change process. The next stage involves the commitment of all players to the idea of change and the philosophical underpinnings of the management strategies selected to help bring about the change. Next, the leaders need to encourage creativity in the workforce and promote innovation. These factors will change not only the way people work but also the way public health organizations look.

It is not necessary to accept the third-wave theory. Much more important is to accept the changes that are occurring in our society since September 11, 2001. This is clearly a time of major change in which leaders from all segments

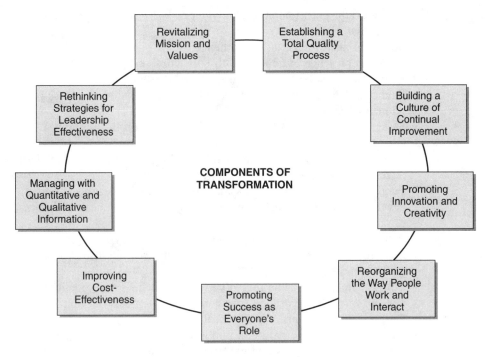

**FIGURE 19-1    Components of Transformation**
*Source:* Reprinted with permission from E. Murszalek-Gaucher and R. J. Coffey,
*Transforming Healthcare Organizations,* p. 57, © 1990, Jossey-Bass Inc., Publishers.

of our society will need to address the issues that are causing the change and
arising out of the change. It is clear that there may be more waves in the future. Maynard and Mehrtens have defined an emerging fourth wave.[8] The
fourth wave moves beyond the collaboration approaches defined by Toffler to
a more complexity-based approach that unifies us as a society and creates an
environment in which we co-create our future out of our beliefs about what
we want the future to be. Leadership will be different in the future where
global stewardship and a view of the world that ignores boundaries will guide
our leadership activities. Protection of our environment and our communities
will also guide our activities. Quality-of-life issues will also be a dominant factor in our thinking and work. Shechtman has viewed the fourth wave as a
communication-intensive social system.[9] As he looks forward to a fifth wave,
he points to a period of personal transformation where we take more responsibility for our actions. Exercise 19-1 presents an opportunity to explore wave
theory from the perspective of a public health problem.

In terms of the practical applications necessary for our work today, public health leaders will need to answer the call for a new form of public health
that is based on the following principles:

- Public health must clarify its mission, its vision, and its parameters
  and sell its vision to the public.
- Public health must become proactive rather than reactive.
- In a mostly private health system, public health must become the voice
  of the public. Public health should not be privatized.

- Public health must remain the provider of last resort (although *last* means *last*).
- Boards of health must be strengthened.
- A federal presence in public health must continue.
- Prevention must be stressed and marketed.
- Environmental health and occupational health must be treated as public health partners.
- State laboratories need to be involved in setting up the public health agenda.
- Assessment activities must be strengthened through the use of modern technology and applied epidemiological methods.
- Public health leaders need to work with their public health partners to develop a stronger infrastructure for addressing public health concerns of our communities.
- Public health professionals must become policy makers.
- Leadership development must not only be stressed but also be financially supported.
- Stronger links need to be forged between academics and practitioners. The links need to incorporate the core academic fields of public health and the core functions of public health.
- The multidisciplinary nature of public health must be strengthened at the same time that a unified perspective on public health must be promoted among public health's constituencies.
- State-level public health agencies must remain largely independent.
- The partnership between state-level health agencies and local health agencies must be strengthened.
- Public health agencies must think globally but act locally.
- Public health agencies must teach the public about public health.
- Coalitions, including public-private partnerships, must be built.
- Assurance must be redefined on a regular basis.
- Public health must sell its best practices.
- Public health leaders need to be prepared for any emergencies that may arise.
- Public health leaders should run for and hold elected office.

## The Leaders Speak

Case Study 2-A discussed a study done by the author from 1996 to 1998. In the study, 100 American public health leaders and 30 public health leaders from England, Scotland, and Ireland were interviewed. In the American portion of the study, the leaders were asked about an agenda for public health in the 21st century. Some leaders predicted that certain potential health-related problems, such as new infectious diseases and increased resistance of microorganisms to antibiotics, might erupt and affect the overall tasks of public health agencies. Some were also concerned about the aging of the American population.

The leaders did not fully agree on what public health is and what it does. The lack of consensus was probably partly due to the multidisciplinary background of the leaders and the specific emphasis of the programs they oversaw. Although many leaders believed that the mission of public health was to promote health and prevent disease, some found this mission statement too simplistic. Without a clear mission and a well-formulated vision, it becomes difficult to talk to others about public health. Thus, public health leaders jointly should explore the governing public health paradigms and revise them as necessary, develop a consensus on a mission and a vision for public health, and sell the mission, vision, and paradigms to community constituents.

During the last few decades of the 20th century and even more since the terrorist events of 2001, public health leaders have tended to respond to health crises rather than plan public health agendas likely to prevent crises. The goal for the 21st century is for public health leaders to take charge of their destiny and devise action plans directed toward improving the health of community residents. Proactive approaches should be the order of the day and the century.

Public health leaders will continue to act as the voice of the public in matters of health. Because public health agencies perform oversight activities, complete privatization of public health will not occur, and public health agencies will need to be integrated into the health care system. Because the development of a national health system in the United States remains a remote possibility, oversight by public health leaders is critical.

Boards of health and local and state departments of health should act as partners rather than adversaries. Board members are community gatekeepers and have an obligation to promote the community's priorities. Because of the importance of their role, board members need training in how to do their job. If boards become strengthened, the whole infrastructure of public health will become strengthened as well. It would help if board members would network with other board members, with all boards of health in the state (if a board of health structure exists), and with the public health practitioners at the local and state levels. Public health leaders are aware of the lack of connection between the federal health agencies, the state health department (or, in some states, the human services agency), and local public health agencies. It is important to create strong links among these three levels of government, and public health leaders, among others, will have to take the initiative in forging these links. A federal presence is critical if policy is to be formulated for the nation.

Public health leaders need to push a primary prevention agenda. In many places, although prevention constitutes a major portion of the public health agenda, the public health leaders do little to promote the agenda. Public health agencies and their leaders need to address primary prevention in a strategic manner and come up with approaches for improving the health of the public through the prevention of disease.[10] Prevention includes actions that reduce susceptibility or exposure to health threats (primary prevention), detect and treat disease in early stages (secondary prevention), and alleviate the effect of disease and injury (tertiary prevention).[11]

During the late 20th century, local public health agencies concentrated their efforts on secondary and tertiary prevention programs. A shift to primary prevention initiatives, in which people become responsible for their own health, is needed.

Public health encompasses occupational health and safety as well as environmental health. Unfortunately, these disciplines tend to be neglected by public health leaders with a strong personal services orientation. Environmental health and occupational health specialists need to be given the same standing as other public health professionals. Also meriting a seat at the table are state and local laboratory directors, many of whom have been trained in a number of areas, including public health science. The professional diversity that characterizes public health is not a weakness but one of its strengths.

The public health leaders interviewed by the author recognized the importance of the community assessment process and argued that assessment techniques need to be improved. One recommendation was to train public health partners in the basics of epidemiological methods in order to combine community assessment and epidemiology. Without question, public health leaders must acquire good computer skills and become acquainted with new information technologies as they emerge. Sharing epidemiological and other types of data with public health leaders across the country will become the norm.

Public health leaders will need to become more versed in policy development. As experts, these leaders can influence elected officials and thereby promote the public health agenda at the local, state, and federal levels. In addition, public health agencies, like other human services organizations, need money to operate and carry out their mandate. Financial support is critical, and public health leaders will need to seek funding from multiple sources. State funding will cover only part of a health department budget, and so public health leaders will need to act as entrepreneurs in getting outside funding.

Public health leaders need to share ideas with their academic partners. Faculty members are often excluded from the strategic-planning process, yet they bring to the table a knowledge of health-related sciences, an understanding of the core disciplines of public health, and a knowledge of emerging health problems—all of which can be extremely important for addressing the problems that public health leaders face.

As noted, public health professionals come from many different disciplines, and although the diversity in educational background is an important strength, public health leaders must create a unified perspective to present to the public. To put it one way, while speaking with many voices to each other, public health leaders must speak with a common voice when dealing with community partners.

The public health leaders interviewed were intrigued, to varying degrees, with three models for the future of public health: a situation in which independent public health agencies exist, an integrated system in which public health is one of the players, and an integrated system in which public health is the organizer of the system. Although some of the leaders liked each of the three models, they generally believed that it is necessary to maintain an independent public health presence in the community. Maintaining independent agencies will be critical if the United States does not develop a national health service.

There is a caution here. Public health leaders in other countries pointed out that public health often gets lost in a national health system. In England, the public health leaders found much of their time was spent purchasing services for their districts. American public health leaders were concerned about the possibility that the state health department would get absorbed into a state human services superagency. They believed that the state health department should be maintained as a separate entity within state government.

Public health agencies at different governmental levels must act as partners and cease to be antagonistic. Public health leadership programs are a means of creating partnerships between state and local agencies because the trainees come from all levels of government. Local public health leaders should communicate with state leaders and understand their concerns, and they should also be aware of the current activities of the World Health Organization and, where necessary, incorporate international health concerns into their planning efforts. Local leaders also need to communicate to the proper authorities information about local health issues that may eventually have a national or international impact.

Despite the efforts to promote public health, the public still does not understand the nature of the field. Without the support of the public, public health leaders will have difficulty planning for the future. The solution is for public health leaders to develop a multipronged approach to both health communication and social marketing. They also need to get out into the community, forge partnerships in the public and private sectors, and educate their partners about public health.

It is through assurance activities that creative intervention strategies will be tested and evaluated. Yet assurance itself will have to be redefined regularly, as new techniques are developed and tested. Assurance in the year 2020 will be different from assurance in the year 2050.

Finally, the public health leaders interviewed by the author emphasized the importance of selling public health's best practices and not being shy about it. If public health leaders do not market themselves well, the public health field as a whole suffers. However, one thing I noticed about public health leaders was their passion and strong belief in the issues that they support. Case Study 19-A is the story of Ardell Wilson, a public health leader and her crusade on behalf of asthmatic children.[12]

---

## Case Study 19-A
## Story of Ardell Wilson

*The Faces of Public Health. Pfizer.*

When *The New York Times* reported in May 2003 that one in four school-age children in central Harlem had asthma, even longtime asthma researchers were surprised. This New York City neighborhood had one of the highest rates of asthma ever documented in the United States. High rates of asthma are not limited to inner-city neighborhoods like Harlem, however. Dr. Ardell A. Wilson, chief of the Bureau of Community Health at the Connecticut Department of Public Health, knows this all too well. Born and raised in New York City—and living with asthma herself—Ardell confronted the disease and made Connecticut the first state in the nation to standardize the treatment protocol for asthma for school-age children.

A graduate of Washington Irving High School in Manhattan, Ardell enrolled at Bronx Community College to earn her associate's degree. While still at Washington Irving, Ardell's guidance counselor pushed her to take college prep courses in advanced biology and advanced algebra even though she intended, like her elder sister, to stick with secretarial studies. That encouragement helped her do well at Bronx

*(continues)*

**Case Study 19-A** *continued*

Community College. After graduating, and by this time married with a young son, she attended City College of the City University of New York part time, earning her bachelor's degree in 1976. She planned to major in elementary education but after one semester switched to biology, which she found more interesting.

As she completed her degree at City College, Ardell knew she wanted to work in health care. She chose dentistry because she felt it was the most stable health-related field—with a young son at home, she needed her work hours to be predictable. Ardell attended the Columbia University School of Dental and Oral Surgery for four years with the idea that she would start her own dental practice. During the last two years, she enlisted with the U.S. Public Health Service. In return for help with her tuition costs, she committed to practice in underserved areas for three years after graduation.

Upon graduation, Ardell joined the Boriken Neighborhood Health Center, a community health center in East Harlem, and spent three years there in an all-female dental service. She also worked at Columbia one day a week, teaching preventive dentistry. Ardell believed that the preventive aspects of dentistry were more critical to a population's long-term health than corrective dentistry. During her final year at Boriken, and based on positive feedback from her preventive dentistry students, Columbia recruited Ardell to join the Division of Community Health as a faculty member. She taught ethics, jurisprudence, and statistics and, at the same time, began a private practice in lower Manhattan, working there part time with a colleague from Columbia. Her work at Columbia was fulfilling because she could make an impact teaching those who in turn would serve the underserved. She also discovered in her private practice that she preferred the community health center setting, where she served those who were truly in need.

In 1984, the Robert Wood Johnson (RWJ) Health Services Research Scholars Program awarded Ardell a fellowship to study at Harvard. The program was intended to train academics to become leaders in health services research. Dr. Howard Bailit, then at the Columbia University School of Public Health and now at the University of Connecticut, encouraged Ardell to apply for the RWJ program to broaden her perspective on health care delivery systems. At Harvard she worked with mentors outside of dentistry and was especially grateful for the training she received from Dr. Laurence Branch, a specialist in geriatrics, survey research, and aging. During her fellowship, Ardell earned her master's degree in public health from the Harvard School of Public Health with a concentration in maternal child health and aging. Although she lived apart from her family for two years—her husband and son remained in New Rochelle and they saw each other only on weekends—she would gladly choose to do those two years over again. She credits her experience at Harvard for preparing her to do what she does today.

At Harvard, Ardell geared her research activities toward becoming a diplomate (specialist) of the American Board of Dental Public Health (ABDPH). She involved herself in learning everything she could about the aging of America, including health insurance and the delivery of services.

She received a certificate in geriatrics from the Harvard School of Medicine Geriatric Education Center. With her mentor, Dr. Branch, she turned her attention to the most vulnerable elderly population, those living in nursing homes. Her work in this area resulted in the documentation of the oral health problems of the elderly living in nursing homes in Massachusetts and earned her the James M. Dunning Award in Health Services Research. She also became the first African-American woman diplomate of the ABDPH.

Upon completing her fellowship in 1986, Ardell returned to Columbia to direct the Division of Community Health and the joint degree program in public health and dentistry. In 1988, Connecticut recruited her to become the state's oral health director.

Ardell rose through a series of positions in Connecticut as the state restructured its government agencies numerous times. She served as the state's oral health director for only two months and then combined that position with community health programs involving school-based health centers, community health centers, maternal child health, and substance abuse. In 1991, she became deputy director of the Connecticut Drug and Alcohol Abuse Commission. She oversaw four state hospitals serving substance abusers and collaborated with community-based agencies. Her greatest contribution, she believes, was expanding services for women by creating residential facilities where the women's children could join them.

In 1993, the Alcohol and Drug Abuse Commission merged into the newly named Connecticut Department of Public Health and Addiction Services, and Ardell reassumed some of her previous responsibilities in community health. In 1995, she became bureau chief of Community Health within a reconstituted Department of Public Health, a position she still holds. She supervises 150 to 200 people in a wide range of public health endeavors, including epidemiology, infectious disease, chronic disease, family health, and risk assessment for environmental and occupational health. She also oversees the State Loan Repayment Program, which encourages young health professionals (physicians, dentists, hygienists, nurses) to practice in underserved areas while the state repays their school loans. Ardell also develops relationships with funders, mostly at the federal level, a key responsibility of her position.

In 2000, Ardell turned her attention to the issue of asthma, a chronic respiratory disease that affects an estimated 10.4% of Connecticut's children under age 18, or more than 86,000 children statewide. She collaborated with the New England Regional Task Force on Asthma as well as stakeholders from Connecticut—managed care organizations, community organizations, and public health professionals—on a Pediatric Asthma Management Initiative. Those collaborations resulted in a model Asthma Action Plan for Connecticut. The Asthma Action Plan, a color-coordinated management tool, is developed in conjunction with a health care provider to help people manage asthma by teaching them to recognize when they are in the green zone (under control), yellow zone (need to improve control), or red zone (need immediate care). The Asthma Action Plan is available in both English and Spanish. Copies were distributed to clinical practices and managed care organizations throughout the state.

In 2001, on the heels of the Asthma Action Plan, Ardell convened a statewide Asthma Summit to publicize the extent of the asthma problem documented in the newly released "Asthma in Connecticut Report." The summit led to a Statewide Asthma Task Force charged with developing a Comprehensive Statewide Asthma Plan and Implementation Process. Numerous activities were initiated to address asthma—from public education and awareness campaigns and provider education to clinical management and surveillance activities. Because children spend a significant part of their day in school and school-related activities, a tool kit called "Managing Asthma in Schools" for school nurses (and school administrators) was developed with the help of school nurses. Shortly afterward, the Department of Public Health helped daycare providers develop their own kit called "Managing Asthma

*(continues)*

in Childcare Facilities." The tool kits—three-ring binders with inserts that can be reproduced as needed—addressed the facts of asthma triggers, asthma management, and the administration of medications in simple and accessible terms. Although the approach and materials were low-tech, they worked.

In 2003, the Connecticut Legislature responded to the advocacy efforts of Ardell and the task force and passed legislation that gave the Department of Public Health the ability to collect data from schools and implement a statewide surveillance system for schoolchildren with asthma. This added to the department's ongoing hospital inpatient and outpatient surveillance activities. As someone with asthma herself, Ardell found the calendar sent by her managed care organization, based on the Asthma Action Plan materials, to be proof of the success of this initiative. The red, yellow, and green indicators for the severity of an attack, matched to recommended interventions, are quick and handy references for anyone suffering from asthma.

The Association of State and Territorial Health Officials recognized Connecticut's Asthma Action Plan as a program of vision, the first of its kind in the nation and still leading the way. In addition to schools, Connecticut authorized daycare personnel to administer medicine to treat asthma attacks as they occur, the first state to do so, making possible a continuum of care. The Connecticut Asthma Program distributes easy-to-use, understandable materials to all levels of the public health system— parents, school nurses, daycare providers, physicians, clinics, and hospitals. In fact, the department produced 10 educational pediatric asthma management vignettes (with an interactive Web site) entitled "Natalie Says," directed at young children and their parents. The vignettes (in English and Spanish) review the importance of asthma management in a child-friendly way. The comprehensive array of asthma materials standardize asthma management protocol and help patients and caregivers understand what makes asthma worse and how to adjust medications and physical activities accordingly. The materials lead to effective management of asthma in children and are a testament to Ardell Wilson's vision and leadership.

Ardell believes this is an excellent time for young people to go into public health. For the first time, the human genome project offers hope that the genetic causes of some diseases can be discovered and the course of those diseases altered. The issue of health care access has come under greater scrutiny, with workforce studies and evaluations of the fairness of insurance and delivery systems. Environmental health will continue to be at the center of public health, encouraging people to consider what they can do to make home and work environments safer. Yet another issue, public health systems that are needed to address health emergencies, has emerged front and center in the public eye.

Ardell believes that public health will be very different 10 years from now. Technologies now being perfected will make computer/Internet-based training the preferred method, replacing conferencing. A focus on the elderly population will be more pronounced, and research should advance treatment for Alzheimer's disease, falls, and other perils of old age. The growing elderly population will require big increases in health care delivery systems, especially nursing homes and assisted living facilities. Ardell sees a bright future for prevention and health promotion after education strategies that limit the growth of health care costs are recognized to work.

For Ardell Wilson, the journey from New York to Connecticut has been long but enjoyable. Along the way, she has made her mark as a dentist and public health specialist. Perhaps most significantly, she has been a literal breath of fresh air for the children and families of Connecticut. Her leadership in asthma management is a model for communities throughout the United States.

## Summary

This chapter reviewed the main challenges facing public health leaders in this century. All of these challenges have been discussed in greater detail in various places throughout the book. The strategies that public health leaders will need to use in order to meet these challenges are both numerous and diverse in kind. Among the most important, at least if public health leaders are themselves to be believed, is to return to public health's traditional focus on primary prevention. Another is to work at educating the public about public health, because it is clear there is general ignorance about what public health practitioners do. By pushing a prevention agenda and publicizing public health successes, along with the other strategies listed, public health leaders will go a long way toward ensuring that public health has the future it deserves and that the public deserves it to have.

### Discussion Questions

1. What current public health challenges do you see as most needing the attention of public health leaders?
2. What strategies might public health leaders use to meet some or all of these challenges?
3. What are some new characteristics of public health predicted to occur in the so-called third wave?
4. Why is there a lack of consensus on what public health is, even among public health practitioners?
5. How can public health leaders promote a prevention agenda?
6. How can public health leaders support the creation of an integrated health care system?
7. Will government public health agencies exist in 2050? Why or why not?

### Exercise 19-1:   Infant Mortality and Wave Theory

*Purpose:* to examine how public health leaders would address a public health issue in five scenarios based on wave theory

*Key concepts:* wave theory, scenario-building, leadership

*Procedure:* Divide the class or training group into smaller groups of five to eight people. Looking at infant mortality, develop a scenario for addressing this public health problem from the five waves of change discussed in the chapter.

Wave 1: Hunting and gathering to an agriculture-based society
Wave 2: Agricultural-based society to an industrial one
Wave 3: Industrial society to an information and knowledge-based society

Wave 4: Information and knowledge-based society to a complexity society that is communication intensive

Wave 5: Complexity-based society to one based on personal transformation

## References

1. P. F. Drucker, "Management's New Paradigms," *Forbes,* October 5, 1998, 152–156.
2. Drucker, "Management's New Paradigms."
3. D. P. Lenihan, *Strategic Management in Public Health: A Leadership Approach* (Sudbury, MA: Jones and Bartlett, in preparation).
4. L. Rowitz, *Public Health for the 21st Century: The Prepared Leader* (Sudbury, MA: Jones and Bartlett, 2006).
5. Rowitz, *Public Health for the 21st Century: The Prepared Leader.*
6. A. Toffler, *The Third Wave* (New York: Morrow, 1980).
7. J. Kotter, *Leading Change* (Boston: Harvard Business School Press, 1996).
8. H. B. Maynard Jr. and S. E. Mehrtens, *The Fourth Wave* (San Francisco: Berrett-Kohler Publishers, 1993).
9. M. R. Shechtman, *Fifth Wave Leadership: The Internal Frontier* (Tempe, AZ: Facts on Demand Press, 2002).
10. B. J. Turnock, *Public Health: What It Is and How It Works,* 4th ed. (Sudbury, MA: Jones and Bartlett, 2009).
11. Turnock, *Public Health: What It Is and How It Works.*
12. Pfizer Public Health Group, *The Faces of Public Health* (New York: Pfizer Global Pharamaceuticals, 2004).

# CHAPTER 20

# TRADITIONAL AND CRISIS PUBLIC HEALTH LEADERS

Crisis leadership [is] planning for the unthinkable.

Ian Mitroff

September 11, 2001, changed our perspective on public health because it changed many of our views of life in America in the 21st century. Being a leader today is quite different than it was just a few short years ago. However, I have tried in this book to demonstrate that leadership is a complex process. Leaders need to learn many things, but most of all they need to commit themselves to lifelong learning. In order to be a successful leader, leaders need to master most of the tools and techniques discussed throughout this book. Crisis leaders not only need to master these tools and techniques, but many other tools as well.[1] Traditional public health leaders have worked well in environments that have some emergencies occur, but the emergencies and crises of this first decade of the 21st century have put new demands on our public health leaders. We now live in a public health environment that emphasizes preparedness and our ability as leaders to address any crisis that may occur from a natural disaster like Hurricane Katrina to terrorist acts and economic crises that affect our ability to do our work in an effective and efficient manner. In this final chapter, we will look at some of these issues and also discuss briefly the importance of public health leaders taking a global perspective on public health in the future.

## Transition from Traditional to Community-Based Organizations

As I have pointed out in several chapters of this book, public health leaders have led their agencies from a traditional agency-based linear approach to public health to a systems-based community focus. Table 20-1 presents some of these changes, from starting with a traditional organization in a fairly stable environment to some form of community or societal disruption that affects the agency directly. During this chaos phase, many of the tools and techniques discussed in this book are utilized to restore some equilibrium in the agency. However, the changes brought about through the period of disruption push the organization into a transition phase.

For the organization in transition, the core functions and essential public health services provide a foundation on which to create change as the

**Table 20-1   A Systems Approach to Public Health Organizational Change**

| Traditional Organization | Chaos I | Organization Transition | Chaos II | Community Organization |
|---|---|---|---|---|
| 1) Organizational planning | 1) Evaluation | 1) Core functions (system) | 1) Systems thinking (transition to outside the agency) | 1) Community building |
| 2) Organizing | 2) Communication | 2) Essential services | 2) Collaboration | 2) Preparedness and response |
| 3) Heading internally | 3) Strategic planning | 3) Public health law | 3) Public/private | 3) Community engagement |
| 4) Motivating stuff | 4) CQI | 4) Health communication | 4) Partnerships | 4) Tipping awareness |
| 5) Controlling activities | 5) Re-engineering | 5) Complexity | 5) Cultural competency | 5) Learning organization |
| 6) Organizational practices | 6) Reinvention | | 6) Performance measurement | 6) Meta-leadership |
| 7) Budgeting | 7) Turnaround | | | |
| 8) Development | 8) Goal realignment | | | |
| 9) Cultural diversity | 9) Problem solving | | | |
| 10) Mentoring/coaching | 10) Decision making | | | |
| 11) Linear thinking | 11) Conflict resolution | | | |
| | 12) Negotiation | | | |
| | 13) Emotional intelligence | | | |
| | 14) Risk communication | | | |
| | 15) Change | | | |
| Steady state | Disruption | Steady state | Disruption | Steady state |

organization moves to a more community-based approach to public health. This transition phase is often short-lived, and the organization enters into another period of disruption. Leaders will need to use systems thinking skills, collaboration, public-private connections, culture competency learning, and performance measurement techniques to move to its next level of development. Eventually, the agency will be much more community-based and will use many new skills to relate to its community. In crisis, leaders will also use these tools and techniques to aid their agencies to deal with the disruption due to these emergency events.

Clearly, different skills as well as the utilization of traditional leadership skills tied to the severity of the change in the environment are required by leaders in different phases of organizational change. Exercise 20-1 presents a chance to look at the skills needed to maintain the organization internally in a traditional day-to-day organization pattern, externally in a noncrisis-affected organization, and finally in crisis situations.

## The Crisis Cycle

Since September 11, 2001, public health leaders have been involved in the development of emergency preparedness and response activities in their communities. This model of preparedness appears to be affecting the overall orientation of public health leaders to the work of public health in a crisis-oriented society. I have discussed elsewhere the importance of public health leaders understanding that the effectiveness and efficiency of the work they do is dependent on the organization of the public health system as well as on the strong foundation of principles guided by public health practice. These practice principles are critical in addressing all types of public health issues. It is imperative for public health leaders to integrate their knowledge of public health with the changing environment in which they work.

Since the disaster caused by Hurricane Katrina in the summer of 2005, there has been a renewed interest in public health and natural disasters. Between 1963 and the end of 2007, there have been an average of 31 declared disasters per year.[2] The Federal Emergency Management Agency (FEMA) data in Table 20-2 show the number of declared disasters for each of these years

**Table 20-2    Declared Disasters by Year or State**

**By Year**

| Year | Number of Disaster Declarations |
| --- | --- |
| 2008 | 9 |
| 2007 | 63 |
| 2006 | 52 |
| 2005 | 48 |
| 2004 | 68 |
| 2003 | 56 |
| 2002 | 49 |
| 2001 | 45 |
| 2000 | 45 |

*(continues)*

**Table 20-2** *continued*

**By Year**

| Year | Number of Disaster Declarations |
|---|---|
| 1999 | 50 |
| 1998 | 65 |
| 1997 | 44 |
| 1996 | 75 |
| 1995 | 32 |
| 1994 | 36 |
| 1993 | 32 |
| 1992 | 45 |
| 1991 | 43 |
| 1990 | 38 |
| 1989 | 31 |
| 1988 | 11 |
| 1987 | 23 |
| 1986 | 28 |
| 1985 | 27 |
| 1984 | 34 |
| 1983 | 21 |
| 1982 | 24 |
| 1981 | 15 |
| 1980 | 23 |
| 1979 | 42 |
| 1978 | 25 |
| 1977 | 22 |
| 1976 | 30 |
| 1975 | 38 |
| 1974 | 46 |
| 1973 | 46 |
| 1972 | 48 |
| 1971 | 17 |
| 1970 | 17 |
| 1969 | 29 |
| 1968 | 19 |
| 1967 | 11 |
| 1966 | 11 |
| 1965 | 25 |
| 1964 | 25 |
| 1963 | 20 |
| 1962 | 22 |
| 1961 | 12 |
| 1960 | 12 |
| 1959 | 7 |
| 1958 | 7 |
| 1957 | 16 |
| 1956 | 16 |
| 1955 | 18 |
| 1954 | 17 |
| 1953 | 13 |

**By State and Territory**

| | State | Number of Disaster Declarations |
|---|---|---|
| 1 | Texas | 81 |
| 2 | California | 73 |
| 3 | Florida | 59 |
| 4 | New York | 56 |
| 5 | Oklahoma | 54 |

| | State | Number of Disaster Declarations |
|---|---|---|
| 6 | Louisiana | 53 |
| 7 | Alabama | 46 |
| 8 | Kentucky | 45 |
| 9 | Ohio | 43 |
| 10 | Illinois | 43 |
| 11 | Pennsylvania | 42 |
| 12 | Missouri | 42 |
| 13 | Mississippi | 42 |
| 14 | Arkansas | 42 |
| 15 | Washington | 41 |
| 16 | West Virginia | 40 |
| 17 | Minnesota | 40 |
| 18 | Virginia | 39 |
| 19 | Tennessee | 39 |
| 20 | Iowa | 38 |
| 21 | Kansas | 37 |
| 22 | North Dakota | 36 |
| 23 | Nebraska | 36 |
| 24 | North Carolina | 35 |
| 25 | Indiana | 34 |
| 26 | Wisconsin | 31 |
| 27 | Maine | 31 |
| 28 | Georgia | 31 |
| 29 | Alaska | 31 |
| 30 | South Dakota | 27 |
| 31 | Oregon | 25 |
| 32 | Vermont | 24 |
| 33 | New Jersey | 24 |
| 34 | Michigan | 24 |
| 35 | Federated States of Micronesia | 24 |
| 36 | Hawaii | 23 |
| 37 | Massachusetts | 21 |
| 38 | Puerto Rico | 20 |
| 39 | New Mexico | 20 |
| 40 | Idaho | 20 |
| 41 | Arizona | 20 |
| 42 | New Hampshire | 19 |
| 43 | Maryland | 18 |
| 44 | Nevada | 17 |
| 45 | Montana | 17 |
| 46 | South Carolina | 15 |
| 47 | Colorado | 15 |
| 48 | Northern Mariana Islands | 14 |
| 49 | U.S. Virgin Islands | 13 |
| 50 | Connecticut | 13 |
| 51 | Guam | 12 |
| 52 | Delaware | 12 |
| 53 | American Samoa | 10 |
| 54 | Wyoming | 7 |
| 55 | Utah | 7 |
| 56 | Rhode Island | 7 |
| 57 | Marshall Islands | 7 |
| 58 | District of Columbia | 7 |
| 59 | Palau | 1 |
| **Total Disaster Declarations** | | 1,743 |
| **Average** | | 30 |

*Soruce:* FEMA, Annual Major Disaster Declaration Totals. Available at http://www.fema.gov/news/disaster_totals_annual.fema. Accessed February 18, 2008.

and the total for each state during this period. It is important to note that the years since 1989 have shown above-average designated disasters, with major increases since 2000.

Since 2001, much discussion and deliberation has occurred about natural and human-made disasters and the importance of public health response in many of these disasters. Crisis can best be seen in terms of a cycle approach. Figure 20-1 shows one model of a crisis cycle. First, we ask public health agencies and their partners to do a risk audit to determine our disaster history and what we have learned from them. The risk audit also addresses the concern of probability of similar events in the future. This knowledge requires the use of this information to mitigate the occurrence of future events or to lessen the impact of these events in the future. This knowledge will affect the preparedness planning activities of the public health agency or community partners working together on a community-wide emergency preparedness plan. When the local community emergency preparedness plan was printed in our local newspaper, I undertook a very unscientific survey of my neighbors and found many were not even aware that our community had an emergency plan.

> **Leadership Tip**
>
> *The best time to return calls is before lunch or at the end of the day. The calls will be shorter.*

Once a plan is developed and before a disaster or emergency occurs, mitigation issues once again become important. Local crisis management teams will want to explore ways to avoid various categories of crisis or to lessen the effects of one if it occurs. Another issue involves whether the plan's operational aspects are clear. When and if a crisis occurs, it is important to move to the response phase as quickly as possible in order to lessen the effects of the event. Mitigation strategies are once again important. If the response is immediate and effective, recovery will occur more quickly. After-action plan-

**FIGURE 20-1  Crisis Cycle**

The Crisis Cycle  **551**

ning activities as well as mitigation strategies are once again critical to the recovery phase. Even though recovery may take time depending on the severity of the crisis event, the cycle will begin again with another risk audit.

Mitigation actions involve four types of measures.[3] First, there are engineering and construction issues related to whether buildings are constructed to prevent damage and whether there are appropriate building codes. The second set of mitigation actions relate to physical planning, which is affected by the understanding of the physical environments where people live and land use issues. The third category of mitigation measures relates to the economic factor. Strong economies seem to respond better to disasters than poor economies. The final set of mitigation actions is related to the society or community as a whole. Public awareness is an important factor. If people know what to do if a disaster will soon occur or if one does occur, this will help in response and speed up recovery. Exercises and drills are important here as well.

From a public health perspective, leaders will utilize many skills and techniques to manage and lead in a crisis situation. Figure 20-2 graphically shows some of the leadership skills necessary in preparedness activities are different from the skills developed at other levels of the pyramid.[4] By strengthening the public health system and its infrastructure, we can better respond to a disaster when it occurs. These crisis skills must be combined with many of the skills described in this book.

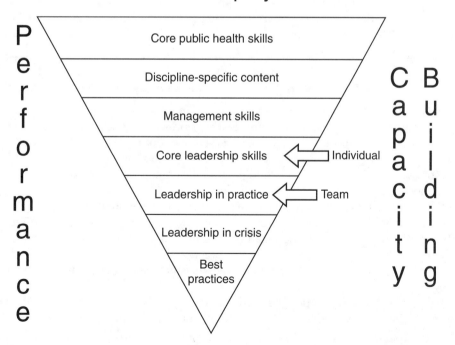

**FIGURE 20-2    The Skills of the Prepared Public Health Leader in Crisis**

## Next Steps

The requirements associated with successful leadership seem to present leaders with a moving target. Our world is ever changing. As the world changes, public health leaders need to be flexible enough to adjust to these changes. Not only is public health leadership important to build the public health infrastructure in the United States, but leadership is also important in building public health infrastructure around the world.[5] With the health issues in the world becoming more complex, the number of agencies addressing these issues appears to be increasing as well. Leadership is critical for this growing response to health and disease around the world. Public health leaders are needed for policy development, development and formulation of innovative public health programs, monitoring of global health issues, and evaluation. Leadership development programs similar to those in the United States are needed throughout the world. If these programs can be collaborative with the leadership development programs in the United States, coordinated global public health initiatives become more possible. As we look forward, we discover the necessity of understanding people throughout the world.

Global issues such as global warming, pandemic influenza, child survival initiatives, human immunodeficiency virus/acquired immune deficiency syndrome, and other emerging global infections become more and more important.[6] Public health leaders need to remove the barriers between countries to work in partnership with our public health colleagues all over the world. Hesselbein has stated that the time for partnership is now.[7] A world vision related to healthy families and children, excellent schools, decent and available housing work opportunities, and health equity is necessary for international public health to become a reality. Leaders are needed to make this happen.

The International Health Regulations provide a blueprint for some of this work. Case Study 20-A by Judith Munson, the executive director of the International Collaborative for Public Health Emergency Preparedness (ICPHEP), explores some of these issues.

---

### Case Study 20-A
### A Public Health Practice Quiz for Judith W. Munson

***What are the emergency preparedness leadership issues in global public health?***
This is an important question, because leadership in emergency preparedness in a globalized world requires a significant broadening of our knowledge. In global public health, knowledge is required about the world we live in and about the earth we live on. We need to be alert to where the threats are and how to contain or to prevent them. These are the most essential elements.

How to pursue this knowledge; where to start? Before embarking upon this adventure, consider your own personal background and your own depth of experience. This search will guide your entrance onto the international platform. Find that one country or that one region or that area of practice that has formed your life or has informed your career path. Then pursue the issues that are connected to those countries, regions, or areas of practice.

If that exercise does not provide the necessary guidance to you, then pursue one or more of the many media outlets for information. Suggestions include:

- Select and review daily online publications of international reach, for example, the *Economist*, the *International Herald Tribune*, the *Financial Times*, the *New York Times World*, or, simply, Reuters and CNN International.

- Access Web sites devoted to public health internationally, for example, the World Health Organization http://www.who.int/en/, the European Union Commission on Health and Consumer Protection http://ec.europa.eu/dgs/health_consumer/index_en.htm, the European Centre for Disease Prevention and Control http://ecdc.europa.eu/, and the Pan American Health Organization http://www.paho.org/.
- Subscribe to daily e-mail updates from Web sites with topics of interest to you (many, if not most, are free of charge).

As you use these resources, news of public health emergencies around the globe will come into your purview. They could be disease outbreaks, natural disasters, environmental contaminants, or other phenomena such as nuclear incidents, toxic spills, or the reemergence of a highly infectious communicable disease. You will also be instantly knowledgeable about the response and recovery capabilities of the public health agencies and their practitioners wherever the incident may have occurred. You will be well-informed concerning threats to public health around the globe and knowledgeable about public health leadership models that work, as well as those that do not.

### How do we develop relationships with public health leaders in other countries?

Developing relationships with public health leaders in countries other than the United States takes time, effort, and attention. Relationships start first with a meeting and then proceed according to mutual needs and perceived benefits. To begin, it is essential to meet the other individual, at least initially, "in person." The best place to meet public health leaders from other countries is at conferences, seminars, or other professional gatherings. But even in these familiar settings, it takes an effort to make an acquaintance and to establish a rapport. It is rare for the individual from the foreign country to initiate a conversation. More typically, it is the person who is a citizen of the host country who engages others who are in attendance. This is not surprising, because one accepts the role of host and the other accepts the role as guest. If a rapport is established and a common collegial interest has been discussed and acknowledged, an exchange of calling cards signals the potential for developing a relationship.

Still rare, but more and more possible as technology provides even greater (and more cost-effective) options, the "in person" requirement can take place by other than face-to-face conventional meetings. Technological innovations have been used more and more in establishing and enhancing personal contacts internationally because of the cost savings. Some examples are participating in an online chat room, posting regularly on a blog, or actively participating in an online continuing education offering. Internet-based course offerings, conference calls initiated by international professional associations that make use of VOIP (voice over internet protocol, also known as Internet telephony) mechanisms such as Skype (http://about.skype.com/), provide opportunities to "meet" public health leaders from other countries without leaving your office. When the conference call for the meeting uses the VOIP telephony mechanism with webcams, these audio and video conferencing mechanisms provide a close approximation of an in-person meeting or a face-to-face introduction with colleagues in foreign jurisdictions—and often the entire service is free.

Typically, however, technological enhancements are more effective after the "in person" meeting has taken place and a baseline of interaction has been set. The

*(continues)*

**Case Study 20-A** *continued*

conversations that take place among the participants in an Internet-based forum provide opportunities to hear a colleague express expertise on a topic of interest to you. This may prompt you to make the effort to follow up on that introductory mechanism.

But to maintain a relationship—and even to nurture it into a friendship—requires patience and understanding. E-mail is a quick and commonplace method of communicating, but there are some potential problems. Often, a name of a person e-mailing from a foreign country will incorporate accents and other diacritical marks that can throw an e-mail message or e-mail response into the spam folder where it can sit for days or weeks without being read. The time lags occasioned by such events can often be the death knell to a developing international relationship if communication is based solely on e-mail. Making calls to a land line or to a cell phone by using the Internet (VOIP offerings) are inexpensive and can save a relationship.

### What are the leadership and emergency preparedness issues in the application of the International Health Regulations?

The most recent version of the International Health Regulations (IHR 2005) came into force on June 15, 2007 (http://www.who.int/csr/ihr/en/). This revision represents the most important treaty to emerge from the community of nations interested in protecting the health of the world's populations. In large measure a response to the severe acute respiratory syndrome (SARS) epidemic that shook the world of public health when it circled the globe in 2003, this revision is geared toward international public health security.

The virus—which was the causative agent of the newly emerging disease—perplexed and confounded the public health practitioners and laboratory scientists around the globe because of four factors: (1) they did not know where it came from; (2) they did not know how it was transmitted; (3) they did not know how to cure it; and (4) they did not have a vaccine that could prevent it. Air travelers, exposed to the emerging virus while in Hong Kong, returned to their home countries with this new disease, which at that point did not even have a name. The name ultimately given to it described the symptoms of its victims.

The World Health Organization (WHO) and its governing body, the World Health Assembly (WHA), had been in the process of redrafting and updating the International Health Regulations (IHR 1969) even before SARS emerged. Applicable to only three diseases since 1969—cholera, plague, and yellow fever (smallpox having been declared eradicated by 1980)—the IHR (1969) were not beneficial during the SARS epidemic. Nonetheless, WHO had to step into the leadership role. It did so by issuing the first global travel alert, and shortly thereafter it issued the first emergency travel advisory. There followed a series of travel recommendations (e.g., postpone all but essential travel) until all affected destinations were removed from the list and the areas with recent transmissions were finally given the all-clear.

The SARS experience prompted more focused attention at WHO headquarters on the need to update the IHR (1969). Results came quickly. The revisions were adopted at the WHA meeting of June 2005 and came into force two years later on June 15, 2007. Instead of being applicable only to named diseases, activation of this new international framework hinges upon reporting a "public health emergency of international concern" to the National Focal Point (NFP) office. As of August 15, 2007, 179 state parties had designated an NFP office. The U.S. NFP office is located within the Department of Health and Human Services, at its operations center.

Leadership issues with regard to the implementation of the IHR (2005) abound. WHO published the IHR (2005) Areas of Work for Implementation in June 2007 (http://www.who.int/csr/ihr/area_of_work/en/index.html).

The primary leadership concern that must be addressed now is this: the need to educate our public health workforce on the provisions of the IHR and their importance to public health preparedness in every sector. This is essential. Likewise, public health faculties must make them a part of the curriculum so that the future leaders—those who are students now—graduate ready to assume their roles on the international platform.

### Can you give an example of a successful partnership in global public health leadership?

Yes. There are several outstanding examples of successful partnering in global public health leadership. The one that is spotlighted here, however, is the "Knowledge Management for Public Health" program (also known as KM4PH) launched by WHO and its partners, including the World Federation of Public Health Associations (WFPHA), within the last couple of years (http://www.who.int/km4ph/en/).

It is an example of a working partnership between a public health agency of global reach—WHO—and its technology partner located in the heart of the American Midwest—the University of Iowa College of Public Health. The college provides the Global Public Health Campus software that allows the KM4PH's activities to be brought to public health practitioners around the globe, even countries where connectivity to the Internet is slow. The knowledge transfer opportunities and benefits are greatest under these circumstances.

KM4PH features an online discussion portal that provides an opportunity for public health practitioners, students, and academics to participate in real-time, live, Web-based conferences. Held weekly, the online conferences are conducted in several languages (different languages at different times) and can accommodate 150 participants at any one time. Those signing in are from many different countries. Participants can see the list of participants and can send e-mail messages to any one (or all) of them during the conference. The presentations are visible on the computer screen, and the voice of the presenter is heard. At times the presenter is seen as well, depending upon the availability of camera (webcam) capability. Participants can raise their hands online and be heard by using the microphone icon. Participants can even applaud!

The software the KM4PH network uses through the University of Iowa Global Campus is called Elluminate Live! It provides the online collaborative learning forum. The KM4PH program collaborates with the WFPHA, which has official relationship status with WHO. WFPHA is an organization of public health associations around the globe. It seeks to enhance international understanding among international nongovernmental, multiprofessional, and civil society organizations dedicated to developing and promoting effective global policies, all directed to improving the health of populations. WFPHA's governing members are national and regional public health associations, currently numbering more than 70. Members also include regional associations of schools of public health. The KM4PH network is an integral part of the WFPHA Strategic Plan 2007–2012.

Here in the United States, in one state, a successful organization known as ICPHEP (http://www.ICPHEP.org) has been mounted between and among public health and law schools in Illinois and a law school and a medical school—as well

*(continues)*

**Case Study 20-A** *continued*

as governmental entities—in the Czech Republic. Although originating in academia, the practice community has quickly signed on and the benefits of establishing collaborative relationships are resulting in increased interest in international affairs and its possibilities on both sides of the Atlantic. One example is the participation of the First International Fellow, the Senior Officer for Pandemic Preparedness at the Czech Ministry of Health, in the Mid-America Regional Public Health Leadership Institute at the University of Illinois, School of Public Health.

### What are the connections between law and public health practice in a global context?

This is such an important question, because law is the foundational element of public health practice. The International Health Regulations (IHR 2005) are an excellent example of what can be achieved when the legal framework for a public health initiative has been processed, vetted, and adopted by all the members of the international community. The same can be said about the WHO Framework Convention on Tobacco Control (WHO FCTC). There are currently 168 signatories to the WHO FCTC (http://www.who.int/tobacco/framework/countrylist/en/index.html). These two instruments represent major strides in the practice of public health in a global context. But there are also others that are of equal importance but in a regional or cross-border context.

The United States has been reaching out beyond its borders for the purpose of establishing significant relationships grounded in legal instruments or in legislative enactments. One initiative is the Early Warning Infectious Disease Surveillance (EWIDS) Program Activities on the Northern and Southern Border States (http://www.bt.cdc.gov/surveillance/ewids/). Another initiative consists of the four regional public health collaborations that have been established across the border areas between the United States and Canada and the United States and Mexico. Two of the many activities that are now underway are the drafting of memoranda of understanding to share data, personnel, and equipment between jurisdictions during an infectious disease public health emergency; another is expanding the Laboratory Response Network into Canada and Mexico. See Progress Areas at http://www.bt.cdc.gov/surveillance/ewids/.

Recently, the United States Senate and House of Representatives passed a joint resolution granting consent to the International Emergency Management Assistance Memorandum (IEMAMOU), which states:

> The purpose of this compact is to provide for the possibility of mutual assistance among the jurisdictions entering into this compact in managing any emergency or disaster when the affected jurisdiction or jurisdictions ask for assistance, whether arising from natural disaster, technological hazard, manmade disaster, or civil emergency aspects of resources shortages.

The IEMAMOU had been agreed upon by Connecticut, Maine, Massachusetts, New Hampshire, Rhode Island, and Vermont and the Canadian provinces of New Brunswick, Newfoundland, Nova Scotia, Prince Edward Island, and Quebec. The joint resolution can be found at http://www.govtrack.us/congress/billtext. xpd?bill=sjll0-13.

---

Public health leaders gain from lifelong learning. Public health cannot do its job effectively without a well-trained public health workforce. The best next step is a strong commitment to public health professionals who dedicate their lives to serving others.

We must be the change we want to see in the world.

Mahatma Ghandi

## Discussion Questions

1. Describe the crisis cycle and how different types of crisis and their aftermath fit the cycle.
2. What effect does the operational definition of a local health department have on understanding how public health responds to a disaster?
3. Why are mitigation strategies important in crisis?
4. How would you develop a global public health leadership development initiative?

### Exercise 20-1:   Traditional and Crisis Leadership

*Purpose:* to explore the skills necessary for traditional public health leaders inside their agency and outside with crisis leadership skills to determine similarities and differences in the skills necessary to be an effective public health leader

*Key concepts:* traditional leadership skills, crisis leadership skills

*Procedure:* Divide your class or training group into groups of eight to ten people. One third of the groups will create a traditional (day-to-day) inside-the-agency set of skills. You can put the list on a flip chart sheet of paper. Another third of the groups will create a skill list for a traditional leader with external partners and constituents. The final third will create a list of crisis leadership skills. Each group will present its list and then all participants will discuss what they discovered.

## References

1. L. Rowitz, *Public Health in the 21st Century: The Prepared Leader* (Sudbury, MA: Jones and Bartlett, 2006).
2. Federal Emergency Management Agemcy, Declared Disasters by Year and State, http://www.fema.gov
3. A. W. Coburn, R. J. S. Spence, and A. Pomonis, *Disaster Mitigation,* 2nd ed. (Geneva, Switzerland: United Nations Disaster Management Training Programme, 1994).
4. Rowitz, *Public Health in the 21st Century: The Prepared Leader.*
5. W. L. Roper and J. Porter, "Creating Public Health Leaders: Public Health Leadership Institutes," in W. H. Foege, N. Daulaire, R. E. Black, and C. E. Pearson (eds.), *Global Health Leadership and Management* (San Francisco: Jossey-Bass, 2005).
6. W. H. Foege, "Preface," in W. H. Foege et al. (eds.), *Global Health Leadership and Management* (San Francisco: Jossey-Bass, 2005).
7. F. Hesselbein, "Leadership and Management for Improving Global Health," in W. H. Foege et al. (eds.), *Global Health Leadership and Management* (San Francisco: Jossey-Bass, 2005).

# INDEX